Clinical Practice
of the
Dental Hygienist

Clinical Practice
of the
Dental Hygienist

ESTHER M. WILKINS, B.S., R.D.H., D.M.D.

Department of Periodontology, Tufts University, School of Dental Medicine, Boston, Massachusetts; formerly Associate Professor and Director, Department of Dental Hygiene, School of Dentistry, University of Washington

FOURTH EDITION

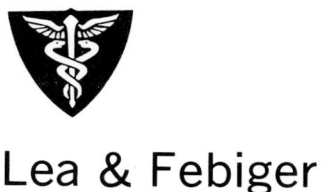

Lea & Febiger   PHILADELPHIA

Library of Congress Cataloging in Publication Data

Wilkins, Esther M
  Clinical practice of the dental hygienist.

  Includes bibliographies and index.
  1. Dental hygiene.   I. Title.
RK60.5.W5   1976   617.6′01   76-7018
ISBN 0–8121–0540–0

Published in Great Britain by Henry Kimpton Publishers, London

Printed in the United States of America

Print No.   5   4   3

Preface

In this fourth edition of *Clinical Practice of the Dental Hygienist,* chapters have been altered substantially and new material has been added to bring the book up-to-date with current concepts of oral health and patient care. The primary purpose of the book is to present content that is fundamental to clinical dental hygiene practice. For comprehensive preventive, therapeutic, and educational services the dental hygienist must be prepared to evaluate dental hygiene aspects of the oral health needs of each patient, and to plan immediate and long range dental hygiene care within the framework of total dental care supervised and conducted by the dentist.

The material in the book is sequenced in a general way to follow the steps in patient care starting with preparation for appointments in Part II, and patient evaluation in Part III. Those who have used the previous editions will find one important chronologic change. The section on prevention, Part IV, precedes Instrumentation, Part V. This is in keeping with the necessary approach to patient care, namely, that initial plaque control and other phases of the patient's self-care logically precede professional treatment.

Professional services make a limited long range contribution to the patient's continuing oral health unless accompanied by daily personal treatment by the patient.

The need for consistent, thorough, efficiently applied technical skills for examination and treatment procedures is emphasized. An attempt is made to stress follow-up and observation of the outcome of treatment. The dental hygienist must understand the factors which limit or delay the attainment of optimum health. Whereas in the past many oral prophylaxes were performed as isolated procedures, the aim of dental hygiene periodontal instrumentation today is to complete the definitive treatment for certain patients, while for others the preparatory phase for additional complex periodontal therapy is accomplished.

New chapters have been added to include material on vital signs, dental and periodontal indices, dental hygiene treatment planning, sealants, periodontal dressings, and sutures. There are new chapters on the care of patients with complete oral rehabilitation, acute necrotizing ulcerative gingivitis, and oral cancer.

Separate chapters have been prepared to expand and emphasize material formerly included within other chapters, for example, the extraoral and intraoral inspection, gingival examination, examination instruments and procedures, inspection of the teeth, disclosing agents, and gingival curettage. There is also new content in many chapters such as sections on the use of pulp testers, panoramic radiography, automatic and accelerated processing, interpretation of radiographs, clinical signs of trauma from occlusion, and the immediate application of the patient history particularly with respect to the identification of patients who require prophylactic premedication.

The references and suggested readings for each chapter have been carefully revised to provide selected bibliographies from the current literature. All books require continuing supplemental reading to learn new research findings.

Sincere thanks are expressed to all who have used the previous editions of this book and to those who have taken the time to offer constructive criticisms. Much support and inspiration have been received from students, practicing hygienists, and teachers. Insofar as possible, their recommendations for additions and improvements have been incorporated. The author is especially indebted to those who reviewed whole chapters and identified essential content for inclusion. In this regard a special note of gratitude goes to Mrs. Anna Pattison, University of Southern California, for specific contributions to Chapters 11 and 12, The Gingiva and Examination Procedures, as well as parts of many other chapters; to Mrs. Connie Bonvecchio, Palm Beach Junior College, for assistance with Chapter 6, Patient Histories; to Miss Barbara Wilson, University of Rhode Island for reviewing

Chapter 7, Vital Signs; to Dr. Stanley Schwartz, Tufts University School of Dental Medicine, for the review of the section on blood pressure; Dr. Nicholas Darzenta, Tufts University, for Chapter 9, Radiographs; Miss Marjorie Short, Middlesex Community College, for Chapter 19, Periodontal and Dental Indices; Miss Edna Bradbury and Dr. Albert J. Kazis, Harvard University School of Dental Medicine, for Chapter 25, The Patient with Complete Rehabilitation; Drs. Israel L. Dogon and Myron J. VanLeeuwen, Harvard University School of Dental Medicine, for Chapter 30, Sealants; Miss Carol Reid, Middlesex Community College, for Chapter 54, Emergency Care; and Dr. James B. Gallagher, Tufts University School of Dental Medicine, for patiently reading all newly prepared drafts, for reviewing material on care of removable dentures, and for countless practical suggestions related to format and illustrations.

The practicing dental hygienist will require ever increasing knowledge, understanding, and overall sophistication in order to achieve professional standards of competence. The student of dental hygiene must learn to observe and evaluate signs of oral health and disease, assess patient reaction and learning, and be able to apply principles from the biologic, physical, social, behavioral, and dental sciences in the care of patients. It is hoped that the approach to dental hygiene used in this book will increase understanding and clinical expertise as the dental hygienist engages in the most challenging and rewarding of tasks, that of providing safe and effective individualized patient care.

Boston, Massachusetts   ESTHER M. WILKINS

Contents

I

Orientation to Clinical Dental Hygiene Practice

Chapter 1

The Professional Dental Hygienist

The registered dental hygienist is a licensed, professional, oral health educator and clinical operator who, as an auxiliary to the dentist, uses preventive, therapeutic, and educational methods for the control of oral diseases to aid individuals and groups in attaining and maintaining optimum oral health. The services of the dental hygienist are utilized in general and specialty dental practices, the armed services, and in programs for research, professional education, public health, school health, industrial health, and institutional care.

The term *dental hygiene care* is used to denote all integrated preventive and treatment services administered to the patient by the dental hygienist. This term is parallel to the commonly used term *dental care* which refers to the services performed by the dentist.

Clinical services, both dental and dental hygiene, have limited long range probability of success if the patient does not understand the need for cooperation in daily procedures of personal care and diet, and for regular appointments for professional care. Educational and clinical services are, therefore, mutually dependent and inseparable in the total dental hygiene care of the patient.

Dr. Alfred C. Fones, who initiated the active use of the dental hygienist and founded the first formal course of professional study in 1913, emphasized the important role of education. In the first textbook for dental hygienists he wrote:

> It is primarily to this important work of public education that the dental hygienist is called. She must regard herself as the channel through which dentistry's knowledge of mouth hygiene is to be disseminated. The greatest service she can perform is the persistent education of the public in mouth hygiene and the allied branches of general hygiene.[1]

Dental hygiene has been studied and the scope of practice has developed from Dr. Fones' original concept. Scientific information about the prevention of oral diseases is accumulating steadily. The need for dental hygiene care and oral health instruction is being emphasized. The clinical practice of the dental hygienist integrates specific care with instructional services required by the individual patient.

I. Role in Patient Care

The dental hygienist may be responsible for gathering and assembling information for use by the dentist in diagnosis and treatment planning. The personal, medical, and dental histories, the radiographic survey, study casts, photographs, and charts of oral conditions observed during the oral inspection, and dental and periodontal examinations may be prepared. These data become part of the patient's permanent record and are used by the dentist and the dental hygienist throughout the treatment procedures and for comparison during continuing recall evaluations.

The role of the dental hygienist is to implement and coordinate the treatment and preventive program prescribed for each patient. Specific clinical services are required and the dental hygienist teaches and guides the patient in his performance of measures for disease control. The success of each phase of treatment, whether periodontic, orthodontic, restorative, or prosthodontic, depends on the patient's cooperative daily performance of the recommended measures. Dental hygiene care as provided by the dental hygienist becomes an integral part of the total care of the patient.

II. Factors Influencing Clinical Practice

A. Legal

The law of a state must be studied and respected by each dental hygienist practicing within that state. Although the various practice acts have basic similarities, there are differences. Changes may be made from time to time.

All states are consistent in the provision that a dental hygienist may practice only under the direction and supervision of a licensed dentist. Terminology varies, but each practice act regulates the patient services which may be delegated by the dentist to auxiliary personnel.

B. Ethical

Professional people in the health services are set apart from others by virtue of the dignity and responsibility of their work. Service is the primary objective of the dental hygienist and is the reason for the existence of the profession. Others look to the professional person for leadership and expect more than ordinary demonstration of good human relations. Being professional requires interpersonal, professional, interprofessional, and community relationships of a high standard.

The American Dental Hygienists' Association has defined the principles of ethics for the professional dental hygienist. Understanding of and loyalty to these principles is essential to successful practice.

PRINCIPLES OF ETHICS OF THE AMERICAN DENTAL HYGIENISTS' ASSOCIATION[2]

Each member of the American Dental Hygienists' Association has the ethical obligation to subscribe to the following principles:

To provide oral health care utilizing highest professional knowledge, judgment, and ability.

To serve all patients without discrimination.

To hold professional patient relationships in confidence.

To utilize every opportunity to increase public understanding of oral health practices.

To generate public confidence in members of the dental health professions.

To cooperate with all health professions in meeting the health needs of the public.

To recognize and uphold the laws and regulations governing this profession.

To participate responsively in this professional Association and uphold its purposes.

To maintain professional competence through continuing education.

To exchange professional knowledge with other health professions.

To represent dental hygiene with a high standard of ethical conduct.

C. Personal

Each dental hygienist may represent the entire profession to the patient being served. The dental hygienist's expressed or demonstrated attitudes toward dentistry, dental hygiene, and other health professions, as well as toward health services and preventive measures, are very apt to be reflected in the subsequent attitude of the patient toward other dental hygienists, and dental hygiene care in general.

Members of health professions need to exemplify the traits which they hold as objectives for others if response and cooperation are to be expected. There are many personal factors of general physical health, oral health, cleanliness, appearance, and mental health to be considered. A few of these are mentioned below.

1. *General Physical Health.* A routine plan for complete physical examination is important since the maintenance of personal health is a necessity to continued service. Optimum physical health depends primarily upon a well-planned diet, a sufficient amount of sleep, and an adequate amount of exercise.

2. *Oral Health.* The maintenance of a clean, healthy mouth demonstrates by example that the dental hygienist follows the teachings of the dental and dental hygiene professions relative to prevention and control of disease. Freedom from offensive odors is important because the hygienist works in close proximity to patients.

3. *Cleanliness and Appearance.* A professional appearance includes a fresh uniform, and clean hose and shoes. Hair must be worn in a neat arrangement to prevent it from falling toward the patient or the instruments while working.

Jewelry other than a professional pin should be avoided since the crevices of pieces such as rings and watchbands harbor microorganisms and make thorough hand washing and scrubbing impossible. A trim dental hygiene cap and moderation in make-up contribute to increased respect for the female dental hygienist.

From the point of view of avoiding infection for both the operator and the patient, daily care of the hands and the fingernails is required. The nails are trimmed short and the hands protected by lotions to keep them soft and smooth.

The skin should be clear and impressively clean. Frequent baths and hair shampoos prevent bodily odors and aid in maintaining cleanliness.

4. *Mental Health.* The mental health of the dental hygienist is reflected in interpersonal relationships and the ability to inspire confidence through a display of professional and emotional maturity. Adequate physical health, recreation, and participation in professional and community activities contribute to optimum mental health.

III. Objectives for Practice

The hygienist's self-analysis is essential in attaining goals of perfection in service to the patient and assistance to the dentist in the total dental and dental hygiene care program. Personal objectives need to be outlined and reviewed frequently in a plan for continued self-improvement. The goal with respect to patients was included in the definition of the dental hygienist at the beginning of this chapter: *to aid individuals and groups in attaining and maintaining optimum oral health.* Other objectives are related to this primary one.

The professional dental hygienist will:

A. Strive toward the highest degree of professional ethics and conduct.
B. Plan and carry out effectively the dental hygiene services essential to the total care program for the patient.
C. Apply knowledge and understanding of the basic and clinical sciences in the intelligent recognition of oral conditions and prevention of oral diseases during clinical practice.
D. Apply scientific knowledge and skill to all clinical techniques and instructional procedures.
E. Recognize each patient as an individual and adapt techniques and procedures accordingly.
F. Identify and care for the needs of patients who have unusual general health problems which affect dental hygiene procedures.
G. Demonstrate interpersonal relationships which permit attending the patient with assurance and presenting dental health information effectively.
H. Provide a complete and individualized instructional service for each patient.
I. Practice safe and efficient procedures pertaining to the care and sterilization of instruments and to general clinical routines.
J. Apply a continuing process of self-evaluation in clinical practice throughout professional life.
   1. Be objective and critical of procedures used in order to perform the best possible service.
   2. Appreciate the need for acquiring new knowledge and skills as current advancements merit it.

IV. Factors to Teach the Patient

A. The role of the dental hygienist as an auxiliary in the dental profession.

B. The scope of service of the dental hygienist as defined by state practice acts.
C. The interrelationship of instructional and clinical services in dental hygiene care.

References

1. Fones, A C., ed.: *Mouth Hygiene*, 4th ed. Philadelphia, Lea & Febiger, 1934, p. 248.
2. American Dental Hygienists' Association, House of Delegates: *Professional Code of Ethics for the Dental Hygienist*, Revised November, 1974.

Suggested Readings

Dental Hygiene Services

American Dental Association, Council on Dental Education: Report on the Education and Utilization of Dental Auxiliaries, *J. Am. Dent. Assoc.*, 88, 1039, May, 1974.
Blau, M. A.: Expanded Use of Auxiliary Personnel in Orthodontic Practice, *Am. J. Orthod.*, 64, 137, August, 1973.
Inter-Agency Committee on Dental Auxiliaries, *J. Am. Dent. Assoc.*, 84, 1025, May, 1972.
Lobene, R. R., Berman, K., Chaisson, L. B., Karelas, H. A., and Nolan, L. F.: The Forsyth Experiment in Training of Advanced Skills Hygienists, *J. Dent. Educ.*, 38, 369, July, 1974.
Motley, W.: The Traditional Dental Hygienist: A Factual Review, *Dent. Hyg.*, 47, 368, November-December, 1973.
Myers, S. E.: Operating Dental Auxiliaries, *WHO Chronicle*, 26, 511, November, 1972.
O'Leary, T. J., Koerber, L. G., and Catherman, J. L.: Preparing Dental Hygiene Students for Expanded Functions, *J. Dent. Educ.*, 36, 18, October, 1972.
Poupard, J. M.: Projecting the Future of Dentistry and Its Auxiliaries, *Dent. Hyg.*, 47, 159, May-June, 1973.
Romcke, R. G. and Lewis, D. W.: Use of Expanded Function Dental Hygienists in the Prince Edward Island Dental Manpower Study, *J. Can. Dent. Assoc.*, 39, 247, April, 1973.
Schmidt, P.: Expanded Duties of Auxiliaries: a Hygienist's Viewpoint, *Am. J. Public Health*, 62, 54, January, 1972.
Schwerin, U.: The Maturation Crisis of a Profession, *Dent. Hyg.*, 48, 145, May-June, 1974.
Sisty, N. L.: The University of Iowa Experimental Program in Dental Hygiene, *Dent. Hyg.*, 47, 79, March-April, 1973.
Sisty, N. L. and Henderson, W. G.: A Comparative Study of Patient Evaluations of Dental Treatment Performed by Dental and Expanded-Function Dental Hygiene Students, *J. Am. Dent. Assoc.*, 88, 985, May, 1974.

Professionalism and Ethics

Alper, M. N.: Ethics and the Dental Hygienist, *J. Am. Dent. Hyg. Assoc.*, *40*, 157, 3rd Quarter, 1966.

Alstadt, W. R.: Ethics—Of What Value? *J. Am. Dent. Hyg. Assoc.*, *41*, 15, 1st Quarter, 1967.

American Dental Association, Council on Judicial Procedures, Constitution and Bylaws: American Dental Association Principles of Ethics with Official Advisory Opinions as Revised, *J. Am. Dent. Assoc.*, *90*, 184, January, 1975.

Fenn, M.: Factors in Interpersonal Relations, *J. Am. Dent. Hyg. Assoc.*, *42*, 138, 3rd Quarter, 1968.

Fleming, W. C.: The Attributes of a Profession and Its Members, *J. Am. Dent. Assoc.*, *69*, 390, September, 1964.

Hine, M. K.: The Professional Concept—Its History and Meaning to Health Service, *J. Am. Coll. Dent.*, *37*, 19, January, 1970.

MacQuarrie, E. E.: Factors in the Development of Professional Attitude, *J. Am. Dent. Hyg. Assoc.*, *45*, 86, March-April, 1971.

Martin, J. G.: The New Professionalism, *J. Am. Dent. Hyg. Assoc.*, *45*, 182, May-June, 1971.

Motley, W. E.: *Ethics, Jurisprudence and History for the Dental Hygienist*. Philadelphia, Lea & Febiger, 1972, pp. 37-50.

Schnurr, B. J.: The Characteristics of Maturity in Dental Hygiene, *Dent. Hyg.*, *47*, 226, July–August, 1973.

Chapter 2

Planning Dental Hygiene Care

The dental hygienist participates with the other members of the dental team in the care of the patient. Together they must help the patient learn about his or her oral health needs, how these needs can be dealt with to bring the health of the oral cavity to an optimum level, and then how to maintain the optimum level to prevent future disease. As an operating auxiliary with formal training and licensure for performing intraoral procedures, the dental hygienist has a key position in the total care of the patient.

I. Types of Services

The services which the dental hygienist performs can be divided into three basic categories, namely, preventive, therapeutic, and educational. The three are inseparable and overlapping as patient care is planned and accomplished.

A. Preventive

Preventive services fall into two groups, primary and secondary. *Primary prevention* refers to measures carried out so that disease does not occur and is truly prevented. *Secondary prevention* involves the treatment of early disease to prevent further progress of potentially irreversible conditions which, if not arrested, may lead eventually to extensive rehabilitative treatment or loss of teeth. An example of a primary preventive measure is the application of a topical agent for dental caries prevention. Removal of submarginal calculus and smoothing the root surface in a relatively shallow pocket is an example of a secondary prevention procedure in that the treatment of a small pocket contributes to the prevention of a deep pocket with marked bone loss.

B. Educational

Educational aspects of dental hygiene service permeate the entire patient care system. The preparation for specific treatment, the success of treatment, and the long-term success of both preventive and therapeutic services are dependent on the patient's understanding and daily care of the oral cavity.

C. Therapeutic

Dental hygiene treatment services are an integral part of the total treatment procedures. All scaling, root planing, and curettage procedures, along with the steps in postoperative care, are parts of the therapeutic phases in the treatment of periodontal diseases. Restorative procedures are involved in the treatment of dental caries.

II. Purposes in Planning Care

Planning dental hygiene care for a patient means preparing a schedule to guide the therapeutic and preventive activities prescribed by the dentist and delegated to the dental hygienist. Initially the dental hygienist plays a major role in the collection of data to be used by the dentist in formulating the diagnosis on which the total treatment plan is based.

The dental hygienist must have a clear understanding of the patient's needs, the nature of his oral illness, and the principles relating to the treatment of the illness. The dental hygienist should be aware of the patient's emotional needs and psychological reactions to his oral conditions. It is important to create an atmosphere in which the patient can respond to instruction, carry out the necessary procedures to supplement professional treatment, and cooperate during dental and dental hygiene appointments for the specific services.

STEPS IN PATIENT CARE

A purpose of this chapter is to bring into focus aspects to be considered in the planning and execution of competent dental hygiene care. Because much of the text is concerned with details of how to perform services for the patient, it is important to keep services and techniques in their proper perspective. There is much more involved in dental hygiene than the performance of technical procedures.

In general the sections of the book are arranged in an order to correspond with a sequence in which dental hygiene ser-

vices may logically be performed. A brief descriptive outline of the sequence is presented here.

I. Preliminary Preparation for Appointments

Supervision of the operatory, equipment, instruments, and all measures for the prevention of disease transmission constitutes a basic essential phase in patient care. A neat clean operatory contributes to the development of confidence and appreciation on the part of the patient.

Clean, sanitized equipment and sterile instruments are prerequisite to the patient's safety. Dental personnel must make every effort to prevent disease transmission.

II. Diagnostic Work-up

The diagnostic work-up is a name applied to the collection of data about the patient which is to be used by the dentist for the diagnosis and treatment plan, and by the dentist and dental hygienist as a guide to treatment and its follow-up. The diagnostic work-up is discussed in more detail on pages 57–58.

The initial step is to determine the present state of the patient's general and oral health. The medical and dental histories, oral inspection, radiographic examination, and other sources of information are used. The findings of dental and periodontal examination are charted, study casts are made, vital signs recorded, and other tests made as indicated.

III. Treatment Plan

The dentist uses the data collected to formulate a diagnosis and outline a treatment plan. The many factors taken into consideration in treatment planning are described in Chapter 21, pages 293–300. It is necessary to plan a sequence of treatment that will assure elimination of etiologic factors of disease and restoration to health.

Within the overall treatment plan, the dental hygiene plan is organized with preventive, educational, and therapeutic phases, all designed to supplement parts of the treatment carried out by the dentist. The plan, then, is an outline of the essential procedures to be followed by the dentist, dental hygienist, and the patient.

IV. Preventive Services

Preventive measures needed are revealed during the collection of data for the diagnostic work-up. The history, examinations, dietary analysis, and radiographs can point up the specific prevention related to dental caries, periodontal diseases, oral habits, or other area that is needed. The preventive plan is outlined for those measures to be carried out in the dental office and those for the patient to conduct on a daily basis. Suggestions for the preventive plan may be found on page 302.

V. Educational

In conjunction with the preventive and therapeutic programs, the patient needs to become well-informed concerning the disease process, and how it can be arrested. Specific measures for the prevention of recurrence have to be demonstrated and practiced, redemonstrated, and reviewed as much as needed until appropriate habits of self-care have been established. Education may extend beyond the single patient, to the family, as well as into the community.

VI. Treatment

The therapeutic phase encompasses all of the dental hygiene techniques, and, depending on the state in which the hygienist practices, may include restorative and periodontal procedures. The procedures may involve *preliminary* treatment in which the teeth and gingiva are prepared for the additional treatment performed by the dentist, or *definitive* treatment. With definitive treatment, the hygienist's procedures may be the total treatment required, as is often the case in a young patient with gingivitis, when a combination of preventive, educational and therapeutic treatment is conducted by the dental hygienist. Follow-up treatment procedures are essential, and recall at appropriate intervals is directed at the preservation of the healthy state acquired during initial phases.

VII. Recall

Upon completion of the initial treatment phase, each patient's recall program is determined and future appointments reserved. The recall appointment is for the purpose of evaluation of the present state of oral health, and the steps follow the same pattern as the original diagnostic work-up. Each finding is charted, recorded, and reported to the dentist for re-evaluation. A new treatment plan is outlined. Preventive and educational phases are evaluated and renewed.

VIII. The Challenge of Planning Patient Care

Advancement in dental science has made it imperative for the professional dental hygienist to be able to adapt dental hygiene care to changing concepts with understanding and flexibility. Dental hygiene care needs to be modified intelligently according to the patient himself, his oral condition and disease, and his personal problems. Each patient is an individual with specific problems of oral care which need consideration. Good dental hygiene care is patient-centered.

The professional dental hygienist must be a self-directed person who can apply scientific knowledge to problem solving. The questions are: What is the status of this patient's oral health? Why and how did it happen? What can I do to supplement that which the dentist does for the patient? What can the patient do for himself that I can help him learn? What will be the outcome?

In the effort to deliver more effective and comprehensive health service, a set pattern of dental hygiene care, one which was memorized or learned by rote, cannot always be used. Knowledge must be applied to meet the individual needs of each patient.

II

Preparation for Dental Hygiene Appointments

Chapter 3

The Operating Room and Instruments

The cleanliness and neatness of the operating room reflect the character and conscientiousness of the dental personnel. The patient, with his limited knowledge of dental science, may judge the ability of the dental personnel by the appearance of the office.

The patient's attitude is important but more important is the relationship of cleanliness to the presence of microorganisms and the need for performing techniques in a hygienic situation. In addition, when equipment receives adequate care it will operate more efficiently and maintain its attractive appearance longer.

Fastidiousness in housekeeping duties and care of equipment and instruments appreciably increase the value of a dentist's auxiliary. The dental hygienist participates as a member of the dental team in contributing to the overall office cleanliness and tidiness.

A schedule for housekeeping contributes to effective work simplification. Certain duties must be carried out at the completion of each patient appointment, some once or twice daily, whereas others

are weekly or biweekly. Operating room and equipment care is a continuing process.

I. Objectives

Effective care of instruments and equipment contributes to the following:
A. Control of the spread of microorganisms.
B. An increase in the operating efficiency of the office personnel.
C. An atmosphere of cleanliness and orderliness which will contribute to the patient's well-being.
D. An increase in the patient's confidence in the ability of the dental personnel.
E. The maintenance of the working efficiency of office equipment and instruments which will prolong their span of usefulness.
F. A decrease in the occurrence of unpleasant odors in the office.

CARE OF OPERATING ROOM FURNITURE AND EQUIPMENT

The orderliness and immaculate cleanliness of the operatory result from continuing care. An excellent test for the effects of care and any minor oversights is for the dentist or hygienist to sit in the dental chair occasionally and look around at what the patient sees from that vantage point.

I. Furniture

Exterior surfaces of the dental chair, cabinets, dental unit, mobile stand or operating assembly, x-ray machine, operating stools, dental light, and any other fixed or movable furniture or equipment must be cleaned and polished on a regular basis. They should be wiped after each appointment, and receive a spot washing daily and a thorough cleaning weekly. A mild soap and water or agents indicated by the manufacturer to preserve the finish should be used. The walls near the sink, door knobs, window sills, and other well-used surfaces need attention.

II. Evacuation Equipment

Sanitation of evacuation equipment is essential to both function and esthetics. Oral evacuation equipment, whether central or for the individual room, must be effectively cleaned and a disinfecting spray utilized. Following each use, the oral tip is removed for autoclaving unless a disposable tip is used, and water is run through the connecting hose. A collection tank that is not emptied through the main system needs emptying regularly depending on use.

A cuspidor must be wiped clean and the rim rubbed vigorously with a surface disinfecting solution before each appointment. It must be thoroughly cleaned daily with removal of the catch basket and cleaning of metal or enamel parts. The saliva ejector needs at least two cups of water run through it following each use, since saliva is sticky and tends to coat the linings of the tubings. At least daily, the head of the tubing must be removed and the small mesh trap cleaned.

CARE OF MOTOR-DRIVEN INSTRUMENTS

Because the prophylaxis angle and handpiece contain intricate moving parts, they require regular cleaning and lubrication. Specific care is important first for the patient's safety as related to the transmission of microorganisms which is described in Chapter 4, page 25. Care of these instruments is also necessary because polishing agents, saliva, and oral debris can become lodged within the casing and damage the instrument.

Constant exposure to foreign particles and frictional movement contribute to aging of these instruments. The original cost and the cost of repairs are high; therefore routine care on a preventive basis is essential to all handpieces and angles.

Manufacturers of the instruments enclose instructions for their care. These should always be followed carefully with attention to directions which are specific for the individual make or brand.

I. The Prophylaxis Angle

The prophylaxis angle is a potential source for cross-contamination because of its close, direct contact with oral fluids during use. Selection of a prophylaxis angle can be significant. The instrument of choice is one which has an inner seal whose purpose is to prevent penetration of saliva into the working parts. It has been shown that culturing of two types of prophylaxis angles revealed internal contamination in over 50 percent of conventional angles, but fewer than five percent of those with an internal seal were contaminated.[1]

It cannot be overemphasized that the prophylaxis angle must be cleaned, lubricated, and sterilized soon after each use. To accomplish this, it is necessary to maintain several prophylaxis angles. Immediately following an appointment, the prophylaxis angle which was used needs to be wiped vigorously with a gauze sponge moistened with an effective disinfectant so that saliva and debris cannot dry on the surface.

A. **Manual Cleaning**
1. Attach prophylaxis angle to handpiece.
2. Separate rubber cup attachment and removable gears in accord with manufacturer's specifications, using the wrench or screw driver provided for the specific instrument.
3. Run forward and backward in cleaning fluid.
4. Scrub inside of head (opening into main body of angle) with end of pipe cleaner.
5. Again, run forward and backward in cleaning fluid.
6. Clean the parts which were separated: use a small soft brush dipped in the cleaning agent.
7. Wipe off cleaning fluid.

B. **Ultrasonic Cleaning** (page 20)
1. Disassemble rubber cup attachment and removable gears.
2. Place in ultrasonic tank solutions in sequence specified by manufacturer's directions.
3. Time: approximately one minute immediately after use; three to five minutes when postponed.

C. **Sterilization**
1. Use sterilization procedure indicated by the manufacturer. Autoclaving procedure is outlined on page 30 and hot oil on page 33.
2. Use a corrosion-preventive agent to coat the prophylaxis angle prior to autoclaving.[2,3]

D. **Lubrication**[4]
1. Lubricate prophylaxis angle after sterilization by autoclave.
2. Apply sterile oil with sterile swab.
3. Place a drop of oil under cap (rubber cup attachment).
4. Fill head with petrolatum.
5. Reassemble parts carefully, allowing gears to mesh so that the shaft turns easily.

II. **Belt-Driven Handpiece**

A. **Cleaning**
1. Remove outer sheath (figure 3–1).

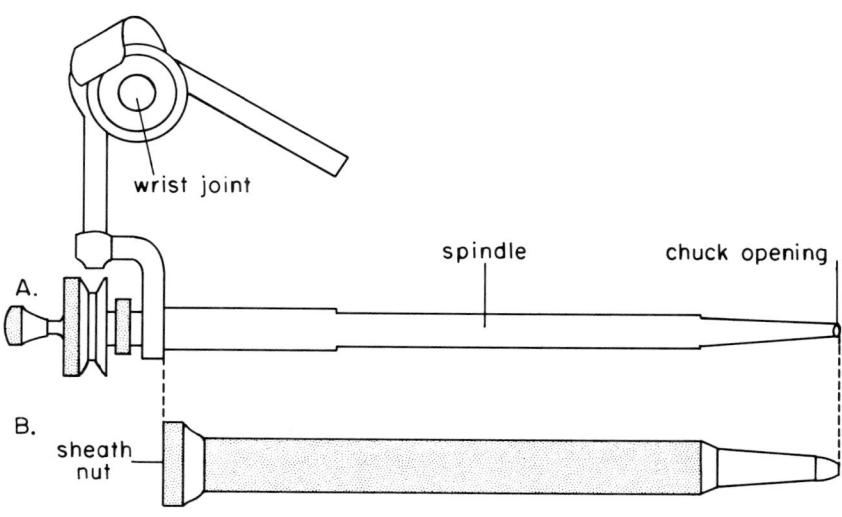

Figure 3–1.   Parts of a belt-driven dental handpiece. **A.** Handpiece with sheath removed. **B.** Sheath.

2. Wipe spindle (covering of inner part) with a clean dry cloth.
3. Ultrasonic cleaning may be used.

B. **Sterilization**
1. Use method in keeping with manufacturer's instructions. Autoclave or hot oil are indicated for many belt-driven handpieces (pages 30 and 33).
2. Use corrosion-preventive agent to coat the handpiece prior to autoclaving.[2,3]

C. **Lubrication**
Ordinarily the handpiece should be lubricated each morning as the oil will drip out while it hangs overnight. When the handpiece is laid flat, it may be lubricated at the end of the day. Caution should be used when applying oil as an excessive amount causes increased heat production and unnecessary wear.
1. Lubricate handpiece after sterilization by autoclave.
2. Apply sterile oil with sterile swab or pipe cleaner.
3. Oil chuck opening (at working end of spindle) with pipe cleaner dipped in oil. Insert pipe cleaner into the opening as far as it will go.
4. Hold handpiece with chuck opening up, and apply two drops of oil to tip of spindle. Draw the oil-moistened pipe cleaner across the back of the spindle once.
5. Apply a small amount of oil to wrist joint of handpiece attachment with cotton pliers; press ball of joint as oil is applied.
6. Replace sheath slowly to avoid splashing oil.

III. Dental Motor and Arm

A. **Daily Care**
Wipe arm, including pulleys.

B. **Weekly Care**
Oil pulley with end of pipe cleaner dipped in oil.

C. **Monthly Care**
Place *one* drop of oil in each oil hole of motor in accord with the manufacturer's specifications.

D. **Belt**
1. Adjust tension of belt for smooth running.
2. Replace belt when it begins to fray to avoid its breaking during an appointment.

IV. Air-Driven Handpiece[5]

There are a number of air-driven straight handpieces which can be operated at a speed low enough for dental hygiene polishing procedures. The care of these handpieces varies and *the manufacturer's specifications must be followed explicitly.*

A. **Oiling**
Some air-driven handpieces require no oiling; others have a centralized self-lubricating system which requires at least one daily check and refill from the outside box with special oil.

B. **Conditioning or Special Cleaning Fluid**
Required for certain handpieces.

C. **End of Day**
Most require that the water line be closed off and air run through for 30 seconds.

D. **Sterilization**
Because of the construction of the handpiece, known and proven sterilization methods cannot be used; therefore disinfection is the best that can be accomplished.
1. Characteristics which exclude usual techniques of sterilization include: the plastic (nylon) sleeve in the inner mechanism cannot be

heated to sterilizing temperature; the whole handpiece cannot be immersed in liquids which may be damaging to internal parts.

2. Sterilization by autoclave of the outer sheath is possible with some brands. Before it is replaced, the inner surface must be thoroughly dried.

E. **Disinfection:**
Between Appointment Care

1. Principles for action of a disinfectant: a quick, however vigorous, wiping of the outer sleeve of the handpiece is not adequate to satisfy requirements for chemical disinfection since the contact with the solution is too brief.

2. The film of saliva and debris if allowed to dry can form a protective covering for viable microorganisms. Immediately after use of the handpiece, this film should be removed.

3. Procedure[6]
   a. Wipe vigorously and thoroughly with two separate sterile gauze sponges saturated with an effective disinfectant solution.
   b. Recommended disinfectants
      (1) Isopropyl alcohol (70%)
      (2) Isopropyl alcohol (70%) mixed with .05 to 0.5% iodine (iodophore) surgical scrub. Prepare by adding one part iodine scrub to one part 70% alcohol. Remove excess iodine with plain alcohol.[6]
      (3) Phenolic compound such as two percent Staphene or Lysol.
      (4) Glutaraldehyde (two percent)[7]

4. After the mechanical cleansing, wrap a third 4" by 4" sterile gauze sponge saturated in the disinfectant around the handpiece and cover with a clean finger cot. The cot prevents volatilization of the disinfectant and maintains the gauze in place. The cot should remain in place a minimum of 15 minutes but preferably up to 30 minutes in accord with disinfection procedures.[8]

CARE OF MANUAL INSTRUMENTS

I. Handling

A transfer or handling forceps (figure 4–1, page 37) should be kept especially for use during the handling of unsterile instruments to eliminate the necessity for direct contact with the hands. Rubber gloves should be worn.

During processing for cleaning and sterilization careless handling of instruments with delicate working ends such as scalers and explorers can lead to fracture of the tips. Rubbing or rough contact of blades or tips with other instruments contributes to their dullness. Pressure or bending will distort various instruments, a problem which could be crucial to the use of explorers or periodontal probes.

Attention to glassware such as dappen dishes is necessary to prevent chipping or breakage. In addition, during careful handling, prevention of injury to the hands is of particular importance since before sterilization the instruments are contaminated.

To prevent rusting or discoloration, instruments should be cleaned as soon as possible after use. Even stainless steel can acquire a tarnish which is difficult to remove. If there is an unavoidable delay, or when instruments are accumulated to be cared for after a series of appointments, they should be rinsed with cold water to remove blood and debris and then immersed in warm water containing a blood solvent or detergent.

II. Manual Cleaning[9]

A. Rinse

Rinse or soak in cold water to remove blood and debris.

B. Decontaminate

Immerse in trisodium phosphate solution (one tablespoon per quart of water). Rinse thoroughly under running water.

C. Dismantle Instruments

Dismantle instruments with detachable parts such as the porte polisher and the mouth mirror with handle, and open instruments with joints such as scissors.

D. Clean by Scrub Technique

1. Apply a solvent to remove greases or oils.
2. Scrub with a stiff brush with detergent and running water to remove all particles of dried blood or debris.
3. Use a detergent, not ordinary soap.
   a. Soap can form insoluble alkalies in hard water which can enmesh and protect the bacteria from the sterilizing effect later.
   b. Cake soap can harbor microorganisms and become a potential source of transfer.
   c. Avoid use of abrasives or sharp cleaners as they may roughen the instrument surface and affect the stainless properties of the metal.
4. Apply individual measures for problem areas.
   a. Grooves and joints where debris can collect and harden, for example, the mouth mirror with grooves at the attachment of the shank as well as around the mirror rim.
   b. Saliva ejector. Slide a pipe cleaner dipped in detergent through a wide opening, or use a fine twisted wire through a narrow opening; use an instrument tip such as a broken explorer to clean around the small openings in the receiving end.

E. Rinse

Rinse in hot water to remove all detergent.

F. Dry

1. Purposes
   a. To prevent instrument discoloration if there is an interval before sterilization.
   b. Water will dilute the pre-autoclaving emulsion or cold disinfection solution.
   c. To prepare for sharpening.
2. Air dry. Prevents need for extra handling and added possibility of contamination of fingers.
3. Dry carefully with paper towels when time does not permit air drying. Care must be taken to protect the fingers. Dispose of towels.

G. Care of Scrub Brushes

1. Wash contaminated brushes in detergent, rinse thoroughly, and autoclave.
2. Label brushes or identify by using a specific size or shape only for instrument care to prevent inadvertent mixing with hand scrubbing brushes.

III. Ultrasonic Cleaning[10,11,12]

Ultrasonic cleaning prior to sterilization is safer than manual cleaning. Risk of injury to hands and infection is not as great.

Manual cleaning of instruments is a difficult and time-consuming procedure with numerous disadvantages. When ultrasonic equipment is adjusted for optimum performance and those using it are properly informed and adhere to the manufacturer's instructions, the quality of cleaning is much better than by the hand scrub technique. *Ultrasonic processing is not a substitute for sterilization: it is only a cleaning process.*

A. **Advantages**

Benefits from the use of ultrasonic cleaning include the following:

1. Increased efficiency in obtaining a high degree of cleanliness.
2. Reduced potential danger to operator from direct contact with serum hepatitis virus and other pathogens.
3. Improved effectiveness for disinfection.
4. Elimination of possible dissemination of microorganisms through release of aerosols and droplets which can occur during the scrubbing process.
5. Penetration into areas of the instruments where the bristles of a brush are too coarse to contact.
6. Removal of tarnish.

B. **Principles of Action**

Ultrasonic vibrations initiate cavitation in the cleansing solution. Cavitation means that minute bubbles are generated which expand until they are unstable, then they collapse by bursting inward. This creates minute vacuum areas which are responsible for the cleaning process by dislodging, dispersing, or dissolving the material which has adhered to the surface of the instrument.

Cleaning is accomplished by both the physical agitation and chemical dissolution. Soluble material goes into solution and heavier material sinks to the bottom of the cleaning tank.

C. **Procedure**

1. Various concentrates of the solution are available from the manufacturers. Selection is based on the specific use, for example, one solution is prepared for general instrument cleaning and another for removal of denture stains.
2. Wear rubber gloves to protect against infection and chemicals.
3. Instruments are placed in the carrier tray or basket, and submerged in the solution.
   a. Guard against overloading and crowding which can prevent the solution from reaching all surfaces.
   b. Open jointed instruments; dismantle detachable parts.
   c. Space instruments to avoid contacts between easily damaged surfaces which may lead to bending or dulling.
   d. Do not mix various metals in the same bath; for example, separate stainless steel, aluminum, copper, and brass.
4. Timing varies from one to ten minutes depending on the unit, the solution, and the material being treated. Consult manufacturer's chart.
5. Drain on removal, then rinse thoroughly with warm water.
6. Dry in air thoroughly.

D. **Care of Unit**

Filter or change solution and clean the unit regularly to maintain its efficiency.

PREPARATION FOR STERILIZATION

Methods for sterilization and disinfection will be described in the next chapter, along with other means for preventing the transmission of disease such as the proper handling of sterile supplies, handwashing, and the use of a face mask. In this chapter, preliminary procedures have been described for cleaning the instruments prior to sterilization.

Instruments may be arranged for the autoclave in a number of ways. For example, they may be placed on cloth or paper in the tray of the autoclave and covered with another paper or cloth, or they may be grouped by sets needed for an individual appointment and then packaged in an autoclave bag or a canister-type holder.

After sterilization, the instruments can be transferred with a sterile transfer forceps to an operating tray which has been covered with a sterile towel and then covered with a second sterile towel for transfer to the chairside. Gauze sponges, cotton rolls, and other accessories to the appointment can be packaged in small lots for individual appointments. Whichever system is used, the maintenance of sterility is the first consideration.

The system for use of preprepared trays described below has a number of advantages. With analysis and experiment, each dental hygienist can adapt a tray system to the specific needs of an individual practice.

I. Preprepared Trays

Preprepared trays are preplanned trays, arranged to contain all of the items usually needed for a particular appointment, and sterilized and assembled, ready for delivery at the dental chair at the time of the appointment. The trays are prepared in advance so that either a half day's or an entire day's appointments may be conducted without the confusion frequently related to the preparation for individual appointments.

A. **Characteristics**
1. Trays should be as large as possible but small enough for sterilization in the autoclave.
2. Instruments should be arranged in an orderly manner on the tray, in sequence for use, with accessory materials conveniently placed. Instruments and materials to be used throughout the appointment are grouped in contrasting position to those such as floss or cotton roll holders, which may be used once or twice during the appointment.
3. An excess of instruments should be avoided. Double-ended instruments conserve space and limit the need for repeated changing. The basic tray should meet the basic needs.
4. Extra instruments to replace a dulled or dropped instrument, or to supplement when a particular problem requires a special instrument, are autoclaved in labeled autoclave bags, and kept in a convenient place within reach of the operating position.
5. Trays should be marked for identification of contents, for examples, *Adult Scaling and Curettage; Small Child Examination.*
6. Specially designed cabinets with slots for sterile trays are available or may be constructed for storage purposes.
7. When a number of similar trays are prepared in advance, it is best to use them in sequence to maintain sterility.

B. **Advantages**
1. Instruments can be sterile at the time of use; when instruments are handled several times, first to transfer from the sterilizer to a cabinet, then back to a tray or bracket table, sterility is destroyed.
2. Preserves sharpness of instruments since they can be arranged and kept apart from other instruments, in an orderly manner. When placed in a bag or canister, contact with other instruments can dull them.
3. Increases efficiency and conserves time:
   a. Between-appointment preparation is minimized; delays for the patient are lessened.

b. Instruments needed are at the fingertips.

4. Trays may be positioned at the convenience of the dental hygienist working alone, or the assistant in a team plan (pages 54–55).

5. Sterilizing procedures can be systematized.

II. Preprepared Tray Arrangements

Suggested contents for trays are listed here. Specific names and numbers for explorers, probes, scalers, curets, or other instruments are not included because of individual variation. However, specific lists should be made and posted near the tray content lists for dental operations, so that all concerned with tray preparations can have immediate reference.

Variations in tray contents vary with the type of practice. In a specialty practice as, for example, periodontics, trays for dressing and suture removal would be needed more frequently than in a general practice; therefore more trays would be prepared in advance.

A. Initial Appointment: Examination Tray

Mouth mirror
Explorers
Probe
Cotton pliers
Saliva ejector tip
Air syringe tip
Gauze sponges
Applicator
Impression trays for study casts
X-ray film holder if made of a material which can be autoclaved.

B. Adult Scaling and Root Planing

Mouth mirror
Explorers
Probe
Cotton pliers
Scalers
Curets
Dappen dishes
Polishing cups
Porte polisher; wood points
Aspirator or evacuator tip
Air syringe tip

Saliva ejector tip
Gauze sponges
Dental floss lengths
Cotton rolls
Applicator

C. Topical Fluoride Application

Cotton roll holders
Cotton rolls cut to appropriate lengths
Cotton pellets and cotton pliers, or applicators
Dappen dish
Saliva ejector tip
Air syringe tip

TECHNICAL HINTS

I. Wash handpiece belt occasionally with mild soap and water to remove grease and oil. Grease and oil cause loss of traction and attract dust. Replace belt while it is still partially dry.

II. Do not leave mandrel-mounted cutting or polishing instruments in a handpiece overnight or other extended period of time. Steel shanks may rust and corrode and plastic chucks are subject to distortion.

III. Keep prophylaxis angles and handpiece protected from dust and debris.

References

1. Stewart, R. T. and Levin, B. G.: A Source of Iatrogenic Infection, *J. Am. Dent. Hyg. Assoc.*, 45, 169, May–June, 1971.
2. Charbeneau, G. T., and Berry, G. C.: A Simple and Effective Autoclave Method of Handpiece and Instrument Sterilization Without Corrosion, *J. Am. Dent. Assoc.*, 59, 732, October, 1959.
3. Bertolotti, R. L. and Hurst, V.: Inhibition of Corrosion during Autoclave Sterilization of Carbon Steel Dental Instruments, *J. Am. Dent. Assoc.*, 97, 628, October, 1978.
4. Charbeneau, G. T. and Peyton, F. A.: Evaluation of Lubricants for Dental Handpieces and Contra-Angles, *J. Dent. Res.*, 36, 479, June, 1957.
5. Sockwell, C. L.: Dental Handpieces and Rotary Cutting Instruments, *Dent. Clin. North Am.*, 15, 219, January, 1971.
6. Crawford, J. J.: *Clinical Asepsis in Dentistry: Advanced Instruction Concerning Causes and Prevention of Infections in Dental Practice.* Chapel Hill, University of North Carolina, 1978.

7. Neugeboren, N., Nisengard, R. J., Beutner, E. H., and Ferguson, G. W.: Control of Cross-contamination, *J. Am. Dent. Assoc.*, 85, 123, July, 1972.
8. Larato, D. C.: Sterilization of the High Speed Dental Handpiece, *Dent. Dig.*, 72, 107, March, 1966.
9. Perkins, J. J.: *Principles and Methods of Sterilization in Health Sciences*, 2nd ed. Springfield, Charles C Thomas, 1969, pp. 237–239, 262–263.
10. Charbeneau, G. T.: Use of Ultrasonic Techniques for Cleaning Instruments and Appliances, *J. Prosthet. Dent.*, 11, 573, May–June, 1961.
11. Perkins: op cit., pp. 245–253.
12. Shaner, E. O.: Acoustical-Chemical Parameters for the Ultrasonic Sterilization of Instruments, *J. Oral Thera. and Pharm.*, 3, 417, May, 1967.

Suggested Readings

American Dental Association, Council on Dental Materials and Devices, Peyton, F. A.: Status Report on Dental Operating Handpieces, *J. Am. Dent. Assoc.*, 89, 1162, November, 1974.

Litchfield, N. B.: A Sterile Tray Storage System for Dental and Medical Use, *Aust. Dent. J.*, 13, 135, April, 1968.

Raskin, E. R.: A Handpiece Sterilization Procedure, *J. Prosthet. Dent.*, 14, 990, September–October, 1964.

Simon, W. J.: *Clinical Dental Assisting*. Hagerstown, Maryland, Harper & Row, 1973, pp. 185–188.

Sinnett, G. M. and Wuehrmann, A. H.: Dental Operatory of the Future, in Peterson, S., ed.: *The Dentist and His Assistant*, 3rd ed. St. Louis, Mosby, 1972, pp. 392–401.

Chapter 4

Prevention of Disease Transmission

Transmission of disease is an insidious process. When a patient is known to have a condition which involves communicable pathogenic microorganisms, special precautions can be taken before instruments and other nondisposable items are used for another patient. The presence of disease-producing organisms is not always known; therefore, there is a need for application of protective, preventive procedures prior to, during, and following *all* patient appointments.

Pathogenic (disease producing), potentially pathogenic, or nonpathogenic microorganisms may be present in the oral cavity of each patient. Pathogenic organisms may be transient. Patients may be carriers of certain diseases. Inadvertent transmission to subsequent susceptible patients or to dental personnel may occur as a result of careless handwashing or inadequate sterilization or handling of sterile instruments.

The intact mucous membrane of the oral cavity protects against infection to a degree. However, when the gingival tissues are manipulated during instrumentation, microorganisms can be introduced into the underlying tissues.

I. Microorganisms of the Oral Cavity

At birth the oral cavity is sterile, but within a few hours to one day a simple oral flora develops. In a mature mouth, bacterial counts of the saliva are close to six billion per milliliter and are composed of at least 30 species.[1] Most of the salivary bacteria come from the dorsum of the tongue, while some are from other mucous membranes.[2] Much larger counts, up to 200 billion microorganisms per milliliter, are found in dental plaque.

A. Pathogens

The organisms of many communicable diseases enter the body by way of the oral cavity. A few infectious diseases have specific oral manifestations such as the chancre and mucous patches of syphilis and the Koplik's spots of measles. Pathogens can be present within the oral cavity without an oral manifestation, a fact which is of particular importance to the total consideration of disease transmission.

Certain pathogens may reside regularly in the oral cavity in small numbers. A few of the pathogens which may be found in the oral cavity, along with their pathologic manifestations, are:

1. *Staphylococcus aureus* (abscesses, postoperative infections).
2. Hemolytic streptococcus (rheumatic fever, subacute bacterial endocarditis).
3. *Candida albicans* (Candidiasis or thrush, skin infections).
4. Herpes simplex virus (fever blisters, herpetic stomatitis).
5. *Mycobacterium tuberculosis* (tuberculosis).
6. *Treponema pallidum* (syphilis).
7. *Diplococcus pneumoniae* (pneumonia).
8. Hepatitis viruses (Type A, Infectious hepatitis; Type B, Serum hepatitis).

B. **Hepatitis**[3,4,5]

The incidence of hepatitis has increased significantly over the past 20 years. Among professional personnel, both medical and dental, the incidence has reached startling proportions to the point where the use of strict sterilization and self-protection measures are mandatory.

1. *Types.* At least two types of hepatitis have been identified. No cross immunity has been demonstrated between the two.
   a. Type A. Short incubation or infectious hepatitis has an incubation period usually two to six weeks.
   b. Type B. Long incubation or serum hepatitis has a variable incubation period usually about two months after parenteral exposure and about three months after oral exposure, and up to six months.
2. *Route of Transmission.* Either type may be transmitted by an oral-fecal or a parenteral route. Parenteral refers to a route other than oral, for example, intravenous or subcutaneous by way of a break in the skin. Transmission by saliva and blood present the greatest hazards.
3. *Course of Disease and Symptoms.* Hepatitis is characterized by inflammation of the liver in both types. With either, there may or may not be jaundice. Recovery may take two to four months. The viruses have been demonstrated in the blood stream and saliva, and excreted in the feces, several months after symptoms have disappeared.
4. *Carrier.* Many people carry hepatitis without having had disease symptoms. Approximately five percent of those who have just had acute hepatitis become carriers. There may be a much higher percentage in people who have an impaired immune response associated with certain disorders such as Down's syndrome (Mongolism), leukemia, and uremia managed by dialysis. Dental personnel need to be tested to determine whether or not they are carriers.
5. *Gamma Globulin.* Gamma globulin injections can prevent or reduce symptoms of infectious hepatitis. The injections are recommended following exposure to infectious hepatitis.

C. **Prevention of Transmission**[7]

The following list of procedures for dental personnel pertains in particular to hepatitis, but the same basic principles are important to all disease prevention. Other pathogenic microorganisms may have unique characteristics which require special measures.

1. Prepare a comprehensive patient history. Refer suspected patients for laboratory tests available for

symptomless carriers. When a patient has a history of jaundice within three months, treat the patient as a carrier.

2. Use disposable covers wherever possible. Cover lamp handles and other surfaces where contact may be made.
3. Wear a mask and a hair cover.
4. Use a thorough scrub technique for preparation of the hands. Cover all skin breaks. Wear rubber gloves.
5. Use disposable injection needles and other disposables when treatment involves penetration of tissue.
6. Keep needles capped on the instrument tray at all times to avoid accidental penetration or self-inoculation.
7. Destroy injection needles when disposing of them so that no unauthorized person can have access to them.
8. Dispose of all partially emptied carpules of anesthetics.
9. Wash instruments promptly following oral procedures to prevent blood and other organic material from drying on and therefore interfering with subsequent sterilization.
10. Wear gloves when preparing instruments for sterilization.
11. Avoid use of instruments which create aerosols (ultrasonic scaler, handpiece at high speed) when necessary to treat a patient known to be carrier.
12. Use only steam under pressure or dry heat sterilization for instruments, never methods that only disinfect.
13. Apply careful techniques and sterilization procedures for all, not just suspected or known carriers.
14. Perform surface disinfection for all possible contacts of the hand which have had contact with the oral cavity of a patient.
15. Develop habits which minimize

contacts with switches and other parts of the dental unit and chair, light, and operating stool.

II. Microorganisms of the Air

Transmission of microorganisms occurs by direct droplets from patient to operator or operator to patient, by way of hands and instruments which have made contact with the patient's oral cavity, or indirectly from the hands to other objects, such as the equipment or records, from which organisms may be picked up and brought to an oral cavity or skin break.

In addition, organisms enter the air of the operatory and thus provide another means for indirect transmission to a susceptible person, a subsequent patient, or a member of the dental team.

A. Dust-borne Organisms

Clostridium tetani (tetanus bacillus), *Staphylococcus aureus*, and enteric bacteria may travel in the dust brought in from outside and which moves in and about dental operatories. When doors are opened and closed and people pass in and out, dust is set into motion which can settle on instruments, other objects, or people.

Infectious microorganisms also reach dust from the oral cavities of patients by way of airborne particles. Dust-borne organisms can be sources of contamination for dental instruments and the hands of dental personnel.

General cleanliness of the operatory has already been discussed in the previous chapter. Surface disinfection of all equipment contacts during a dental appointment contributes to control of dust-borne pathogens. Agents for surface disinfection are described on page 19.

B. Aerosol Production

1. *Definition.* An aerosol is an artificially generated collection of particles suspended in air and capable of

causing an airborne infection. Airborne particles vary in size. Those less than 50 micrometers (μm) in diameter are considered true aerosols. They are biologic contaminants that occur in solid or liquid form, are invisible, and remain suspended in air for long periods. Heavier, larger airborne particles drop and splatter on objects, people, or the floor.

2. *Origin.* Aerosols are created during breathing, speaking, coughing, or sneezing. They are produced during all intraoral procedures including examination and manual scaling. When produced by air-spray, air-water-spray, polishing the teeth, or other handpiece activity, the number of aerosols increases to tremendous proportions.[8]

3. *Contents*
   a. Single microorganism.
   b. Clump of microorganisms adhered to a dust or debris particle.
   c. One or more organisms in a liquid droplet.
   d. Aerosols created during cavity preparation may contain tooth fragments, microorganisms resident in the saliva, plaque, and/or oropharynx or nasopharynx, oil from a handpiece, water droplets.
   e. Aerosols produced during the use of an ultrasonic scaler have been shown to contain great numbers of organisms including hemolytic and nonhemolytic *Staphylococcus albus,* alpha, beta, and gamma streptococci, pneumococci, and diphtheroids.[9]

4. *Concentration.* Bacteria-laden aerosols are in greater concentration close to the scene of operation, and the quantity decreases with distance.[10]

C. **Prevention of Transmission**

The control of airborne infection depends on elimination or limitation of the organisms at their source, interruption of transmission, and protection of the potentially susceptible recipient.[11]

1. Limitation of organisms
   a. Postpone elective treatment for a patient known to have specific communicable organisms in the oral cavity.
   b. Use preoperative oral hygiene measures. Toothbrushing with water or a mouthwash or rinsing with water or a mouthwash have been shown to reduce the bacteria contained in aerosols. Rinsing with an antibacterial mouthwash was slightly more effective than the other procedures.[12]
   c. Introduction of antibacterial agent into the water supply to the handpiece.[13] By this method, the antibacterial agent becomes a part of the droplet nuclei, thus having a longer working period to kill the microorganisms.

2. Interruption of transmission
   a. Use rubber dam, high volume evacuation, and hand instrumentation as much as possible.[14]
   b. Install air control methods to supply adequate ventilation, filtration, and relative humidity.
   c. Employ vacuum cleaning to remove dirt and microorganisms rather than dust-arousing housekeeping methods. The cleaner must have a filter to prevent the escape of organisms after they are suctioned.[11]

3. Protection of the recipient
   a. Masks. Dental personnel need an impermeable mask; patient needs a protective shield for nose and eyes[15] (pages 38–39).
   b. Eyeglasses. When corrective

lenses are not needed by dental personnel, large plain glass eyeglasses must be worn to protect from the aerosols and splatter.

STERILIZATION

I. Sterilization Clarified

Clarification of terms is important to understanding the objectives to be attained in the use of various methods applied for the control of disease transmission. Definitions included here are for comparison of results which can be expected when various methods and/or materials are applied. Other terms are defined in the glossary.

A. **Sterilization**

The process by which all forms of life, including bacterial spores and viruses, are destroyed.

B. **Disinfection**

Any process, chemical or physical, by means of which pathogenic agents or disease-producing microorganisms can be destroyed. *Disinfectants* are applied to inanimate objects in contrast to *antiseptics* which are applied to living tissues. As ordinarily employed, disinfection may or may not destroy tubercle bacilli or inactivate viruses, particularly the hepatitis viruses.

C. **Sanitization**

The process by which the number of organisms on inanimate objects are reduced to a safe level. It does not imply freedom from microorganisms and generally refers to a cleaning process.

D. **Surface Disinfection**

The process by which microorganisms which contaminate surfaces of implements and equipment are removed by wiping with a sterile sponge soaked in a disinfectant.

E. **Contamination**

The presence of microorganisms on a body surface or on inanimate articles or substances.

II. Control Program

The program for the control of microorganisms in a dental clinic or office needs to be planned around destruction of the most resistant, dangerous microorganisms. Adequacy of a particular procedure or agent is generally based on its effectiveness in killing all vegetative forms of pathogenic organisms including spores, *Mycobacterium tuberculosis*, and the hepatitis viruses.

The success of a planned system for disease transmission control depends on the cooperative effort of each member of the dental health team. *The objective should be to provide the most complete degree of sterile technique possible and practical in order to break any chain of infection.* The factors involved in attaining this objective in the preparation for and during the appointment include the following:

A. Adequate housekeeping and maintenance.
B. Cleanliness of the air.
C. Surface disinfection of equipment and disinfection of items impossible to sterilize.
D. Consistent, thorough handwashing procedures and protection of skin breaks.
E. Sterilization and effective handling of instruments.
F. Use of disposable packaged and presterilized items when available and when their use means safer procedures.
G. Protection of dental personnel with mask and glasses or eye protector.
H. Reduction of aerosols by preparation of patient with antiseptic mouthwash rinse or other oral hygiene measure,

and surface disinfection for the field of operation in the oral cavity.

I. Definitive postoperative decontamination and cleaning of instruments.

METHODS OF STERILIZATION

The elected process of sterilization must provide quick and complete destruction of all microorganisms, viruses, and spores, must not damage instruments and other materials, and must be capable of being carried out efficiently. Before sterilization, attention must be directed to insure that all instruments have been thoroughly cleaned. Oil, grease, and blood or organic matter which have been allowed to dry on the instruments can harbor spores and resistant microorganisms and protect them from sterilization. Instrument preparation for sterilization has been described on pages 21–23.

The two principal agents capable of producing sterility are moist heat and dry heat. Destruction of microorganisms by heat takes place as a result of inactivation of essential cellular proteins or enzymes. Moist heat causes coagulation of protein whereas with dry heat the action is one of oxidation.

I. Moist Heat: Steam Under Pressure[16,17,18]

A. **Use**

Moist heat may be used for all materials except oils, waxes, and powders which are impervious to steam, or materials which cannot be subjected to high temperatures, such as plastics.

B. **Principles for Action**

1. Sterilization is achieved by action of heat and moisture; pressure serves only to attain high temperature.
2. Sterilization depends on the penetrating ability of steam.
   a. Air must be excluded, otherwise steam penetration and heat transfer are prevented.
   b. Space between objects is essential to assure access for the steam.
   c. Materials must be thoroughly cleaned since adherent material can provide a barrier to the steam.
   d. Air discharge occurs in a downward direction; load must be arranged for free passage of steam toward bottom of autoclave.

C. **Preparation of Materials**

Linens are laundered; instruments are scrubbed or cleaned in ultrasonic cleaner and dried (pages 20–21).

1. *Protection of Metal Instruments from Corrosion.* Use corrosion inhibitor.[19] Immerse, drain, and wrap or place in tray. This procedure is needed primarily for carbon steel instruments.
2. *Wrapping.* Bundles may be made with paper, muslin, or cellulose dialysis tubing.[20] Steam will not penetrate canvas, cellophane, plastic cloth, or aluminum foil. Tie or seal with autoclave tape; do not use pins for fastening paper because the holes made leave openings for contamination. Label with date and list of contents.
3. *Autoclave Tape.* Bundle is sealed with tape which develops colored stripes at 250° F.
4. *Autoclave Bags.* These are commercially available; they should not be overloaded.
5. *Tray.* Trays are perforated to permit steam to pass through.
6. *Packing Autoclave.* Pack loosely to permit steam to reach all instruments in all packages; place jars or tall vessels on their sides to permit air to leave as steam enters.

D. **Operation**

Follow manufacturer's specifications for use of autoclave.

1. *Temperature.* 250° F (121° C) which is usually attained at 15 to 20 pounds pressure.
2. *Time.* Minimum 15 to 20 minutes after the temperature reaches 250° F; 30 minutes for materials to be stored.

E. **Cooling**
   1. *Dry Materials.* Release steam pressure, turn operating valve, and open the door; required time for drying about 15 minutes.
   2. *Liquids.* Reduce chamber pressure slowly at an even rate over 10 to 12 minutes to prevent boiling or escape of fluids into the chamber; preferable to turn off the autoclave and let the pressure fall before opening the door. Check heat sensitivity of solution and avoid prolonged exposure as indicated.

F. **Care of Autoclave**
   1. *Daily.* Maintain proper level of distilled water; wash trays and interior surfaces of chamber with water and a mild detergent; clean removable plug, screen or strainer.
   2. *Weekly.* Flush chamber discharge system with an appropriate cleaning solution such as hot trisodium phosphate.

G. **Sterilization or Spore Test**
   Autoclave tape color change is related to temperature, not time, so for a real test of sterilization, a weekly spore test is recommended. A test should also be made on a new machine or following repairs.
   Ampules containing living, resistant spores plus a color indicator are available. Sources are listed in the Technical Hints at the end of this chapter. An ampule is placed in the center of a load of packages to be autoclaved. After sterilization has been completed by the usual time-temperature, the ampule and one which was not auto-

claved are incubated according to the manufacturer's directions. Unautoclaved spores will change the color indicator, whereas the autoclaved spores will not germinate.

H. **Evaluation**
   1. *Advantages*
      a. All microorganisms, spores, and viruses destroyed quickly and efficiently.
      b. Wide variety of materials may be treated; most generally economical.
   2. *Disadvantages*
      a. May corrode carbon steel instruments if precautions are not taken; tends to reduce cutting edges slightly.
      b. Unsuitable for oils or powders that are impervious to heat.

II. **Dry Heat**[16,17,21]
A. **Use**
   1. Primarily for materials which cannot safely be sterilized with steam under pressure.
   2. Oils and powders when they are thermostabile at the required temperatures.
   3. For small metal instruments enclosed in special containers or which might be corroded or rusted by moisture, such as endodontic instruments.

B. **Principles for Action**
   1. Sterilization is achieved by heat which is conducted from the exterior surface to the interior of the object; the time required to penetrate varies between materials.
   2. Sterilization can result when the whole material is treated for a sufficient length of time at the specified temperature: timing for sterilization must therefore start when the entire contents of the sterilizer have reached the peak temperature needed for that load.

3. Oil, grease, or organic debris on instruments insulates and protects microorganisms from the sterilizing effect.

C. **Preparation of Materials**
   1. *Instruments,* glassware, or other materials must be thoroughly cleaned and dried.
   2. *Packaging or Containers.* Small amounts best, because of access of heat, as well as the practical aspect of sterilizing an amount which will be used for a given purpose.
   3. *Packing the Sterilizer.* Allow space for access of heat around each item; never load to the limit.

D. **Operation**
   1. *Temperature.* 320° to 325° F (160° to 163° C) held for at least one hour, preferably longer. Timing must start after the desired temperature has been reached.
   2. *Penetration time* varies with different materials, and the nature and properties of various materials must be considered.
   3. *Care* must be taken not to overheat as certain materials can be affected: temperatures over 320° F may destroy the sharp edges of certain instruments.
   4. *Spore tests for sterilization* are available. Procedures are similar to those for autoclave (see **I.**G above).

E. **Evaluation**
   1. *Advantages*
      a. Useful for materials which cannot be subjected to steam under pressure.
      b. When maintained at correct temperature, it is well-suited for sharp instruments.
      c. No corrosion as found with steam under pressure.
   2. *Disadvantages*
      a. Long exposure required; penetration slow and uneven.

b. High temperatures critical to certain materials.

METHODS OF DISINFECTION

Disinfection does not accomplish complete destruction of all forms of microorganisms; therefore it is not a substitute for sterilization but rather a supplement to it. Physical or chemical means are used for disinfection. The effect produced is one of coagulation, precipitation, or denaturation of the protein, particularly the enzymes, of microorganisms.

I. Boiling Water[16,22]

A. **Use**
   Boiling water may be used for the disinfection of metal instruments, glassware, or other materials which can be subjected to water.

B. **Principles for Action**
   1. Disinfection is accomplished by heat.
   2. Objects must be completely submerged for a sufficient length of time.
   3. Bactericidal effect is increased by the addition of an alkali such as two percent sodium carbonate.
   4. Use distilled water to supply the boiler.

C. **Preparation of Materials**
   1. Scrub thoroughly, or use ultrasonic cleaner (pages 20–21).
   2. Disassemble or open jointed instruments.
   3. Arrange items carefully in metal basket of boiler to protect delicate and sharp edges and provide access of the boiling water; instruments must be completely submerged.

D. **Operation**
   1. Minimum of 20 minutes at boiling (212° F or 100° C at sea level).
   2. When instruments are added to those already boiling, the time cycle must be repeated.

3. An increase of heat does not increase the temperature of boiling water. Action is more vigorous and evaporation is increased.
4. Instruments should be removed with transfer forceps while hot and dried promptly to prevent rusting.

E. **Care of unit**

To decrease corrosive action on instruments and the formation of scaly deposit on the sides of the unit, use distilled water and add an antirust agent such as trisodium phosphate, sodium carbonate, or borax. Daily cleaning is necessary for units in constant use. Add a small amount of acetic acid (vinegar) and boil for 10 minutes to loosen the scale, then apply scrub brush and water, and rinse before filling.

F. **Evaluation**

1. *Advantages.* Relatively short time required for disinfection and the preparation of materials is simple.
2. *Disadvantages.* Limited usefulness in a dental office because of the resistance of certain organisms, reduction in sharpness of instruments, and the tendency for instruments to corrode.

II. Hot Oil[16]

A hot oil unit which utilizes a hydrocarbon or silicone oil has been used for jointed instruments and for certain handpieces, provided the manufacturer has so designated.

A. **Principles for Action**

1. Disinfection is achieved by heat.
2. Instrument must be completely submerged for a sufficient length of time.

B. **Preparation of Materials**

See pages 16 and 19 for handpiece and instrument cleaning.

C. **Operation**

1. *Temperature and time.* Disinfection can be attained at 300° F (149° C) for 15 minutes or at 260° F (125° C) for 20 to 30 minutes. Using 320° F (160° C) spore-formers will also be destroyed if held for a minimum of one hour. Timing must start after the desired temperature has been reached. Since some prophylaxis angles may be destroyed at high temperatures, the highest temperature possible should be used and the expected results evaluated.
2. *Handpiece care.* When a handpiece is removed from the oil bath, it must be drained, a towel should be held around the handpiece, and the power turned on so that excess oil can be removed before use to prevent splashing a patient.

D. **Evaluation**

1. *Advantages.* Sharp edges are not dulled; hot oil does not rust or corrode metal.
2. *Disadvantages.* The long exposure required can reduce the hardness of metal instruments; oil may produce unpleasant odors while heated; cleaning of the unit is inconvenient and unpleasant.

III. Chemical Solutions[23,24]

The term "cold sterilization," which is rather commonly used, is a misnomer which can be misleading. There is no cold chemical agent at the present time which can be considered a substitute for complete sterilization accomplished by steam under pressure or dry heat.

Chemical agents which have been tried in the past or are in current use have not been shown completely effective in killing resistant tubercle bacilli, hepatitis viruses, or bacterial spores. Many of the chemical solutions are only bacteriostatic which, for certain preparations, may depend on concentration since some agents are bactericidal at one concentration and bacteriostatic at another. Since chemical solutions do not destroy certain pathogens, viruses, and spores, it is important to recognize that the solution itself can become contaminated and thus contaminate instruments placed in it.

The American Dental Association has outlined provisions for acceptance of chemicals proposed for the disinfection of instruments, and lists those approved in the *Accepted Dental Therapeutics*. For acceptance a disinfectant must be effective in killing vegetative forms of pathogenic organisms, influenza and enteroviruses and the tubercle bacillus within 30 minutes. The label must include statements to clarify the inability of the agent to kill spores and hepatitis viruses, the unsuitability for disinfection of hyperdermic needles, and other specific regulatory information.[6]

A. **Uses**
1. For stop-gap measure to use only until sterilizable instruments can be obtained: disinfection of instruments or other items which cannot be sterilized because of their incompatibility with heat. This does not imply disinfection for items intended to be disposable.
2. For surface disinfection of immovable attachments contacted during an appointment.
3. For disinfection of dental appliances prior to insertion into the patient's mouth. Selection of a disinfectant depends on compatibility with oral tissues, although thorough rinsing with water after use of disinfection is indicated. Solution is used for one patient only.
4. Acts as the active ingredient in surgical handwashing preparations.

B. **Principles for Action**
1. Disinfection is achieved by coagulation, precipitation, or oxidation of protein of microbial cells or denaturation of the enzymes of the cells.
2. Disinfection depends on the contact of the solution at the known effective concentration for the optimum period of time.
3. Items must be thoroughly cleaned and dried since action of the agent is altered by foreign matter and dilution.
4. Solutions have specific shelf life. Some may change their pH, or the active ingredient may decrease. Length of time may depend on amount of use; check manufacturer's directions.

C. **Preparation of Materials**
1. *Scrub* thoroughly or use ultrasonic cleaner (pages 20–21) to eliminate organic matter (blood, debris, oil, grease) which interferes with the action of the chemical. Use wire brush for grooved metal instruments such as files or burs.
2. *Dismantle* or open jointed instruments to permit direct contact of solution with each surface.
3. *Rinse* thoroughly to eliminate soap or detergent which is incompatible with the chemical.
4. *Dry* thoroughly. Dilution of the chemical solution will lessen or eliminate its effect. Place on paper towels to blot dry. Care must be taken not to puncture rubber gloves.

D. **Operation**
1. Place instruments in solution and immerse completely; solution must contact all parts. Care must be taken to prevent overloading.
2. Temperature: usually room temperature.
3. Time: follow manufacturer's instructions. Time varies from 20 to 60 minutes.

4. Do not add other instruments without starting timing over again.
5. When time is complete, drain the instruments, remove with sterile transfer forceps, and dry with a sterile towel. When a solution is known to be irritating to tissue or distasteful, instruments should be rinsed to remove the chemical.
6. Aluminum-capped anesthetic carpules may react with chemical agents such as preparations of formaldehyde, mercury, phenols, or quaternary ammonium compounds. With corrosion of the aluminum, the anesthetic inside can be considered contaminated.

E. **Care of Equipment**
1. Keep the container covered to prevent contamination of the solution from dust- or airborne microorganisms.
2. Clean the container and change the solution on a regular schedule to maintain its cleanliness, proper dilution and potency in accord with the shelf life of the chemical.

F. **Types of Chemical Agents**

Chemical agents used as disinfectants include compounds or derivatives of phenol, iodine, chlorine, formaldehyde, alcohols, organic mercurials, and quaternary ammonium compounds. Combination germicides have been prepared and show that in certain instances the combination is more effective than any one chemical alone.

There are many disinfectants, some of which are appropriate for use in the dental office for disinfection and sanitation. A few of the more widely used ones are described briefly below.
1. *Glutaraldehyde*
   a. Action. Buffered 2% glutaraldehyde has a two-week shelf life. It is effective against fungi, some viruses (not hepatitis), and bacteria including the tubercle bacillus in 10, preferably 15, minutes, and against spores when the time is extended to 10 hours.
   b. Precautions. Buffered 2% glutaraldehyde can cause irritation of the eyes and skin, and should be handled to prevent skin contact. Rinsing with water immediately following contact is necessary. Carbon steel instruments may corrode if left in the solution over 24 hours.
   c. Clinical care. Rinse instruments with sterile water or 70% isopropyl alcohol after removing from the disinfecting solution to prevent contact of the solution with the patient's oral cavity.
   d. Examples: Cidex (buffered 2% glutaraldehyde); Sonacide (a new acid 2% glutaraldehyde).[25]
2. *Phenolic Compounds*
   a. Action. The 1 percent solutions are effective for destroying vegetative bacteria and fungi, and the 2 percent are effective against the tubercle bacillus. They serve primarily in the germicide-cleaning capacity.
   b. Examples: Amphyl, O-syl, San Pheno X, Staphene, and hexachlorophene.
3. *Iodine Complex: Iodophors*
   a. Action. Free iodine in a preparation or the liberation of iodine provides effective antibacterial action. Povidone-iodine has been shown to be effective in a surgical soap preparation, as a mouthwash for use prior to surgical procedures to reduce bacteremia and aerosols, and as a solution for topical application.[26,27]
   b. Example: Betadine.

4. *Quaternary Ammonium Com-*
   pounds
   a. Action: will not destroy spores, tubercle bacilli, or hepatitis viruses but will kill most vegetative cells if instruments are clean and smooth; not dependable for instruments that penetrate tissue. They are relatively nonirritating to tissue.
   b. Limitations. Solutions containing benzalkonium chloride are effective against a narrow range of microorganisms and viruses. They are inactivated by soap and are reduced in effectiveness in the presence of organic matter. They are removed from solution by cotton and gauze; therefore sponges for surface disinfection must be freshly soaked with the solution just before use.
   c. Examples: Cetylcide, benzalkonium chloride (Zephiran), and benzethonium chloride (Phemerol).
5. *Alcohols*
   a. Action: will not destroy spores or hepatitis viruses but are effective against other viruses and most vegetative cells including the tubercle bacillus.
   b. Ethyl alcohol: has been used extensively as a germicide. In 70 percent concentration it is generally considered more effective for skin disinfection than at higher concentrations. It acts to denature proteins and may precipitate a protective coat around microorganisms in blood, pus, or mucus, therefore it should not be applied without first thoroughly scrubbing the instrument.
   c. Isopropyl alcohol: used in 50 to 70 percent concentration, it is generally considered at least as effective as ethyl alcohol for skin disinfection. Not recommended for continued use because it is a fat solvent and can defat the skin leaving it dry and scaly.

OPERATING PROCEDURES

The rules for conduct for the prevention of the transmission of disease are based on knowledge of the types and sources of microorganisms and the steps of cross-contamination. The two major routes of cross-contamination are the direct route by means of instruments from one mouth carried without sterilization to the next patient, and the indirect route whereby contaminated hands, surfaces, and other go-between objects provide the opportunity for organisms to be picked up and carried to the next patient.

Some of the basic preventive steps have been listed on page 26 in connection with the transmission of the hepatitis viruses, and other steps have been described on page 28 in relation to contamination from aerosols. Once a procedural system has been worked out, a safe and comfortable routine can be followed by all dental personnel working together.

To outline a procedural system, the terms *surgically sterile* and *surgically clean* need to be understood. Hospital operating room procedure follows the strictest aseptic techniques, that is, free from all types of microorganisms. To accomplish such a state, a surgical hand scrub, a mask, gown, and glove dress procedure for all operating personnel and assistants, a completely draped patient, and presurgical preparation of the patient, particularly the site of operation, are parts of the total hospital routine. This represents the closest possible to a truly *surgically sterile* situation.

A *surgically clean* procedure maintains the sterile condition at as high a degree as possible. All materials and techniques are sterile. Handwashing and other preparatory routines are planned to minimize bacterial counts. Because of the incidence of microorganisms on the tongue, in the saliva, in carious lesions, in dental plaque, and in gingival and periodontal pockets, only a lessening of the total counts in the field of operation can be accomplished, and that only on a temporary basis. The handling of sterile instruments, the wearing of a face mask and protective glasses, hand washing, the preparation of the patient with an antiseptic mouth rinse, and the use of an antiseptic on oral tissue surfaces are essential routine procedures. Whether an oral treatment procedure is considered major or minor or long or short does not make it any less involved in disease transmission.

CARE OF STERILE INSTRUMENTS

Instruments must be sterilized prior to each appointment. Direct transmission of microorganisms because of use of unsterile instruments is inexcusable.

After the effort has been made to sterilize and disinfect, procedures are then conducted to prevent contamination and to control the transfer of pathogenic microorganisms. Although a strict procedure for sterile technique such as is practiced in a hospital operating room would be difficult or even impossible in a dental office, it is possible to preserve the chain of sterility through effective handling and storage procedures.

I. Handling

A. **Opening the Sterile Package**
1. Do not open instrument packages until ready to use.
2. Touch only the outer surface of the wrapper and remove contents with a sterile transfer (handling) forceps.

B. **Use of Transfer Forceps**
1. Keep ends of forceps sterile during use: avoid touching sides and rims of container when removing the forceps or returning (figure 4–1).
2. Handle forceps with ends down to prevent solution on sterile ends

from passing over upper unclean portion. If that is done, when the forceps are again turned down, the contaminated solution will run down and render the ends unsuitable for handling sterile items.

3. Care of transfer forceps
   a. Holding solution. The disinfectant solution used in the container for the transfer forceps (figure 4–1A) is intended to hold the forceps in a sterile state. A strong stable disinfectant such as an aldehyde is recommended.[24]
   b. Scrub and autoclave the forceps and container daily. Keep covered to prevent airborne organisms from contaminating the forceps and solution.
   c. Change solution frequently in accord with the shelf life of the solution used.

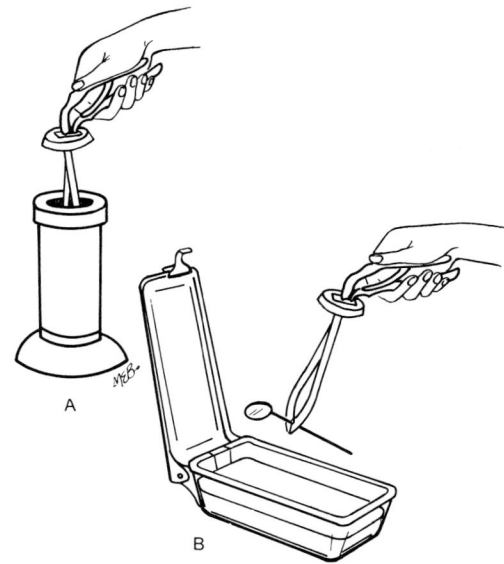

A

B

Figure 4–1. Use of transfer forceps. **A.** To keep ends of forceps sterile during use, avoid touching sides and rims of container when removing the forceps or returning them. **B.** Handle forceps in a vertical position with ends down to prevent the chemical disinfectant solution from passing to upper unclean portion of the forceps and then back over the sterile portion when the forceps is turned down again.

4. Handle only sterile articles with the sterile forceps. A second forceps must be kept in the sterilizing area for handling contaminated instruments.

C. **Transfer of Sterile Items from a Closed Container**

   1. Hold cover of container in left hand in a downward direction while using the transfer forceps to remove item from inside. Return cover promptly.
   2. When it is necessary to place the cover down, turn it up with sterile inside surface away from the tabletop to prevent contamination to the inner surface (figure 4–2).

II. Storage

A. **Preprepared Trays**

   Trays may have fitted covers which are autoclaved with them, or they may be covered with a sterile towel when preset for comparatively short periods.

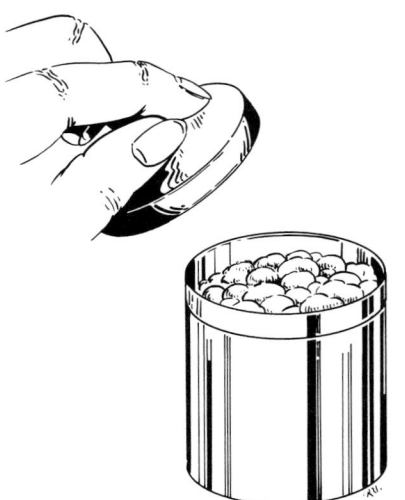

Figure 4–2. Removing the cover from a container of sterile supplies. When the cover is held while contents of the container are removed with a sterile transfer forceps, the cover should be held with inner surface downward as shown. When the cover must be placed on the table, the outer surface is placed downward to prevent contamination to inner surface.

Trays should be kept in a closed cabinet to exclude dust, aerosols, or other contaminants.

B. **Individual Instrument Packages**

   Individual instrument packages are labeled prior to sterilization and kept in a closed cabinet or other container unless for immediate use. Paper bags must be handled carefully to prevent puncture.

C. **Dating**

   All stored sterile packages should be dated and used in rotation.

D. **Factors Affecting Contamination of Sterile Wrapped Supplies:**[28]

   1. Porosity of the wrapper.
   2. Method of wrapping.
   3. Changes in atmospheric conditions surrounding the package.
   4. Handling the package so that air is forced in and out.

E. **Resterilize stored packages at least every 30 days.**

   Packages are exposed to the hazards of dust, excessive handling, and accidental contamination.

USE OF FACE MASK

In the attempt to control airborne infections, it has been common practice to wear a mask when either the patient or the operator has been known to have an acute respiratory infection. Such a practice has its own value but does not take into account the incubation period of certain diseases, or the transient and potentially pathogenic microorganisms which may not manifest disease in one individual but can be pathogenic for another.

Dispersion of particles of debris, pumice, water, all of which are contaminated by the patient's oral flora, occurs regularly during all instrumentation, with the greatest aerosols created following the use of a handpiece and ultrasonic scaler. Evidence of the spread of particles appears on the splashed face, glasses, and uniform of the dental hygienist and on the coverall placed over the patient for protection from the spray. Aerosol production was described on pages 27–28.

I. Mask Efficiency

A. Essential Characteristics

Undesirable characteristics which minimize the comfort with which a mask will be worn are the ability to create irritation to the nose, heat leading to perspiration, and pressure or a tight feeling about the ears and face which may leave marks on the face. Unfortunately discomfort is a common reason for neglect in wearing a mask which can make an important contribution to the total disease control plan.

The shape, material, and degree of absorption will influence the efficiency. A scientifically effective mask will

1. Prevent inward and outward passage of microorganisms or filter particles produced during dental and dental hygiene procedures.
2. Have minimal marginal leakage.

B. Materials

A variety of materials have been used for masks, including gauze and other cloth, plastic foam, fiberglass, synthetic fiber mat, and paper. In one research study, foam, paper, and cloth were found to be the least adequate filters of aerosols.[29] Fiberglass masks were shown to be the most effective.

II. Recommendations

A. Wear a well-fitted mask and large protective glasses (whether or not correction for a sight problem is needed) when in the presence of aerosol production (figure 4–3).
B. Keep the mask on after completing a procedure, while staying in the operatory in the presence of aerosols.

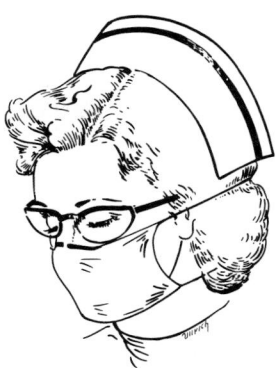

Figure 4–3. Face mask with protective glasses. The mask fits over nose and chin and is tied securely to prevent slipping. A mask should be worn only once for a short period of time and changed for each patient appointment. Glasses are worn over the edge of the mask to help prevent fogging of the glass. When a prescription is not required, clear glass eyeglasses are essential for protection from aerosols and general debris from the patient's mouth.

Particles under five micrometers remain suspended longer (up to 24 hours) than larger particles and can be inhaled directly into terminal lung alveoli. Removal of a mask in the operatory immediately following the use of aerosol-producing procedures permits direct exposure to airborne organisms.

C. Use a clean fresh mask for each patient.

HANDWASHING

Hands, through direct contact with a patient's mouth, become contaminated and therefore are sources for cross-infection. Cross-contamination can be prevented by making a conscious effort to keep the hands from touching objects other than the instruments and disinfected parts of equipment prepared for the immediate patient, and to rewash during and at the completion of each oral procedure.

Emphasis has always been placed on the need for thorough washing or scrubbing prior to starting; now increased emphasis must also be placed on immediate postappointment washing. Through contact with the patient's record, the dental chair, operating stool, telephone, or a multitude of possible other items, many opportunities occur for contamination and spread of microorganisms.

With understanding of the bacteriology of the skin, with use of a degerming agent to reduce the number of microorganisms on the skin, and with attention to a conscientious handwashing routine, a high degree of control of cross-contamination can be attained. Handwashing is of prime importance to the dental hygienist, dentist, and patient.

I. Bacteriology of the Skin

A. Resident Bacteria

Large numbers of relatively stable bacteria inhabit the surface epithelium or deeper areas in the ducts of skin glands or depths of hair follicles; they are ultimately shed with the exfoliated surface cells, or with excretions of the skin glands. They may be altered by newly introduced pathogens, or reduced by washing and disinfection procedures.

B. Transient Bacteria

These reflect the continuous contamination by routine contacts: some are pathogens and may act temporarily as residents, may be washed away, or in the event that a skin break exists, may cause disease. Most transients can be readily removed with soap and water.

C. Handwashing

Effective and frequent handwashing can reduce the overall bacterial flora of the skin and prevent the organisms acquired from the patient from becoming skin residents. It is impossible to sterilize the skin, but every attempt must be made to reduce the bacterial flora to a minimum.

II. Principles for Handwashing

A combination of mechanical friction under running water and the application of a germicide can be effective in lessening the surface bacterial flora.

A. Purposes of the Scrub

An effective scrub procedure can be expected to accomplish the following:
1. Removal of surface dirt and bacteria.
2. Dissolution of the normal greasy film on the skin.
3. Destruction of surface bacteria when an antiseptic accompanies or follows the scrub.
4. Reduce bacterial flora of the hands to an absolute minimum.

B. Facilities
1. Use a sink with a foot pedal for water flow control to avoid contamination from faucet handles.
2. Adaptation for regular sink: turn on water at the beginning and leave on throughout the entire procedure. Turn faucets off with the towel after drying hands.
3. Use a liquid soap or detergent dispenser with foot pedal control to avoid contamination to and from a hand-operated dispenser or cake soap.
4. Use a sink of sufficient size so that contact with the inside of the wash basin can be avoided easily. A sink cannot be sterilized and is highly contaminated.
5. Prevent contamination of uniform by not leaning against the sink.

C. Scrub Brushes
1. Clean brushes with a detergent and autoclave.
2. Avoid over-vigorous use of the brush to minimize skin irritation; utilize mechanical motion and friction, and rinse with moderately warm water.

3. Identify brushes by label for hand-washing only to assure no mixing with instrument cleaning brushes.

D. **Hand Care**

1. Maintain clean, smoothly trimmed fingernails with well-cared-for cuticles to prevent breaks where microorganisms can enter.
2. Remove hand and wrist jewelry. Microorganisms can become lodged in crevices of rings, watches, watchbands where scrubbing is impossible.
3. Use sterile finger cots or rubber gloves to protect breaks in the skin. Always wear gloves when there is known infection present. Complete the wash or scrub, then place gloves.

III. Surgical Scrub

Each hospital or oral surgery clinic will have rules and regulations for scrub procedures. These should be posted over the scrub sinks. The directions outlined here have been compiled from several sources.[30-32]

A. The *stroke-count method* is preferred because there is greater consistency of thoroughness. With a timed procedure there is much more chance for individual variation.

B. Put on eyeglasses and face mask before beginning wash.

C. Wash hands and arms over the elbows with disinfectant scrub soap specified by the hospital or clinic (Betadine may be recommended) to remove gross dirt before taking the brush. Use strong rubbing motions, 10 on each side of hand, wrist, arm. Interlace fingers and thumbs to clean proximal surfaces.

D. Rinse under cool running water. Direct water from fingertips toward hand, wrist, then elbow.

E. Use orangewood stick to clean about and under the fingernails, and rinse under running water.

F. Apply liquid scrub soap and scrub with brush using the following number of strokes: 20 strokes to nails, 10 to fingers and hands, and 6 to arm surfaces. Maintain a good lather. Fingers, hands, and arms have four surfaces each, and overlapping strokes are needed to cover the entire anatomy. When circular strokes are used, make certain that each area receives 10 strokes.

G. Rinse: fingertips first, then hand, arm, elbow. Rinse the brush and transfer it to the other hand.

H. Scrub other hand and arm in the same sequence as before. Rinse thoroughly. Discard the brush in receptacle designated for presterilization.

I. Repeat the procedure for each arm using another sterile brush. Rinse well. Take care not to contaminate the clean hands on faucets or edge of sink since that indicates the need to start from the beginning again.

J. Hold hands up and away from body; proceed to the operating room.

K. Receive sterile towel.

1. Dry fingers first, then hand, wrist, forearm.
2. Do not reapply towel to hands after drying arms; do not touch towel to unwashed areas.

L. Hold hands up or grasped together to maintain effects of the scrub.

IV. Short Scrub

In a hospital or other surgical clinic, a short scrub is permitted between cases depending on the degree of contamination and infectiousness of the case. In certain instances gloves may be washed if they have not been punctured. A similar procedure as followed for the surgical scrub is used, with fewer strokes.

The short scrub procedure may be recommended for the initial handwashing in a dental office or clinic before the first appointment of a day. A two-minute wash is used before each succeeding appointment.

One procedure for a short scrub is abbreviated here.[33]

A. Rinse hands and arms to elbows.
B. Wash, using surgical scrub soap, starting from fingers and moving to elbows. Hold hands up.
C. Rinse, starting from finger tips, to hands, arms, elbows.
D. Remove scrub brush from sterilized package, keeping hands high.
E. Using several measures of scrub soap on the brush, begin the scrub:
   1. Hold brush in right hand and brush back and forth across nails of left hand five times.
   2. Beginning with left thumb, work up and down (five strokes in each area) on all sides of each finger, then palm, and back of hand (approximately two minutes).
   3. Scrub left wrist to elbow with up and down motion. Do not go back to fingers and wrist once they have been scrubbed (approximately one minute).
   4. Rinse well, from fingers to hand, wrist, arm.
F. Rinse brush and transfer to other hand.
G. Repeat entire procedure starting with other hand.
H. Dry hands.
   1. Paper towels are preferred, using a separate towel for each hand.
   2. Cloth towels: use one end of a large towel for one hand and other end for the other, taking care not to drag the towel over unwashed parts; or use a separate smaller towel for each hand.

V. Hand Washing

Instead of a short scrub, another procedure used before the initial appointment of the day is a vigorous three-minute wash, which consists of at least three latherings.[34] An iodine soap is the preferred antiseptic washing liquid. Such a procedure is inadequate prior to oral surgery or in preparation for a patient with a known infection for which a scrub technique is indicated.

A. Use cool water. Wet hands and arms to elbows.
B. Apply Betadine, and lather hands and forearms. Clean nails with disposable wooden or plastic stick.
C. Use a brush to clean away visible dirt during the first lathering.
D. Rinse thoroughly from finger tips toward wrists, then arms.
E. Lather vigorously for 30 seconds and rinse at least three times.
F. Dry with paper towels, one for each hand. Dry hand first, then arm. Use the paper towel to turn off faucet when that is not foot or knee controlled.
G. Succeeding patients. Wash vigorously for one to two minutes, lathering at least three times. Rinse and dry as above. Clasp hands or hold them up to prevent recontamination.

PATIENT PREPARATION

At the beginning of this chapter the incidence of organisms in the mouth was described (page 25). The oral microorganisms contaminate the field of operation and exist in infected aerosols which permit cross-contamination to subsequent patients as well as to dental personnel. Aerosol production was described on page 27. The use of preoperative mouthwash, irrigation, and toothbrushing has been shown to lower the numbers of oral bacteria, and hence to lower the numbers of infected aerosols created during instrumentation.[12,35,36]

Oral procedures which penetrate tissues such as giving anesthesia by injection, or scaling and curetting submarginal pocket surfaces, can introduce bacteria into the tissues. Enough organisms injected into the tissue could multiply and create an abscess. Because of natural resistance, the body can handle and destroy invading microorganisms provided the numbers can be kept to a minimum.

When bacteria are introduced into the gingival tissues, particularly in a pocket, the bacteria can enter the blood stream and create a bacteremia (page 496). Bacteremia has been demonstrated following various types of surgery including tooth removal and periodontal surgery. A bacteremia may also result from scaling and root planing. Research studies have shown that bacteremias occur less frequently following the use of an antiseptic mouthwash prior to treatment.[37-40]

The numbers of bacteria on the gingival or mucosal surfaces can be reduced by the use of a strong antiseptic. In two studies using povidone-iodine mouthwash, the counts of bacteria were reduced before and during scaling and gingivectomy.[37,41] Reduction of surface and total oral bacteria during oral procedures can contribute to surgical cleanliness and more favorable healing following treatment.

Practical procedures for the preparation of a patient include preoperative oral hygiene measures and the application of a surface disinfectant. These contribute to the prevention of disease transmission.

A. **Preoperative Oral Hygiene Measures**
1. *Toothbrushing.* Toothbrushing disturbs and removes microorganisms. When a patient is being trained in plaque control measures and needs supervision at each appointment, a double purpose can be accomplished. Demonstration of plaque removal from the teeth and gingiva contributes to the surface degerming prior to treatment procedures.
2. *Rinsing.* A strong antiseptic mouthwash should be used.
3. *Irrigation.* Irrigating around each tooth to reduce numbers of pocket organisms. The power of the irrigating stream should not be strong enough to force organisms deep below a pocket and hence into the bloodstream.[42]

B. **Application of a Surface Disinfectant**
1. Prior to injection of anesthetic. As a needle is introduced into the mucosa for penetration to deeper tissues, microorganisms on the surface can be carried into the tissue. During positioning of the instrument for injection the needle might accidentally contact a tooth surface and pick up some plaque which could be carried to and into the injection site. Reduction of surface microorganisms can reduce the hazards related to the injection of bacteria with a needle.
2. Prior to scaling and other dental hygiene instrumentation.
   a. Instrumentation in the sulcus or pocket and around the gingival margin can create breaks in the tissue where bacteria can enter. Submarginal instrumentation in a pocket with broken down sulcular epithelium can contribute to the entrance of bacteria into the underlying tissues. Local infection or bacteremia can be created.
   b. Procedure. Dry surface and swab area prior to instrumentation. Use the antiseptic solution to irrigate the sulci and pockets carefully to prevent forcing the solution into the tissues. Research has shown povidone-iodine to be a prophylactic germicide.[41,42]

TECHNICAL HINTS

I. **Sources for Spore Tests for Sterilization**

American Sterilizer Corporation, 2424 West 23rd Street, Erie, Pennsylvania, 16512

Attest Biological Monitoring Systems, 3M Company, Medical Products Division, St. Paul, Minnesota, 55119

Bioquest, P. O. Box 243, Cockeysville, Maryland, 21030

Unispore, Castle Company, Division of Sybron Corporation, 1777 East Henrietta Road, Rochester, New York, 14623

II. Inadvertent Disease Transmission

A. Watch for ways for coincidental disease transmission.
B. Check the toys and other objects in the reception area. Washable toys should be used.
C. Wash hands before and after using a telephone during a patient appointment.
D. Clean a patient's denture with a surgical soap after receiving the denture for scaling and polishing during an appointment. When the denture is to be adjusted, the dentist should use sterile burs and stones, a sterile ragwheel, and sterile pumice (page 550).
E. Sterilized disposable covers for light handles may be prepared. A removable handle for the operating light has been invented and described.[43]

FACTORS TO TEACH THE PATIENT

I. Importance of the patient's complete history to the protection of both the patient and the operator.
II. Facts about the normal oral flora and the factors which influence an increased number of bacteria on the tongue, mucosa, and in the plaque.
III. Methods for personal daily control of the oral bacteria through plaque control and tongue brushing.
IV. Reasons for preoperative brushing, rinsing, and irrigating.
V. Method for thorough rinsing (page 342).

References

1. Burnett, G. W. and Schuster, G. S.: *Pathogenic Microbiology.* St. Louis, Mosby, 1973, p. 123.
2. Gibbons, R. J., Kapsimalis, B., and Socransky, S. S.: The Source of Salivary Bacteria, *Arch. Oral Biol.*, 9, 101, January-February, 1964.
3. Beeson, P. B. and McDermott, W., eds.: *Textbook of Medicine*, 14th ed. Philadelphia, Saunders, 1975, pp. 1336–1340.
4. Burnett and Schuster: op. cit., pp. 419–422.
5. World Health Organization: *Viral Hepatitis.* Technical Report Series, No. 512. Geneva, World Health Organization, 1973, 52 pp.
6. Council on Dental Therapeutics: Quaternary Ammonium Compounds not Acceptable for Disinfection of Instruments and Environmental Surfaces in Dentistry, *J. Am. Dent. Assoc.*, 97, 855, November, 1978.
7. British Dental Association, Dental Health Committee: The Prevention of Transmission of Serum Hepatitis in Dentistry, *Brit. Dent. J.*, 137, 28, July 2, 1974.
8. Micik, R. E., Miller, R. L., Mazzarella, M. A., and Ryge, G.: Studies on Dental Aerobiology: I. Bacterial Aerosols Generated During Dental Procedures, *J. Dent. Res.*, 48, 49, January-February, 1969.
9. Larato, D. C., Ruskin, P. F., and Martin, A.: Effect of an Ultrasonic Scaler on Bacterial Counts in Air, *J. Periodont.*, 38, 550, November-December, 1967.
10. Hausler, W. J. and Madden, R. M.: Microbiologic Comparison of Dental Handpieces. 2. Aerosol Decay and Dispersion, *J. Dent. Res.*, 45, 52, January-February, 1966.
11. Pokowitz, W. and Hoffman, H.: Dental Aerobiology, *N.Y. Dent. J.*, 37, 337, June-July, 1971.
12. Wyler, D., Miller, R. L., and Micik, R. E.: Efficacy of Self-Administered Preoperative Oral Hygiene Procedures in Reducing the Concentration of Bacteria in Aerosols Generated During Dental Procedures, *J. Dent. Res.*, 50, 509, March-April, 1971.
13. Grayson, B. H., Li, W. K. P., and Benjaminson, M. A.: Viability of Bacteria in High-Speed Dental Drill Aerosols with Antimicrobial Agents in the Water Coolant System, *J. Dent. Res.*, 52, 7, January-February, 1973.
14. Brown, R. V.: Bacterial Aerosols Generated by Ultra High-Speed Cutting Instruments, *J. Dent. Child.*, 32, 112, 2nd Quarter, 1965.
15. Travaglini, E. A., Larato, D. C., and Martin, A.: Dissemination of Organism-Bearing Droplets by High-speed Dental Drills, *J. Prosthet. Dent.*, 16, 132, January-February, 1966.
16. American Dental Association, Council on Dental Therapeutics: *Accepted Dental Therapeutics*, 36th ed. 1975, pp. 53–58.
17. Ernst, R. R.: Sterilization by Heat, in Lawrence, C. A. and Block, S. S.: *Disinfection, Sterilization, and Preservation.* Philadelphia, Lea & Febiger, 1968, pp. 703–737.
18. Perkins, J. J.: *Principles and Methods of Sterilization in Health Sciences*, 2nd ed. Springfield, Charles C Thomas, 1969, pp. 95–121, 256–267.
19. Bertolotti, R. L. and Hurst, V.: Inhibition of Corrosion during Autoclave Sterilization of Carbon Steel Dental Instruments, *J. Am. Dent. Assoc.*, 97, 628, October, 1978.

20. Crump, M. C.: Cellulose Dialysis Tubing for the Sterile Storage of Dental Instruments, *Oral Surg.*, 22, 658, November, 1966.
21. Perkins: op. cit., pp. 286–311.
22. Ibid, pp. 312–316.
23. American Dental Association, Council on Dental Therapeutics: op. cit., pp. 58–61, 200–211.
24. Perkins: op. cit., pp. 327–344.
25. Lyon, T. C. and Keselyak, J.: Evaluation of Sonacide as a New Liquid Sterilant, *I.A.D.R. Program and Abstracts of Papers*, February, 1974, p. 213.
26. Crowder, V. H., Welsh, J. S., Bornside, G. H., and Cohn, I.: Bacteriological Comparison of Hexachlorophene and Polyvinylpyrrolidone-iodine Surgical Scrub Soap, *Amer. Surg.*, 33, 906, November, 1967.
27. American Dental Association, Council on Dental Therapeutics: op. cit., p. 204.
28. Perkins: op. cit., pp. 407–408.
29. Micik, R. E., Miller, R. L., and Leong, A. C.: Studies on Dental Aerobiology: III. Efficacy of Surgical Masks in Protecting Dental Personnel from Airborne Bacterial Particles, *J. Dent. Res.*, 50, 626, May-June, 1971.
30. Douglas, B. L. and Pirok, D. J.: Inpatient Procedure, in Douglas, B. L., ed.: *Introduction to Hospital Dentistry*, 2nd ed. St. Louis, Mosby, 1970, pp. 25–27.
31. Peers, J.: The Surgical Hand Scrub, in Hooley, J. R.: *Hospital Dentistry*. Philadelphia, Lea & Febiger, 1970, pp. 94–98.
32. Price, P. B.: Surgical Scrubs and Preoperative Skin Disinfection, in Perkins: op. cit., pp. 345–361.
33. University of Vermont, Program in Dental Hygiene: Standard Scrub Procedure, D. H. 001, 1974.
34. Crawford, J. J.: *Clinical Asepsis in Dentistry: Advanced Instruction Concerning Causes and Prevention of Infections in Dental Practice*. Chapel Hill, University of North Carolina, 1974, p. 15.
35. Litsky, B. Y., Mascis, J. D., and Litsky, W.: Use of Antimicrobial Mouthwash to Minimize the Bacterial Aerosol Contamination Generated by the High-Speed Drill, *Oral Surg.*, 29, 25, January, 1970.
36. Mohammed, C. I. and Monserrate, V.: Preoperative Oral Rinsing as a Means of Reducing Air Contamination During Use of Air Turbine Handpieces, *Oral Surg.*, 29, 291, February, 1970.
37. Brenman, H. S. and Randall, E.: Local Degerming With Povidone-iodine. II. Prior to Gingivectomy, *J. Periodont.*, 45, 870, December, 1974.
38. Francis, L. E., deVries, J., and Lang, D.: An Oral Antiseptic for the Control of Post-extraction Bacteraemia, *J. Can. Dent. Assoc.*, 39, 55, January, 1973.
39. Jones, J. C., Cutcher, J. L., Goldberg, J. R., and Lilly, G. E.: Control of Bacteremia Associated With Extraction of Teeth, *Oral Surg.*, 30, 454, October, 1970.
40. Scopp, I. W. and Orvieto, L. D.: Gingival Degerming by Povidone-iodine Irrigation: Bacteremia Reduction in Extraction Procedures, *J. Am. Dent. Assoc.*, 83, 1294, December, 1971.
41. Randall, E. and Brenman, H. S.: Local Degerming with Povidone-iodine. I. Prior to Dental Prophylaxis, *J. Periodont.*, 45, 866, December, 1974.
42. Crawford: op. cit., p. 9.
43. Tolman, D. E.: Modification of Operating Light: Addition of Removable Handle for Use During Surgical Procedures, *J. Oral Surg.*, 31, 353, May, 1973.

Suggested Readings

Crawford, J. J.: Sterilization and Disinfection, in Richardson, R. E., Barton, R. E., and Brauer, J. C., eds.: *The Dental Assistant*, 4th ed. New York, McGraw-Hill, 1970, pp. 145–157.

Crawford, J. J. and Oldenburg, T. R.: Practical Methods of Office Sterilization and Disinfection, *J. Oral Med.*, 22, 133, October, 1967.

Crawford, J. J., Parker, W. D., and Parker, N. H.: Asepsis in Periodontal Surgery, *I.A.D.R. Program and Abstracts of Papers*, February, 1974, p. 99.

Custer, F. and Addington, L.: Physical Changes of Instruments During Sterilization, *J. Periodont.*, 36, 382, September-October, 1965.

Custer, F. and Coyle, T.: Instrument Changes During Sterilization, *J. Dent. Res.*, 49, 487, May-June, 1970.

Firtell, D. N., Moore, D. J., and Pelleu, G. B.: Sterilization of Impression Materials for Use in the Surgical Operating Room, *J. Prosthet. Dent.*, 27, 419, April, 1972.

Glaze, S. and White, S. C.: Interpatient Microbiological Cross-Contamination Via Dental X-Ray Machines, *I.A.D.R. Program and Abstracts of Papers*, February, 1974, p. 214.

Hill, W. J., Malveaux, F. J., and Whitehurst, V. E.: Comparable Bactericidal Activity of Two Chemosterilizers, *J. Dent. Res.*, 53, 338, March-April, 1974.

Hoffman, H.: Control of Infectious Disease Agents in Dental School Clinics, *J. Dent. Educ.*, 39, 169, March, 1975.

Johnson & Johnson, Dental Division: *Handbook of Dental Practice Asepsis*, New Brunswick, 1967.

Katberg, J. W.: Cross-contamination Via the Prosthodontic Laboratory, *J. Prosthet. Dent.*, 32, 412, October, 1974.

Larato, D. C.: Disinfection of Pumice, *J. Prosthet. Dent.*, 18, 534, December, 1967.

Lyon, T. C.: Quaternary Ammonia Compounds: Should They Be Used for Disinfection in the Dental Office? *Oral Surg.*, 36, 769, November, 1973.

Malveaux, F. J., Whitehurst, V. E., and Magerman, L. A.: Relative Effectiveness of Certain Chemosterilizers on Selected Microbial Species, *J. Dent. Res.*, 51, 62, January-February, 1972.

McEntegart, M. G. and Clark, A.: Colonisation of Dental Units by Water Bacteria, *Br. Dent J.*, *134*, 140, February 20, 1973.

Miller, C. H., Lu, D. P., and Crimmel, J. E.: Bactericidal Efficiency of Some Antimicrobial Chemicals, *J. Dent. Res.*, *52*, 184, January-February, 1973.

Neugeboren, N., Nisengard, R. J., Beutner, E. H., and Ferguson, G. W.: Control of Cross-contamination, *J. Am. Dent. Assoc.*, *85*, 123, July, 1972.

Nolte, W. A., ed.: *Oral Microbiology*, 2nd ed. St. Louis, Mosby, 1973, pp. 339–341, 347–375.

Nubar, E.: Fallacy of Cold Sterilization, *J. Am. Dent. Hyg. Assoc.*, *46*, 172, May-June, 1972.

Walsh, R. F. and Ames, M. I.: Reinforcing the Aseptic Chain in Hospital Dental Practice, *J. Hosp. Dent. Pract.*, *6*, 57, April, 1972.

Aerosols

Abel, L. C., Miller, R. L., Micik, R. E., and Ryge, G.: Studies on Dental Aerobiology: IV. Bacterial Contamination of Water Delivered by Dental Units, *J. Dent. Res.*, *50*, 1567, November-December, 1971.

Hoffman, H.: Air Hygiene in Dental Practice, *Oral Surg.*, *11*, 1048, September, 1958.

Mazzarella, M. A. and Flynn D. D.: Dental Aerosols, in Dimmick, R. L. and Akers, A. B., eds.: *An Introduction to Experimental Aerobiology*. New York, Wiley-Interscience, 1969, pp. 437–462.

Miller, R. L., Micik, R. E., Abel, C., and Ryge, G.: Studies on Dental Aerobiology: II. Microbial Splatter Discharged from the Oral Cavity of Dental Patients, *J. Dent. Res.*, *50*, 621, May-June, 1971.

Pollok, N. L., Williams, G. H., Shay, D. E., and Barr, C. E.: Laminar Air Purge of Microorganisms in Dental Aerosols, *J. Am. Dent. Assoc.*, *81*, 1131, November, 1970.

Shreve, W. B., Wachtel, L. W., and Pelleu, G. B.: Air Cleaning Devices for Reduction in Number of Airborne Bacteria, *J. Dent. Res.*, *49*, 1078, September-October, 1970.

Williams, G. H., Pollok, N. L., Shay, D. E., and Barr, C. E.: Laminar Air Purge of Microorganisms in Dental Aerosols: Prophylactic Procedures with the Ultrasonic Scaler, *J. Dent. Res.*, *49*, Suppl., 1498, November-December, 1970.

Face Masks

Bailey, R., Giglio, P., Blechman, H., and Nunez, C.: Effectiveness of Disposable Face Masks in Preventing Cross Contamination During Dental Procedures, *J. Dent. Res.*, *47*, 1062, November-December, 1968.

Stark, M. M., Nicholson, R. J., and Augsberger, R. H.: Aerosol Hazards and Face Mask Protection, *J. Calif. Dent. Assoc.*, *44*, 513, December, 1968.

Travaglini, E. A. and Larato, D. C.: A Disposable Dental Face Mask with a Plastic Eye Shield for Operating with the Air Turbine Drill, *J. Prosthet. Dent.*, *15*, 525, May-June, 1965.

Hands

Bartels, H. A., Gilbert, L., and Yee, J.: Further Observations on Oral Microbial Contamination of the Fingers, *N.Y. State Dent. J.*, *36*, 231, April, 1970.

Bartels, H. A.: Oral Microbial Contamination of the Dentist's Fingers, *New York Dent. J.*, *35*, 531, November, 1969.

Bhaskar, S. N., Cutright, D. E., Gross, A., and Hunsuck, E. E.: The Army Medical Irrigator and the Hydroscrub Device, *J. Am. Dent. Assoc.*, *84*, 854, April, 1972.

Cutright, D. E., Bhaskar, S. N., Gross, A., and Mulcahy, D. M.: A New Method of Presurgical Hand Cleansing, *Oral Surg.*, *33*, 162, February, 1972.

Hoffman, H.: Hygiene of the Hands in Dental Practice, *Oral Surg.*, *11*, 216, February, 1958.

Hepatitis

Crawford, J. J.: New Light on the Transmissibility of Viral Hepatitis in Dental Practice and Its Control, *J. Am. Dent. Assoc.*, *91*, 829, October, 1975.

Donaldson, D.: Homologous Serum Hepatitis and the Dental Treatment of Renal Dialysis and Kidney Transplant Patients, *Br. Dent. J.*, *132*, 391, May 16, 1972.

Glazer, R. I., Spatz, S. S., and Catone, G. A.: Viral Hepatitis: A Hazard to Oral Surgeons, *J. Oral Surg.*, *31*, 504, July, 1973.

MacFarlane, T. W. and Mason, D. K.: The Dentist and the Prevention of Serum Hepatitis, *Br. Dent. J.*, *132*, 487, June 20, 1972.

Mosley, J. W. and White, E.: Viral Hepatitis as an Occupational Hazard of Dentists, *J. Am. Dent. Assoc.*, *90*, 992, May, 1975.

Redeker, A. G.: Viral Hepatitis: Current Concepts, *Postgrad Med.*, *53*, 77, January, 1973.

Chapter 5

Patient Reception and Positioning in the Dental Chair

The patient's well-being is an important consideration throughout the appointment. At the same time, the operator must function effectively and efficiently by applying work simplification principles to reduce stress and fatigue.

The physical arrangement and interpersonal relationships provide the setting for specific services to be performed. The patient's presence in the office is an expression of confidence in the dentist and the auxiliary personnel. This confidence is inspired by the reputation for professional knowledge and skill, the appearance of the office, and the action of the workers in it.

I. Preparation for the Patient

A. Instruments and Supplies

These should be ready before the patient enters. Preprepared tray (page 23) should be uncovered in the presence of the patient.

B. Records

Open record for review and place radiographs in viewbox.

C. Equipment

1. Surface Disinfection. All objects which are touched while treating a patient must be wiped vigorously with a disinfectant following each appointment in preparation for the next. Spraying a disinfectant does not penetrate or remove the film of organisms; vigorous rubbing with pressure is needed.[1]

   a. Two applications of disinfectant should be applied to handpieces and water syringe (page 19).

   b. All parts of the unit which are touched during an appointment need disinfection. These include:

   Light handles
   Handpiece hose attachment
   Water and air syringe (use disposable or autoclavable tips)
   End of saliva ejector hose (use disposable or autoclavable tip)
   Evacuator hose
   Control knobs for all parts including the unit, chair, and cabinet
   Edges and surface of bracket tray or other place where instruments will be placed
   Pens, pencils, telephone

2. Position Chair

   a. Upright, in low position.

   b. Chair arm adjusted for access.

   c. Pre-adjustment of traditional chair when size of patient is known will contribute to ease while making final adjustments.

3. Place cover over headrest.
4. Clear pathway to chair of obstacles: rheostat, operating stool.

II. Patient Reception

A. **Introductions**
   1. The dental assistant or the dentist may introduce the new patient to the dental hygienist, but more frequently a self-introduction is in order. The patient is greeted by name and the hygienist's name is clearly stated, for example, "Good morning, Mr. Smith; I am Miss Jones, the dental hygienist." Wearing a name-tag for the patient's convenient observation is helpful.
   2. Procedure for introducing the patient to others:
      a. A lady's name always precedes a gentleman's.
      b An older person's name precedes the younger person's (when of the same sex and when the difference in age is obvious).
      c. In general, the patient's name precedes that of a member of the dental personnel.

B. **Procedures**
   1. Invite patient to be seated.
      a. For the average patient, stand ready to adjust the chair.
      b. Assist the elderly, infirm, or very small children; guide into the chair with support to the patient's arm.
      c. Wheelchair patient: bring wheelchair directly beside the dental chair and provide support when indicated.
   2. Place female patient's handbag within her view.
   3. Have patient remove eyeglasses and place in case, handbag, or other safe place.

4. Apply drape and towel. Female patient's legs may be draped when she is in a contour chair.
5. Receive prosthetic removable appliances and place in water in a protective container.

POSITION OF THE DENTAL HYGIENIST

The adjustment for the position of the patient is contingent upon the position of the dental hygienist. Attention to the patient's comfort must always be foremost, but when the working arrangement is considered it is realistic to remember that the patient's position will be assumed for a relatively short time compared with that of the dental hygienist who may conduct a major portion of professional activity in close proximity to the chairside. The patient, therefore, is positioned to permit the dental hygienist to accomplish a thorough, biologically oriented dental hygiene service conveniently and efficiently within a reasonable length of time.

I. Objectives

Objectives concern the health of the dental hygienist, the service to be performed, and the effect on the patient. The *preferred* working position is one which will attempt to accomplish the following:

A. Contribute to rather than detract from the health of the dental hygienist.
B. Provide physical comfort and mental tranquility.
C. Apply principles of body mechanics which will reduce fatigue and maintain stamina for prolonged periods of peak efficiency.
D. Contribute to ease and efficiency of performance which will produce complete, thorough results for effective treatment; this, in turn, will have long-range benefits for the patient.
E. Transmit to the patient a sense of well-being, security, and confidence,

as well as a need for cooperation with dental personnel.

F. Develop better patient-dental hygienist relationships because of greater comfort, lessened physical stress, and reduced appointment time.

G. Be flexible in relation to individual needs of patients with special health problems where limitations of physiological or pathological conditions require variations in chair positions.

H. Be flexible in relation to studying and utilizing, where applicable, new concepts of patient care and new developments in dental equipment which will contribute to all objectives of service.

II. The Seated Dental Hygienist

In keeping with current day concepts, it is expected that the dental hygienist will utilize an operating stool. Benefits to the dental hygienist can result which relate to general health, productivity, and the manner in which work is accomplished. Greater comfort and opportunity to relax is afforded the patient when the dental hygienist is seated and the patient must necessarily be lowered back to a reclining or supine position.

A. **Characteristics of an Acceptable Operating Stool**[2,3]

1. *Base.* Broad and heavy for stability.
2. *Mobility.* Completely mobile; not connected to other dental equipment; built with free-rolling casters; without tipping hazards.
3. *Seat.* Relatively large to provide complete body support; padded firmly yet not too hard; without a welt on the leaning edge which could dig into the upper part of the thigh.
4. *Rotating Support.* May be applied to the operator's back, side, or abdomen for support.

5. *Height.* Adjustable to provide exactly the correct level for the individual so that feet can be flat on the floor and thighs parallel with the floor.
6. *Assistant's Stool.* Needs additional support at the base with at least five casters recommended for maximum stability; should be freely adjustable for height. A footrest is needed at the base of the chair since the assistant is positioned four to six inches higher than the operator, and generally the feet could not reach the floor.

B. **Use of the Operating Stool**

Once the operating stool is adjusted for the individual, it does not need changing, unless other personnel also use it. Once adjusted, the height remains constant, and other dental equipment is arranged to accommodate for optimum usage at the convenience of the seated dental hygienist. Positioning which incorporates principles of good body mechanics will benefit both dental hygienist and patient. Basic positioning includes the following features related to posture and the field of operation.[4,5]

1. Feet are flat on the floor; thighs parallel with the floor (figure 5–1 A).
2. Back is straight; head is relatively erect; shoulders are relaxed and parallel with floor.
3. Body weight is completely supported by the chair; balancing on the edge of the stool should be avoided (figure 5–1 B).
4. Eyes are directed downward in a manner which prevents neck strain and eye strain; it is not necessary to bend the head.
5. Operating distance from the patient's mouth to the eyes of operator should be 14 to 16 inches.

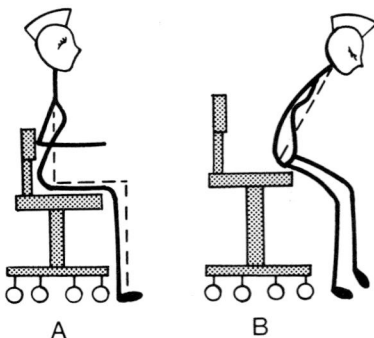

Figure 5–1. Use of operating stool. **A.** Correct position with feet flat on the floor, thighs parallel with floor, and body weight supported by chair. **B.** Incorrect position with seat high, body balanced on the edge of the stool, and back bent forward.

6. With elbows close to the sides, the field of operation (patient's mouth) is adjusted close to elbow height.

III. The Standing Dental Hygienist

As in the seated position, the standing posture also requires application of principles of good body mechanics.

A. Distribution of Balance

1. Both feet are flat on the floor with toes forward.
2. Back is straight; head relatively erect; shoulders relaxed and parallel with floor.
3. Weight is centered over the balls of the feet and distributed evenly to both feet; knees are slightly flexed.

B. Relation to Field of Operation

1. With elbows close to sides, the field of operation (patient's mouth) is adjusted close to elbow height.
2. Eyes are directed downward in a manner which prevents neck strain and eye strain; it is not necessary to bend the head.
3. Operating distance from the patient's mouth to the eyes of operator should be 14 to 16 inches.

DENTAL CHAIR POSITION

Once the height of operation is established by the height of the dental hygienists's elbow, dental chair positioning relates directly to the type of dental chair. The sequence of procedures for effective, efficient adjustment of the traditional or conventional dental chair and the contour chair is outlined here.

I. Traditional Dental Chair

The back of the chair is adjusted first, then the headrest, the chair is inclined to adjust the seat, and finally the whole chair lowered or raised to bring the field of operation to the correct level and angulation. For most patients, the footrest remains in a constant position, but it should be adjusted to meet individual needs.

A. Prepositioning for Patient Reception

1. Seat parallel with floor.
2. Back slightly inclined back and away from the upright position.
3. Headrest tilted back to prevent its bumping the patient as he is seated.
4. Location of base of chair on the floor should permit access to the dental unit when chair is inclined (figure 5–2).

B. Backrest

1. Raise or lower until the curvature of the chair back corresponds with the curvature in the middle of the patient's back.
2. When correctly positioned, the top border of many traditional chairs will be at a level approximating the lower third of the patient's scapulae. Other chairs have taller backs which may reach nearer the upper third of the scapulae.

C. Headrest

1. Request the patient to hold the head erect with chin slightly up.
2. Bring the headrest to a position almost touching the back of the

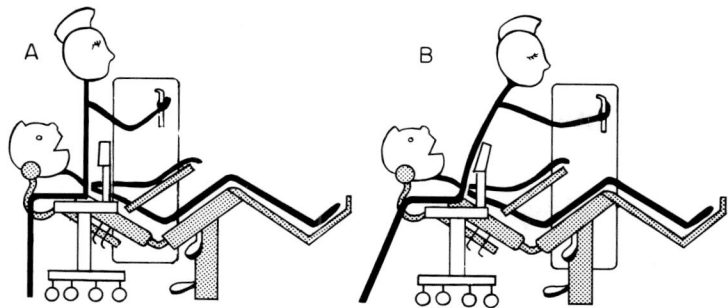

Figure 5-2. Relation of patient in dental chair to traditional dental unit and seated dental hygienist. **A.** Correct position with patient's mouth at elbow height, convenient to unit without stretching, **B.** Incorrect position with dental chair too far removed. Dental hygienist must stretch across patient to reach unit.

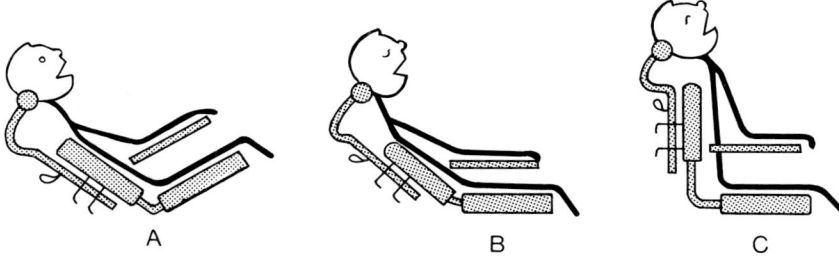

Figure 5-3. Traditional dental chair adjustment, **A.** Correct position with backrest and headrest adjusted so that the body is straight from hip to top of head and the whole chair is tilted back. **B.** Incorrect position with headrest too far forward and chair seat flat which encourages the patient to slide forward. **C.** Incorrect with headrest too far back.

head under the occipital protuberances before securing it.

D. **Chair Seat**

1. Incline the whole chair back as a unit. For the correct position, usually the chair will be tilted as far as it will go.
2. The "V" formed between the seat and the back prevents the patient from sliding forward (figure 5-3 A).

E. **Final Adjustment**

1. *The Seated Dental Hygienist*
   a. Lower the chair to its lowest level and incline the chair back as far as it will go.
   b. To lower the field of operation further, it may be necessary to lower the back of the chair.

2. *The Standing Dental Hygienist*
   With the chair inclined as far back as possible, raise or lower the whole chair until the patient's mouth is at elbow height.
3. *Basic Position of the Patient.* When correctly positioned, the spinal cord of the patient should be straight from the brain to the hips. An imaginary straight line can be drawn from the top of the ear to the hips to test this.

F. **Effects of Chair Maladjustment**

1. *Backrest Too Low or Too High.* Curvature of the spine will cause muscle tension, restlessness, and the patient will attempt to slide into a more comfortable posture which

may move him out of appropriate operating position.

2. *Headrest Too High or Too Far Forward.* Chin moves toward chest, there is difficulty in maintaining accessibility and vision; dental hygienist must lean forward and bend neck sidewards (figure 5–3 B).

3. *Headrest Too Low or Too Far Back.* Patient's neck muscles can be stretched and become fatigued; swallowing may be difficult; patients will slide down (figure 5–3 C).

4. *Chair Seat Parallel with Floor.* Patient will slide forward and down (figure 5–3 B).

II. Contour Dental Chair

The contour chair differs from the traditional chair in many ways. Its adjustment is easier than for the traditional chair with its many separate parts. Once the basic goal is learned, contour chair adjustment does not vary for different sized patients as much as does traditional chair adjustment.

A. **Characteristics of a Contour Chair for Efficient Utilization**[2,6]

1. Provides complete body support.
2. Seat and leg support work as a unit; back and headrest work as a unit; both are power controlled.
3. Has a thin back without protruding adjustment devices so that the chair may be lowered close to the dental hygienist's lap for proper positioning of the field of operation.
4. Has supports which hold the patient's arms as the chair is lowered into the supine position; otherwise the hands hang down or the patient must hold them up forcibly.
5. Chair base should be as shallow as possible to permit the chair to be lowered as close to the floor as needed for correct operating.
6. Chair base should be motor-driven

with pedal access from the working position on the dental operating stool. Likewise, the switches for the back and seat should be readily available to both the assistant and operator.

B. **Prepositioning for Patient Reception**

1. Chair at low level; back upright.
2. Chair arm raised on side of approach.

C. **Adjustment Steps**[2]

1. Patient is first seated with back upright.
2. Female patient's legs are draped.
3. Chair seat and foot portion is raised first to help the patient settle back.
4. Backrest is lowered until the patient reaches the supine position.
5. Patient is requested to slide up until the head is at the upper edge of the backrest and on the side next to the dental hygienist. Note patient position in figure 5–5.

D. **Final Adjustment**

1. Lower or raise the total chair until the field of operation (patient's mouth) is at hygienist's elbow level as previously described.
2. Basic position of patient: back level and parallel with floor; for maxillary instrumentation, complete supine position with feet slightly higher than the head (figure 5–4)

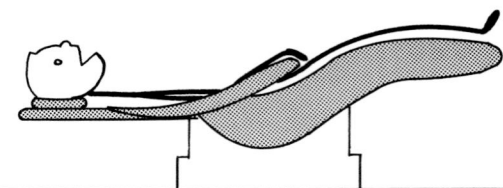

Figure 5–4. Contour chair. For maxillary instrumentation, patient is in supine position with back of chair parallel with floor and feet slightly higher than the head. For mandibular instrumentation, adjust chair back to a 20-degree angle with the floor.

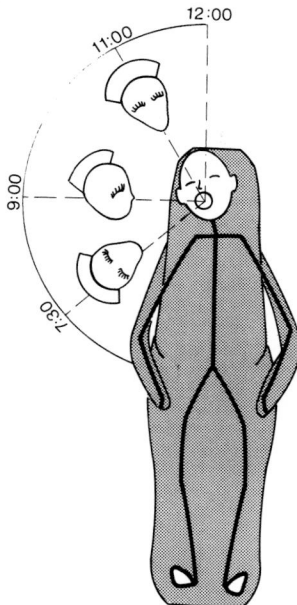

Figure 5–5. Operating positions. Patient's head is placed at the upper edge of the backrest and on the side next to the dental hygienist. The right-handed dental hygienist is positioned between 7:30 and 11:00 for access to the patient's oral cavity from the side-front, side, or side-back. The left-handed hygienist is positioned between 1:00 and 4:30.

3. When working on the mandibular arch from the 9:00 or 7:30 position (figure 5–5), it is sometimes helpful to raise the back of the patient slightly. The whole chair must then be lowered to bring the field of operation back to elbow height.

E. **Conclusion of Appointment**
  1. Raise backrest slowly.
  2. Tilt chair forward.
  3. Have patient sit in upright position briefly to avoid possible effects of postural hypotension. Symptoms of dizziness and faintness may occur.

III. Chair Position for Small Child

A. **Traditional Chair**
  1. Use a portable seat or a large firm cushion to raise seat level.

2. Cover the seat with a cloth to protect the finish from the child's shoes.
3. Lower back and headrest to lowest levels with back at right angles to chair seat.
4. Incline chair back.
5. Final adjustment: child's head will rest as near the headrests as possible; legs may be crossed to give support.

B. **Contour Chair**

Adjustment the same as for an adult. Child will slide up so that the head is near the top of the backrest and on the side toward the dental hygienist (figure 5–5).

FUNCTIONAL FACTORS

I. Lighting[2,5,7]

During treatment, visibility of specific tooth surfaces or areas for instrumentation is prerequisite to thoroughness without undue trauma to the adjacent tissues. With inadequate light, inefficiency increases and leads to prolonged operating time which reduces patient cooperation.

The position of the dental light or lights and the intensity of the beam affect the illumination. A study of the operating room, with measurement of the total light at the patient's face in working position, and selection of an operating light which meets certain standards can assure intensity sufficient for good visibility and yet safe for the eyes.

A. **Dental Light: Requirements**
  1. Ratio of intensity of dental light to room light should not exeed four to one.[7] With the recommended dental light of 1200 foot-candles, the room light should be 300 foot-candles, measured at the patient's mouth. A foot-candle is the unit of measure of the intensity of light.
  2. Intensity of room light should be

sufficient to prevent too great a contrast between it and the illuminating beam.

3. The light should be readily adjustable both vertically and horizontally and the beam capable of being focused.

4. It should be filtered to reduce glare and heat.

5. The size must be small enough so that it may be brought close to the operating area without being in the way, blocking the room light, or being a hazard for movement of people in its vicinity.

B. **Dental Light: Location**

1. *Attachment.* To unit, chair, or ceiling. Chair attachment has advantage in moving when the chair is moved; ceiling attachment has greater versatility for use over patient in supine position.

2. *Dual Lighting.* With the use of the supine patient position in a contour chair, advantages to the use of two operating lights have been demonstrated.[5,7] One light directed from the front of the patient illuminates the maxillary arch; the other light from over and behind the patient's head directs light to the mandibular arch.

C. **Dental Light: Adjustment**

1. Direct the light first on the towel under the patient's chin, then rotate light up to the mouth to avoid flashing light in the patient's eyes.

2. Disposable eye protectors may be provided for the patient to prevent glare.[7]

II. Working Positions

A. **Objectives**

1. The operator must see the field of operation clearly without having to assume body positions which are harmful if held over long periods.

2. When an assistant participates, the field of operation must be accessible and visible to both dental hygienist and dental assistant.

3. Instruments and equipment must be within reach without stretching.

B. **Basic Zone for Operation**

The dental hygienist may perform patient services from a position which permits access to the patient's oral cavity from the side-front, the side, or the side-back. The hours of a clock have been used effectively to designate positions at the dental chair and zones of operation. With 12:00 directly over the top of the patient's head and 6:00 toward the feet, the side-front position is 7:30 to 8:00, the side is at 9:00, and the side-back at 11:00 (figure 5–5). Certain procedures require positions between these numbers. The left-handed dental hygienist operates between 1:00 and 4:00 to 4:30.

C. **Dental Hygienist without Assistant**

1. Arrange necessary items for immediate access without leaving operating stool.

2. Movable cabinet with preprepared tray may be placed at 12:00, 3:00, or 8:00 depending on the convenience to the operating positions.

3. Cervical tray may be used and positioned conveniently around the patient.

4. Height of tray for instruments should be at or slightly below the elbow of the dental hygienist so that no effort need be expended when instruments are changed.

D. **Dental Hygienist with Assistant**[2,4,5]

1. Position of assistant: seated with eye level four to six inches above the dental hygienist's eye level and facing toward the head of dental chair (figure 5–6).

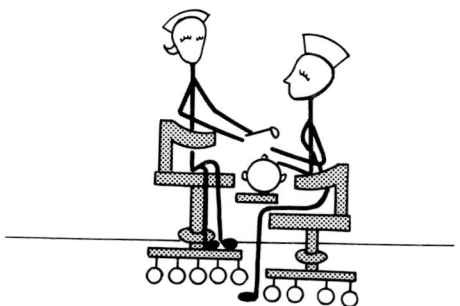

Figure 5–6. Dental hygienist with dental assistant. The dental assistant is seated with eye level four to six inches above the dental hygienist's eye level. The sterile preprepared tray is placed on a portable cabinet in front of the assistant within easy reach for passing instruments.

2. Assistant applies principles of good body mechanics: body weight supported by operating stool; feet are rested on the base of the operating stool.

3. Instruments and other essential materials are kept within arm's length and the portable cabinet with sterilized preprepared tray is in front of the dental assistant.[8]

4. Four-handed dentistry procedures are practiced with instrument transfers and evacuation during operations.

TECHNICAL HINTS

I. In the supine position, a patient is ideally situated for support of his circulation; very rarely could a patient faint while lying with his feet slightly higher than his head.[9]

II. The face of the dental hygienist should not be in close proximity to that of the patient. If it is difficult to keep working distance at 14 to 16 inches, an eye examination may be indicated.

III. Keep body contact at an absolute minimum. A good operator does not lean on the patient or rest the forearms on the patient's shoulders, or his hands on the patient's face or forehead. Unnecessary contact can be very unpleasant to a patient and, in addition, is unsanitary.

IV. Conditions which contraindicate use of the supine position include congestive heart, cerebral vascular insufficiency, and any condition associated with breathing difficulty such as severe asthma or sinusitis.

FACTORS TO TEACH THE PATIENT

I. Orientation of patients, particularly previous patients, is important when a contour chair and changes in operating procedures are introduced.

   A. Explain advantages; complete body support for the patient, better positioning for better access, light, and vision; therefore a smoother, more efficient operation may be performed; increases patient relaxation which in turn contributes to the speed and success of services.

   B. Give specific instruction on the parts of the chair or other equipment which will be of concern to the patient to prevent embarrassment or adverse reactions.

II. Research has shown that astronauts withstand the most stress in the supine, contoured, body-supported position.[9]

References

1. Crawford, J. J.: *Clinical Asepsis in Dentistry. Advanced Instruction Concerning Causes and Prevention of Infection in Dental Practice.* Chapel Hill, University of North Carolina, 1974, pp. 18–21.
2. Sinnett, G. M. and Wuehrmann, A. H.: The Dental Operatory of the Future, in Peterson, S., ed.: *The Dentist and His Assistant*, 3rd ed. St. Louis, Mosby, 1972, pp. 392–401.
3. Anderson, J. A.: The Selection and Use of Operator's Stools and Contour Chairs, *Dent. Clin. North Am.*, p. 303, July, 1965.
4. Robinson, G. E., Wuehrmann, A. H., Sinnett, G. M., and McDevitt, E. J.: Four-handed Dentis-

try: the Whys and Wherefores, *J. Am. Dent. Assoc.*, 77, 573, September, 1968.

5. Spahn, V. and Kilpatrick, H. C.: Functional Work Habits, *J. Am. Dent. Hyg. Assoc.*, 43, 82, 2nd Quarter, 1969.
6. Kilpatrick, H. C.: Present and Future Functional Dental Equipment, *J. Am. Dent. Assoc.*, 72, 1348, June, 1966.
7. Miller, E. M. and Miller, J. S.: Oral Lighting, *J. Am. Dent. Assoc.*, 71, 856, October, 1965.
8. Sinnett, G. M., McDevitt, E. J., Robinson, G. E., and Wuehrmann, A. H.: Four-handed Dentistry: a New Mobile Dental Cabinet Design, *J. Am. Dent. Assoc.*, 78, 305, February, 1969.
9. Tarsitano, J. J.: Contour Configuration, *J. Am. Dent. Assoc.*, 70, 1194, May, 1965.

Suggested Readings

Bomba, J. L.: Fiber Optic Lighting Systems: Their Role in Dentistry, *Dent. Clin. North Am.*, 15, 197, January, 1971.

Crowley, P. I.: Backache, Tension and Fatigue, *J. Am. Dent. Hyg. Assoc.*, 41, 207, 4th Quarter, 1967.

Cureton, T. K., Jr.: Physical Fitness and Dynamic Health, in Bernier, J. L. and Muhler, J. C., eds: *Improving Dental Practice Through Preventive Measures*, 2nd ed. St. Louis, Mosby, 1970, pp. 397–431.

Forsyth, W. D., Allen, G. D., and Everett, G. B.: An Evaluation of Cardiorespiratory Effects of Posture in the Dental Outpatient, *Oral Surg.*, 34, 562, October, 1972.

Glenner, R. A.: The Dental Chair—A Brief Pictorial History, *J. Am. Dent. Assoc.*, 86, 38, January, 1973.

Hilborn, L. B., Campbell, E. M., and Hall, W. R.: Facility Design and Equipment Considerations for the Team Practice of Dentistry, *Dent. Clin. North Am.*, 18, 873, October, 1974.

Meade, J. B.: Dentist-patient Comfort in Sit-down Dentistry, *J. Am. Dent. Assoc.*, 76, 804, April, 1968.

Tarasoff, G. J.: Postural and Kinaesthetic Considerations in Modern Sit-down Dentistry, *J. Can. Dent. Assoc.*, 35, 154, March, 1969.

Thompson, E. O.: Principles of Efficient Dental Equipment Use, *J. Am. Dent. Assoc.*, 74, 708, March, 1967.

Weinert, A. M.: An Evaluation of the Modern Dental Lounge Chair, *Dent. Clin. North Am.*, 15, 129, January, 1971.

Four-Handed: Instrument Transfer

Castano, F. A. and Alden, B. A., eds.: *Handbook of Expanded Dental Auxiliary Practice*. Philadelphia, Lippincott, 1973, pp. 16–21.

Cooper, T. M.: Four-handed Dentistry in the Team Practice of Dentistry, *Dent. Clin. North Am.*, 18, 739, October, 1974.

Handelman, S. L., Kwasman, R., MacIntyre, B. A., and Barrett, G. V.: Factors Affecting Dental Team Performance, *J. Am. Dent. Assoc.*, 89, 880, October, 1974.

Kryger, L. K.: Putting Four Hands To Work, in Peterson, S. ed.: *The Dentist and His Assistant*, 3rd ed. St. Louis, Mosby, 1972, pp. 145–157.

Pipe, P., Kryger, L. K., Underwood, B., and MacIntyre, M.: *Introduction to Four-handed Dentistry, A Multi-media Self-instructional Program for Dental Assistants*. Philadelphia, Lippincott, 1974.

Paul, E.: A Practical Guide to Assisted Operating. 1. Principles of Assisted Operating, *Brit. Dent. J.*, 133, 258, September 19, 1972; 2. Aspiration, *Brit. Dent. J.*, 133, 305, October 3, 1972; 3. Instrument Handling (1), *Brit. Dent. J.*, 133, 348, October 17, 1972; 4. Instrument Handling (2), *Brit. Dent. J.*, 133, 384, November 7, 1972; 5. Instrument Handling (3), *Brit. Dent. J.*, 133, 437, November 21, 1972.

Robinson, G. E., McDevitt, E. J., Sinnett, G. M., and Wuehrmann, A. H.: *Four-Handed Dentistry Manual*, 2nd ed. Birmingham, University of Alabama School of Dentistry, 1971.

Schmid, W. and Stevenson, S. B.: Dynamic Instrument Placement, and Operator's and Assistant's Stool Placement, *Dent. Clin. North Am.*, 15, 145, January, 1971.

Simon, W. J.: *Clinical Dental Assisting*. Hagerstown, Maryland, Medical Department, Harper & Row, 1973, pp. 198–201.

Spencer, P. R.: Chairside Procedures for the Dental Assistant, in Park, V. R., Ashman, J. R., and Shelly, G. J.: *A Textbook for Dental Assistants*, 2nd ed. Philadelphia, Saunders, 1975, pp. 394–422.

Strickland, W. D.: Operative Dentistry, in Richardson, R. E., Barton, R. E., and Brauer, J. C., eds.: *The Dental Assistant*, 4th ed. New York, McGraw-Hill, 1970, pp. 432–439.

III

Patient Evaluation

INTRODUCTION

Before treatment begins, information must be obtained about the patient's general and oral health from which a diagnosis and treatment plan can be formulated. The gathering, organizing, and assembling of all data from observations, patient questioning, and clinical and radiographic examination may be called a *diagnostic work-up*. Basically, it is a collection of all pertinent facts and materials for the dentist to use during diagnosis and treatment planning and for use during all treatment as a guide.

The chapters in this section, *Patient Evaluation*, include descriptions for the preparation of materials which make up a diagnostic work-up. While a dental hygienist prepares specific parts of the work-up, comments on or reactions to any findings must be withheld until after the diagnosis and treatment plan are finalized by the dentist. Even a simple well-intentioned remark can be misleading to the patient and create misunderstandings which can be difficult to clarify later.

I. Parts of a Diagnostic Work-up

A. Basic Procedures

The essential information for evaluation of a patient prior to formulation of the diagnosis and treatment plan by a dentist is derived from the following:

1. Patient histories (personal, medical and dental).
2. Determination of vital signs.
3. Extraoral and intraoral inspection.
4. Radiographic survey.
5. Study casts.
6. Examination of the gingival and periodontal tissues including clinical signs of disease involvement, pocket measurement and charting, and mobility evaluation.
7. Examination of the teeth to determine and record deposits, restorations, carious lesions, other structural defects, pulp vitality, and occlusion factors.

B. Diagnostic Work-up for Preventive Treatment Plan

A preventive program is planned to meet individual needs. Therefore information to be obtained depends on the particular oral problems and could include:
1. Dental or periodontal indices.
2. Dietary analysis.
3. Caries activity test.

C. Additional Procedures

In addition to the basic procedures, other parts of a diagnostic work-up will be selected depending on the individual needs of a patient, as well as the specialty area and special emphasis of the dentist. Selection of procedures to be used is influenced by the age group to which the patient belongs, and on the results of preliminary findings from the histories and examinations made in the basic procedures listed above.

Certain procedures may be of an emergency examination category. For example, if during the intraoral inspection of the oral mucosa a suspicious lesion was found for which a biopsy was indicated, such a diagnostic procedure would take precedence over any other.

In accord with the policy or special request of the dentist, a diagnostic work-up may include some or all of the following:

1. Photographs.
2. Biopsy or cytologic smear.
3. Tests for suspected systemic conditions such as bleeding tendencies, sickle cell anemia, or diabetes.
4. Special consultations or referrals to a physician.

II. Purposes

The diagnostic work-up can benefit the patient, aid the dentist, and provide an overall perspective from which the dental hygienist can conduct a patient-oriented dental hygiene care program. Basic objectives of a diagnostic work-up prepared by the dental hygienist are to

A. Organize information and materials for the dentist to use while making the diagnosis and outlining the treatment plan for the patient.
B. Aid the dental hygienist in
   1. Planning dental hygiene preventive care and instruction for the patient.
   2. Guiding techniques during dental hygiene appointments.
   3. Correlating dental hygiene care with dental care.

C. Provide a permanent, documented, continuing record of the patient's oral and general health for
   1. Evaluating the response to treatment which may be compared with future observations at follow-up and recall appointments.
   2. Protecting the dental practice in case of misunderstandings or evidence in legal matters should questions arise.
D. Increase the scope of contribution of the dental hygienist to comprehensive patient care by the dental health team.

EXAMINATION PROCEDURES

A specific objective of patient examination as a part of the total diagnostic work-up is the recognition of deviations from normal which may be signs and symptoms of disease. The importance of careful, thorough examination cannot be overstressed. Concentration and attention to detail are necessary in order that each slight deviation from normal may be entered on the record for review by the dentist. Signs and symptoms of disease are the deviations from normal which must be recorded.

I. Symptoms

A symptom is a perceptible change from the normal. It is a phenomenon or change of condition arising from and accompanying a disease, which constitutes an indication of the disease. Some symptoms are general and may occur during various disease states. Other symptoms are pathognomonic which means that the symptom is unique to a particular disease and can distinguish it from other diseases. There are subjective and objective symptoms.

A. *Subjective symptoms* are those which the patient experiences and describes or are brought out by questioning. Examples: pain, tenderness, itching.

B. *Objective symptoms* are those which are observed by clinical examination. Examples: changes in color, size, contour of a tissue (not noted by the patient) or a finding revealed by use of a probe, explorer, or radiograph.

II. Types of Examination

A. Complete

A complete examination means that a thorough comprehensive diagnostic work-up is prepared.

B. Screening

Screening implies a brief examination using only parts of the complete diagnostic work-up. Screening is used for initial evaluation and classification of patients in clinical situations. In a community health program when a survey of a population is made to single out people with a particular condition, it is called screening.

C. Limited

A limited examination is usually made for an emergency. It is used primarily in the management of acute conditions.

D. Follow-up

A follow-up examination is a type of limited examination. It is used to observe the effects of treatment after a period of time during which the tissue or lesion could recover and heal. Indications for the need for additional or alternate treatment would be apparent.

E. Recall

A recall examination is made after a specified period of time following the completion of treatment and the restoration to health. A recall examination is a complete examination with a comprehensive diagnostic work-up. The purpose of the recall examination is for evaluation of the maintenance of health.

III. Examination Methods

A patient is examined by various visual, tactile, manual, and instrumental methods. General types are defined briefly here, and other specific methods are found throughout the book as they apply to a certain area under consideration.

A. Visual inspection

1. *Direct observation.* Visual examination is made in a systematic order to note surface appearance (color, contour, size, etc.) and to observe movement and other evidence of function.
2. *Radiographic inspection.* The use of x-ray can reveal deviations from the normal not notable by direct observation.
3. *Transillumination.* A strong light directed through a soft tissue or a tooth to enhance inspection is especially useful for detecting irregularities of the teeth and locating calculus.

B. Palpation

Palpation is examination using the sense of touch through tissue manipulation or pressure on an area with the fingers or hand. The method used depends on the area to be investigated. Types of palpation are described on page 92.

C. Instrumentation

The use of the instruments of examination such as the explorer and probe are for specific examination of the teeth and the periodontal tissues. They are described in detail on pages 183–201.

D. Percussion

Percussion is the act of tapping or striking a surface or tooth with the fingers or an instrument. Information about the status of health of the part is determined either by the response of the patient or by the sound. Example: A metal mirror handle is used to tap each tooth successively. When a tooth is known to be painful to movement, percussion should be avoided.

E. **Electrical test**

The electrical pulp vitality tester is used to detect the presence or absence of vital pulp tissue. The technique for use is described on page 218.

F. **Auscultation**

Auscultation is the use of sound. An example is the sound of clicking or snapping of the temporomandibular joint when the jaw is moved.

TOOTH NUMBERING SYSTEMS

There are three tooth designation systems in general use. They are the *Continuous Numbers 1 through 32* as adopted by the American Dental Association[1]; the *F.D.I. Two-digit*, adopted by the Federation Dentaire Internationale[2]; and the use of *Quadrant numbers 1 through 8*. Since dentists have learned different systems, it behooves each auxiliary person to be familiar with all.

I. Continuous Numbers 1 through 32

A. **Permanent Teeth**

Start with the right maxillary third molar (Number 1) and follow around the arch to the left maxillary third molar (16); descend to the left mandibular third molar (17), and follow around to the right mandibular third molar (32). Figure III–1 shows the crowns of the teeth with the corresponding numbers.

B. **Primary or Deciduous Teeth**

Use continuous upper case letters A through T in the same order as described for the permanent teeth: right maxillary second molar (A) around to left maxillary second molar (J); descend to left mandibular second molar (K), and around to the right mandibular second molar (T).

II. F.D.I. Two-Digit

A. **Permanent Teeth**

The first digit indicates the quadrant; starting with the maxillary right (quadrant 1) to maxillary left (quadrant 2), mandibular left (quadrant 3) and mandibular right (quadrant 4). The

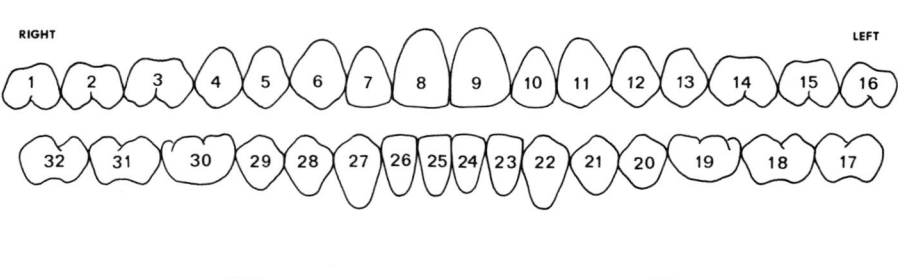

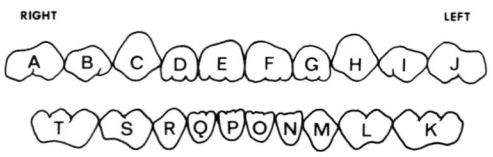

Figure III–1.   Tooth Numbering System: Continuous Numbers 1 through 32. Each tooth is designated by a specific number starting with the right maxillary third molar (Number 1), and following around to the left maxillary third molar (Number 16), to the left mandibular third molar (17), back around to the right mandibular third molar (32). Primary teeth are designated by letters.

second digit indicates the number of the tooth within the quadrant, starting with number one at the midline and counting to number eight, the third molar (figure III–2).

It is recommended that the digits be pronounced separately. For example, "two-five" means the maxillary left second premolar, and "four-two" is the mandibular right lateral incisor.

B. Primary or Deciduous Teeth

The quadrants for the primary teeth are numbered to continue with the permanent teeth. The maxillary right quadrant is Number 5, maxillary left is 6, mandibular left is 7, and mandibular right is 8. Second numbers are 1 through 5 to correspond with the primary teeth from the midline (figure III–2). For example, "eight-three" is

PERMANENT TEETH

Maxillary right								Maxillary left							
1–8	1–7	1–6	1–5	1–4	1–3	1–2	1–1	2–1	2–2	2–3	2–4	2–5	2–6	2–7	2–8
4–8	4–7	4–6	4–5	4–4	4–3	4–2	4–1	3–1	3–2	3–3	3–4	3–5	3–6	3–7	3–8
Mandibular right								Mandibular left							

PRIMARY TEETH

Maxillary right					Maxillary left				
5–5	5–4	5–3	5–2	5–1	6–1	6–2	6–3	6–4	6–5
8–5	8–4	8–3	8–2	8–1	7–1	7–2	7–3	7–4	7–5
Mandibular right					Mandibular left				

Figure III–2. Tooth Numbering System: F.D.I. Two-digit. Each quadrant is numbered 1 through 4, Number 1 the maxillary right, Number 2 the maxillary left, 3 the mandibular left, and 4 the mandibular right. Each tooth is numbered by the quadrant number and by the number of the tooth within the quadrant, starting with number 1 at the midline, to 8 the third molar. The quadrants of the primary teeth continue with the permanent teeth, from 5 (maxillary right) through 8 (mandibular right).

PERMANENT TEETH

Maxillary right								Maxillary left							
8	7	6	5	4	3	2	1	1	2	3	4	5	6	7	8
8	7	6	5	4	3	2	1	1	2	3	4	5	6	7	8
Mandibular right								Mandibular left							

PRIMARY TEETH

Maxillary right					Maxillary left				
E	D	C	B	A	A	B	C	D	E
E	D	C	B	A	A	B	C	D	E
Mandibular right					Mandibular left				

Figure III–3. Tooth Numbering System: Quadrant Numbers 1 through 8. With Number 1 for each central incisor, the teeth in each quadrant are numbered to 8 the third molar. See text for quadrant designation method. Primary teeth are identified by upper case letters A through E.

the mandibular right primary canine, and "six-five" is the maxillary left second primary molar.

III. Quadrant Numbers 1 Through 8

A. Permanent Teeth

With Number 1 for each central incisor, the teeth in each quadrant are numbered to 8, the third molar (figure III–3). To identify individual teeth, horizontal and vertical lines are used, drawn to indicate the quadrant. For example, the left maxillary first premolar is ⌊4, the right mandibular first and second molars are 76⌉. An entire quadrant may be represented by the use of the letter Q, for example the maxillary right quadrant is Q⌋.

B. Primary Teeth

Upper case letters A through E are used instead of the numbers. Examples are the mandibular left canine ⌈C, and the maxillary right first primary molar D⌋.

References

1. American Dental Association: System of Tooth Numbering and Radiograph Mounting, Approved by the American Dental Association House of Delegates, October, 1968.
2. New F.D.I. Two-Digit Tooth-Recording System, *F.D.I. Newsletter* (London), No. 74, 1971.

Suggested Readings

Allen, D. L., McFall, W. T., and Hunter, G. C.: *Periodontics for the Dental Hygienist*, 2nd ed. Philadelphia, Lea & Febiger, 1974, pp. 87–115.
American Dental Association, Council on Dental Care Programs: Code on Dental Procedures and Nomenclature, *J. Am. Dent. Assoc.*, 85, 789, October, 1972.

Brown, W. T., and Burns, R. L.: Comprehensive Oral Examination, *J. Am. Soc. Prev. Dent.*, 2, 18, September-October, 1972.
Foster, J.: Case Histories, Charting and Diagnosis, in Peterson, S., ed.: *Clinical Dental Hygiene*, 4th ed. St. Louis, Mosby, 1972, pp. 37–52.
Goldman, H. M. and Cohen, D. W.: *Periodontal Therapy*, 5th ed. St. Louis, Mosby, 1973, pp. 298–326.
Keller, S. E. and Manson-Hing, L. R.: Diagnosis and Treatment Planning for the Child Patient, in Finn, S. B.: *Clinical Pedodontics*, 4th ed. Philadelphia, Saunders, 1973, pp. 71–91.
Kerr, D. A., Ash. M. M., and Millard, H. D.: *Oral Diagnosis*, 4th ed. St. Louis, Mosby, 1974, pp. 5–15, 79–83.
Little, J. W. and King, D. R.: The Significance of Physical Diagnosis, Patient History, Data, and Medical Screening in the Dental Office, *Ann. Dent.*, 31, 42, Fall, 1972.
Mitchell, D. F., Standish, S. M., and Fast, T. B.: *Oral Diagnosis/Oral Medicine*, 2nd ed. Philadelphia, Lea & Febiger, 1971, pp. 1–2, 93–100.
Romanow, I.: Examination, Charting and Diagnosis, in Ward, H. L., ed.: *A Periodontal Point of View*. Springfield, Charles C Thomas, 1973, pp. 29–52.

Dental Photography

Dahlberg, W. H.: Photography in Periodontics, *Dent. Clin. North Am.*, p. 763, November, 1968.
Grupe, H. E.: Teleconverter Lenses in Clinical Photography, *Dent. Radiogr. Photogr.*, 43, 39, No. 2, 1970.
Hetherington, W. I. and Freehe, C. L.: Single Lens Reflex Cameras and Associated Equipment for Use in Dental Photography, *Dent. Clin. North Am.*, p. 699, November, 1968.
Hurtgen, T. P.: Visual Aid Technics, *Dent. Radiogr. Photogr.*, 46, 40, No. 2, 1973.
Hurtgen, T. P.: Kodak Pocket Instatech Close-up Camera, *Dent. Radiogr. Photogr.*, 47, 9, No. 1, 1974.
Rao, S. R. and Sweitzer, H.: Multple-view Photographs for Dental Visual Aids, *Dent. Radiogr. Photogr.*, 44, 40, No. 2, 1971.
Smith, G. E. and Hodson, J. T.: Serial Photography for Operative Dentistry, *J. Am. Dent. Assoc.*, 88, 1004, May, 1974.
Wilk, C. M.: Optimum Dentistry Through Oral Photography, *Dent. Radiogr. Photogr.*, 46, 63, No. 3, 1973.

Chapter 6

Personal, Medical, and Dental History

For safe, scientific dental and dental hygiene care, a meaningful, complete patient history is necessary. The history directs and guides procedures to be taken in preparation for, during, and following appointments.

At least a part of the history is needed before oral examination procedures with periodontal probe and explorer are carried out. The use of instruments which would manipulate the soft tissue around the teeth may be contraindicated in certain instances until after a medical consultation to determine whether protective, precautionary measures are needed.

When there is a question about the medical history as described by the patient or when an unusual or abnormal condition is observed, consultation with the patient's physician, or referral for examination of the patient who does not have a physician, is mandatory. Even emergency treatment such as for the relief of pain should be postponed or kept to a minimum until the patient's status is determined.

The significance of the history cannot be overestimated. Oral conditions reflect the general health of the patient. Dental procedures may complicate or be complicated by existing pathological or physiological conditions elsewhere in the body. General health factors influence response to treatment such as tissue healing and thereby affect the outcomes which may be expected from oral care.

The state of the patient's health is constantly changing. Therefore the history represents the period in the patient's life in which the history was made. With successive recall appointments the history must be reviewed and considered along with other new findings.

I. Purposes of the History

Carefully prepared personal, medical, and dental histories are used in comprehensive patient care to

A. Provide information pertinent to the etiology and diagnosis of oral conditions and the total treatment plan.

B. Reveal conditions which necessitate precautions, modifications, or adaptations during appointments to assure that dental and dental hygiene procedures will not harm the patient and that emergency situations will be prevented.

C. Aid in the identification of possible unrecognized conditions for which the patient should be referred for further diagnosis and treatment.

D. Permit appraisal of the general health and nutritional status which in turn contributes to the prognosis of success in patient care and instruction.

E. Give insight into emotional and psychological factors, attitudes, and prejudices which may affect present appointments as well as continuing care.

F. Document records for reference and comparison over a series of appointments for periodic follow-up.

G. Furnish evidence in legal matters should questions arise.

II. History Preparation

The general methods in current use are the *interview,* the *questionnaire,* or a combination of the two. There are several systems for obtaining the history.

A. **Alternative Appointment Procedures**
1. *Complete history* made at the initial visit: may be a combination of interview and questionnaire.
2. *Brief history* of vital items obtained at the initial visit; complete history obtained at a succeeding appointment.
    a. Purposes of brief history: to prepare for emergency care and to learn of any condition which may contraindicate instrumentation in and around the gingival sulcus during dental and periodontal examinations.
    b. Brief history may be in the form of a questionnaire, while an interview for follow-up provides opportunity for individual evaluation.
3. *Self-history* prepared at home: the patient is given a form to complete between appointments. Such a form might include some checking as in a questionnaire, and some space to allow free expression by the patient.

B. **Record Forms**
1. *Types.* Many varying forms are in current use. Forms are available commercially or from the American Dental Association,[1] but many dentists prefer to prepare their own design and have the form printed to their specifications.
2. *Characteristics of an Adequate Form.* The number of items or questions included is not necessarily indicative of the value of the form. The extensive and involved form may be as practical or impractical as the brief checklist which permits no detailed description. Success in use depends on function and a clear common understanding of the meaning of the recorded information to all who will refer to it.

    Some characteristics of an adequate form are that it should
    a. Provide for convenient notation of important details in a logical sequence.
    b. Permit quick identification of special needs of a patient when the history is reviewed prior to each appointment.
    c. Allow ample space to record the patient's own words whenever possible in the interview method, or for self-expression by the patient on a questionnaire.
    d. Have space for notes concerning attitudes and knowledge as stated or displayed by the patient during the history making or other later appointments.
    e. Be of a size consistent with the complete patient record forms for filing and ready availability.

C. Introduction to the Patient

The patient needs to realize why the information requested in the histories is essential before treatment can be undertaken. Dental personnel must convey the idea that oral health and general health are interrelated, without creating undue alarm concerning potential ill effects or harmful sequelae from required treatment.

For building rapport, children may participate in their history preparation, but most of the information will need to be supplied by a parent. The signature of the responsible adult on the record is advisable.

III. The Questionnaire

Positive findings on a completed questionnaire need supplementation in a personal interview. A questionnaire by itself cannot be expected to satisfy the overall purposes of the history but can be adapted best to phases of the personal history, some aspects of the dental history, and factual information in the medical history.

A. Types of Questions

The Health Questionnaire available from the American Dental Association (figure 6–1) provides useful examples of questions essential to patient evaluation.[1] In addition there is a short form available in which questions are directed to provide information on drug use, allergies, and current medical treatment for preliminary or emergency use.*

1. System-oriented questions

Direct questions or topics for the patient to check whether or not he has had a disease of, for example,

*Copies of the questionnaires are obtainable in quantity. Request the A.D.A. Catalog and order form from the Order Department, American Dental Association, 211 E. Chicago Ave., Chicago, Ill. 60611. The catalog numbers are: Health Questionnaire P1-HQ (Long Form) and P1-HQ 1 (Short Form).

the digestive system, respiratory system, or urinary system may be used. The questions may contain specific body parts, for example the stomach, lungs, kidneys. Specific questions can then be directed to the specific disease state and the dates of duration.

2. Disease-oriented questions

A typical set of questions for the patient to check may start with "Do you have, or have you had, any of the following diseases or problems?" A listing under that question contains items such as diabetes, asthma, rheumatic fever, arranged alphabetically or grouped by systems or body organs. Follow-up questions can determine dates of illness, severity, and outcome.

3. Symptom-oriented questions

In the absence of previous or current disease states, questions may lead to a suspicion of a condition which in turn can give the opportunity to recommend and encourage the patient to schedule a physical examination with a physician. Samples of the symptom-oriented question appear in figure 6–1, for example, "Are you thirsty much of the time?" "Does your mouth frequently become dry?" or "Do you have to urinate (pass water) more than six times a day?" the positive answers for which could lead to tests for diabetes detection.

B. Advantages of a Questionnaire

1. Broad in scope: useful during the interview to identify positive areas which need additional clarification.
2. Time saving.
3. Consistent: all selected questions are included, and none omitted because of time or other factors.

HEALTH QUESTIONNAIRE

Date_____

Name_____Address_____
      Last   First   Middle   Number & Street

_____
      City   State   Zip Code   Home & Business Phone

Age_____Sex_____Height_____Weight_____Occupation_____

Married_____Spouse_____Single_____

Closest Relative_____Phone_____

In the following questions, circle yes or no, whichever applies. Your answers are for our records only and will be considered confidential.

1. Has there been any change in your general health within the past year............YES   NO

2. My last physical examination was on_____

3. Are you now under the care of a physician..YES   NO
   a. If so, what is the condition being treated_____

4. The name and address of my physician is_____
   _____
   _____

5. Have you had any serious illness or operation. ....YES   NO
   a. If so, what was the illness or operation _____

6. Have you been hospitalized or had a serious illness
   within the past five (5) years...YES   NO
   a. If so, what was the problem_____

7. Do you have or have you had any of the following diseases or problems.
   a. Rheumatic fever or rheumatic heart disease................................YES   NO
   b. Congenital heart lesions...YES   NO
   c. Cardiovascular disease (heart trouble, heart attack, coronary insufficiency,
     coronary occlusion, high blood pressure, arteriosclerosis, stroke)..........YES   NO
     1) Do you have pain in chest upon exertion................................YES   NO
     2) Are you ever short of breath after mild exercise........................YES   NO
     3) Do your ankles swell..YES   NO
     4) Do you get short of breath when you lie down, or do you require extra pillows
       when you sleep ....YES   NO
   d. Allergy..YES   NO
   e. Asthma or hay fever...YES   NO
   f. Hives or a skin rash...YES   NO
   g. Fainting spells or seizures..YES   NO
   h. Diabetes..YES   NO
     1) Do you have to urinate (pass water) more than six times a day..........YES   NO
     2) Are you thirsty much of the time......................................YES   NO
     3) Does your mouth frequently become dry..............................YES   NO
   i. Hepatitis, jaundice or liver disease...YES   NO
   j. Arthritis...YES   NO
   k. Inflammatory rheumatism (painful swollen joints)........................YES   NO
   l. Stomach ulcers..YES   NO
   m. Kidney trouble..YES   NO
   n. Tuberculosis..YES   NO
   o. Do you have a persistent cough or cough up blood ....YES   NO
   p. Low blood pressure..YES   NO
   q. Venereal disease..YES   NO
   r. Other_____

Figure 6–1. Health Questionnaire. From *Accepted Dental Therapeutics.* Copyright by the American Dental Association. Reprinted by permission.

8. Have you had abnormal bleeding associated with previous extractions, surgery, or trauma..YES NO
   a. Do you bruise easily..YES NO
   b. Have you ever required a blood transfusion...YES NO
     If so, explain the circumstances_____

9. Do you have any blood disorder such as anemia...YES NO

10. Have you had surgery or x-ray treatment for a tumor, growth, or other condition of your mouth or lips...YES NO

11. Are you taking any drug or medicine...YES NO
    If so, what _____

12. Are you taking any of the following:
   a. Antibiotics or sulfa drugs...YES NO
   b. Anticoagulants (blood thinners)...YES NO
   c. Medicine for high blood pressure..YES NO
   d. Cortisone (steroids)..YES NO
   e. Tranquilizers...YES NO
   f. Aspirin...YES NO
   g. Insulin, tolbutamide (Orinase) or similar drug...YES NO
   h. Digitalis or drugs for heart trouble...YES NO
   i. Nitroglycerin...YES NO
   j. Other_____

13. Are you allergic or have you reacted adversely to:
   a. Local anesthetics..YES NO
   b. Penicillin or other antibiotics...YES NO
   c. Sulfa drugs..YES NO
   d. Barbiturates, sedatives, or sleeping pills...YES NO
   e. Aspirin...YES NO
   f. Iodine..YES NO
   g. Other_____

14. Have you had any serious trouble associated with any previous dental treatment..YES NO
    If so, explain_____

15. Do you have any disease, condition, or problem not listed above that you think I should know about...YES NO
    If so, please explain_____

16. Are you employed in any situation which exposes you regularly to x-rays or other ionizing radiation...YES NO

WOMEN
17. Are you pregnant..YES NO
18. Do you have any problems associated with your menstrual period....................YES NO

Remarks:

_____
SIGNATURE OF PATIENT

_____
SIGNATURE OF DENTIST

Figure 6–1. (Continued)

4. Patient has time to think over the answers: not under pressure, nor under the eyes of the interviewer.
5. Patient may write information which he might hesitate to express directly in an interview.
6. Legal aspect of a written record with patient's signature.

C. **Disadvantages of a Questionnaire** (if used alone without a follow-up interview)
1. Impersonal: no opportunity to develop rapport.
2. Inflexible: no provision for additional questioning in areas of specific importance to an individual patient.

IV. The Interview

In long-range planning for the patient's health, much more is involved than asking questions and receiving answers. The rapport established at the time of the interview contributes to the continued cooperation of the patient.

A. **Participants**

The dental hygienist is alone with the patient or parent of the child patient. The history should never be taken in a reception room when other patients are present.

B. **Setting**
1. The consultation room or office is preferred; the patient should be away from the atmosphere of the operatory where his thoughts would be on the techniques to be performed.
2. Operatory: may be the only available place where privacy is afforded.
   a. Seat patient comfortably in upright position.
   b. Turn off running water and dental light, and close the door.
   c. Sit on operating stool to be at eye level with the patient.

C. **Pointers for the Interview**

Interviewing involves communication between individuals. Communication implies the transmission or interchange of facts, attitudes, opinions, or thoughts through words, gestures, or other means. Through tactful but direct questioning, communication can be successful and the patient will give such information as he knows. Frequently the patient is unaware of a health problem.

The attitude of the dental hygienist should be one of friendly understanding, reassurance, and acceptance. Genuine interest and willingness to listen when a patient wishes to describe symptoms or complaints not only aids in establishing the rapport needed but frequently provides insight into the patient's real attitudes and prejudices. By asking simple questions at first, and more personal questions later after rapport has developed, the patient will be more relaxed and frank in answering.

Self-confidence and gentle efficiency on the part of the dental hygienist give the patient a feeling of confidence and help put him at ease. Skill is required since tact, ingenuity, and judgment are taxed to the fullest in the attempt to obtain both accurate and complete information from the patient.

D. **Interview Form**

The interviewer may use a structured form with places to check and fill in, or record on blank sheets from questions created from a guide list of essential topics. Either may involve reference to the positive or negative answers on a previously completed questionnaire. Familiarity with the items on the history will permit the interviewer to be direct and informal without reading from a fixed list of topics, a method which may lack the personal touch necessary to gain the patient's confidence. When appropriate, the patient's own words are recorded.

E. **Advantages of the Interview**
1. Personal contact contributes to development of rapport for future appointments.
2. Flexibility for individual needs: details obtained can be adapted for supplementary questioning.

F. **Disadvantages of Interview**
1. Time-consuming when not prefaced with questionnaire.
2. Unless a list is consulted, items of importance may be omitted.
3. Patient may be embarrassed to talk about personal conditions and may hold back significant information.

V. Items Included in the History

Information obtained by means of the history is directly related to how the goals of dental and dental hygiene care can and will be accomplished. In tables 6–1, 6–2, and 6–3, items are listed with suggested influences on appointment procedures. Objectives for the items to include in the various parts of the history are listed below.

In specialized practices objectives may require increased emphasis on certain aspects. The age group most frequently served would influence the material needed. Parental history and pre- and postnatal information may take on particular significance for the treatment of a small child; in a pedodontist's practice a special form could be devised to include all essential items.[2,3]

Insight and awareness shown while preparing the patient history depends on background knowledge of the oral manifestations of systemic diseases, medications for various conditions, and drug–drug interactions.[4,5] Interpretation of

findings and alertness to immediate needs for application are described on page 70.

A. **Personal History** (table 6–1)

The basic objectives in gathering the personal information about the patient are:
1. Data essential for appointment planning and business aspects.
2. Approval of care of a minor, and other legal aspects.
3. Patient's physician: for consultation relative to interrelations between general and oral health.

B. **Medical History** (table 6–2)

Objectives of the medical history are to determine whether the patient has any conditions in the following categories.[6]
1. Diseases which may contraindicate certain kinds of dental and dental hygiene treatment.
   Examples. Leukemia because of lowered resistance to infection; congestive heart failure requires treatment before stressful procedures, particularly surgery, can be performed.
2. Diseases which require special precautions or premedication prior to treatment.
   Examples. Antibiotic coverage for patient with a history of rheumatic fever or congenital heart defect to prevent subacute bacterial endocarditis; epileptic who may need increased sedation to prevent a seizure if treatment is to be stressful.
3. Diseases under treatment by a physician which require medicating drugs which may influence or contraindicate procedures of the dental hygiene appointments.
   Examples. Tranquilizers in daily use could contraindicate premedication with sedatives; anticoagu-

lant therapy requires consultation with physician.

4. Allergic or untoward reactions to drugs.

    Examples. All drugs which may possibly be used or recommended to the patient for postoperative care should be checked with the patient as to previous use and reaction.

5. Diseases and drugs with manifestations in the mouth.

    Examples. Hematological disorders, Dilantin–induced hyperplasia.

6. Diseases which endanger the dental personnel.

    Examples. Active tuberculosis; history of hepatitis.

7. Physiological state of the patient.

    Examples. Pregnancy, puberty, menopause.

C. **Dental History** (table 6–3, page 77)

The dental history should contribute to knowlege of:

1. The immediate problem, chief complaint, cause of present pain, or discomfort of any kind in the oral cavity.

2. The previous dental care as described by the patient including extent of restorative and prosthetic replacement, as well as any adverse effects.

3. The attitude of the patient toward oral health and care of the mouth as may be indicated by previous periodic dental and dental hygiene treatment.

4. The personal daily care exercised by the patient as evidence of his knowledge of the purposes of continuing care and of the value placed on the teeth and their supporting structures.

VI. Review of History

Periodically updating the history at recall evaluation appointments is essential. Changes in health status revealed by interim medical examinations or evidenced by reported illness or hospitalizations must be recorded and considered during continuing treatment.

Following a review of the previously recorded history, the questions can be directed to the patient to compare the present condition with the previous one and to determine at least the following:

A. Interim illnesses: changes in health.

B. Visits to physician: reasons and results.

C. Laboratory tests performed and the results: blood, urine, or other analyses.

D. Current medications.

E. Changes in the oral soft tissues and the teeth observed by the patient.

IMMEDIATE APPLICATION OF PATIENT HISTORIES

Together with information from all other parts of the diagnostic work-up, the patient histories are essential to the treatment plan. Treatment planning for an individual patient is described on pages 293–299.

Prior to that, immediate evaluation of the histories is necessary before proceeding to succeeding steps in the preparation of materials for the complete diagnostic work-up. Any one of the objectives for the medical history (V., B., page 69) could alter the procedures to be accomplished.

The list which follows is not intended to be exhaustive, but rather suggestive. From these items, it is expected that the dental hygienist will be alerted to precautions which may be needed.

I. Identification of Conditions Which Require Medical Consultation

A. Dentist and physician need immediate consultation relative to current therapy, medications, or health status of the patient.

B. Patient referred for physical examination when signs of possible disease condition are apparent.

C. Patient referred for laboratory tests.

II. Communicable Disease

A history of communicable disease, either current, in the past, or recent past, requires attention to the prevention of disease transmission through direct contact, instruments, and other materials used during examination. Methods for precautions related to hepatitis and other diseases were described on pages 26–27. Self-protection restrictions by all dental personnel are mandatory.

III. Prophylactic Premedication

Patients susceptible to bacterial endocarditis must have antibiotic premedication prior to any tissue manipulation during the examination which could create a bacteremia. Tissue manipulation, particularly the use of a probe and an explorer submarginally, must be withheld until the condition has been discussed with the patient's physician. Bacteremia created by instrumentation is described on page 496 and bacterial endocarditis on page 680.

Other patients who may need prophylactic premedication are those with marked reduced capacity to resist infection. There is no indication for generalized use of antibiotics in healthy persons for the purpose of preventing infection.[7,8]

A. Indications for Prophylactic Premedication to Prevent Bacterial Endocarditis

1. Rheumatic and congenital heart disease.[9]
2. Rheumatic fever and other febrile disease which predisposes to valvular damage. When a patient has a heart murmur, it is necessary to determine from the patient's physician whether the murmur is considered functional or organic. A functional murmur does not require premedication, whereas an organic murmur which is based on a defect in the structure of the heart does require antibiotic coverage.[10]
3. Prior cardiac surgery and valvular prosthesis. The patient with intracardiac prosthesis requires extensive antibiotic coverage and should be managed only under orders of the attending physician. Coverage also is usually indicated for a patient with a pacemaker which has implanted wires.

B. Other Indications for Prophylactic Premedication

1. Uncontrolled, unstable diabetes. Controlled diabetics are treated as healthy patients (pages 689, 698).
2. Grossly contaminated traumatic facial injuries.
3. Reduced capacity to resist infection.
   a. Anticancer chemotherapy.
   b. Blood disease, particularly acute leukemia and agranulocytosis.
   c. Irradiation.
   d. Corticosteroid or immunosuppressive therapy.
4. Renal transplant and hemodialysis; glomerulonephritis or other active renal disorder.[11–13]

IV. Conditions Which Contraindicate Certain Procedures

A. Radiation

When a patient is under radiation therapy, or has had recent radiation for other purposes, a complete oral radiographic survey may be contraindicated. Conference with the physician involved may be necessary to determine the quantity of radiation received.

B. Allergies

Although not many agents used during the diagnostic work-up are involved, there is a possibility.

Table 6–1.   Items for the Personal History

Items to Record in Patient History	Considerations	Influences on Appointment Procedures
1. Name Addresses: Residence and Business Telephone Numbers Sex Marital Status For Child: Name of Parent or Guardian For Parent: Ages and Sex of Children	Accurate recording necessary for business aspects of dental practice	Aids in establishing rapport Instruction applicable to entire family Advice concerning fluorides for children
2. Birthdate	Whether of age or a minor Oral conditions related to age changes: diseases, healing, and other possible characteristics	Approval of parent or guardian necessary for care of minor or mentally handicapped person; signature must be obtained Approach to patient instruction
3. Birthplace and Residence in Early Years	Presence of fluoride in drinking water. Food and eating patterns Conditions endemic to certain areas	Effects of fluoride on teeth Instruction in dietary needs adapted to cultural practices
4. Occupation: Present and Former Spouse's Occupation For Child: Parent's Occupation	May be a factor in etiology of certain diseases, dental stains, occlusal wear May affect diet, oral habits, general health	Instruction applied to specific needs Dexterity in use of self-care devices related to dexterity gained from occupation Influence on oral care of entire family For child: which parent will supervise and assist child in oral care
5. Physician	Name, address, and telephone number For consultation	Consultation indicated: (1) for condition which may require premedication (2) when disease symptoms are suspected but patient does not state (3) in an emergency
6. Referred by and Address	To whom to send referral acknowledgement and appreciation	Contribution to rapport with patient Patient referred by another patient may have concept of the office procedures.

Table 6–2.   Items for the Medical History

Item to Record in the History	Considerations	Influences on Appointment Procedures
1. General Health and Appearance	Disabilities Overall impression of well-being Patient's appraisal of his own health	Response, cooperation and attitude to expect during appointments
2. Medical Examination	Date most recent examination Reason for the examination Tests performed; results Anticipated surgery	May need verification with the physician if questions exist Need for superior state of oral health in advance of surgery (a) when long recovery is expected and patient may miss recall (b) prior to transplant, heart surgery or prosthesis
3. Major Illnesses and Hospitalizations	Causes of illness Type and duration of treatment Anesthetics used Convalescence Course of healing: normal, not normal	Influence of illnesses on health and care of the oral cavity Anesthetic choice Healing to anticipate following gingival treatments
4. Height and Weight	Weight changes over past years or months Obesity Undernourishment Child growth pattern	Marked weight change may be a symptom of undiagnosed disease; suggest referral for medical examination Influence on dietary instructions for oral health
5. Current Treatment by Physician	Nature and duration of illness	Effects on dental and dental hygiene procedures and personal care
6. Radiation Therapy	Reason, location, duration Head and neck radiation: susceptibility to osteo-radionecrosis	Effect on oral radiographic survey: prevention of over-exposure
7. Medication: prescribed by physician	Drugs, medicine, injections, tonics, vitamins, pills: past and present, purpose Drug–drug interactions with possible dental prescriptions Effects on oral tissues	Consultation with physician concerning adjustments in dosage for dental or dental hygiene appointments Indications for premedication Problem of xerostomia associated with many drugs (diuretics, tranquilizers, estrogens, antihistamines are examples) Inhibition of inflammatory response (steroid therapy, for example)

Table 6–2, *Continued*

Item to Record in the History	Considerations	Influences on Appointment Procedures
8. Self-medication	Type and frequency Drug abuse	Information not revealed by patient could complicate treatment. Lack of interest in oral health, only pain relief
9. Familial Medical History	Predisposition to certain diseases (example: diabetes) History of diseases which occur in the family	May help patient seek medical examination when symptom suggests possible disease
10. Daily Diet	Recommendations of patient's physician, past and present Vitamin supplements Appetite Regularity of meals Food likes and dislikes	Instructions to be given relative to oral health Prognosis for healing after treatment Need for dietary review and analysis (page 402)
	Use of alcohol: frequency	Excessive use: effect on anesthesia Poor nutritional state is common; lack of oral care May result in poor patient cooperation
11. Communicable Disease	Stage of disease; current therapy Degree of communicability; susceptibility of dental personnel	Reappointment to a future date Wear face mask, gloves, or other precautionary measure. Consultation with physician
A. Hepatitis	If patient had jaundice within past three months, whether diagnosed as hepatitis or not, treat as a carrier Date of termination of disease Likelihood of carrier state	Postpone elective treatment when possible Attention to skin breaks, sterile procedures, wear rubber gloves (page 27)
B. Venereal Disease	Oral lesion may be present May not obtain history	Wear gloves for oral inspection (pages 93, 103).
C. Tuberculosis	Active or passive Current treatment	Passive: use supplementary aseptic technique; wear face mask. Active: techniques performed under hospital sterile procedures
12. Allergies	Determine substances to which the patient is allergic: Anesthetics Penicillin Medicaments Foods Iodine	Avoid use of substances to which the patient is allergic. Consider allergies when planning dietary recommendations

Table 6–2, *continued*

Item to Record in the History	*Consideration*	*Influences on Appointment Procedures*
13. Respiratory Problems Asthma Bronchitis Bronchiectasis Emphysema	Agents which may bring on attack Prevention measures Breathing problems Coughing spells	Chair position for appointments Anesthesia choice
14. Diabetes	Uncontrolled requires antibiotic premedication. Ask patient when insulin was taken. Diet and medication requirements Family incidence: identification of susceptible but undiagnosed	Appointment time related to insulin therapy and mealtime Avoid tissue trauma Need frequent recall Preparation for emergencies (pages 693, 731)
15. Cardiovascular Diseases	Category and history of disease (pages 676–677) Type of treatment; medication Consultation with physician	Short appointment to prevent fatigue Selection of anesthesia; premedication Preparation for emergencies Emphasis on preventive oral care measures
A. High Blood Pressure	May be a symptom of other disease state Current therapy Choice of anesthetic	Length of appointment Allay fears to prevent apprehension
B. Congenital Heart Disease and Rheumatic Heart Disease	History of rheumatic fever Current therapy Consultation with physician	Prophylactic antibiotic to prevent subacute bacterial endocarditis (pages 680–681)
16. Blood Diseases	Type and duration Current therapy Consultation with physician Need for high level of oral health	Serious condition: palliative treatment may be all that is possible. Frequent recall to prevent long, tiring appointments and to administer preventive service (pages 683–684)
17. Bleeding	Previous experiences: causes, treatment History of disorder with coagulation problem Check use of aspirin (relation to bleeding tendency) Laboratory tests for bleeding time, coagulation, may be needed	Emergency prevention through pre-appointment precautions Avoid tissue trauma May need to apply dressing after scaling to provide pressure

Table 6–2, continued

Items to Record in the History	Considerations	Influences on Appointment Procedures
18. Eyes	Purpose for correction with eyeglasses, contact lenses Manifestations of systemic disease	Protection of eyes during instrumentation, especially handpiece and ultrasonic scaler Adaptations for blind or partially blind (pages 669–671) Use of glasses during patient instruction
19. Ears	Deafness or degree of deafness Infections, operations	Adaptations for instruction (pages 671–672)
20. Nasal Sinuses, Tonsils, Adenoids	Mouthbreathing as a possible factor in gingival disease Breathing problems during appointment	Chair positioning for gagging prevention Personal care emphasis for effects of mouthbreathing
21. Gastrointestinal Disease	Nature and treatment of the disease Diet restrictions prescribed by physician	Patient instruction in accord with prescribed diet and medication
22. Epilepsy	Frequency of seizures Medications prescribed Consultation may be indicated Minimize stress during appointment	Gingival hyperplasia from Dilantin therapy (page 635) Preparation for first aid (pages 638, 732)
23. Endocrine Influences	Nature of possible problem related to age group Possible oral manifestations Current therapy Effect of birth control pills, estrogens	Emphasis on high level of plaque control Adaptations of procedures during appointments (pages 703–711)
24. Pregnancy	Month, parturition date Possible oral manifestations History of previous pregnancies	Adjust physical arrangements for patient comfort Adapt techniques (pages 716–718) Need for frequent recall

25. Physical Disabilities	Extent of disability
	Nature, cause, treatment
	  Cerebral palsy
	  Multiple sclerosis
	  Arthritis
	  Poliomyelitis
	  Other (pages 657–668)
	Consult physician for special precautions; possible effects related to current medications
		Adjustment of physical arrangements
		Adaptations of techniques and instruction needs (pages 655–657)

26. Mental, psychiatric, psychological	Emotional problems expressed by patient Medications	Mental retardation: special adaptations (pages 646–650) Attitudes toward personal care

Table 6-3. Items for the Dental History

Items to Record in the History	Considerations	Influences on Appointment Procedures
1. **Reason for Present Appointment**	Chief complaint in patient's own words Pain or discomfort Onset, symptoms, duration of an acute condition	Need for immediate treatment Attitude toward dentistry and preventive care
2. **Previous Dental Appointments**	Date last treatment Services performed Regularity	Patient knowledge concerning regular dental care Cooperation anticipated
3. **Anesthetics Used**	Local, general Adverse or allergic reactions	Choice of anesthetic
4. **Radiographs**	Date most recent survey Availability from previous dentist Amount of exposure considered with exposure for medical purposes	Amount of exposure: limitations Patient's appreciation for need and use of radiographs
5. **Family Dental History**	Parental tooth loss or maintenance	Attitude toward saving teeth and preventive dentistry
6. **Previous Treatment**	Type of treatment; frequency of recall Whether referred to specialist	Attitude toward specialized care Previous familiarity with role of dental hygienist
A. Periodontal	History of acute infection (acute necrotizing ulcerative gingivitis, page 597) Surgery; postoperative healing	Attitude toward self-care and disease control
B. Orthodontic	Age during treatment; completion Previous problem Habit correction	For current treatment, consultation with orthodontist needed to determine instructions.
C. Endodontic	Dates, etiology	Periodic recheck
D. Prosthodontic	Types of prostheses	Care of prostheses and abutment teeth
E. Other	Extent of restorations	Understanding toward prevention
7. **Injuries to Face or Teeth**	Causes and extent Fractured teeth or jaws	Limitation of opening
8. **Temporomandibular Joint**	History of discomfort, disease, dislocation Previous treatment	Effect on opening; accessibility during instrumentation

Table 6–3, continued

Items to Record in the History	Considerations	Influences on Appointment Procedures
9. Habits	Clenching, bruxism, doodling Mouth breathing Biting objects: fingernails, pipe stem, thread, other Cheek or lip biting Patient awareness of habits	Tension of patient Instruction relative to effects of habits
10. Smoking	Form of tobacco, amount used Frequency Knowledge of effects on oral tissues	Instruction concerning oral effects Need for frequent observation to detect tissue changes if patient continues at same rate Tooth stains; dentifrice selection
11. Fluorides	Systemic, topical, dates Residences during tooth development years Amount of fluoride in drinking water	Current preventive procedures and need for reevaluation
12. Plaque Control Procedures	Toothbrushing: current procedures Type of brush (manual or automatic) Texture of bristles Frequency of use Age of brush; frequency of having a new brush Dentifrice Name How selected; reason Additional cleansing devices and frequency of use Dental floss Water irrigation Perio-aid, rubber tip, or other Mouthwash or other agents: frequency, purpose. Source of instruction in care of oral cavity	Present practices and previous instruction New instruction needed; reception by patient Relation of techniques to prevention of dental caries and periodontal diseases Supervision of child by parent: current practices Problems of habit change

TECHNICAL HINTS

I.   Date all records.

II. Keep permanent records in ink.

III. The completed history for a minor should be signed by a parent or guardian.

IV. All information obtained for a patient history must be maintained in strictest confidence.

V.   For patients with special health problems which require premedication or other adaptation of procedure, print in red ink with a fine pen in ½ to ¾ inch letters diagonally across all permanent record pages the identifying word such as DIABETIC, HEPATITIS, CARDIAC, or RHEUMATIC.

VI. Analyze the usefulness of items on the patient history form periodically and plan for revision as scientific research reveals new information which must be applied.

FACTORS TO TEACH THE PATIENT

I.   The need for having the personal, medical, and dental history prior to performance of dental and dental hygiene procedures.

II. The relationship between oral health and general physical health.

III. The interrelationship of medical and dental care.

IV. Advantages of cooperation in furnishing information which will help dental personnel to interpret observations accurately and to assure the dentist that the correct diagnosis and treatment plan have been made.

V.   All patients who require antibiotic premedication need special emphasis on the importance of preventive dentistry, the imperative need for regular dental care, and the necessity for precautions to be taken whenever dental or dental hygiene treatment is to be given.

References

1. American Dental Association, Council on Dental Therapeutics: *Accepted Dental Therapeutics*, 36th ed. Chicago, American Dental Association, 1975, pp. 3–7.
2. Keller, S. E. and Manson-Hing, L. R.: Diagnosis and Treatment Planning for the Child Patient, in Finn, S. B.: *Clinical Pedodontics*, 4th ed. Philadelphia, Saunders, 1973, pp. 72–79.
3. Mink, J. R., Spedding, R. H., and Gellin, M. E.: Pedodontics in General Practice, in Morris, A. L. and Bohannan, H. M., eds.: *The Dental Specialties in General Practice*. Philadelphia, Saunders, 1969, pp. 113–124.
4. American Dental Association, Council on Dental Therapeutics: op. cit., 4–16, 34–40.
5. Pallasch, T. J.: *Clinical Drug Therapy in Dental Practice*. Philadelphia, Lea & Febiger, 1973, pp. 206–216.
6. Millard, H. D.: Techniques of Clinical Diagnosis of Importance to the Dentist, *Dent. Clin. North Am.*, p. 21, March, 1963.
7. Pallasch: op. cit., pp. 122–128.
8. McCallum, C. A.: Antimicrobial Agents, in Finn, S. B.: *Clinical Pedodontics*, 4th ed. Philadelphia, Saunders, 1973, pp. 71–91.
9. American Dental Association, Council on Dental Therapeutics: op. cit., pp. 9–10, 169.
10. Kerr, D. A., Ash, M. M., and Millard, H. D.: *Oral Diagnosis*, 4th ed. St. Louis, Mosby, 1974, p. 354.
11. Bottomley, W. K., Cioffi, R. F., and Martin, A. J.: Dental Management of the Patient Treated by Renal Transplantation: Preoperative and Postoperative Considerations, *J. Am. Dent. Assoc.*, 85, 1330, December, 1972.
12. Hooley, J. R. and Petersen, W. M.: Dental Management of Patients with Renal Failure Being Treated by Hemodialysis, *Oral Surg.*, 28, 660, November, 1969.
13. Kruger, G. O.: *Textbook of Oral Surgery*, 4th ed. St. Louis, Mosby, 1974, p. 146.

Suggested Readings

Bahn, S. L.: Drug-Related Dental Destruction, *Oral Surg.*, 33, 49, January, 1972.

Barrett, R. A.: Diagnostic Laboratory Test—Who Needs It? *J. Am. Soc. Prev. Dent.*, 3, 26, November-December, 1973.

Bennett, C. R.: *Monheim's Local Anesthesia and Pain Control in Dental Practice*, 5th ed. St. Louis, Mosby, 1974, pp. 209–231.

Brasher, W. J. and Rees, T. D.: Systemic Conditions in the Management of Periodontal Patients, *J. Periodont.*, 41, 349, June, 1970.

Burket, L. W.: *Oral Medicine*, 6th ed. Philadelphia, Lippincott, 1971, pp. 7–16.

Ellinger, C. W., Kanner, I., Wesley, R., Frazier, Q., and Rahn, A.: Are Your Patients as Healthy as You Think They Are, Doctor? *J. Am. Soc. Prev. Dent.*, 3, 36, November-December, 1973.

Foster, J.: Case Histories, Charting, and Diagnosis, in Peterson, S., ed.: *Clinical Dental Hygiene*, 4th ed. St. Louis, Mosby, 1972, pp. 37–48.

Grant, D. A., Stern, I. B., and Everett, F. G.: *Orban's Periodontics*, 4th ed. St. Louis, Mosby, 1972, pp. 300–306.

Halpern, I. L.: Patient's Medical Status—A Factor in Dental Treatment, *Oral Surg.*, 39, 216, February, 1975.

Hooley, J., R.: *Hospital Dentistry*. Philadelphia, Lea & Febiger, 1970, pp. 33–46.

Hussar, D. A. : Interactions Involving Drugs Used in Dental Practice, *J. Am. Dent. Assoc.*, 87, 349, August, 1973.

Kerr, D. A., Ash, M. M., and Millard, H. D.: *Oral Diagnosis*, 4th ed. St. Louis, Mosby, 1974, pp. 36–70, 348–360.

Mitchell, D. F., Standish, S. M., and Fast, T. B.: *Oral Diagnosis/Oral Medicine*, 2nd ed. Philadelphia, Lea & Febiger, 1971, pp. 16–19, 82–91.

Morris, A. L.: The Medical History in Dental Practice, *J. Am. Dent. Assoc.*, 74, 129, January, 1967.

Myall, R. W. T. and Gregory, H. S.: Current Trends in the Prevention of Bacterial Endocarditis in Susceptible Patients Receiving Dental Care, *Oral Surg.*, 28, 813, December, 1969.

Parsons, J. R.: The Principles of Diagnosis, *Dent. Clin. North Am.*, 18, 3, January, 1974.

Picozzi, A. and Neidle, E. A.: Medical Status of Adult Dental Patients, *J. Am. Dent. Assoc.*, 86, 858, April, 1973.

Poulsom, R. C.: An Anaphylactoid Reaction to Periodontal Surgical Dressing: Report of Case, *J. Am. Dent. Assoc.*, 89, 895, October, 1974.

Rees, T. D. and Brasher, W. J.: Incidence of Certain Systemic Conditions Among Patients Presenting for Periodontal Treatment, *J. Periodont.*, 45, 669, September, 1974.

Rothwell, P. S. and Wragg, K. A.: Assessment of the Medical Status of Patients in General Dental Practice. A Comparative Survey of a Questionnaire and Verbal Inquiry, *Br. Dent. J.*, 133, 252, September, 1972.

Sabes, W. R. and Blozis, G. G.: The Clinical Laboratory—What It Means to You and Your Patients, *J. Am. Soc. Prev. Dent.*, 3, 33, November-December, 1973.

Shafer, W. G., Hine, M. K., and Levy, B. M.: *A Textbook of Oral Pathology*, 3rd ed. Philadelphia, Saunders, 1974, pp. 566–619.

Tarsitano, J. J.: The Use of Antibiotics in Dental Practice, *Dent. Clin. North Am.*, 14, 697, October, 1970.

Tarsitano, J. J.: Never Treat a Stranger, *J. Am. Dent. Assoc.*, 73, 856, October, 1966.

Tocker, J. and Weibert, E.: The Dental Significance of Corticosteroids, Antihypertensive Drugs and Anticoagulants, *Dent. Hyg.*, 49, 11, January, 1975.

Tolas, A. G.; Medical Problems Which Influence Choice of Anesthetic, *Dent. Clin. North Am.*, 17, 211, April, 1973.

Interview

Palmer, C.: The Art of Communication and Counseling, in Nizel, A. E.: *Nutrition in Preventive Dentistry: Science and Practice*. Philadelphia, Saunders, 1972, pp. 343–355.

Zaki, E. and Mangold, M. M., eds.: Garrett, A., *Interviewing. Its Principles and Methods*, 2nd ed. New York, Family Service Association of America, 1972, 209 pp.

Chapter 7

Vital Signs

The vital signs are the body temperature, pulse and respiratory rates, and blood pressure. Recording vital signs contributes to the proper systemic evaluation of a patient in conjunction with the complete medical history. Treatment planning and appointment sequencing are directly influenced by the findings. Proficiency in determination of the vital signs is essential during emergency treatment (pages 723–733).

Abnormal vital signs must be regarded with suspicion since they may indicate previously undetected systemic problems. For example, a patient's life may be saved because of treatment initiated after diagnosis of hypertension made during a follow-up of blood pressure determination.

When vital signs are not within normal range, the patient should be informed and consent obtained to discuss the findings with a physician. When the patient does not have a personal physician, a recommendation for referral for additional diagnostic procedures is indicated.

BODY TEMPERATURE

While preparing the patient history and making the extraoral and intraoral examinations, the need for taking the tempera-ture may become apparent, or the dentist may have requested this procedure based on information obtained prior to the patient's present appointment. When the temperature is to be taken along with the other vital signs, the pulse and respiratory rates are determined concurrently while the thermometer is in the patient's mouth.

A temperature above the normal range indicates the presence of infection. Patients can have an elevated body temperature due to oral causes such as an apical or periodontal abscess, pericoronitis, or acute necrotizing ulcerative gingivitis. Determination of the temperature of a patient with an oral infection may be necessary for diagnosis and treatment planning.

For the protection of the health of the personnel in the dental office or clinic, to prevent loss of working time due to illness, as well as for the protection of subsequent patients who may be indirectly exposed, it is important to detect the presence of a systemic, contagious condition. Screening for elevated temperature among patients may have particular significance during certain seasons or epidemics. When a definite increase in temperature is found, the patient can be dismissed by the dentist to prevent further contamination of the office or clinic, and advised to consult a physician.

I. Maintenance of Body Temperature

A. **Normal Adult:** 98.6° F (Fahrenheit) or 37° C (Centigrade)
B. **Increased Temperature:** values over 99.0° F are considered indicative of fever.
C. **Factors Which Influence Body Temperature**
   1. Time of day: highest in late afternoon and early evening; lowest during the night.
   2. Temporary increase: caused by exercise, application of external heat such as a hot bath, and use of hot drinks.
   3. Decrease: during hemorrhage, starvation, or physiologic shock.
   4. Pathology: sustained increase during infection.

II. Methods for Determination of Temperature

A. **Oral:** most commonly used.
   1. Indications for use. An oral thermometer is used for the patient who
      a. Can follow instructions.
      b. Can keep the mouth closed to hold the thermometer.
      c. Will not bite or otherwise break the thermometer (which could happen with small children or confused patients of any age).
      d. Has no mouth injuries or problems breathing through the nose.
   2. Contraindications: The oral thermometer cannot be used for a patient who is unconscious, confused, irrational or restless, infants or small children, or a patient with a very dry mouth.
B. **Rectal:** generally applicable when the oral thermometer is contraindicated.
C. **External:** Axillary and groin positions are the least accurate but occasionally the oral or rectal methods are impossible to use.

D. **Types of Thermometers**
   1. Mercury-column clinical thermometer: consists of a bulb containing mercury which, when heated by the body temperature, expands and rises in the hollow center of the glass stem. The bulb of the oral thermometer is usually tapered, whereas the rectal thermometer has a blunt, round mercury bulb.
   2. Electronic: some hospitals use electronic thermometers which require less time for taking the temperature, are more easily cared for because of their disposable tips, and which prevent cross-contamination.
E. **Comparison of Readings**
   Rectal readings are about 1° F above oral readings, and oral readings are about 1° F above axillary or groin readings.

III. Procedure

A. **Equipment:** clinical thermometer, tissues, clock or watch with second hand.
B. **Prepare Patient**
   1. Tell patient what is to be done.
   2. Wait 15 minutes for the patient who has just had a hot or cold beverage or has smoked within 10 minutes, as the surface temperature of the oral mucosa can alter the accuracy of the thermometer reading.
C. **Prepare the Thermometer**
   1. Hold the thermometer only by the stem, never by the bulb.
   2. Wipe with a tissue.
   3. Check the reading: it must be below 96° F (35.6° C).
   4. Shake down the mercury level if not already below 96° F. The thermometer maintains the highest temperature previously registered, and remains there until the force of shaking lowers the mercury level.
      a. Move away from furniture or other hard objects to prevent accidental forceful contact of the thermometer.

b. Grasp stem firmly and shake with a firm, even, downward motion one or two times.

c. Recheck the reading and reshake when indicated.

D. Take the Temperature

1. Insert the bulb under the patient's tongue, with stem outside of the mouth.

2. Instruct patient to hold the thermometer gently with the lips, to avoid biting, and to breathe through the nose.

3. Observe watch or other timer, and remove thermometer after three clocked minutes.

4. Wipe off the thermometer; throw away the tissue.

E. Read and Record

1. Stand with back to light source and hold the thermometer by the stem at eye level to read.

2. Roll the thermometer slowly between the fingers to find the solid column of mercury.

3. Read at the point where the mercury ends. Each long line represents a degree of temperature, and short lines between are at two-tenths (0.2) of a degree.

4. Retake the temperature when the reading is unusually high or low.

   a. Reshake the mercury column down.

   b. Watch the patient to make certain that the thermometer is in position during the three minutes.

5. Record date, time of day, and temperature on the patient's record.

6. Inform the dentist of a temperature over 99.0° F.

F. Care of the Thermometer

1. Disposable: need for sterilization is eliminated and cross-contamination prevented.

2. Conventional

   a. Wash with soap and slightly warm water; rinse with clear cool water; dry. Hot water can raise the temperature and force the mercury to break the thermometer.

   b. Soak in disinfectant solution, completely covered, at least 20 minutes.

   c. Rinse with water and dry before placing in container or using again. Container should be autoclavable.

PULSE

The pulse is the intermittent throbbing sensation felt when the fingers are pressed against an artery. It is the result of the alternate expansion and contraction of an artery as a wave of blood is forced through by the heartbeat. The pulse rate is the count of the heartbeats. Irregularities of strength, rhythm, and quality of the pulse should be noted while counting the pulse rate.

I. Maintenance of Normal Pulse

A. Normal Pulse Rates

1. Children: At birth the pulse rate is between 130 and 160 beats per minute, and in the young child it is usually over 100 until about the third year. Older children will range from 80 to 100.

2. Adults: There is no absolute normal. The adult range is 60 to 80 beats per minute, slightly higher for women than men.

B. Factors Which Influence Pulse Rate

An unusually fast heartbeat (over 150 beats per minute in an adult) is called tachycardia; an unusually slow beat (below 50) is bradycardia.

1. Increased pulse: caused by exercise, stimulants, eating, strong emotions, extremes of heat and cold, and some forms of heart disease.

2. Decreased pulse: caused by sleep, depressants, fasting, quieting emotions, and low vitality from prolonged illness.

3. Emergency situations: listed in table 54–1, pages 729–733.

II. Procedure for Pulse Rate Determination

A. **Sequence:** the pulse rate is conveniently obtained at the same time that the thermometer is in the patient's mouth to determine body temperature. Respirations are counted immediately following the pulse rate.

B. **Sites:** the pulse may be felt at several points over the body. The one most commonly used is on the radial artery at the wrist, and is called the *radial pulse* (figure 7–1). Other sites convenient for use in a dental office or clinic would be the *temporal* artery on the side of the head in front of the ear, or the *facial* artery at the border of the mandible.

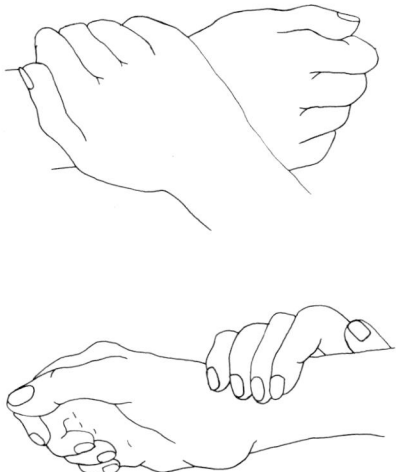

Figure 7–2. Determination of pulse rate. **Upper,** correct position of hand. **Lower,** the tips of the first three fingers are placed over the radial pulse located on the thumb side of the ventral surface of the wrist.

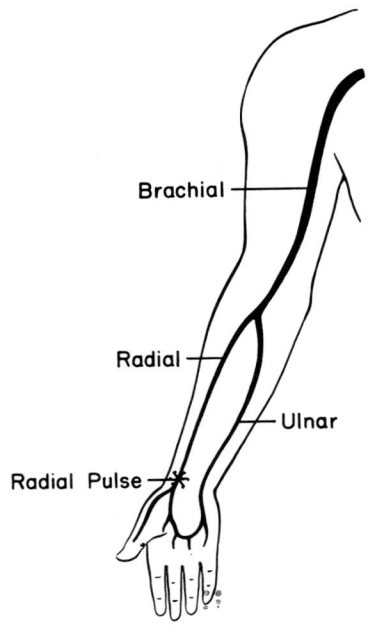

Figure 7–1. Arteries of the arm. Note location of radial pulse. The brachial pulse may be felt just before the brachial artery branches into the radial and ulnar arteries.

C. **Prepare the Patient**
1. Tell the patient what is to be done.
2. Have the patient in a comfortable position with arm and hand supported, palm down.
3. Locate the radial pulse on the thumb side of the wrist with the tips of the first three fingers (figure 7–2). Do not use the thumb as it contains a pulse which may be confused with the patient's pulse.

D. **Count and Record**
1. When the pulse is felt, exert slight pressure. Too much pressure could cause syncope, particularly pressure on the carotid pulse.
2. Count for one clocked minute. Use the second hand of a watch or clock. Check with a repeat count.
3. While taking pulse, observe the following:
   a. Rhythm: regular, regularly irregular, irregularly irregular.
   b. Volume and strength: full, strong, poor, weak, thready.
4. Record on patient's record: date, pulse rate, other characteristics.

5. Call to the dentist's attention when unusual findings are noted.

RESPIRATION

The function of respiration is to supply oxygen to the tissues and to eliminate carbon dioxide. Variations in normal respirations may be shown by characteristics such as the rate, rhythm, depth, and quality and may be symptomatic of disease or emergency states.

I. Maintenance of Normal Respirations

A respiration is one breath taken in and breathed out.

A. **Normal Respiratory Rate**
1. Children: The number of respirations per minute may be as high as 80 at birth. During the first year the normal range is considered from 20 to 40.
2. Adults: The adult range is from 14 to 20 per minute, slightly higher for women.

B. **Factors Which Influence Respirations**

Many of the same factors which influence pulse rate also influence the number of respirations. A rate of 12 per minute or fewer is considered subnormal for an adult; over 28 is accelerated; and rates over 60 are extremely rapid and dangerous.
1. Increased by work and exercise, excitement, nervousness, strong emotions, pain, hemorrhage, shock.
2. Decreased by sleep, certain drugs, pulmonary insufficiency.
3. Emergency situations: listed in table 54–1, pages 729–733.

II. Procedures for Observing Respirations

A. **Determine Rate**
1. Make the count of respirations immediately after counting the pulse.

2. Maintain the fingers over the radial pulse.
3. Respirations must be counted so that the patient is not aware, as the rate may be voluntarily altered.
4. Count the number of times the chest rises in one clocked minute. It is not necessary to count both inspirations and expirations.

B. **Observe Depth.** Describe as shallow, normal, or deep.

C. **Observe Rhythm.** Describe as regular (evenly spaced) or irregular (with pauses of irregular lengths between).

D. **Observe Quality.** Describe as strong, easy, weak or labored, noisy. Poor quality may have an effect on body color; for example, a bluish tinge of the face or nailbeds may mean an insufficiency of oxygen.

E. **Note Sounds.** Describe deviate sounds made during inspiration, expiration, or both.

F. **Observe Position of Patient.** When the patient assumes an unusual position to secure comfort during breathing or prefers to remain seated upright, mark records accordingly.

G. Record all findings on the patient's record.

H. Call to the attention of the dentist any unusual findings.

BLOOD PRESSURE

Information about the patient's blood pressure is essential during dental and dental hygiene appointments, since special adaptations may be needed. Screening for blood pressure in dental offices has been shown to be an effective health service.[1,2] Many people may make regular visits to their dentists but see their physicians infrequently.[2]

I. Components of Blood Pressure

Blood pressure is the force exerted by the blood on the blood vessel walls. When the left ventricle of the heart contracts, blood is forced out into the aorta and travels through the large arteries to the smaller arteries, arterioles, and capillaries. The pulsations extend from the heart through the arteries and disappear in the arterioles. During the course of the cardiac cycle the blood pressure is changing constantly.

A. **Systolic Pressure.** Systolic pressure is the peak or the highest pressure. It is caused by ventricular contraction.

B. **Diastolic Pressure.** Diastolic pressure is the lowest pressure. It is the effect of ventricular relaxation.

C. **Boundaries.** More than one reading is needed within a few minutes to determine an average and assure a correct reading. That should be followed by serial readings at least every six months and always before surgery or other stressful treatment.

II. Factors Which Influence Blood Pressure

A. **Maintenance of Blood Pressure.** Blood pressure depends on
   1. Force of the heart beat (energy of the heart).
   2. Peripheral resistance; condition of the arteries; changes in elasticity of vessels which may occur with age.
   3. Volume of blood in the circulatory system.

B. **Factors Which Increase Blood Pressure**
   1. Exercise, eating, stimulants, and emotional disturbance.
   2. Menopause: In general, women have recorded blood pressure 4 to 5 mm. Hg less than men until menopause when there is usually an abrupt rise to slightly more than the average male.

C. **Factors Which Decrease Blood Pressure:** fasting, rest, depressants, and quiet emotions.

D. **Pathology**
   1. Hypertension: sustained abnormal elevation
      a. Age and history need consideration when classifying normal and abnormal for an individual.
      b. Systolic pressure over 140 and diastolic over 95 bear watching and rechecking. Pressures over 150 systolic and 100 diastolic are reportable and the patient must be referred to a physician for examination.
      c. Increased diastolic is more significant than increased systolic.
   2. Hypotension: abnormally low blood pressure. In shock the systolic pressure may drop to 70 or 80 mm. Hg (pages 725, 729).

III. Equipment for Blood Pressure Determination

A. **Sphygmomanometer** (blood pressure machine): consists of an *inflatable cuff* and *two tubes,* one connected to the *pressure hand control bulb,* and the other to the *pressure gauge.*
   1. Types of pressure gauges
      a. Aneroid: round dial.
      b. Mercury manometer: column of mercury.
   2. Reading the gauge
      a. Gauges are marked with long lines at each 10 mm. Hg with shorter lines at 2 mm. intervals between each long line.
      b. The level of the column of mercury of the manometer should be at eye level for accurate reading and must not be tilted.
   3. Position of gauge: keep out of sight of patient to alleviate anxiety.

B. **Stethoscope** (a listening aid that magnifies sound): consists of an *endpiece* which is connected by tubes to carry the sound to the *earpieces.*

1. Types of endpieces: bell-shaped or flat (diaphragm). The bell shape is used for medical examinations, particularly for chest examination.
2. Care of earpieces: clean by rubbing with gauze sponge moistened in disinfectant.

IV. Procedure for Blood Pressure Determination

A. Prepare Patient
1. Tell patient briefly what is to be done. Detailed explanations are to be avoided since they may excite the patient and change the blood pressure.
2. Seat patient comfortably with arm slightly flexed and forearm supported on a level surface at the level of the heart.
3. Use either arm unless otherwise indicated by, for example, a handicap. Repeat blood pressure determinations should be made on the same arm as there may be as much as 10 mm. Hg difference between arms.
4. Take pressure on bare arm, not over clothing. A tight sleeve should be loosened or the garment removed.

B. Apply Cuff
1. With the patient's arm resting on the arm of the dental chair with the elbow at or below the level of the heart, apply the completely deflated cuff snugly and evenly. The lower edge of the cuff is placed one inch above the antecubital fossa (figure 7–3).
2. Adjust the position of the gauge for convenient reading.
3. Palpate one inch below the antecubital fossa to locate the brachial artery pulse (figure 7–1). The stethoscope endpiece will be placed over the spot where the brachial pulse is felt.

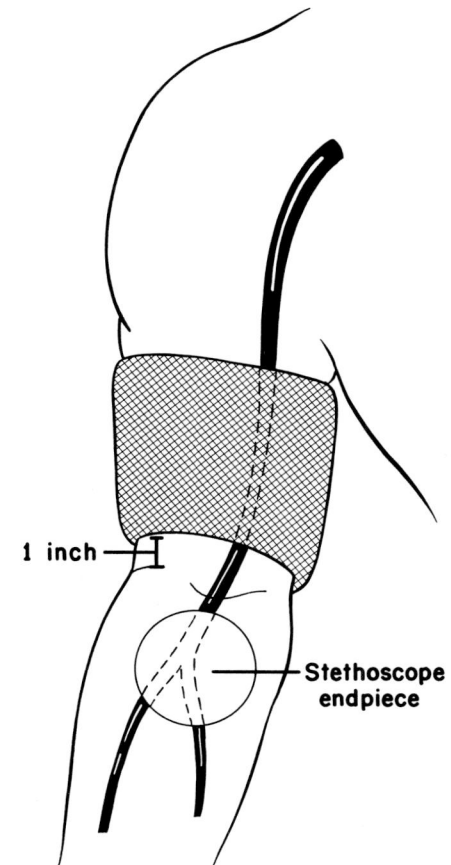

1 inch

Stethoscope endpiece

Figure 7–3. Blood pressure cuff in position. The lower edge of the cuff is placed approximately one inch above the antecubital fossa. The stethoscope endpiece is placed over the palpated brachial artery pulse point approximately one inch below the antecubital fossa and slightly toward the inner side of the arm.

4. Position the stethoscope earpieces in the ears with the tips directed forward.

C. Take the Radial Pulse for One Minute.
Hold fingers on the pulse.

D. Inflate the Cuff
1. Close the needle valve (air lock) attached to the hand control bulb firmly but so it may be readily released.
2. Pump quickly to inflate the cuff until the radial pulse stops.

3. Look at the dial, and pump to 30 mm. Hg beyond where the radial pulse was no longer felt. This means that the brachial artery is collapsed by the pressure of the cuff and no blood is flowing through.

E. **Position the Stethoscope Endpiece.** Place the endpiece over the palpated brachial artery, one inch below the antecubital fossa, and slightly toward the inner side of the arm (figure 7–3). Hold lightly in place.

F. **Deflate the Cuff Gradually**
   1. Release the air lock slowly (2 to 3 mm per second) so that the dial drops very gradually.
   2. Listen for the first sound: *systole* ("tap tap"). Note the number on the dial which is the *systolic pressure.*
   3. Continue to release the pressure slowly. The "tap" diminishes in intensity and is surrounded by a murmuring. This is followed by an increased intensity of the murmur and a decrease in the intensity of the tap.
   4. First diastolic sound: a definite change from the sharp tap to a muffled tap. Note the number on the dial where the last distinct tap was heard. That number is the *diastolic pressure.*
   5. Release further (about 10 mm) until there is a cessation of all sounds. That is the second diastolic point. In some clinics and hospitals the last sound is taken as the diastolic pressure.
   6. Let the rest of the air out rapidly.

G. **Repeat for Confirmation.** Wait 30 seconds before inflating the cuff again.

H. **Record**
   1. Write date and arm used.
   2. Record blood pressure as a fraction, for example 120/80. When both diastolic points are recorded it can be written 120/80/72.

I. Call to the prompt attention of the dentist any unusual variation from normal or from previous readings noted in the patient's permanent record.

TECHNICAL HINTS

I. For an extremely obese patient the application of the cuff around the forearm and placing the stethoscope endpiece over the radial artery may give a truer measurement of blood pressure than the upper arm usual procedure.

II. Blood pressure cuffs of various widths may be obtained. In a pedodontic practice, a narrower cuff can be used.

III. Sources of Materials

   National High Blood Pressure Education Program
   High Blood Pressure Information Center
   120/80 National Institutes of Health
   Bethesda, Maryland 20014

   American Heart Association
   Material Development Department
   44 E. 23rd St.
   New York, New York 10010

FACTORS TO TEACH THE PATIENT

I. How vital signs can influence dental and dental hygiene appointments.

II. The importance of having a blood pressure determination at regular intervals.

References

1. Berman, C. L., Guarino, M. A., and Giovannoli, S. M.: High Blood Pressure Detection by Dentists, *J. Am. Dent. Assoc.,* 87, 359, August, 1973.
2. Abbey, L. M.: Screening for Hypertension in the Dental Office, *J. Am. Dent. Assoc.,* 88, 563, March, 1974.

Suggested Readings

Berman, C. L., Guarino, M. A., and Giovannoli, S. M.: Letter to the Editor: On High Blood Pressure, *J. Am. Dent. Assoc.,* 88, 1242, June, 1974.
Berman, C. L.: Screening Dental Patients for Hypertension, (Editorial), *Dent. Surv.,* 50, 46, November, 1974.

Borhani, N. O., ed.: *Medical Basis for Comprehensive Community Hypertension Control Programs,* United States Department of Health, Education, and Welfare, DHEW Publication No. (NIH) 75–715, Bethesda, Md.

Chue, P. W. Y.: Hypertension: Implications for Dentistry, *Dent. Surv., 51,* 25, May, 1975.

Chue, P. W. Y.: The Clinical Measurement of Arterial Blood Pressure, *Dent. Surv., 51,* 30, June, 1975.

Merck, Sharp, and Dohme: *Measuring Blood Pressure, A Guide for Paramedical Personnel.* West Point, Pennsylvania.

Chapter 8

Extraoral and Intraoral Inspection

A complete, carefully executed examination of the mouth and adjacent structures is essential to total evaluation prior to treatment. A variety of lesions may be observed for which the patient may or may not report subjective symptoms. Recognition, treatment, and follow-up of these lesions may be of definite significance to present and future general and oral health.

Despite the occurrence of many seemingly minor lesions, the danger of oral malignancies remains a definite possibility.[1] Approximately five percent of all male cancers and two percent of female cancers occur in the area of the oral cavity.[2] Every effort must be made to detect potentially cancerous lesions early.

Each area of the mucous membrane must be examined, and minor deviations from normal must be given prompt attention. A life may depend on a dental hygienist's oral inspection. Routine inspection for each new patient and at each recall appointment provides a realistic approach to the control of oral disease.

The oral tissues are sensitive indicators of the general health of the individual. Changes in these structures may be the first indication of subclinical disease processes in other parts of the body.

Although not legally permitted to diagnose, the dental hygienist has the responsibility to observe, record, and call to the attention of the dentist deviations from the normal appearance of the oral cavity. Prerequisite to accomplishing this are knowledge and understanding of the normal morphology and function (anatomy and physiology) of the oral cavity and the surrounding area which can be applied in the intelligent recognition of oral conditions.

OBJECTIVES

A thorough inspection is essential to the total care of the patient as suggested by the following objectives:

I. To observe all areas in and about the oral cavity and to record and call to the attention of the dentist those areas which appear to deviate from normal and which may be evidence of disease.

II. To screen each patient at least annually for lesions suspicious of cancer.

III. To recognize a need for postponement of the current appointment because of evidence of communicable disease or in deference to the need for urgent medical consultation and/or treatment.

IV. To prevent the development of advanced, irreversible, or untreatable oral disease by early recognition of initial lesions.

V. To detect suspected conditions which will require additional testing or other diagnostic aids which the dentist may use or may direct the dental hygienist to use under supervision.

VI. To identify extraoral and intraoral deviations from normal which are related to and for which dental hygiene care and instruction may need special adaptations.

VII. To provide a means of comparison of individual oral inspections over a series of recall appointments, and thus to determine the effects of dental hygiene care and the success of patient instruction.

VIII. To provide information for continuing records of the patient's diagnosis and treatment plan for legal purposes.

COMPONENTS OF INSPECTION

The current concept of patient care is that the total patient is being treated, not only the oral cavity, and particularly not only the teeth and their immediately surrounding tissues. The inspection must be, therefore, an all-inclusive one to include any detectable physical, mental, or psychological influences of the whole patient on his oral health.

Certain parts of the examination may be carried out by the dentist. Other parts will be delegated to the dental hygienist. Thorough inspection must become a routine part of each patient recall appointment if treatment for the control and prevention of oral diseases is to be effective.

I. Inspection Methods

The various examination methods were described on page 59. The extraoral and intraoral examination is accomplished primarily by direct observation and palpation, but other methods are also used.

A. **Direct Observation.** Patient position, optimum lighting, and effective retraction for accessibility contribute to the accuracy and completeness of the inspection. Visual examination is made in conjunction with other methods.

B. **Palpation.** Fingers or hands are used to move or press tissue to detect changes in consistency and size. Types of palpation include the following:

1. *Digital:* Use of a single finger. Example: index finger applied to inner border of the mandible beneath the canine–premolar area to determine the presence of a torus mandibularis.

2. *Bidigital:* use of finger and thumb of the same hand. Example: palpation of the lips (figure 8–1).

3. *Bimanual:* use of finger or fingers and thumb from each hand applied simultaneously in coordination. Example: index finger of one hand palpates on the floor of the mouth

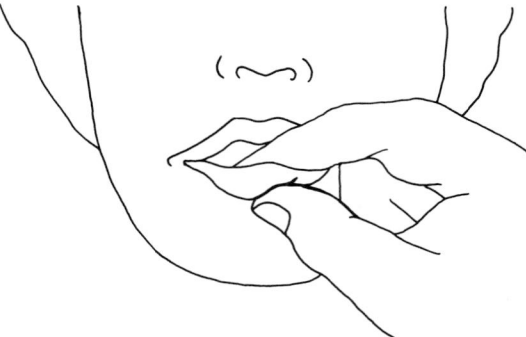

Figure 8–1. Palpation of the lip. Bidigital palpation is applied to detect deviations from normal particularly induration.

inside, while a finger or fingers from the other hand press on the same area from under the chin externally.

4. *Bilateral:* the two hands are used at the same time to inspect corresponding structures on opposite sides of the body. Comparisons may be made. Example: fingers placed beneath the chin to palpate the submandibular lymph nodes (figure 8–2).

II. Order of Inspection

A recommended order for inspection is outlined in table 8–1, in which factors to consider during appointments are related to the actual observations made and recorded. The sequence presented in table 8–1 is adapted from the *Oral Cancer Examination Procedure* available from the American Cancer Society.[3]

A. Systematic Sequence for Examination

The advantages of following a routine order for inspection include:
1. Minimal possibility of overlooking an area and missing details of importance.
2. Increased efficiency and conservation of time.
3. Maintenance of a professional at-

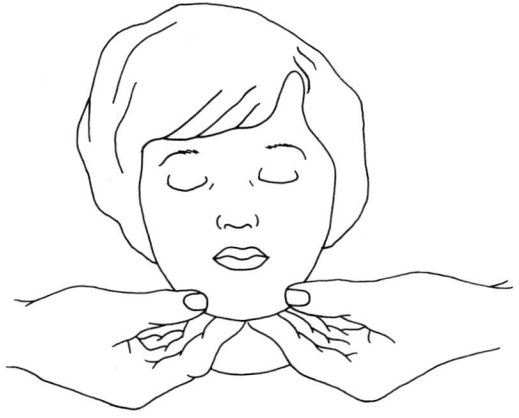

Figure 8–2. Palpation of the submandibular area. Bilateral palpation is used to inspect corresponding structures on opposite sides of the body.

mosphere which will inspire the patient's confidence.

B. Steps for a Thorough Examination (table 8–1)

1. Observe patient during reception and seating to note physical characteristics and abnormalities, and make an overall appraisal.
2. Observe head, face, eyes, and neck, and evaluate the skin of the face and neck.
3. Palpate the salivary glands and lymph nodes.
4. Examine mandibular movement and palpate the temporomandibular joint.
5. Make a preliminary inspection of the lips and intraoral mucosa using the mouth mirror or a tongue depressor. Do not retract directly with ungloved fingers in the event of an open lesion which may be communicable.
6. View and palpate lips, labial and buccal mucosa, and mucobuccal folds.
7. Examine and palpate the tongue including the dorsal and ventral surfaces, lateral borders, and base. Retract to observe posterior third (figure 8–3).
8. Observe mucosa of the floor of the mouth. Palpate the floor of the mouth.
9. Examine hard and soft palates, tonsillar areas, and pharynx. Use mirror to observe oropharynx, nasopharynx, and larynx.
10. Note amount and consistency of the saliva.

C. Compare with expected normal appearance. Note deviations from normal.

D. Corroborate findings with information from the patient's history.

E. Call questionable areas to the dentist's attention promptly.

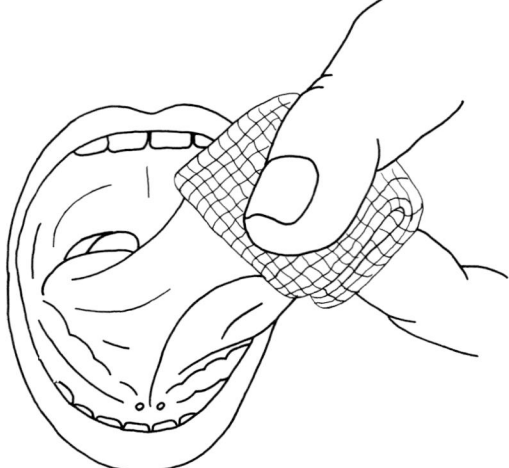

Figure 8–3. Tongue examination. To observe the posterior third of the tongue and the attachment to the floor of the mouth, hold the tongue with gauze, retract the cheek and move the tongue first out to the right, then the left, as each section of mucosa is carefully inspected.

III. Description of Observations

A. Record Form
1. Contain adequate space for complete descriptions of lesions observed; not only a check sheet.
2. Contain spaces for successive examinations at periodic recall intervals.

B. Information to Include
1. Location. The location may be described in words, or use a printed diagram on the record form to mark specific location of deviations from normal (figure 8–4).
2. History
   a. Whether the lesion is known to the patient or not known.
   b. Duration; changes in size and appearance.
   c. Symptomatology.
3. Physical Characteristics
   a. Size: indicate width and depth in millimeters.
   b. Shape or contour: define whether the lesion is elevated (papillary) or depressed (ulcerlike); pedunculated, cracked, fissured.
   c. Color: compared with other areas of the patient's mouth.
   d. Resiliency, consistency: firm, indurated, soft, spongy.
   e. Surface texture: smooth, irregular.

C. Definitions
1. Descriptive Terminology
   a. *Discrete:* separate, not running together or blending.
   b. *Confluent:* running together, blended. Originally separate but subsequently formed into one.
   c. *Pedunculated:* elevated, papillary-type lesion having a narrow part (stem) which acts as a support and connector.
   d. *Verrucose:* covered with or full of wart-like growths.
   e. *Papillary:* small nipple-like elevation or projection.
   f. *Erythema:* red area of variable size and shape.
   g. *Petechia*(e): minute round red spot.
   h. *Induration:* hardened area of tissue.
2. Types of Lesions
   a. *Macule* (macula): circumscribed spot, not elevated above the surrounding level and distinguished by a different color.
   b. *Papule:* small (pinhead to 5 mm.), circumscribed, solid elevated area which may be pointed, rounded, or flattened.
   c. *Vesicle:* small (2 to 5 mm.), circumscribed, elevated lesion having a thin surface covering and containing fluid (small blister).
   d. *Bulla:* large (5 mm. to several cm.) vesicular-type lesion filled with fluid (large blister or bleb).

MUCOSAL ABNORMALITIES

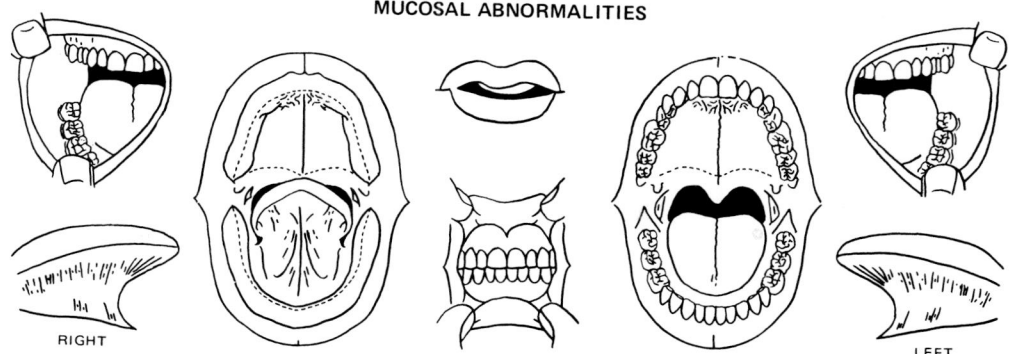

Figure 8–4. Record form for clinical findings. In this section of a clinical examination record form, outline of a deviation from normal may be drawn to show the location and size. (Courtesy, University of Southern California School of Dentistry.)

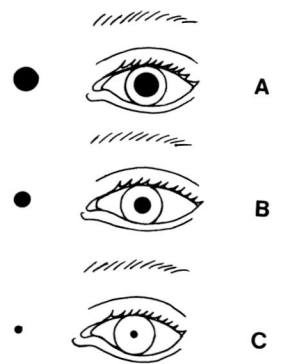

Figure 8–5. Examination of the pupils. **A.** *Dilated*, occurs in shock, heart failure, and other emergencies, and drug overdose of hallucinogens and amphetamines; **B.** *Normal*; **C.** *Pinpoint*, occurs in drug overdose of morphine and related drugs, and barbiturates. (Adapted from American National Red Cross, *Standard First Aid and Personal Safety.*)

A bullous lesion may develop individually or result from the union of several vesicles.

  e. *Pustule:* vesicular-type lesion containing purulent material rather than clear fluid.

  f. *Ulcer:* defect or break in continuity of the epithelium to produce a depressed area. It may result from the rupture of a vesicle or a bulla, and usually has some degree of erythema at the margin.

  g. *Erosion:* shallow defect which does not extend through the epithelium into underlying tissue.

  h. *Nodule:* solid elevated lesion (5 mm. to 2 cm. wide).

  i. *Tumor:* solid growth of varying size which arises from the mucosa and projects out; swelling or overgrowth of cells independent of normal growth.

  j. *Torus:* bony elevation or prominence usually found on the midline of the hard palate (torus palatinus) and the lingual surface of the mandible (torus mandibularis) in the premolar area.

  k. *Leukoplakia:* white keratotic patch-like lesion on the mucosa which cannot be rubbed off.

ORAL CANCER

The objective is to detect cancer of the mouth at the earliest possible stage. Discovered early, it is likely to have a high cure rate, whereas when a cancer extends into adjacent structures and to the lymph nodes of the neck, the prognosis is poor.

Since the early lesions are generally symptomless, they may go unnoticed and unreported by the patient. Observation by the dentist or dental hygienist, therefore,

Table 8–1.   Extraoral and Intraoral Inspection

Order of Inspection	To Observe	Influences on Diagnosis and Appointments
1. Overall Appraisal of Patient	Posture, gait General health status; size Hair Breathing, state of fatigue	Response, cooperation, attitude toward treatment Length of appointment possible
2. Face	Expression: evidence of fear or apprehension Shape, twitching, paralysis Profile for occlusion classification Jaw movements during speech	Need for alleviation of fears Use of face mask when evidence of upper respiratory infection Enlarged masseter muscle may relate to bruxism or clenching habit
3. Skin	Color, texture, blemishes Traumatic lesions Eruptions, swellings Growths, moles	Skin color may relate to systemic factors; need for additional medical history and referral Skin lesions may require referral for biopsy Open lesions need treatment before oral treatment Influence on instruction in diet and health
4. Eyes	Size of pupil (figure 8–5) Color of sclera Eyeglasses	Pupils dilated or pinpoint as a result of certain emergency situations (shock, heart failure, drug overdose, see pages 729–733) Certain disease conditions manifest changes in the eyes Eyeglasses essential during instruction to patient
5. Nodes (figure 8–6) Palpate: a. auricular b. parotid c. submental d. submandibular e. inferior auricular f. upper and lower deep cervical	Induration Coordinate with intraoral examination	Need for referral for biopsy
6. Temporomandibular joint	Limitations or deviations during movement Tenderness, sensitivity Crepitus	Disorder of the joint

Table 8–1, *continued*

Order of Inspection	To Observe	Influences on Diagnosis and Appointments
7. **Lips** a. Observe closed, then open b. Palpate using thumb and index finger (figure 8–1)	Color, texture, size Cracks, angular cheilosis Blisters, ulcers Traumatic lesions Irritation from biting habit Limitation of opening; muscle tone, elasticity Evidences of mouthbreathing or tongue thrusting Induration	Need for biopsy; referral Immediate need for postponement of appointment when lesions could interfere with procedures Care during retraction Difficulty of accessibility or visibility during intraoral procedures Patient instruction: dietary, special plaque procedures for mouthbreather
8. **Breath Odor**	Severity Relation to oral hygiene and overall gingival state	Possible relation to systemic condition Emphasis on oral care and plaque control
9. **Labial and Buccal Mucosa** (left and right examined systematically) a. Observe vestibule, mucobuccal fold, frena, opening to Stensen's duct b. Palpate the entire cheek areas.	Color, size, texture, contour Abrasions, traumatic lesions cheekbite, lip bite Effects of smoking Ulcers, growths Moistness of membranes Relation of frena to free and attached gingiva Flexibility of cheeks Induration	Need for biopsy, referral, or cytologic smear Frena and other anatomical parts that need adaptation of impression tray Avoidance of sensitive areas during retraction, radiographic film placement, or plaque control instruction
10. **Tongue and Floor of Mouth** a. Dorsum (1) at rest with mouth slightly open (2) protruded b. Base of tongue Hold tip of tongue with gauze sponge. Place mirror gently against uvula to view downward. c. Lateral borders Hold tongue with sponge: extend to left then right (figure 8–3).	Color, size, texture, consistency Papillae, fissures Coating Lesions: ulcers, traumatic Deviation or straight Asymmetry Mobility; limitation of movement Attachments to floor of mouth and back to the anterior pillar Swelling, ulceration, color changes	Need for biopsy, referral, or cytologic smear Large muscular tongue affects retraction, gag reflex, and accessibility for instrumentation and film placement Instruction: tongue brushing, dietary factors

Table 8–1, continued

Order of Inspection	To Observe	Influences on Diagnosis and Appointments
10. Tongue, continued d. Ventral Surface Ask patient to touch the palate with the tip of the tongue.	Undersurface of tongue Varicosities Lesions on floor of the mouth Duct openings from sub-mandibular and sublingual glands Lingual frenum attachments Freedom of movement of tongue	Biopsy, referral, cytologic smear Care of sensitive areas during instrumentation Depth of floor of mouth and elasticity influence placement of radiographic films, and cotton roll holders Tonguetie
e. Ask patient to swallow.	Observe with lips slightly apart for evidence of tongue thrust.	
f. Palpate the entire tongue including the base.	Induration, enlargements	
g. Palpate floor of mouth. (Place index finger of one hand in the mouth, other hand outside under the chin.)	Induration, enlargements	
11. Saliva	Quantity Evidence of dry mouth Quality of saliva: watery, ropy, mucoid	Reduced in certain diseases and by certain drugs Corroborate with items from the history Excess can influence instrumentation techniques
12. Hard Palate Observe and palpate.	Height, contour, color Appearance of rugae Tori, growths, ulcers	May need biopsy, referral, or cytologic smear Signs of tongue thrust and deviate swallow Influence radiographic placement.
13. Soft Palate and Uvula a. Observe: depress tongue with mirror or tongue depressor	Color, size, shape Petechiae Ulcers, growths	Biopsy, referral, smear Large uvula can affect gag reflex

Table 8–1, *continued*

Order of Inspection	To Observe	Influences on Diagnosis and Appointments
14. Tonsillar Region a. Depress tongue with mirror or tongue depressor. b. Ask patient to say "Ah" to open the oropharynx. c. Place mirror behind uvula, glass up, to observe naso-pharynx. (Request patient to breathe through the nose and mouth.)	Anterior and posterior pillars Tonsils, size, shape Color, surface characteristics Lesions, trauma	Biopsy, referral, smear may be indicated Adjustment of procedures for effect of enlarged tonsils on gag reflex Need for face mask when patient has a throat infection (or possible postponement of the appointment) Instruction: adapt plaque control procedures in posterior region when patient has sensitivity to gagging

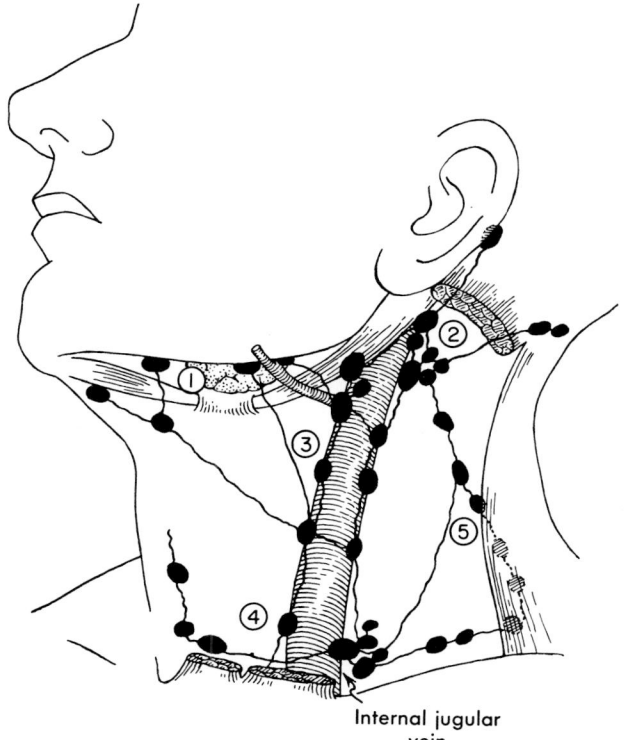

Internal jugular
vein

Figure 8–6. Lymph nodes. Groups of lymph nodes that drain the oral cavity and surrounding structures; **1.** Submandibular group; **2.** Inferior auricular nodes behind the ear; **3.** Upper deep cervical nodes; **4.** Lower deep cervical nodes; **5.** Posterior (spinal accessory) chain group. (From Moore, C.: Synopsis of Clinical Cancer, 2nd ed. St. Louis, Mosby, 1970.)

is the principal method for the control of oral cancer. The first step in accomplishing this is to examine the entire oral mucous membrane for each patient at the initial inspection and at each recall appointment.

The dental hygienist needs to know how to make the oral inspection, where oral cancer occurs most frequently, what an early cancerous lesion may look like, and what to do when such a lesion is found.

I. Location

Tumors may arise at any site in the oral cavity. The most common sites are the floor of the mouth, tongue, lower lip, and the anterior and posterior fauces (pillars). Figure 8–7 diagrams the oral cavity to show the areas where most cancers occur.

Although patients may be instructed in self-examination to watch for changes in oral tissues, it is difficult for a person to see his or her own tissues, particularly the entire floor of the mouth and base of the tongue, by the usual mirror and lighting systems available in a private home.

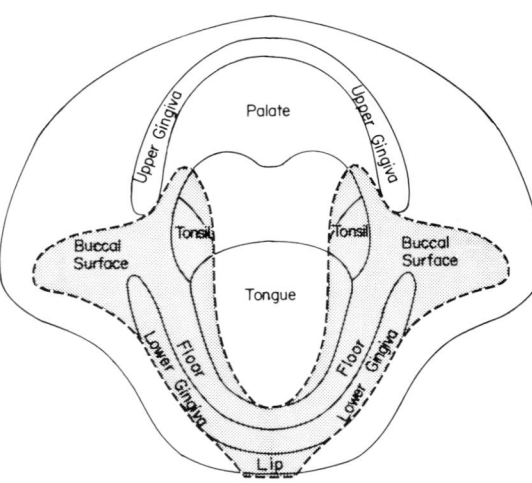

Figure 8–7. Sites of oral cancer. The shaded area represents the most frequent sites of squamous cell carcinoma of the oral cavity. Most of this area is not visible by self-examination and requires regular professional supervision. (From Burket, L. W.: Oral Medicine, 6th ed. Philadelphia, Lippincott, 1971.)

Self-examination needs routine supplementation with professional examination.

II. Appearance of Early Cancer[4]

Early oral cancer takes many forms and may resemble a variety of common oral lesions. All types should be looked at with suspicion. Five basic forms are listed here.
A. **White Areas (leukoplakia).** These may vary from filmy, barely visible changes in the mucosa to heavy, thick, heaped up areas of dry white keratinized tissue. Fissures, ulcers, or areas of induration in the white area are most indicative of malignancy.
B. **Red Areas.** Lesions of red, velvety consistency, sometimes with small ulcers should be identified.
C. **Ulcers.** These may be with flat or raised margins which may appear similar to aphthous ulcers. Palpation may reveal induration.
D. **Masses.** Papillary masses, sometimes with ulcerated areas, occur as elevations above the surrounding tissues. Other masses may occur below the normal mucosa and may be found only by palpation.
E. **Pigmentation.** These occur as brown or black pigmented areas located on mucosa where pigmentation does not normally occur.

III. Procedure for Follow-up of a Suspicious Lesion

As designated by the dentist, a lesion may be biopsied immediately, a cytological smear may be made, or the patient may be referred for additional diagnosis and biopsy.

A. **Biopsy**
   1. Definition. The biopsy technique is the removal and examination, usually by microscope, of a section of tissue or other material from the living body for the purposes of diagnosis.

2. Indications for Biopsy[5]
   a. Any unusual oral lesion which cannot be identified with clinical certainty must be biopsied.
   b. Any lesion that has not shown evidence of healing in two weeks should be considered malignant until proven otherwise.
   c. A persistent, thick, white, hyperkeratotic lesion, and any mass (elevated or not) which does not break through the surface epithelium should be biopsied.

B. **Cytologic Smear**
   1. Definition. The cytologic smear technique is a diagnostic aid in which surface cells of a suspicious lesion are removed for microscopic evaluation for evidence of pathology.
   2. Indications for Smear Technique
      a. An oral smear is an adjunct to a biopsy, not a substitute.
      b. Any lesion for which a biopsy is not planned may be examined by smear.
      c. A lesion which looks like potential cancer should be examined by smear if the patient refuses to have a biopsy specimen taken. A positive report from a smear should convince the patient of the need for treatment or biopsy.
      d. The smear technique is used for periodic examination of treated cases of oral cancer.
      e. In mass screening programs for cancer detection, smears may be taken. However, all lesions of high suspicion should be referred for biopsy.
      f. Research studies to show changes in surface cells, for example the effects of topical agents, may use a smear technique.

3. Limitations of the smear technique
   a. When a clear-cut lesion, recognized as pathologic, is present, treatment must not be delayed by waiting for cytologic smear analysis.
   b. The smear detects only surface lesions.
   c. It is difficult or impossible to scrape deep enough to obtain representative cells from a heavily keratinized lesion.
   d. Treatment cannot be determined by smear technique results only. After a positive smear a biopsy is needed for definitive diagnosis.
   e. Because research has shown that the smear technique is not diagnostically reliable (there can be "false negatives" which turn out to be positive biopsies), a negative report means very little.

EXFOLIATIVE CYTOLOGY

Stratified squamous cells are constantly growing toward the epithelial surface of the mucous membrane where they are exfoliated. Exfoliated cells and cells beneath them are scraped off, and when prepared on a slide, changes in the cells can be detected by staining and studying them microscopically. The cells of a malignant cancer stain differently than normal cells and take on unusual, abnormal forms.

I. Procedure

A. **Materials**
   Gauze sponges
   Glass microscopic slides with frosted end
   Plain lead pencil
   Paper clips
   Blade to scrape lesion (wooden tongue depressor or metal spatula)
   Fixative (95 percent alcohol)
   Protective mailing container
   History form or data sheet

B. **Steps**

1. *Prepare Materials.* Write the patient's name on the frosted ends of two glass slides (two for each lesion), and place a paper clip on the end of one slide to prevent contact between the slides when packaged for mailing to the laboratory.

2. *Prepare the Lesion.* Irrigate the surface to remove debris. Wipe the surface gently with a wet gauze sponge as needed to remove debris or blood. Do not dry.

3. *Scrape the Lesion.* Use a moistened tongue blade (may be moistened in the patient's saliva) or a metal spatula. Scrape the entire surface of the lesion firmly several times (all strokes in the same direction) (figure 8–8A).

4. *Smear the Glass Slide.* Spread the collected material on the glass

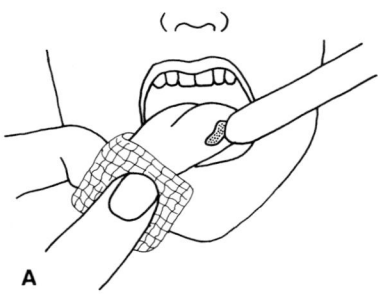

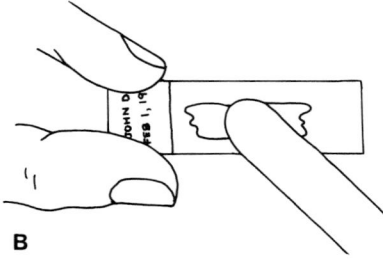

Figure 8–8. Oral cytology technique. **A.** Tongue is held out with gauze sponge while moistened tongue blade or metal spatula is used to scrape a lesion. **B.** Collected material is spread evenly on a glass slide. See text for details.

slide. Start at the center of the clear end of the slide and smear evenly across the surface. Cover an area approximately 20 mm. wide. Handle all glass slides by their edges to prevent finger prints or other contamination (figure 8–8B).

5. *Fix the Cells.* Immediately, to prevent drying of the cells, place the slide on a flat surface and flood with generous drops of 95 percent alcohol.

6. *Obtain Second Smear.* Duplicate previous smear technique using a fresh tongue depressor. Apply fixing agent immediately.

7. *Complete the Fixation.* Leave slides for 30 minutes. After 20 minutes tip the slide to let remaining alcohol run off. Air dry where dust or other foreign material cannot contaminate the smear.

8. *Prepare History or Data Sheet.* Basic information includes the following:

   Dentist: name and address
   Patient: name and address
   Lesion: description (size, color, location, shape, consistency, and duration).
   Other related clinical findings or pertinent history.

9. *Prepare for Mailing.* Wrap slides in facial tissue to prevent breakage. Pack with the history or data sheet.

II. Laboratory Report

The pathologist makes the microscopic examination and classifies the specimen in one of the following categories:

Unsatisfactory Slide is inadequate for diagnosis. The specimen may have been too thick or thin, or the cells may have dried before fixation. Another smear should be made promptly.

Class I	Normal
Class II	Atypical, but not suggestive of malignant cells
Class III	Uncertain (possible for cancer)
Class IV	Probable for cancer
Class V	Positive for cancer

III. Follow-up

A. Report of Class IV or V: refer for treatment of oral cancer.

B. Report of Class III: re-evaluate clinical findings; biopsy usually indicated.

C. Report of Class I or II
1. The patient must not be dismissed until the lesion has healed.
2. When lesion persists, the dentist will either re-evaluate the clinical findings and request a repeat cytological smear, or perform a biopsy.

D. Negative Report
Either biopsy or smear requires careful follow-up when a negative report is obtained for an oral lesion that appears suspicious by clinical examination. It is possible to have a false negative report, that is, a malignancy may be present but the sample examined in the smear or biopsy may not have included cancerous cells.

TECHNICAL HINTS

I. Wear a finger cot or rubber gloves when making the intraoral inspection to avoid contact with infection. It also makes it easier to retract, since the glove may provide more friction.

II. Source of materials for information on cancer is the American Cancer Society, 219 East 42nd Street, New York, New York, 10017. Local or state societies are usually preferable as a direct source.

FACTORS TO TEACH THE PATIENT

I. Reasons for a careful extraoral and intraoral inspection at each recall.

II. The need for reporting any changes in the oral tissues.

III. The Warning Signs of Oral Cancer[3]
A. Sore spot or ulceration of lips, tongue, or other area inside the mouth that does not heal promptly.
B. White scaly area inside the mouth.
C. Swelling of the lips, gums, or other area inside the mouth—with or without pain.
D. Repeated bleeding in the mouth with no apparent cause.
E. Numbness or loss of feeling in any part of the mouth.

IV. General dietary and nutritional influences on the health of the oral tissues.

V. How the oral cavity tends to reflect the general health.

VI. Relationship of smoking, oral health and oral cancer. Booklets for the patient are available from The American Dental Association: *Smoking and Your Oral Health–What You Can Do About It* (G8) and *Smoking and Oral Cancer* (G27). Send for ADA Catalog, Order Department, 211 East Chicago Avenue, Chicago, Illinois 60611.

References

1. Bhaskar, S. N.: Oral Pathology in the Dental Office: A Survey of 20, 575 Biopsy Specimens, *J. Am. Dent. Assoc.*, 76, 761, April, 1968.
2. Cancer Statistics, 1979, *CA—A Cancer Journal for Clinicians*, 29, 6, January-February, 1979.
3. Engleman, M. A. and Schackner, S. J.: *Oral Cancer Examination Procedure.* Published by Oral Cancer Prevention and Detection Center, St. Francis Hospital, Poughkeepsie, N.Y. Distributed by American Cancer Society, 219 E. 42nd Street, New York, N.Y. 10017.
4. Baker, H. W.: Diagnosis of Oral Cancer, in *Oral Cancer*, American Cancer Society, 1972.
5. Kerr, D. A., Ash, M. M., and Millard, H. D.: *Oral Diagnosis*, 4th ed. St. Louis, Mosby, 1974, pp. 322, 327.

Suggested Readings

Bhaskar, S. N.: *Synopsis of Oral Pathology*, 4th ed. St. Louis, Mosby, 1973, pp. 8–58, 339–398, 461–488.

Brown, W. J.: You May Be Seeing Syphilis, *J. Am. Dent. Hyg. Assoc.*, 39, 154, 3rd Quarter, 1965.

Chue, P. W. Y.: Gonorrhea—Its Natural History, Oral Manifestations, Diagnosis, Treatment and Prevention, *J. Am. Dent. Assoc.*, 90, 1297, June, 1975.

Colby, R. A., Kerr, D. A., and Robinson, H. B. G.: *Color Atlas of Oral Pathology*, 3rd ed. Philadelphia, Lippincott, 1971, pp. 91–168.

Glickman, I.: *Clinical Periodontology*, 4th ed. Philadelphia, Saunders, 1972, pp. 488–490.

Kerr, D. A., Ash, M. M., and Millard, H. D.: *Oral Diagnosis*, 4th ed. St. Louis, Mosby, 1974, pp. 79–161.

Marlette, R. H.: Generalized Melanoses and Nonmelanotic Pigmentations of the Head and Neck, *J. Am. Dent. Assoc.*, 90, 141, January, 1975.

Mitchell, D. F., Standish, S. M., and Fast, T. B.: *Oral Diagnosis/Oral Medicine*, 2nd ed. Philadelphia, Lea & Febiger, 1971, pp. 19–22, 106–117.

Rubin, M. P. and Richardson, J. F.: Diagnostic and Therapeutic Considerations in Oral Medicine, in Goldman, H. M., Gilmore, H. W., Irby, W. B., and Olsen, N. H.: *Current Therapy in Dentistry*, Volume Five. St. Louis, Mosby, 1974, pp. 178–219.

Zegarelli, E. V., Kutscher, A. H., and Hyman, G. A., eds.: *Diagnosis of Diseases of the Mouth and Jaws*. Philadelphia, Lea & Febiger, 1969, pp. 1–19, 157–292, 296–297 (color plates).

Drug Signs

American Red Cross: *Standard First Aid and Personal Safety*, New York, Doubleday, 1973, pp. 126–143.

Einstein, S. and Burrell, C. D., eds.: *The Non-Medical Use of Drugs: Contemporary Intervention Issues*. Monograph Series, No. 2, Institute for the Study of Drug Addiction, Farmingdale, N.Y., Baywood Publishing Company, 1973.

United States Department of Justice, Drug Enforcement Administration: *Drugs of Abuse*. Superintendent of Documents, U.S. Government Printing Office, Washington, D.C. 20402.

Oral Cancer

Abrams, A. M. and Melrose, R. J.: Why We Are Failing With Oral Cancer, *J. Am. Soc. Prev. Dent.*, 4, 24, January-February, 1974.

Adams, R. J., Pullon, P. A., and Lee, F.: Expanding the Role of the Dentist in the Detection of Oral and Laryngeal Cancer, *J. Am. Dent. Assoc.*, 89, 607, September, 1974.

Burzynski, N. J.: The Dental Hygienist in Oral Cancer Detection, *J. Am. Dent. Hyg. Assoc.*, 45, 302, September-October, 1971.

Burzynski, N. J., Moore, C., and DeJean, E.: Basic Steps in Mouth–throat Examination for Cancer Detection, *J. Am. Dent. Assoc.*, 81, 932, October, 1970.

Castigliano, S. G.: Oral Cancer, in Burket, L. W.: *Oral Medicine*, 6th ed. Philadelphia, Lippincott, 1971, pp. 581–640.

Christen, A. G.: The Clinical Effects of Tobacco on Oral Tissue, *J. Am. Dent. Assoc.*, 81, 1378, December, 1970.

Drinnan, A. J.: Skin Cancer Detection During Routine Dental Examination, *Dent. Radiogr. Photogr.*, 42, 11, #1, 1969.

Glass, R. T., Abla, M., and Wheatley, J.: Teaching Self-examination of the Head and Neck: Another Aspect of Preventive Dentistry, *J. Am. Dent. Assoc.*, 90, 1265, June, 1975.

Hasler, J. F.: The Dentist and Detection of Skin Cancer of the Head and Neck, *J. Am. Soc. Prev. Dent.*, 4, 30, January-February, 1974.

Kennett, S.: Benign Lesions Simulating Oral Cancer, *J. Can. Dent. Assoc.*, 40, 203, March, 1974.

McCarthy, P. L. and Shklar, G.: *Diseases of the Oral Mucosa*. New York, Blakiston Division, McGraw-Hill, 1964, pp. 270–338.

Moyer, T. A. and Westcott, W. B.: The Role of the Dental Hygienist in Detecting Oral Cancer, *J. Am. Dent. Hyg. Assoc.*, 44, 34, 1st Quarter, 1970.

Nelson, J. F. and Ship, I. I.: Intraoral Carcinoma: Predisposing Factors and Their Frequency of Incidence as Related to Age at Onset, *J. Am. Dent. Assoc.*, 82, 564, March, 1971.

Scholle, R. H.: A Checklist for Clinical Detection of Early Oral Cancer, *J. Am. Dent. Assoc.*, 82, 1298, June, 1971.

United States Department of Health, Education, and Welfare: *The Health Consequences of Smoking*, A Report of the Surgeon General: 1972. Superintendent of Documents, U.S. Government Printing Office, Washington, D.C. 20402.

Biopsy and Exfoliative Cytology

Anderson, D. L. and Hunter, H. A.: The Oral Smear: A Life May Depend on It, *J. Can. Dent. Assoc.*, 36, 148, April, 1970.

Baker, H. W.: Biopsy: Definitive Diagnosis of Oral Cancer, in *Oral Cancer, Diagnosis, Treatment and Rehabilitation*. American Cancer Society, 1973.

King, O. H.: Cytology—Its Value in the Diagnosis of Oral Cancer, *Dent. Clin. North Am.*, 15, 817, October, 1971.

Lange, D. E., Meyer, M., and Hahn, W.: Oral Exfoliative Cytology in the Diagnosis of Viral and Bullous Lesions, *J. Periodont.*, 43, 433, July, 1972.

Mitchell, D. F., Standish, S. M., and Fast, T. B.: *Oral Diagnosis/Oral Medicine*, 2nd ed. Philadelphia, Lea & Febiger, 1971, pp. 172–179.

News of Dentistry: Set Conclusions Pertaining to Oral Cytology, *J. Am. Dent. Assoc.*, 77, 562, September, 1968.

Rickles, N. H.: Oral Exfoliative Cytology: An Adjunct to Biopsy, in *Oral Cancer, Diagnosis, Treatment and Rehabilitation*, American Cancer Society, 1973.

Rovin, S.: Cytology—Its Value in the Diagnosis of Oral Cancer, *Dent. Clin. North Am.*, 15, 807, October, 1971.

Chapter 9

Dental Radiographs

Radiographs are an essential adjunct to other means of oral diagnosis for treatment planning in the dentist's complete care program for the patient. Preparation of the radiographic survey is one of the first procedures to be accomplished for a patient following a partial or complete history and a preliminary extraoral and intraoral inspection. The radiographs are then available for use during the subsequent complete oral inspection and charting. Later during dental hygiene treatment appointments, the radiographs serve to guide instrumentation and to aid in patient instruction.

The objective in radiography is to use techniques which require the least amount of radiation possible to produce radiographs of the greatest interpretive value. This can be accomplished through routine application of known safety measures for the patient and operator, through analysis of techniques to prevent repeated inadequacies, and through continuing study to keep informed of research developments.

Patients ask questions about safety factors and occasionally a patient may refuse to have any radiographs made. The patient must be reassured with confidence, be instructed as to why radiographs are indispensable to oral care, and be informed in how modern equipment and techniques are in accord with minimum radiation.

The American Dental Association has defined the need for radiographic examinations if complete dental care is to be provided and has stated that "Radiographic examination is a diagnostic procedure. The dentist's professional judgment should determine the frequency and extent of each radiographic examination. Determination of the number of film exposures involved in a radiographic examination should be justifiable in terms of the expected yield of diagnostic information."[1] The American Academy of Dental Radiology indicated that "the benefits of the judicious use of x-rays in dentistry far outweigh any conceivable biologic consequences that might be involved."[2]

This chapter is designed to serve as a summary of terminology, fundamentals of x-ray production, techniques of exposure and processing, safety factors, analysis of the completed radiograph, and suggestions for patient instruction. A comprehensive bibliography is provided to allow for additional study.

TERMS USED IN RADIOGRAPHY*

I. Radiology

That branch of medicine dealing with the diagnostic and therapeutic applications of ionizing radiation.

II. Radiation

The emission and propagation of energy through space or a material medium in the form of waves, for example, electromagnetic waves. **Ionizing radiation** is any electromagnetic or particulate radiation capable of producing ions, directly or indirectly, in its passage through matter.

III. Radiography

The art or science of making radiographs.

IV. Radiograph

An image or picture produced on a radiation-sensitive film emulsion, by exposure to ionizing radiation directed through an area or region or substance of interest, followed by chemical processing of the film. (noun) To make a radiograph. (verb)

V. Types of Radiation

A. **Primary**

Radiation coming directly from the target of the x-ray tube. Except for the useful beam, most of this radiation is absorbed in the tube housing.

B. **Useful Beam**

That part of the primary radiation which is permitted to emerge from the

---

*All definitions in this chapter are taken from or adapted from and in accord with the *Glossary of Terms Used in Radiology* prepared by the Committee on Nomenclature, American Academy of Oral Roentgenology, 1962, and revised by John H. Barr, Simon Kinsman, and Albert G. Richards, 1963. Additional definitions to those included in this chapter may be found in the Glossary.

tube housing as limited by the aperture, cone, or other collimating devices.

C. **Leakage**

Radiation other than the useful beam; it escapes through the protective shielding of the x-ray tube housing.

D. **Secondary**

Radiation emitted by any matter being irradiated with x rays. It originates mainly in the irradiated soft tissues of the patient's face, the pointed plastic cone, and the filter.

E. **Scattered**

Radiation that, during the passage through a substance, has been deviated in direction and may have been modified with an increase in wave length. It is one form of secondary radiation.

F. **Stray**

A term used in a broad sense to include all radiation emitted in directions other than that of the useful beam, for example, leakage radiation, secondary radiation, scattered radiation.

VI. Irradiation

The exposure of material to x ray or other radiation. One speaks of radiation therapy but of irradiation of the patient.

ORIGIN AND CHARACTERISTICS OF X RAY

X rays were first dicovered by Wilhelm C. Roentgen in 1895, who called them x rays after the mathematical symbol "x" for an unknown. "Roentgen rays" is a term often applied to mechanically generated x rays.

Professor Roentgen used a Crookes tube and it was not until 1913 that William D. Coolidge designed a tube in which electricity was used instead of gas. Modern x-ray tubes have the same principles of construction as the Coolidge tube. The historical development of the science of radiology and radiography provides a realistic monument to the early research-ers and their efforts.[3,4]

I. Definition and Properties of X Ray

A. X ray

Electromagnetic, ionizing radiation of very short wave length resulting from the bombardment of a material (usually tungsten) by highly acceler-ated electrons in a high vacuum.

B. Properties

1. Short wave length
   a. Hard x rays: shorter wave lengths, high penetrating power.
   b. Soft x rays: relatively longer wave lengths, relatively less penetrating; more likely to be absorbed into the tissue through which the x rays pass.
2. Speed of travel same as visible light.
3. Power to penetrate opaque sub-stances.
4. Invisible.
5. Ability to affect the emulsion of a photographic film.
6. Ability to produce fluorescence on contact with certain crystals.
7. Ability to stimulate or destroy liv-ing cells.

II. How X Rays Are Produced[5-8]

With reference to the definition of x ray above, essential to x-ray production are (1) a source of electrons, (2) a high voltage to accelerate the electrons, and (3) a target to stop the electrons. The parts of the tube and the circuits within the machine are designed to provide these.

A. The X-ray Tube (figure 9–1)

1. *Protective Tube Housing.* X-ray tube enclosure that reduces the primary radiation to permissible exposure levels; highly vacuated glass tube surrounded by a spe-cially refined oil with high insulat-ing powers.
2. *Cathode*
   a. Tungsten filament; which is heated to give off a cloud of electrons.
   b. Molybdenum cup around the filament; to focus the electrons toward the anode.
3. *Anode*
   a. Copper arm containing a tungsten button, the target, positioned opposite the cathode.
   b. Focal spot: that part of the target on the anode which is bom-barded by the focused electron stream when the tube is ener-gized.
4. *Aperture.* Where the useful beam emerges from the tube; is covered with a permanent seal of glass or aluminum.

B. Circuits

1. Autotransformer: voltage compen-sator which adjusts variations in line voltage.

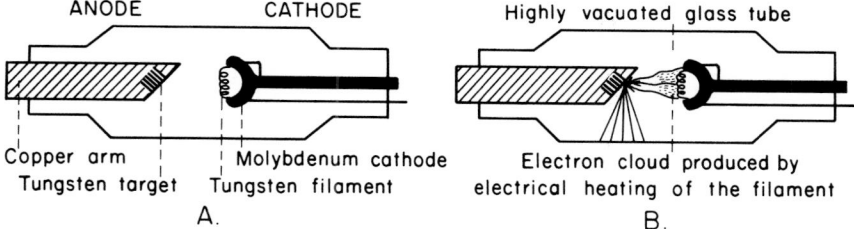

ANODE   CATHODE

Copper arm
Tungsten target   Molybdenum cathode
                   Tungsten filament

A.

Highly vacuated glass tube

Electron cloud produced by
electrical heating of the filament

B.

Figure 9–1. X ray tube. **A.** Inactive, and **B.** In function. Highly accelerated electrons are propelled from the cathode to the anode. X rays are produced as the electrons strike the tungsten target.

2. Filament circuit: step-down.
   a. Voltage of line current is decreased to approximately three volts.
   b. Purpose: heat the tungsten filament to produce electrons.
3. High voltage transformer: step-up.
   a. Voltage of line current (110 volts) is increased to 65,000–90,000 volts (65–90 kVp).
   b. Purpose: give the electrons high speed.
4. Tube circuit: the flow of electrons from the cathode to the anode, activated when the timer button is depressed.

C. **Machine Control Devices**

Machines vary, but in general in operating an x-ray machine there are four factors to control: the line switch (to electrical outlet), the kilovoltage, the milliamperage, and the time. Certain machines operate at a standard kilovoltage (for example, 65 kVp) and milliamperage (10 mA), whereas others permit a range of selection.

1. *Voltage Control* (may be one or two meters, depending on the machine).
   a. Circuit voltmeter; registers line voltage before voltage is stepped up by the transformer (with alternating current this is 110 volts); or may register the kilovoltage that will result after step-up.
   b. KVp selector (kilovoltage peak): to change the line voltage to a selected kilovoltage (65 to 90 kVp).
2. *Milliamperage Control*. Milliammeter: to select the actual current through the tube circuit used during the time of exposure (10 to 20 mA).
3. *Time Control*
   a. X-ray timer: a time switch

mechanism used to complete the electrical circuit so that x rays will be produced for a predetermined time.
   b. Mechanical timer: spring-activated device; range from ¼ to 10 or 15 seconds; does not reset itself.
   c. Electronic timer: vacuum tube device; range from $^{1}/_{30}$ second to 10 seconds; will reset itself automatically; meets needs of modern accelerated techniques.

D. **Steps in the Production of X Rays**[5]
1. Tungsten filament is heated and a cloud of electrons produced.
2. Difference in electrical potential is developed between the anode and the cathode.
3. Electrons attracted to anode from cathode at high speed during the intervals of the alternating current when the anode is charged positive and the cathode negative. (During the alternating half of the cycle the electrons are attracted back into the filament in a self-rectifying tube.)
4. Curvature of the molybdenum cup controls the direction of the electrons and causes them to be projected on the focal spot.
5. Reaction of the electrons as they strike the tungsten target; loss of energy.
   a. Approximately one percent of the energy of electrons is converted to electromagnetic energy of an x ray. (Greater percent at higher kilovoltages.)
   b. Approximately 99 percent of the energy is converted to heat which is dissipated through the copper anode and oil of the protective tube housing.
6. X rays leave the tube through the aperture to form the useful beam.

FACTORS WHICH INFLUENCE THE FINISHED RADIOGRAPH

As the beam leaves the x-ray tube it is collimated, filtered, and allowed to travel a designated source-film (or focal spot-film) distance before reaching the film of a selected speed. The quality or diagnostic usefulness of the finished radiograph as well as the total exposure of the patient and operator are influenced by the collimation, filtration, source-film distance, film speed, kilovoltage, and milliampere seconds. Film processing (pages 133–136) also influences directly the quality of the radiograph, and indirectly the total exposure since re-exposure would be necessary should the film be rendered inadequate during processing.

I. Characteristics of an Acceptable Radiograph

A. *All parts of the image are shown as close to their natural size and shape as possible with a minimum of distortion and superimposition.*
B. *Area to be examined is shown completely with sufficient surrounding tissue included to provide for comparative interpretation.*
C. *Highest Film Quality*
   1. *Density:* the degree of darkening of exposed and processed x-ray film.
   2. *Contrast:* the visual differences in density between adjacent areas on the radiograph.
   3. *Definition:* the property of the projected images relating to their sharpness, distinctness, or clarity of outline.

II. Collimation[9,10]

Collimation is the technique or mechanism for reducing the size and shape of the beam of radiation emitted through the aperture of the tube.
A. **Purposes**
   1. Eliminate peripheral or more divergent radiation.
   2. Minimize exposure to patient's face.
   3. Minimize secondary radiation which can fog the film and expose the bodies of patient and operator.
B. **Method**
   A diaphragm, usually of lead and pierced with a central aperture of the smallest practical diameter for making radiographic exposure is used; located between x-ray tube and cone.
   1. Recommended thickness of lead: ⅛ inch.
   2. Recommended size of aperture: to permit a diameter of the beam of radiation equal to 2¾ inches at the end of the plastic cone next to the patient's face. When a rectangular diaphragm is used, it should be approximately 1½ × 2 inches at the skin. A rectangular diaphragm must be rotated to accommodate for films positioned horizontally or vertically.
C. **Relation to Techniques**
   The dimensions of the largest periapical film are 1¼ by 1⅝ inches. Precise angulation techniques are required to eliminate cone-cut of film.

III. Filtration[9,10]

Filtration is the insertion of layers of aluminum for selective removal of x rays of longer wave lengths from the primary beam.
A. **Purpose**
   To minimize exposure of the patient's skin to unnecessary radiation which will not reach and expose the film.
B. **Methods**
   1. *Inherent filtration:* accomplished by internal barriers built into the x-ray tube, including the glass wall of the tube and the insulating oil surrounding the tube.

2. *Added filtration:* thin, commercially pure aluminum disks inserted between the lead diaphragm and the x-ray tube.
3. *Total filtration:* the sum of the inherent and added filtration.
    a. Recommended total: equivalent of 0.5 mm. (below 50); 1.5 mm. (50–70 kVp); and 2.5 mm. (over 70 kVp) of aluminum.[11]
    b. Check the inherent filtration of the individual x-ray machine; then add a sufficient amount of commercially pure aluminum to bring the total to the recommended level.

C. **Disadvantage of Added Filtration**

Some secondary radiation is produced which scatters in all directions.

IV. Kilovoltage

A. **Amount of Kilovoltage**

Determines the quality of the x radiation.
1. Kilovoltage creates a difference in potential between the anode and the cathode for the production of x rays.
2. The higher the kilovoltage the greater acceleration of the electrons, the greater force with which they bombard the target; therefore, the shorter the wave length.
3. The shorter the wave length, the greater the penetrating power at the skin surface.

B. **Use of High Kilovoltage** (90 kVp)[12,13]

1. Density of the finished radiograph increases with increased kilovoltage (other factors remaining constant).
2. To maintain the proper film density, the milliampere seconds must be decreased as the kVp is increased.
3. Variation in contrast
    a. Low kilovoltage: high contrast, with sharp black-white differences in densities between adjacent areas, but small range of distinction between subject thicknesses recorded.
    b. High kilovoltage: low contrast, with wide range of subject thicknesses recorded: greater range of densities from black to white (more gray tones) which, when examined under proper viewing conditions, provide more interpretive details.
4. Advantages in use of high kilovoltage
    a. Permit shorter exposure time.
    b. Reduce exposure to tissues lying in front of the film packet.
5. Disadvantages
    a. Increased radiation to tissues outside the edges of the film.
    b. More scattered radiation at 90 kVp than at 65 kVp.

V. Milliampere Seconds

A. **Milliamperage**

The measure of the electron current passing through the x-ray tube; it regulates the heat of the filament which determines the number of electrons available to bombard the target.

B. **Quantity of Radiation**

Quantity of radiation is expressed in milliampere seconds (mAs).
1. MAs is the milliamperes multiplied by the time seconds of exposure.
2. Example: at 10 milliamperes for ½ second the exposure of the film is five mAs.

C. **Radiographic Density**

Radiographic density increases with increased milliamperage and/or time of exposure (other factors remaining constant).

VI. Distance[10]

Several distances are involved in x-ray film exposure. The source-surface, the source-film, and the object-film distances must be considered for film placement. In addition, there is the distance which the operator stands from the patient's head during film exposure which is outlined on page 115 in connection with safety factors.

A. **Object-Film Distance**

In a technique where x-ray films are placed against the teeth being radiographed, the object-film distance would be negligible. Close adaptation of the film to the tooth is essential to obtain a sharp image when an eight-inch source-film distance is utilized.

With the paralleling or right-angle technique and use of a longer source-film distance (16–20 inches), there is an increased object-film distance for most radiographs. A collimated beam and increased source-film distance compensate to preserve definition and film quality.

B. **Source-Film Distance**

The directing cone on the x-ray machine is designed to indicate the direction of the central axis of the x-ray beam and to serve as a guide in establishing a desired source-surface and source-film distance. Either an 8- or 16-inch source-film distance is commonly used.

The source-film distance is the sum total of the distance from the source to the cone within the tube housing, the length of the directing cone, and the distance from the end of the cone (at the face) to the film. Directions in technique call for lightly touching the skin with the end of the cone to standardize the source-film distance.

Principles related to source-film distance are:

1. The intensity of the x-ray beam varies inversely as the square of the source-film distance. Example: if a film of the same speed were used at a 16-inch source-film distance as at 8 inches, with all other factors such as kVp and mAs remaining constant, the film at 16 inches would require four times the exposure (time) to maintain the same density in the finished radiograph.
2. The exposure decreases as the distance increases: when the distance is made twice as great, the radiation exposure to the patient is reduced to one-fourth.
3. To maintain film density, an increase in mAs, kVp, or film speed is required when distance is increased.

C. **Advantages in the Use of an Extended Source-Film Distance**

1. Definition or distinctness and clarity of detail improve (because the image is produced by the more central rays).
2. Enlargement or magnification of image decreases (because at shorter distances the outer, more divergent rays tend to enlarge or magnify the image).
3. Skin exposure of the patient is reduced.
4. There is less tissue within the primary beam of radiation since there is less spreading of the x-ray beam.

VII. Films

With optimum filtration, collimation, and fast film, the skin dose to the face can be reduced significantly. Within recent years the manufacture of very slow-speed films has been discontinued, the speed of many films has been doubled, and the use of higher speed films has gained increasing acceptance by the dental profession.

A. **Film**

A thin, transparent sheet of cellulose acetate or similar material coated on one or both sides with an emulsion sensitive to radiation and light.

1. *Emulsion:* gelatin containing countless tiny crystals of silver halide.
2. *Film packet:* small, light-proof, moisture-resistant, sealed paper envelope containing an x-ray film (or two), and a thin sheet of lead foil.
   a. Two-film packet: useful for processing one film differently than the other to make diagnostic comparisons; for sending to specialist to whom patient may be referred; for legal evidence.
   b. Purpose of lead foil backing: prevent exposure of the film by scattered radiation that could enter from back of packet; protection of patient's tissues lying in the path of the x ray.

B. **Speed Groups**[12]
1. Factors in the determination of film speed.
   a. Grain size: smaller grain size the slower the film.
   b. Use of double or single emulsion: slower have single, on one side only. Nearly all present-day films have two emulsions.
2. Film speeds: classified from A (slowest) through F (fastest).

EXPOSURE TO RADIATION

A number of factors influence the biological effects of radiation including the quality of the radiation, the chemical composition of the absorbing medium, the tissues irradiated, the dose (total and rate per unit of time), the blood supply to the tissues, and the size of the area exposed. Generally, radiation of a specific area would be less harmful than whole body radiation. Biological effects of radiation are either somatic (of the general body cells) or genetic (heritable changes, chiefly mutations, produced by the absorption of ionizing radiation by reproductive cells).[17]

I. Ionization

The phenomenon of separation of electrons from molecules which changes their chemical activity is called ionization. The organic and inorganic compounds which make up the human body may be altered by exposure to ionizing radiation. The biological effects following irradiation are secondary effects in that they result from physical, chemical, and biological action set in motion by the absorption of energy from radiation.

II. Permissible Exposure

A. **Exposure**

A measure of the x-radiation to which a person or object, or a part of either, is exposed at a certain place, this measure being based on its ability to produce ionization.
1. *Threshold Exposure.* The minimum exposure that will produce a detectable degree of any given effect.
2. *Entrance or Surface Exposure.* Exposure measured at the surface of an irradiated body, part, or object. It includes primary radiation and backscatter from the irradiated underlying tissue material. The term skin exposure is used with reference to the exposure measured at the center of an irradiated skin surface area.
3. *Erythema Exposure.* The radiation necessary to produce a temporary redness of the skin. The exposure required will vary with the quality of the radiation to which the skin is exposed.

B. **Exposure Units**
1. Roentgen (R): unit of quantity of radiation derived from the ionizing effect of x rays on air.
2. Other units: *rad* (unit of absorbed dose); *rem* (unit of the RBE or Relative Biological Effectiveness).

C. Dose

The amount of energy absorbed per unit mass of tissue at a site of interest. The gonadal dose is the dose of radiation absorbed by the gonads.

D. Permissible Dose

The amount of radiation which may be received by an individual within a specified period without expectation of any significantly harmful result.
1. Assumptions on which permissible doses are calculated[13]:
   a. That no irradiation is beneficial.
   b. There is a dose below which no somatic change will be produced.
   c. Children are more susceptible than older people.
   d. There is a dose below which, even though it is delivered before the end of the reproductive period, the probability of genetic effects will be slight.

E. Radiation Hazard

A condition under which persons might receive radiation in excess of the maximum permissible dose, or radiation damage might be caused to materials.

F. National Council on Radiation Protection and Measurements[11]

1. Limits for dentists and dental personnel (table 9–1).

2. Limits for patients: exposure to x-ray radiation shall be kept to the minimum level consistent with clinical requirements. This limitation is determined by the professional judgment of the dentist.

III. Sensitivity of Cells[14]

A. Factors Affecting

1. Maturity of cell: immature cells are most sensitive.
2. Reproductive capacity: rapidly reproducing are more sensitive; most sensitive when undergoing mitosis.
3. Metabolism: more sensitive in periods of increased metabolism.

B. Radiosensitive Tissues

Blood-forming tissues, reproductive cells, lymphatic tissues, young bone tissue, and skin.

C. Radioresistant Tissues

Most glandular tissues, muscle tissue, nerve tissue, and mature bone tissue.

D. Tissue Reaction

1. *Latent Period.* Lapse between the time of exposure and the time when effects are observed. (May be as long as 25 years, or relatively short as in the case of the production of a skin erythema.)
2. *Cumulative Effect*
   a. Amount of reaction depends on

Table 9–1. Maximum Permissible Dose Equivalent Values (MPD)* to Whole Body, Gonads, Blood-Forming Organs, of Lens of Eye[11]

Average Weekly Exposure†	Maximum 13-week Exposure	Maximum Yearly Exposure	Maximum Accumulated Exposure‡
0.1 R	3 R	5 R	5(N-18)R§

*Exposure of persons for dental or medical purposes is not counted against their maximum permissible exposure limits.
† Used only for the purpose of designating radiation barriers.
‡When the previous occupational history of an individual is not definitely known, it shall be assumed that he has already received the full dose permitted by the formula 5(N-18).
§N=Age in years and is greater than 18. The unit for exposure is the roentgen (R).

dose: less reaction when radiation is received in fractional doses than with one large dose.

b. There will be partial or total repair as long as there is not complete destruction.

c. There may be some irreparable damage which is cumulative as, little by little, more is added (examples: hair loss, skin lesions, falling blood count).

RULES FOR RADIATION PROTECTION

Dental X-ray Protection prepared by the National Council on Radiation Protection and Measurements[11] provides specific information about radiation barriers, film speed group rating, film badge service sources, x-ray equipment data, and operating procedure regulations.

In the application of procedures for protecting the operator and the patient from excessive radiation, particular attention should be paid to unnecessary radiation which may result from the need for an unusual number of retakes due to inadequate technical procedures. Perfecting techniques contributes to the accomplishment of minimum exposure for maximum safety.

I. Protection of Operator

A. Protection from Primary Radiation

1. Avoid the useful beam of radiation. When this is not possible, stand behind a protective barrier.
2. Never hand-hold the film during exposure.
3. Fluorescent mirrors shall not be used in dental examination.

B. Protection from Leakage Radiation

1. Do not hand-hold the tube housing or the directing cone of the machine during exposures.
2. Test machine for leakage radiation. Sur-pak is a film device for surveying dental x-ray machines which

can be obtained at no cost from a State Health Department. The survey determines the size of the beam, the output of the machine, the total filtration, the beam symmetry, and the presence of leakage radiation occurring in a forward direction.

C. Protection from Secondary Radiation

The major sources of secondary radiation are the filter, the pointed plastic cone, and the irradiated soft tissues of the patient's face. The face produces the greatest amount. Methods of protection are related to these three sources.

1. *Minimize total x radiation*
   a. Use high-speed films. When attempting to use high-speed films with older x-ray machines, the original mechanical timers may prove inadequate. Replacement timers are available.
   b. Replace older x-ray machines with modern shockproof equipment.
2. *Use diaphragms or cones to collimate the useful beam* to an area no larger than three inches in diameter when measured at the end of the directing cone. Rectangular collimation has been shown to be more effective than round.[15,16]
3. *Use an open-ended, shielded (lead-lined) cone* in place of the pointed plastic cone. The scattered secondary radiation from the filter and the plastic cone are controlled and eliminated respectively.[17,18]
4. Position of operator while making exposures.
   The operator shall stand behind the patient's head behind the three major sources of secondary radiation, where they cannot directly expose him.
   a. Exposure of the region of the

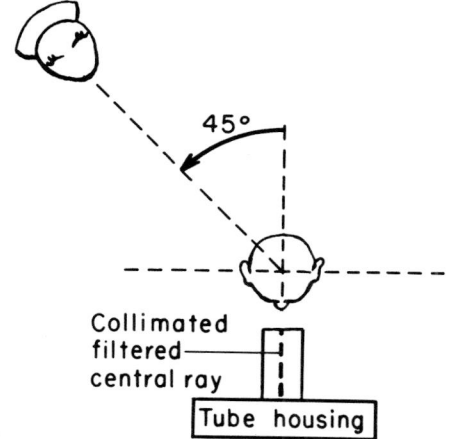

45°

Collimated
filtered
central ray

Tube housing

Figure 9–2. Safer position of operator during film exposure. The operator stands behind the patient's head at a 45° angle to the path of the central ray. The irradiated tissues of the patient's face are the greatest source of secondary radiation.

central incisors: stand at a 45-degree angle to the path of the central ray. This position is approximately behind either the left or the right ear of the patient (figure 9–2).
b. Exposure of other regions: stand behind the patient's head and at an angle of 45° to the path of the central ray of the x-ray beam.
5. *Distance*
a. Safety increases with distance. A long cord on the timer will permit greater freedom of movement.
b. The operator shall stand as far as practical from the patient, at least six feet, and outside the path of the useful beam, or behind a suitable barrier.
c. When space limitations within the dental office prevent occupying the safer positions listed above, the operator should step out of the room and stand behind a thick wall.

D. **Monitoring**

Monitoring refers to the periodic or continuous determination of the amount of ionizing radiation or radioactivity present at a given location, usually for considerations of health protection.

The amount of x-ray radiation that reaches the body of the dentist or dental personnel can be measured economically with a film badge. Badges can be obtained from one of several laboratories. The film badge is worn on the clothing for one, two, or four weeks and is then returned by mail to the laboratory where it was purchased. At the laboratory, the film in the badge is carefully processed and its exposure evaluated. The amount of radiation recorded by the film badge is a measure of the exposure of the wearer who is notified by mail of the amount of exposure.

II. Protection of Patient

A. **Films**

Use high-speed films.

B. **Collimation**

Use diaphragms or cones to collimate the useful beam.

C. **Filtration**

Use filtration of the useful beam to recommended levels (pages 109–110).

D. **Processing**

Process films according to the manufacturer's directions. When a choice of two periods of development is offered, the exposure of the patient can be reduced if the longer development time is employed.

E. **Film Size**

Use the largest intraoral film that can be skillfully placed in the mouth. Maximum coverage is provided in this manner with one exposure, whereas two exposures may be required if smaller films are used to examine the same area of the mouth. This factor is especially important when examining the mouths of children.

F. **Total Exposure**

Do not expose the patient unnecessarily. There must be a good and valid reason for each exposure.

G. **Lead Apron**

A lead apron may be used, particularly for children and pregnant women. When conventional radiographic projections are made, direct exposure of the gonads does not occur.[11]

In California and Wisconsin the use of a lead apron on each patient is required by law.[1] The apron must never be considered a substitute for the other protective measures listed in this section.

H. **High Voltage**

The use of high voltages has been overemphasized. High voltages permit shorter exposure times and reduce the exposure of tissues lying in front of the film packet, but the exposure of the gonads and the tissues lying behind the film packet increases with increased voltage.

TECHNIQUES FOR FILM PLACEMENT AND ANGULATION OF THE RAY

The characteristics of the acceptable finished radiograph have been listed (page 109) and certain technical factors, including collimation, filtration, kilovoltage, milliampere seconds, distance, and films have been described. For consideration next in the procedure for preparation of radiographs is the placement of the film and the angulation of the useful beam.

Intraoral techniques for periapical, bite-wing, and occlusal radiographs are included in this chapter. The principles and uses of panoramic radiographs are also described.

Two fundamental periapical techniques are used in practice, the *paralleling* or right-angle, and the *angle bisection*. The paralleling technique is sometimes referred to as the "long" or "extension cone" and the angle bisection as the "short cone" technique. However, the long cone may be employed with angle bisection procedures.

Operators vary in their application of the principles of the two techniques. Basically, the primary ray should pass through the region to be examined and the film should be placed in relation to the ray so that all parts of the image are shown as close to their natural size and shape as possible with a minimum of distortion in the finished radiograph.

As with other techniques, the development of a systematic procedure is essential. A comfortable, smooth operation saves time and energy for both patient and operator, increases the confidence of the patient in the operator, and allows for consistency in technique which produces consistent results. A basic objective during radiographic technique is to minimize the length of time the film packet remains in the patient's mouth.

I. Intraoral Surveys

A. **Periapical**

1. Purpose: to obtain a view of the entire tooth and its periodontal supporting structures.
2. Films[9]
   a. *Standard* (1¼" × 1⅝"): may be used for all positions.
   b. *Anterior* (¹⁵/₁₆" × 1⁹/₁₆"): for anterior regions where width of arch makes positioning of standard film difficult or impossible.
   c. *Child size* (⅞" × 1⅜"): for primary teeth in small mouths.
3. Number of films used in a complete survey: for the adult mouth it will vary from 14 to 30 depending on the operator's preference, objectives for

showing specific areas, anatomy of the patient's mouth, and the size of the films used. For children see pages 130–131.

B. **Bite-wing (Interproximal)**
1. Purpose: to show the crowns of the teeth, the alveolar crest, and the interproximal area.
2. Films with tab attached
   a. Anterior teeth ($^{15}/_{16}$" × $1^9/_{16}$"): three films are generally used.
   b. Adult posterior teeth, standard film size: four films, one for molar region and one for premolar, each side.
   c. Child posterior teeth, with first permanent molar erupted, standard size film: one on each side.
   d. Adult posterior teeth using longer, narrower film designed to include molars and premolars: one on each side.
3. Commercial tabs: to be attached to standard or child-size films; two types, one a loop to slide over the film packet and the other with an adhesive to attach directly to the film packet.

C. **Occlusal**
1. Purpose: to show large areas of the maxilla, mandible, or floor of the mouth.
2. Film: (2¼" × 3"): for use in self packet or in intraoral cassette.
3. Standard film (1¼" × 1⅝"): for child or individual areas of adult.

II. Preliminary Preparation

A. **Equipment**
1. Surface disinfection of patient surroundings includes wiping the parts of the x-ray machine which are handled in conjunction with oral contact (directing cone, handle of tube housing, timer). Cross-contamination by way of x-ray machines has been demonstrated.[19]
2. Advanced readiness: the patient should not be kept waiting for procedures such as testing the x-ray machine or placing bite-wing tabs on film packets.
3. Timer: check automatic reset or adjust mechanical timer for exposure prior to film placement. Manufacturer's chart is consulted for exposure time at given source-film distance, kilovoltage, and milliamperes.

B. **Patient Preparation**
1. Remove eyeglasses and removable dental appliances.
2. For panoramic radiography, earrings must be removed.

C. **Oral Inspection**
1. Purpose: to determine necessary adaptations during film placement.
2. Factors of particular interest.
   a. Position of teeth and edentulous areas.
   b. Apparent size of teeth as compared to average size of teeth.
   c. Accessibility: height and shape of palate; flexibility of muscles of orifice, floor of the mouth; possible gag reflex, size of tongue.
   d. Unusual features: tori, sensitive areas of the mucous membranes.

III. Patient Cooperation: Prevention of Gagging[20]

Gagging may be the result of psychologic or physiologic factors. It presents some problem in the placement of all films for molar radiographs and may be initiated in the patient who ordinarily does not gag if techniques are not carried out efficiently. Many of the factors related to the prevention of gagging may be applied for the comfort and cooperation of all patients.

A. **Causes of Gagging**
1. Hypersensitive oral tissues, particularly of posterior region of oral cavity.

2. Anxiety and apprehension.
  a. Fear: of unknown, of the film touching a sensitive area.
  b. Previous unpleasant experiences with radiographic techniques.
  c. Failure to comprehend the operator's instructions.
  d. Lack of confidence in the operator.
3. Techniques: film moved over the oral tissues or retained in the mouth longer than necessary.

B. **Preventive Procedures**
  1. Inspire confidence in ability to perform the service.
  2. Alleviate anxiety: explain procedures carefully.
  3. Film placement: firmly and positively without sliding the film over the tissue.
  4. Film retention: use a film holder on which the patient can bite (to distract him).
  5. Instruct patient to breathe through the nose with quick, short breaths during film placement and to hold the breath during exposure.
  6. Use of premedicating agent prescribed by the dentist.
  7. Use of topical anesthetic.
    a. Cold water or ice cube held in the mouth for a short time before film placement dulls the sensory nerve endings.
    b. Salt: one-half teaspoonful placed on the tongue has an anesthetic effect. It may be swallowed or rinsed after radiographs are made.
    c. Prepared topical anesthetics, in the form of an ointment (applied with cotton swab), troche, or rinse give up to twenty minutes of anesthesia (pages 511–513).
  8. Use a panoramic radiographic technique for preliminary examination.

IV. **Definitions and Principles Related to Techniques**

A. **Planes**
  1. *Sagittal or Median.* The plane that divides the body in the midline into right and left sides.
  2. *Occlusal.* The mean occlusal plane represents the mean curvature from the incisal edges of the central incisors to the tips of the occluding surfaces of the third molars. The occlusal plane of the premolars and first molar may be considered as the mean occlusal plane.
     When it is specified in techniques that the occlusal plane of the teeth being radiographed shall be parallel to the floor, at least three head positions are involved for the maxillary: for anterior teeth the head must be tipped forward, for premolars held at the mean occlusal plane, and for molars, tipped back.

B. **Angulation**
  1. *Horizontal.* The angle at which the central ray of the useful beam is directed within a horizontal plane. Inadequate horizontal angulation results in overlapping or superimposition of parts of adjacent teeth in the radiograph.
  2. *Vertical.* The plane at which the central ray of the useful beam is directed within a vertical plane. Inadequate vertical angulation results in elongation or foreshortening in the image.

C. **Long Axis of a Tooth**
  An imaginary line passing longitudinally through the center of the tooth.
  Because of marked variations in tooth position and root curvature, estimation of the long axis of a tooth is difficult. Clinically, it can be considered that the long axis of a posterior

tooth is at right angles to the occlusal surface plane. For single-rooted teeth the long axis would ordinarily pass from the center of the incisal edge to the tip of the apex, but it is not possible to observe this during clinical inspection. It must be remembered that the line from the incisal to the cervical on the labial surface should not be confused with the long axis.

PERIAPICAL SURVEY: PARALLELING TECHNIQUE

The paralleling or right-angle technique is based on the principles that *the film is placed as nearly parallel to the long axis of the tooth as the anatomy of the oral cavity will permit and the central ray is directed at right angles to the film.* In figure 9–3 A the parallel relationship of the film with the long axis of the tooth and the right-angle direction of the central ray are shown.

The distance between the crown of the tooth and the film is increased to attain parallelism. In the majority of positions for individual films, the edge of the film against the soft tissues is approximately in the same position on the palate or the floor of the mouth as when the film is placed against and close to the tooth in, for example, the angle bisection technique. In other words, the distance between the root apex and the film is not materially different in the paralleling technique than in the angle bisection technique. Figures 9–3 A and B show the comparative projection of the parts of the tooth on the film to produce the image in the radiograph.

I. Patient Position

As long as the film is parallel to the long axis of the tooth and the central ray is directed at right angles to the film, the head may be in any position convenient to the operator and comfortable for the patient. Slight modification of positioning may be needed for making radiographs in a supine position.[21,22] With the use of the supine patient position, less radiation to body areas below the neck has been demonstrated.[23]

The use of a film holder facilitates obtaining the correct angulation of the ray, since the directing cone for the central ray can be lined up with the part of the film holder which extends from between the teeth and which is designed to be at right angles to the film.

For the inexperienced operator, horizontal angulation may be visualized more readily when the occlusal plane of the teeth being radiographed is parallel with the floor and the sagittal plane is perpendicular to the floor.

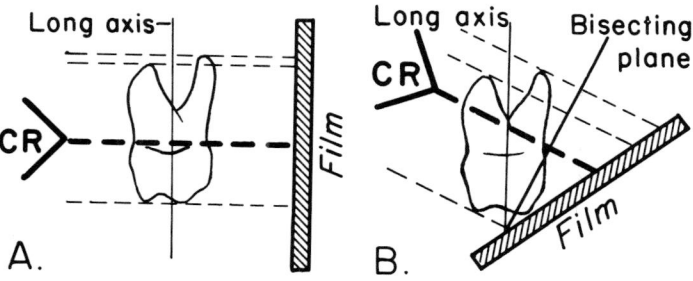

A.   B.

Figure 9–3. Comparison of paralleling and angle bisection techniques. **A.** Paralleling technique. The film is parallel with the long axis of the tooth and the central ray (CR) is directed perpendicular to both the film and the long axis of the tooth. **B.** Angle bisection. The central ray (CR) is directed perpendicular to an imaginary line which bisects the angle formed by the film and the long axis of the tooth.

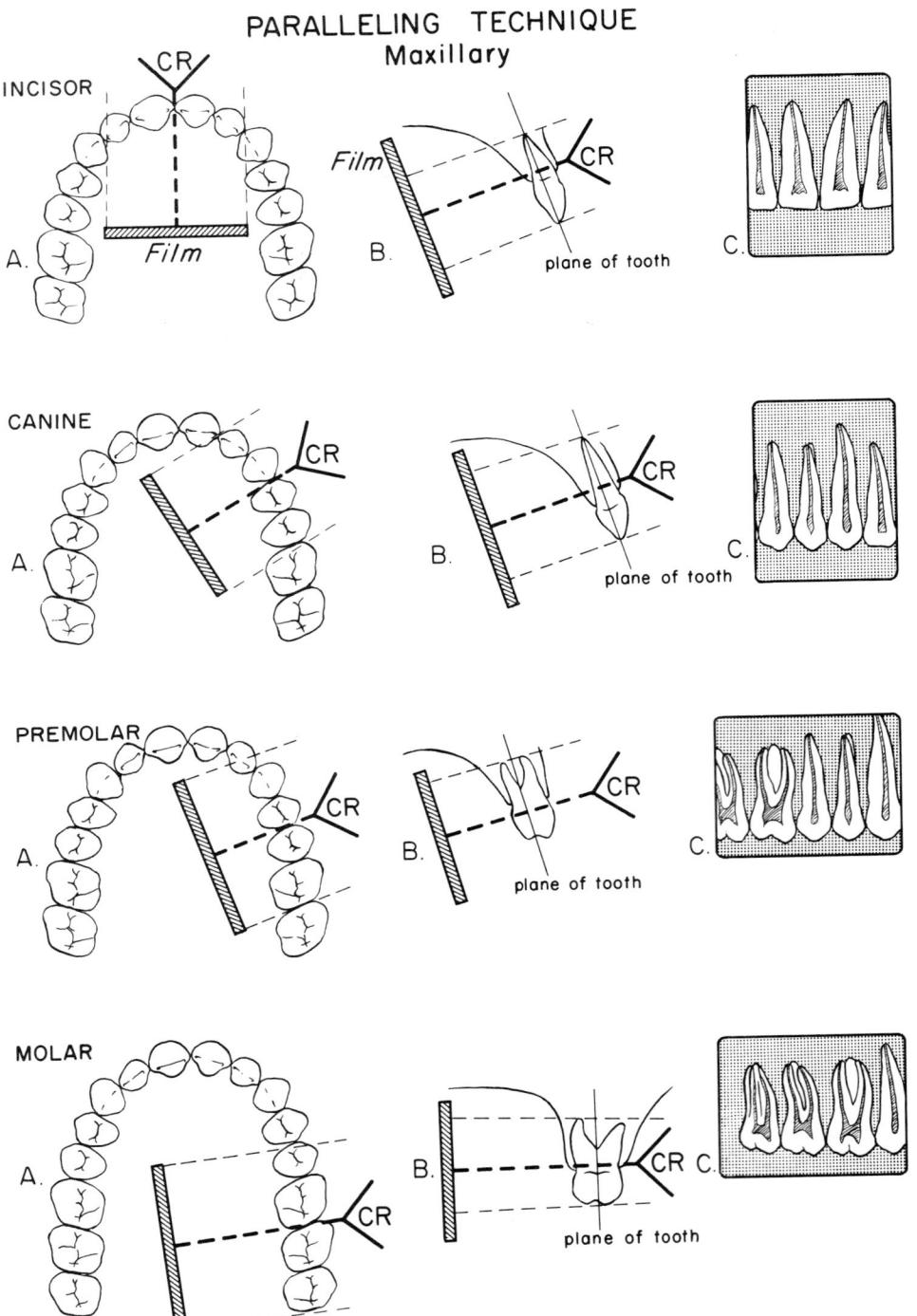

Figure 9–4. Paralleling technique. Film positioning for the four major maxillary positions. Two additional radiographs are frequently made centered at the right and left lateral incisors. **A.** Horizontal angulation with film placed parallel to the long axes of the teeth; central ray (CR) directed parallel with a line through the interproximal. **B.** Vertical angulation with central ray (CR) directed at right angles to the film. **C.** Image objective for the completed radiograph.

PARALLELING TECHNIQUE
Mandibular

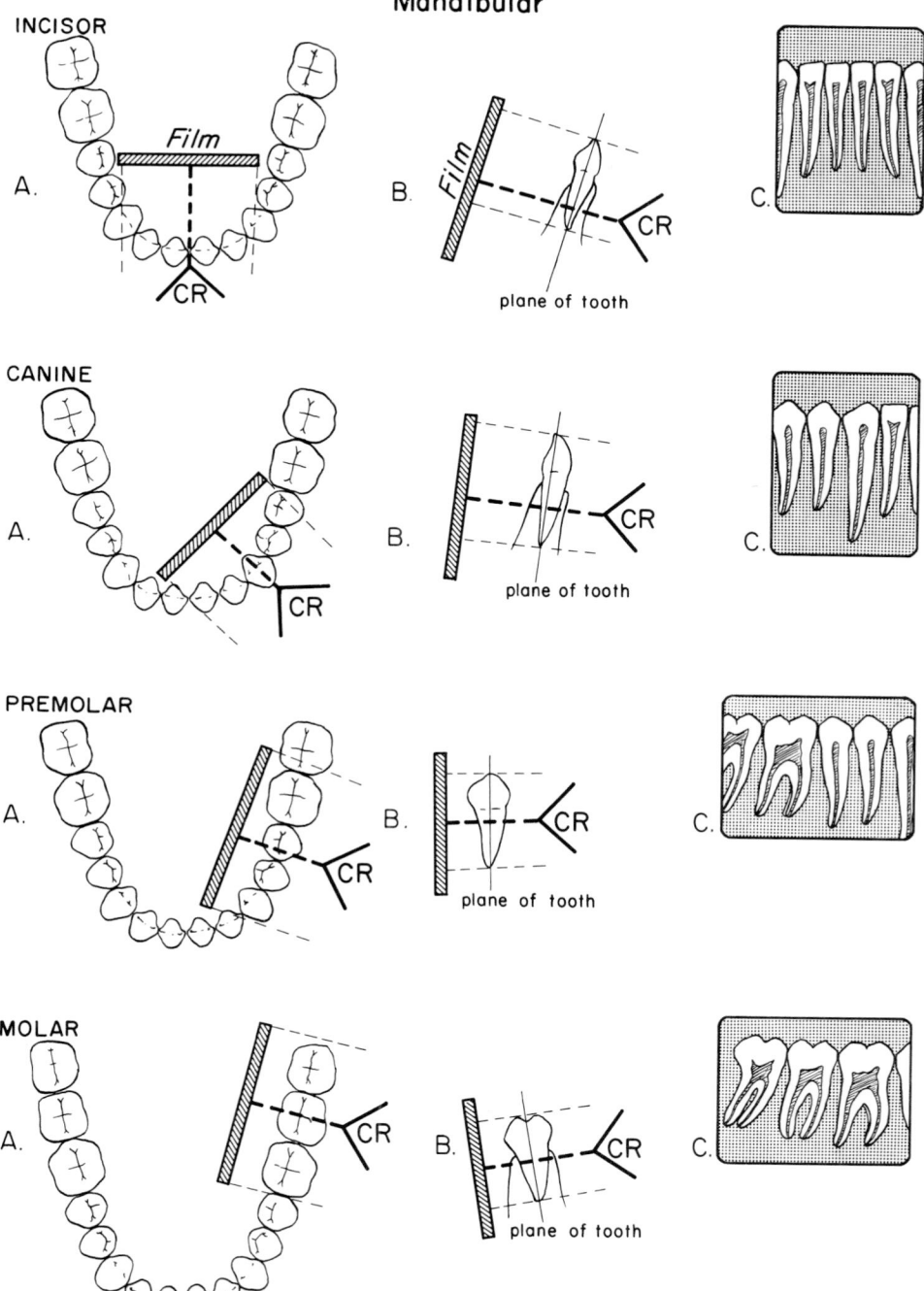

Figure 9–5. Paralleling technique. Film positioning for the four major mandibular positions. Additional radiographs are frequently made centered at the right and left lateral incisors. **A.** Horizontal angulation with film placed parallel to the long axes of the teeth; central ray (CR) directed through the interproximal. **B.** Vertical angulation with central ray (CR) directed at right angles to the film. **C.** Image objective for the completed radiograph.

II. Film Placement

A. Film Position and Angulation of the Central Ray

Instructions for film placement and angulation are included in this section. In addition to the references associated with specific parts of this section, other references will be helpful in studying and perfecting techniques.[24-26]

1. Basic principles for film placement and angulation of the central ray are shown in figures 9–4 and 9–5. The image objective in the completed radiograph is also illustrated.

2. Horizontal angulation: the ray is directed approximately at the center of the film and through the interproximal area.

3. Vertical angulation: the ray is directed at right angles to the film.

B. Film Positioning Devices

Some device for holding the film is essential to a consistent technique accomplished in minimal time without added radiation to the patient from hand-held films. In addition to holding the film, devices may incorporate features to assist in the alignment of the film with the central beam or to contribute to collimation or shielding.

The American Dental Association reviews applications for classification of devices as acceptable, provisionally acceptable, or unacceptable. The list appears in the *Guide to Dental Materials and Devices* and is supplemented between book editions by reports in the *Journal of the American Dental Association.* A number of accessory devices for film positioning, collimation, and shielding are currently listed.[27,28]

1. Characteristics. An effective film positioning device will have characteristics such as the following:

    a. Adaptable to all necessary positions for obtaining diagnostic radiographs of the entire dental arches.

    b. Weight and other properties which do not hinder placement or holding without requiring the patient to hand-hold the device.

    c. Comfortable for the patient during the necessary time interval.

    d. Simplicity of placement; minimal complexity for learning.

    e. Aid in alignment of x-ray beam for correct exposure of film.

    f. Disposable or conveniently sterilized. To this end, more than one device should be maintained to permit sterilization between patients.

2. Types[29]

    a. *Hemostat* is inserted through a rubber bite block and film is positioned and held in claws of the hemostat. The film is positioned in the mouth and held by the patient biting on the bite block.

    b. *Bite blocks:* plastic or wooden (short and long for different areas of the mouth).

    c. *Styrofoam disposable film holder* (Stabe).[30] Simple, comfortable, light weight device; assists in beam alignment by the end which protrudes after the teeth are closed down to hold the device in place (figure 9–6).

    d. *Precision X-ray Device.* Has a facial shield attached to the bar which holds the film in position parallel to the shield. A rectangular hole in the shield permits the passage of only the x rays which will reach the film. (Distributed by the Precision X-ray Company.)

    e. *Snap-A-Ray.* Plastic film holder with two ends for positioning

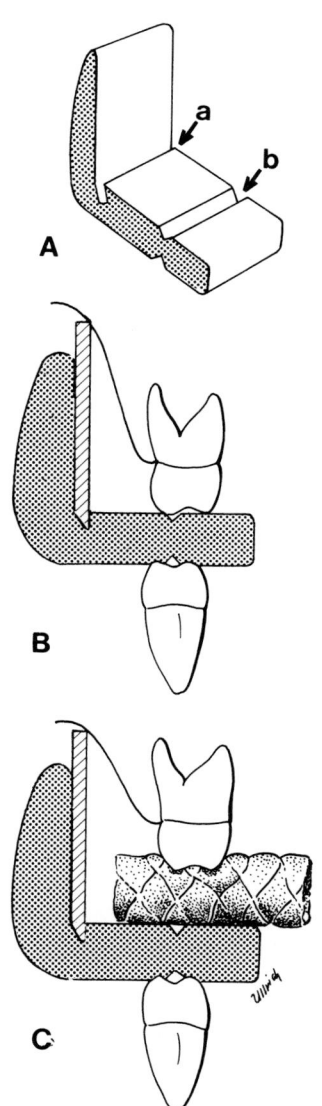

Figure 9–6. Styrofoam disposable film holder. **A.** Empty holder to show **a**, slot for insertion of film, and **b**, break off point to shorten the bite surface for use in mandibular posterior positions; **B.** Film placement for maxillary molar radiograph for patient with high palatal vault; **C.** Film placement for low palatal vault using a cotton roll to lower the film holder.

anterior and posterior films. It is held between the teeth. (Rinn Corporation.)

f. *X-C-P (X-tension C-one P-arallel-ing).* Has an adjustable circular ring which permits film alignment with the primary beam by bringing the open end of the cone in contact with the ring.[31] (Rinn Corporation.)

3. Supplements.

a. Removable denture may be needed in place in opposite jaw to stabilize the film holder.

b. A cotton roll between the film holder or bite block and the biting surface can aid in paralleling when the teeth are short and/or the palatal vault is low.

III. Paralleling Technique: Advantages

A. **Accuracy**

The paralleling technique gives truer size and shape of dental structures with less distortion than when angle bisection is used:

1. Buccal and lingual aspects can be shown in proper relation to each other.

2. Zygomatic bone can be shown in its normal position above the root apices of the molars and premolars.

B. **Bite-wing Radiographs May Not Be Required**

In a complete survey the right angle view of proximal surfaces in paralleling technique radiographs is the same as in the bite-wing. Time and effort as well as radiation to patient are saved.

C. **Simpler to Perform**

Bisection of the angle between the long axis and the film in the bisection technique is difficult to visualize.

D. **Standardized Results Obtained Which Can Be Duplicated**

E. **Horizontal Ray Direction**

No rays are directed toward the pelvis, whereas with angle bisection several radiographs require a relatively steep vertical angulation.

BITE-WING SURVEY

The bite-wing or interproximal survey is used as an adjunct to the periapical survey. It has a special use at the time of periodic patient inspection to detect proximal surface caries between complete periapical surveys, but does not show the periodontium. The complete survey is usually repeated every two to three years, depending on the oral problems of the individual patient.

When the angle bisection technique is used for the periapical radiographs, the bite-wing survey is essential, since an accurate view of all proximal surfaces cannot otherwise be obtained. The angulation for the bite-wing radiographs is based on the same principle as that for periapical surveys made with the paralleling or right-angle technique.

I. Preparation for Film Placement

A. **Patient Position**

1. Traditional. Sagittal plane perpendicular to the floor and occlusal plane parallel with the floor.
2. Patient in Supine Position: the

planes are reversed in their relation to the floor.

B. **Vertical Angulation**

Set at +10 degrees.

C. **Patient Instruction**

Request patient to practice closing on posterior teeth prior to positioning film for posterior bite-wings, and edge-to-edge (figure 14–3 page 223) for anterior.

II. Film Placement and Central Ray Angulation

Figure 9–7 shows in diagram form the position of the molar bite-wing film in relation to the teeth, the horizontal and vertical angulation, and the image objective for both the premolar and molar completed radiographs when standard film is used.

A. **Position of Film**

1. Molar (standard film): mesial border of film at mesial of maxillary second premolar or more distal as needed to include the distal surface of the third molar when it is erupted and in position.
2. Premolar (standard film): mesial border of film at center or mesial of maxillary canine.
3. Anterior: center of film at mesial surface of maxillary canine for the

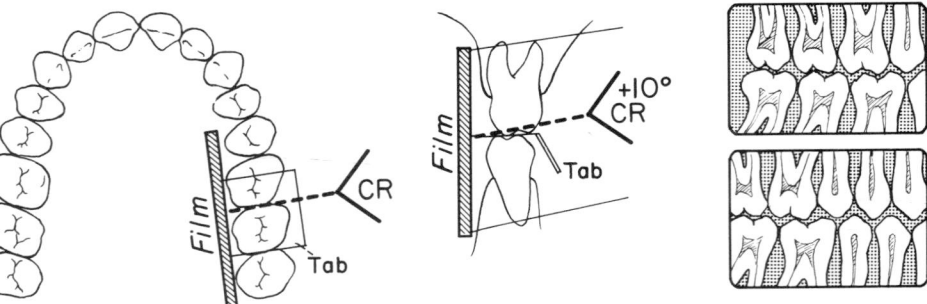

Figure 9–7. Bite-wing radiograph. Left, film position showing horizontal angulation for molar bite-wing with the central ray (CR) directed through the interproximals to the center of the film. Middle, vertical angulation set at +10 degrees. Right, image objective for molar (above) and premolar (below) regions.

two lateral bite-wings; center of film at midline for central bite-wing.

B. **Position of Directing Cone**

With the vertical angulation at +10 degrees, the horizontal angulation is adjusted to direct the central ray to the center of the film. The ray must pass through the interproximals or parallel to a line through the interproximals.

C. **Maintain Film Flat During Exposure**

Although slight curving of the film may be needed for certain patients depending on the oral anatomy and tissue sensitivity, the basic rule is to keep the film as flat as possible to prevent distortion.

PERIAPICAL SURVEY: ANGLE BISECTION TECHNIQUE

The angle bisection technique is based on the geometric principle that *the central ray is directed perpendicular to an imaginary line which is the bisector of the angle formed by the long axis of the tooth and the plane of the film.* Figure 9–3 B illustrates in diagram form the relationship of the long axis of the tooth, the film, and the bisector of the angle formed by these two.

I. Patient Position

A. **Traditional**

1. Sagittal plane: perpendicular to the floor.
2. Occlusal plane: parallel with the floor.

B. **Patient in Supine Position:** the planes are reversed in their relation to the floor.

II. Film Placement and Position

Instructions for film placement and angulation are included in this section.

Additional references will be helpful in studying and perfecting techniques.[32,33]

A. **Basic Considerations**

1. Center of film: at center of teeth being radiographed. The exception to this rule is the maxillary canine film which is placed slightly distal to accommodate film positioning.
2. Border of film: ⅛ to ¼ inches beyond occlusal or incisal.
3. Film must be kept as flat as possible. A cotton roll may be used with the anterior and maxillary molar films to aid in accomplishing this.

B. **Film Position in Relation to Angulation of the Central Ray**

Figures 9–8 and 9–9 show the position of the individual films, the horizontal and vertical angulations, and the image objective in the completed radiograph.

III. Direction of the Central Ray

A. **Direct the Ray through the Apical ⅓ of the Teeth Being Radiographed**

1. *Maxillary.* To determine location of the apices of the teeth draw an imaginary line from the ala of the nose to the tragus of the ear, and the apices will be approximately at that level.
2. *Mandibular.* Apices are located approximately ½ inch above the lower border of the mandible.

B. **Horizontal Angulation**

The ray should pass through the interproximal or parallel to a line through the interproximal, at approximately the center of the area being radiographed.

C. **Vertical Angulation**

Bisect the angle formed by the film and the long axis of the teeth, and direct the ray perpendicular to this line.

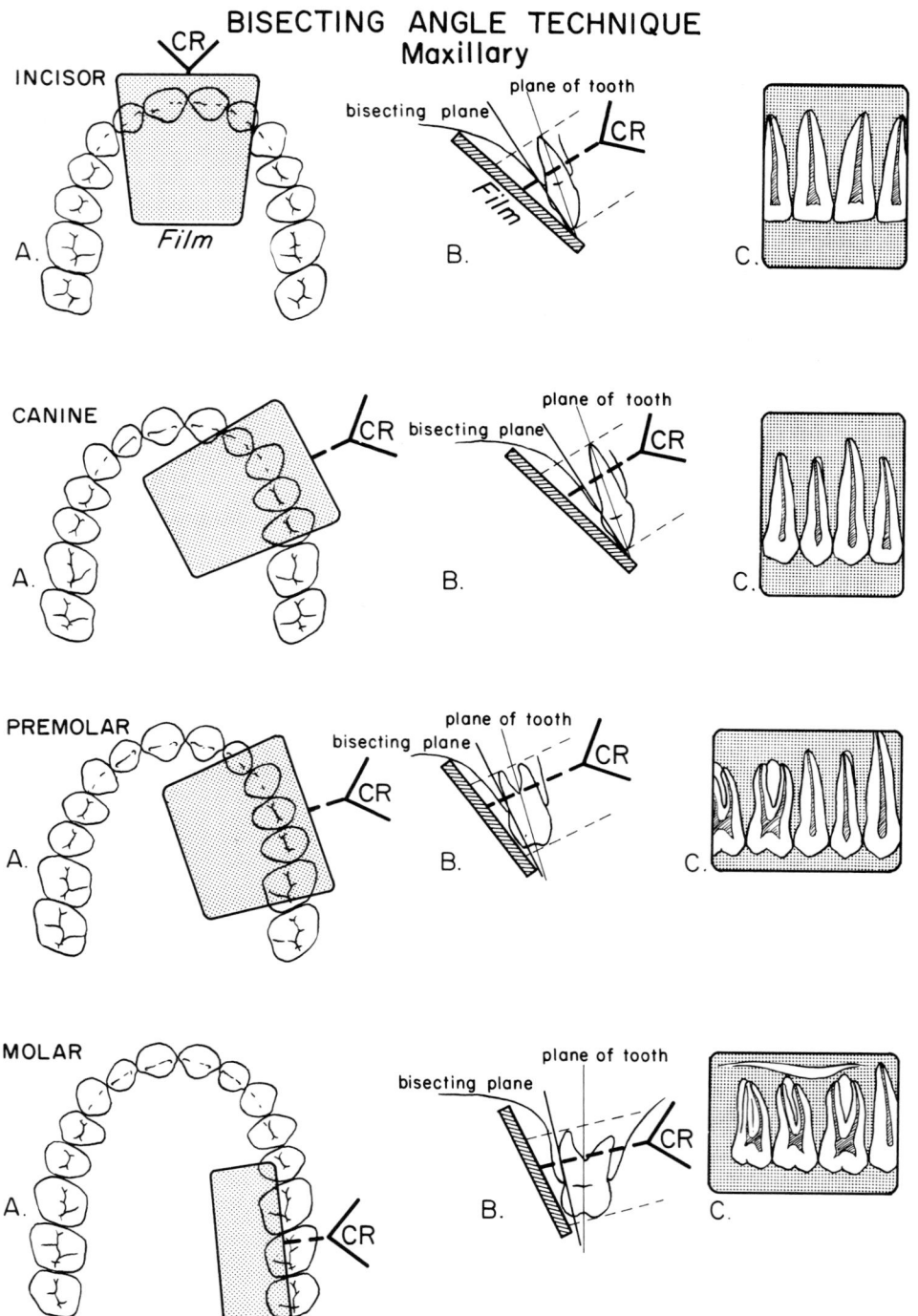

Figure 9–8. Angle bisection technique. Film positioning for the four major maxillary radiographs. Additional radiographs may be made centered at the right and left lateral incisors. **A.** Horizontal angulation with central ray (CR) directed through the interproximal. **B.** Vertical angulation with central ray (CR) directed perpendicular to the bisector of the angle formed by the film and the long axes of the teeth. **C.** Image objective for the completed radiograph.

BISECTING ANGLE TECHNIQUE
Mandibular

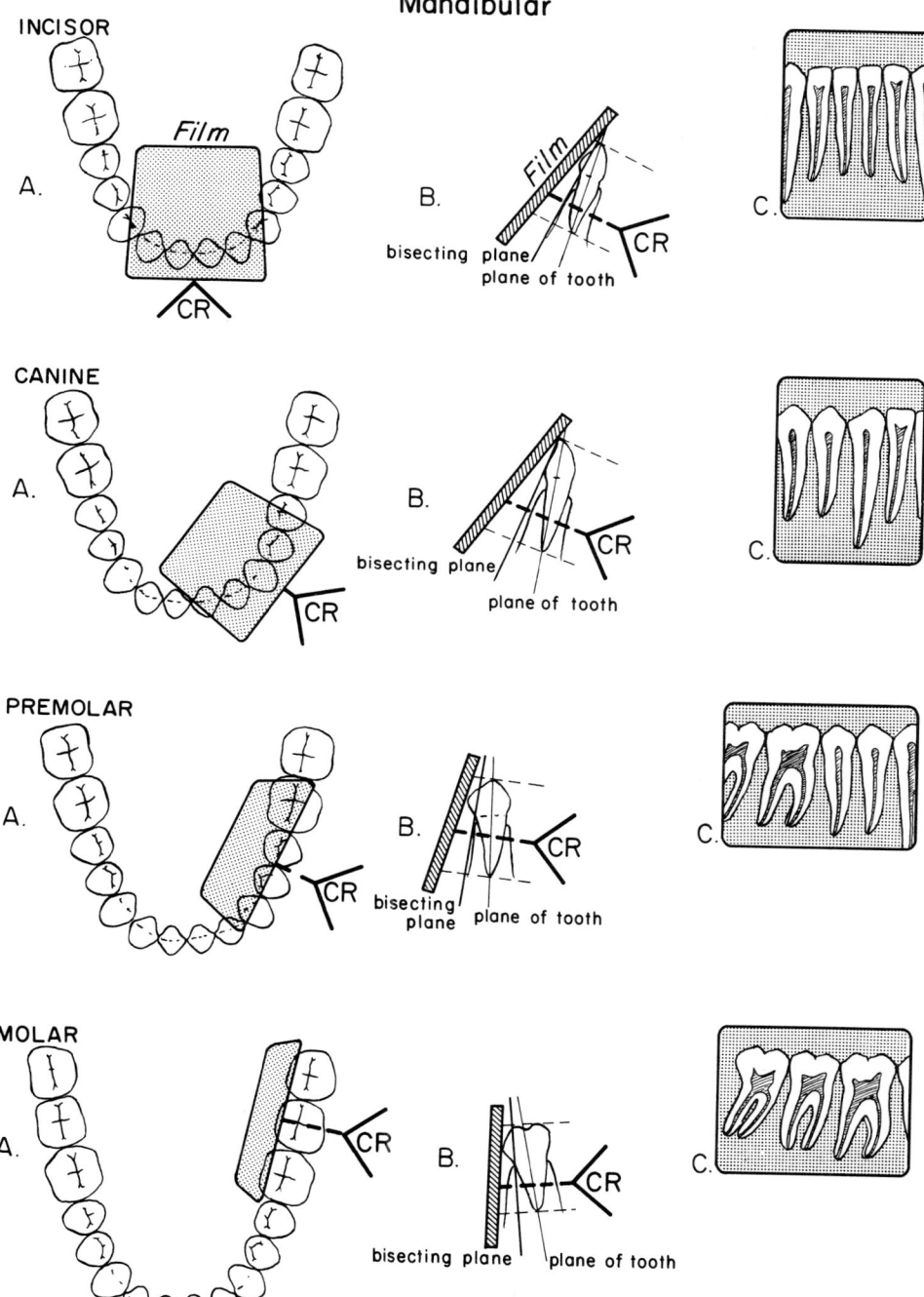

Figure 9–9. Angle bisection technique. Film positioning for the four major mandibular radiographs. Additional radiographs may be made centered at the right and left incisors. **A.** Horizontal angulation with central ray (CR) directed through interproximal. **B.** Vertical angulation with central ray (CR) directed perpendicular to the bisector of the angle formed by the film and the long axes of the teeth. **C.** Image objective for the completed radiograph.

D. **Average Angles for Vertical Angulation**

1. *Uses*

   a. For the anatomically ideal mouth: it would be expected that the average angle and the angle determined by the bisection principle would be the same.

   b. As a point from which to begin when bisecting the angle: usually the angle of the bisection would be within five to ten degrees of the average angle.

   c. As a time saver in angle bisection technique: prior to placing the film in the patient's mouth the cone is positioned at the average angle to facilitate angulation and prevent undue discomfort on the part of the patient.

   d. For the beginner, as a first technique, while he is developing concepts of angle bisection.

2. *The Average Angles*

Maxillary		*Mandibular*	
Central	+40–45	Central	−15–20
Canine	+45–50	Canine	−20–25
Premolar	+30–35	Premolar	−10–15
Molar	+20–25	Molar	− 5– 0

OCCLUSAL SURVEY

The use of occlusal films is particularly important for observing areas which cannot be completely or conveniently shown on other film, in cases where positioning periapical films is difficult or impossible, to supplement the angulation provided by other films for such conditions as fractures, impacted teeth, or salivary duct calculi, and as a specific part of the complete survey for edentulous and very young patients.

In this section the central midline films for maxillary and mandibular are described. A variety of positions for the occlusal films is possible, depending on the area to be examined. Additional references will be helpful as a guide.[34,35]

I. Maxillary Midline

A. **Position of Patient's Head**

The line from tragus of the ear to ala of the nose is parallel with floor.

B. **Film Position**

The emulsion side is toward the palate; posterior border of film is brought back close to third molar region; film is held between the teeth with edge-to-edge closure.

C. **Angulation**

The cone is directed toward the bridge of the nose at a 65-degree angle.

D. **Exposure**

Consult chart of film manufacturer's specifications for exposure related to source-film distance, kilovoltage, and milliamperage. When a cassette is used, exposure time is reduced, an advantage in prevention of movement of the film.

II. Mandibular Midline

A. **Position of Patient's Head**

The head is tilted directly back.

B. **Film Position**

Emulsion side is toward floor of mouth, posterior border of film is in contact with soft tissues of retromolar area; and the film is held between teeth in an edge-to-edge bite.

C. **Angulation**

For incisal region the cone is pointed at the tip of the chin at an angle of approximately 55 degrees. For the floor of the mouth, the cone is directed from under the chin, perpendicular to the film.

D. **Exposure**

Consult chart of film manufacturer's specifications.

PANORAMIC RADIOGRAPHS

Panoramic radiography refers to techniques which produce films showing large areas of the maxillary and mandibular arches with adjacent structures on one or more extraoral films. This type of radiograph is a supplement to a periapical survey but not a substitute.

I. Types of Panoramic Techniques[36-38]

A. **Tomography or Curved-surface Laminagraphy.** Lamina means layer and in this technique a single layer of the teeth and surrounding structures appears in the radiograph. Other structures do not appear superimposed as they do in traditional extraoral techniques. The head is stabilized with a chin support or one of several types of head holders characteristic of each machine. Two methods are used in laminagraphy.
   1. Film and x-ray source rotate around the patient's head. Examples are the Panorex (S. S. White), Panelipse (General Electric), and the Orthopantograph (Siemens).
   2. Patient is rotated between the x-ray source and the film. An example is the Rotagraph (Watson, England).

B. **Still-picture Technique.** An intraoral fine focus x-ray tube is placed within the patient's mouth.
   1. Film in cassette is molded to the face, using separate films for the mandible and the maxilla. An example is the Status-X (Siemens).
   2. Head and film positioner used to make a series of lateral jaw radiographs. An example is the Orthoramix (Dental Corporation of America) which attaches to a conventional x-ray machine. With the Orthoramix four overlapping exposures are made to cover the entire maxillary and mandibular arches.

II. Uses

Because definition and detail are inferior to periapical radiographs and be-cause there is distortion, panoramic radiographs provide an overall view, not a detailed one. They do not show proximal carious lesions except for large cavities, and those can be seen by direct examination. They are also inadequate for examination of the periodontal supporting structures. Some important uses are listed here.[39]

A. **Preliminary Examination.** Panoramic radiographs are helpful for surveying to find areas that require further study.

B. **Oral Pathology.** The scope of an oral examination increases with the use of a panoramic survey.

C. **Supplement to a Periapical Survey** when a complete periapical survey may not be necessary. Child patient and edentulous surveys are examples (pages 130–131).

D. **Orthodontics.** The overall view of growth, development at the beginning of orthodontic observation, diagnosis, and treatment, and during the treatment to assess periodic progress, is beneficial.

E. **Problem Patients.** For patients with handicaps or systemic conditions which hinder cooperation, such as patients with trismus, temporomandibular joint disability, Parkinson's disease, facial paralysis, or patients who are chronic extreme gaggers, examination may not be possible by intraoral techniques.

F. **Oral Surgery.** Use of a panoramic radiograph has been shown to be sufficient for many treatment procedures.

III. Limitations

A. **Inferiority of Definition and Detail.** Causes of poor definition are
   1. Use of intensifying screens.
   2. Increased object-film distance.
   3. Movement of x-ray tube and film.

B. **Distortion**
1. Magnified images are produced because of increased film-object distance.
2. Overlapping. In periapical techniques, each film is angulated with the central ray so that when a tooth is out of line, adjustment is made to prevent overlapping. With panoramic technique, the head and teeth remain fixed, and the ray and film are positioned for the average only.

IV. Technique[40]

Learning to use panoramic equipment is not difficult. Each machine has its own characteristics which can be readily learned from the manufacturer's instructions.

A. **Film.** Film sizes are usually either 5 × 12 or 6 × 12 inches. Speed film should be used to minimize radiation.
B. **Processing.** Regular processing solutions are used for panoramic film development. Special film holders may be obtained.

CHILD PATIENT SURVEY

The frequency for making a radiographic survey of a child, the size and number of films used, and the techniques of film placement may be influenced by several factors. These include primarily the age, cooperation of the patient, and size of the mouth. To be useful the survey must be complete and show all areas.

Aside from the need for radiographs at an early age for accidents or anomalies, the initial survey in the child's life may be made soon after all of the primary teeth are erupted. Adequate oral supervision might suggest a second survey at approximately age six and the third at approximately age ten. Bite-wing surveys at appropriate intervals between complete surveys could be made for dental caries detection

if close contact areas do not permit direct clinical examination.

By the age of nine or ten the size and number of films used for an intraoral survey approximate the adult survey. This section is devoted to a brief consideration of the surveys for the pre-schooler (primary dentition) and the child of six to seven years (initial stage of mixed dentition).

The aim for the young child is to make as thorough an examination of the teeth and their surrounding structures as possible, using a minimum of exposures. The selection of number and types of film is made with the intention to cause the least discomfort possible.

I. Primary Dentition

Various combinations of periapical, bite-wing, occlusal, panoramic, and extraoral films are recommended by the specialists. Film size is suggested which will be consistent with the size of the mouth, the cooperation of the patient, and the ability of the operator. Examples of number and size of films for five effective surveys are listed here.

A. Occlusal views of anterior maxillary and mandibular (standard film) and posterior bite-wings (child or adult anterior film); total of four films.
B. Panoramic radiograph with posterior bite-wing survey.
C. Occlusal views of anterior maxillary and mandibular and maxillary posterior (standard film), posterior bite-wings (child or standard film) and extraoral lateral jaw films (5" × 7") or a panoramic radiograph; total of eight films.
D. Occlusal views of anterior maxillary and mandibular (standard film), posterior bite-wings (two or four, child or standard film), and four extraoral lateral jaw films (8" × 10") or a panoramic radiograph; total of eight or ten films.

E. Periapical views for each posterior quadrant and one each for anterior (child size film); total six films.

II. Mixed Dentition (Six to Nine Years)

Twelve to fourteen exposures using standard film are recommended. These include two posterior bite-wings, four molar (to include first permanent and primary molars), four canine, and two or four incisor periapical views.

III. Technique with Children

A. Orientation to Lessen Apprehension

1. For a young child's first visit to the dental office, making the radiographic survey may be a necessary first procedure. When the child is not able to cooperate the survey may be delayed until the second or even the third visit except in an emergency.
2. Explain procedures carefully; rehearse to show what is to be done; repeat instructions with each film placement.

B. Sequence

Make the easiest, most comfortable exposures first (extraoral, panoramic, occlusal).

C. Periapical Films: use film holder.

D. Use of a Lead Apron

Because of the size of the child, the gonads are closer to the sources of secondary radiation than with an adult.[41] A lead apron should be used (page 116).

EDENTULOUS SURVEY

I. Types of Surveys

Periapical, occlusal, and panoramic surveys have been used alone and together for edentulous patients. The periapical series, usually of 14 films, has been shown to be the most complete and accurate for diagnosis. Radiographic examination of an edentulous mouth is frequently used to detect residual pathology, foreign bodies, and retained teeth or root tips prior to denture construction.

In research to compare three techniques, panoramic, two occlusal films, one maxillary and one mandibular, and a 14-film periapical survey, total residual and potential pathology was found in 37 percent of the periapical surveys, 17 percent in the occlusal radiographs, and 31 percent in the panoramic.[42] A detailed review of the retained root tips in the same study proved that the occlusal films were of little value, whereas the periapical survey revealed 115 tips to only 71 in the panoramic.[43] The research makes it clear that panoramic and occlusal films by themselves cannot be relied upon to provide complete information.

II. Techniques for Periapical Survey

A. Film Placement

1. Paralleling technique. A film holder adjusted to provide a wider biting area is needed.
   a. Rubber bite block on a hemostat: turn bite block around so that the broader dimension is in the vertical plane.
   b. XCP holder can be padded with cotton rolls.[31]
2. Angle bisection technique. Use cotton rolls to aid in positioning the films and increase the angulation to accommodate flattened film.

B. Exposure Time. The time is reduced by approximately 25 percent.[31]

PARACLINICAL PROCEDURES

Supplemental to the chairside clinical procedures are the processing of the films and the mounting of radiographs for diagnostic and clinical use. Standard procedures are outlined in the following sections.

Film processing is the chemical transformation of the latent image, produced in a film emulsion by exposure to radiation, into a stable image visible by transmitted light. The usual procedure is basically a selective reduction of affected silver halide salts to metallic silver grains (development), followed by the selective removal of unaffected silver halide (fixation), washing to remove the processing chemicals, and drying.

CONVENTIONAL PROCESSING

Standardization of processing procedures goes hand in hand with standardized exposure techniques if consistently acceptable radiographs are to be prepared. Processing should be treated as an exacting chemical operation in which each step has specific objectives for the finished product. Fast and extra-fast film are even more sensitive to variations in temperature, light, and processing chemicals than medium and slow film formerly in general use, hence the need for fastidious attention to detail.

I. Essentials of an Adequate Darkroom

Cleanliness and orderliness are mandatory. Since the films are handled in near darkness, materials must be available at the fingertips and each piece of equipment kept in its own place.

The work area must be free from chemicals, water, dust, and other substances which can contaminate the film either by splashing or direct contact should a film touch the bench. The processing room should not be used as a storage room or for other dental procedures in which dust or fumes might be produced.

Convenience and ease in carrying out precision techniques can be provided through good planning for the location and arrangement of equipment.

A. Lighting

1. Darkroom completely void of white light.
   a. All possible light leaks found and eliminated.
   b. Do not use fluorescent overhead light because of afterglow.
2. Safelight[44]
   a. Standard film: Wratten Series 6 B filter with a 7.5-watt bulb placed four feet above the workbench top.
   b. Ester base film: ML-2 filter with a 15-watt bulb placed four feet above bench top.
3. Safe lighting test[45]
   a. Expose a periapical film under usual clinical circumstances.
   b. Unwrap film in totally dark darkroom.
   c. Place film on work tabletop and place a coin on the film.
   d. Turn on safelight and leave for maximum amount of time (such as 20 to 25 minutes) typical of that required when preparing several surveys to be processed together.
   e. Turn off safelight, remove coin, process film.
   f. Observe radiograph: if any evidence of light circle where coin was placed, the darkroom safelight is excessive.
4. Lock on door of darkroom; signal light on outside to show room in use.

B. Basic Equipment and Facilities

1. Tanks for developer and fixer with water bath between.
   a. Removable tanks made of stainless steel with joints welded and polished to prevent reactions with the processing chemicals.[45]
   b. Close-fitting, light-proof cover for tank.
   c. Stirring paddles identified specifically for developer and fixer.
   d. Water bath with connecting water flow and temperature control indicator.

e. Floating tank thermometer (kept in developer tank).
2. Workbench: covered with linoleum or Formica for easy cleaning.
3. Drying facilities: rod to hold hangers over drip pan; electric fan to facilitate drying.
4. Utility sink.
5. Interval timing clock.
6. Storage area beneath workbench for materials to change solutions.
7. Waste receiver: conveniently located for ready disposal of film wrappers to prevent losing films in midst of paper wrappers.

C. **Care of Solution**
1. Factors affecting life of solution.
   a. Original quality (care in preparation).
   b. Age.
   c. Care received (temperature, whether kept covered, contamination).
   d. Number of films processed.
2. Changing solutions: at least every three weeks.
3. Preparation of new solution.
   a. Tanks must be thoroughly scrubbed with water and a soft brush and then thoroughly rinsed.
   b. Label tanks as well as stirrers and mixing jars to prevent possibility of interchange.
   c. Follow manufacturer's specifications and directions precisely.

D. **Protection of Solution**
1. Use same position for tank cover so that same cover routinely is used for the same solution.
2. Purposes for covering tanks
   a. Prevent evaporation: which can change the concentration of the solutions and lower the level so the top film on rack is not covered during processing.
   b. Prevent oxidation: reduces useful life of solution.

c. Prevent contamination: dust, drippings.
3. Temperature: keep cool when not in use: heated solutions can oxidize rapidly.
4. Replenisher: between changing of solutions freshness may be maintained by replenishment according to manufacturer's specifications.

II. **Processing**

A. **Preparation**
1. Stir solutions and check temperature of solutions and water bath: all should be 68° F (20° C) (within 2°).
   a. Lower temperatures: chemical reactions too slow.
   b. Higher temperatures: cause fogging and may soften the emulsion.
2. Check cleanliness of workbench and film racks; wash hands to prevent film contamination.
3. Plan number of films to be processed so that facilities will not be overcrowded: films must hang individually out of possible contact with other films, sides of tanks, or wall in drying area.
4. Prepare labels for identification of radiographs.
5. Extinguish white lights; turn on safelight; lock door.
6. Load film hangers.
   a. Hold film by edges to avoid finger marks, scratches, or bending.
   b. Clip firmly: test by pulling gently on film.

B. **Developing**
1. Set timer. (Refer to time-temperature chart provided by the film manufacturer.*)

*The time-temperature method of processing is the only way to be assured of dependable results. Processing by the "visual inspection" method is not recommended because of the lack of standardization.

2. Completely immerse rack with films in developer; turn on timer.
3. Agitate racks (without splashing) to eliminate air bubbles and assure contact of solution with all film surfaces.
4. When timer rings, remove racks to water or to a stop bath.

C. **Rinsing**
   1. Immerse in freely running water for at least 30 seconds: agitate to provide contact of water with film.
   2. Stop bath: a 10 percent acetic acid may be preferred in place of running water: immerse for 30 to 45 seconds.
   3. Remove and drain for several seconds to prevent carrying an excess of water or acetic acid to the fixing bath.

D. **Fixing**
   1. Immerse completely; set and start timer.
   2. Agitate racks to remove air bubbles and assure contact of the solution with all parts of the film surfaces.
   3. Clearing time: time needed for complete disappearance of white or milky opaqueness.
   4. Total fixing time: minimum of twice clearing time.
      a. Check manufacturer's specifications.
      b. Minimum of ten minutes and maximum of one hour are safe; excess time will produce a light radiograph.
   5. Negatives may be viewed for limited time after clearing when needed for immediate use; return to fixer promptly for completion of fixing process.

E. **Washing**
   1. Place in running water bath for minimum of 20 minutes.
   2. Temperature: 68° F (20° C).

a. Too warm: gelatin will swell, thus hindering diffusion.
b. Drastic temperature changes cause reticulation (network of wrinkles or corrugations in the emulsion); retake necessary.

F. **Drying**
   1. Drain off water and place in dryer.
   2. Radiographs become brittle when left in a heated drying cabinet too long.

III. **How the Image Is Produced**

A. **The Chemistry of Processing**
   1. Film emulsion contains crystals of silver halides (bromide and iodine).
   2. X-ray exposure changes the silver halides to silver and halide ions.
   3. Developer reacts with the halide ions leaving only the metallic silver in a specific arrangement corresponding with the radiolucency and radiopacity of the tissue being radiographed.
   4. Fixer removes only those crystals of silver halide which were not affected by the action of the x rays. Fixer has no effect on the black metallic silver produced by the developer.
   5. End result: a negative showing various degrees of lightness and darkness (microscopic grains of black metallic silver).

B. **Developer Action**
   1. Purpose: to remove the halides from the metallic silver.
   2. Constituents
      a. Developing agents (reducers): *elon* brings out detail and *hydroquinone* reacts slowly and brings out contrast.
      b. Preservative: sodium sulfite: to protect the developing agents from oxidizing rapidly in air.
      c. Restrainer: potassium bromide: inhibits the fogging tendency of

the solution and slows the reaction of the reducers.

d. Activator (alkali): sodium carbonate: initiates the action of the reducers with the halides.

3. Transfer to water bath at completion of developing time: if racks are shaken or allowed to drip over the developer, the solution falling back into the tank will be highly oxidized which will shorten the life of the solution.

C. **Rinsing Purposes**

1. To stop the developing process.
2. To remove the developing solution from the emulsion to reduce carryover of alkaline developer to the acid fixing bath.
3. To preserve the acidity of the fixer and hence make a more efficient, longer-lasting fixing bath.

D. **Fixer Action**

1. Purpose: to remove the undeveloped halide salts.
2. Constituents
   a. Fixing agent: sodium thiosulfate ("hypo"): to dissolve the silver halides.
   b. Acidifier: acetic acid: to neutralize the alkali from the developer.
   c. Hardener: potassium alum: to shrink and harden the emulsion.
   d. Preservative: sodium sulfite: to counteract surface oxidation and stabilize the solution.

E. **Washing Purpose**

To remove residual chemicals from the negative.

AUTOMATIC AND ACCELERATED PROCESSING

Equipment which can provide accelerated or automatic processing (or both) is currently being researched and improved.[46,47] Available units are listed in the Guide to Dental Materials and Devices of the American Dental Association.[46]

I. Objectives and Advantages

Although cost and maintenance factors may be greater than with a traditional darkroom procedure, an automatic and/or rapid processing machine has advantages, including those listed below.

A. Time conservation by dental personnel.
B. Finished radiographs in from 1½ to 8 minutes depending on the machine used. Some have automatic dryers.
C. Consistency of results through automatic control of temperature, time and, in some machines, solution control with infrequent replenishment needed. Some machines require mixing and changing of solutions on a regular basis.
D. Available radiographs for immediate use during diagnosis, which is particularly important in emergencies, during endodontic therapy, and certain surgical procedures.

II. Principles of Operation

Automatic or accelerated processing (or both) is accomplished by one or a combination of the following:

A. **Automatic Film Transport.** Rollers or tracks are used to carry the film through developing, washing, and fixing, washing, and forced drying. Certain machines produce wet films and do not have hot-air drying chambers. The various machines available are built to carry different sizes of film. Some machines may process only standard intraoral films, while others may also accommodate extraoral sizes.
B. **High Temperature.** Increased temperature decreases processing time. Special solutions are needed for the rapid processors because with conven-

tional solutions the excess temperature causes deterioration and fogging of the film. Solution temperatures in the automatic and rapid processors may be from 62° to 100° F and with drying temperatures up to 150° F, the total processing and drying may be cut to 1½ minutes.

C. **Use of Special Films and Processing Solutions**
1. Concentrated processing solution. Solutions with increased chemical reactivity decrease developing time. In one type of machine, a combined developer–fixer is used which eliminates the need for film to pass through two solutions. The film diagnostic quality is less with the special solutions.[48]
2. Films. Films with special emulsions have been developed which process best at higher temperatures and with the special processing solutions.

D. **Agitation.** Mechanically controlled movement of the film and/or movement of the solution is built into some units to provide fresh solution continuously at the film surface. This decreases the processing time.

ANALYSIS OF COMPLETED RADIOGRAPHS

The completed radiographs are mounted and examined at a viewbox or other adequate light source. The characteristics of the acceptable finished radiograph (page 109) serve as a basis for analysis. Nothing less than the ideal should satisfy, and errors must be studied in order to improve techniques for future surveys. Interpretation of radiographs is difficult for the dentist and the determination of pathology requires keen evaluation, but to attempt to base interpretation on inadequate, insufficient radiographs is guesswork rather than true, timely diagnosis.

I. Mounting
A. Legibly mark the mount with the name of patient, date, name of dentist: printing preferred.
B. Handle radiographs only by the edges with clean, dry hands, or wear clean cotton gloves.
C. Keep films clean, free from dust, liquids or other contaminants.
D. Place a clean, dry towel or paper in front of the illuminator where mounting is to be done; arrange radiographs on this, or mount one by one directly as they are removed from the rack.
E. The embossed dot near the edge of the negative is the guide to mounting: the depressed side of the dot is on the lingual.
F. Identify individual negatives by the teeth and other anatomic landmarks.
G. Approved mounting system[49]: looking at the teeth from outside the mouth, the teeth are viewed and mounted in the same manner as the approved numbering system (figure III–1, page 60).

II. Anatomic Landmarks
A. **Definition**

An anatomic landmark is an anatomical structure the image of which may serve as an aid in the localization and identification of the regions portrayed by a radiograph. The teeth are the primary landmarks.

B. **Landmarks Which May Be Seen in the Individual Radiographs**
1. Maxillary molar: maxillary sinus, zygomatic process, zygomatic (malar) bone, hamular process, coronoid process of the mandible, maxillary tuberosity.
2. Maxillary premolar: maxillary sinus.

3. Maxillary canine: maxillary sinus, junction of the maxillary sinus and nasal fossa (Y–shaped, radiopaque).
4. Maxillary incisors: incisive foramen, nasal septum and fossae, anterior nasal spine (V–shaped), median palatine suture, symphysis of the maxillae.
5. Mandibular molar: mandibular canal, internal oblique line, external oblique ridge, mylohyoid ridge.
6. Mandibular premolar: mental foramen.
7. Mandibular incisors: lingual foramen, mental ridge, genial tubercles, symphysis of the mandible. Nutrient canals are seen most frequently in this radiograph.

III. Identification of Inadequacies in Radiographs

Inadequacies are related to film placement, angulation, exposure, processing, care and handling of the film, and, indeed, any step in the entire procedure. Errors appear as problems of inadequate density, contrast, incomplete or distorted images, fogging, artifacts, or stains. Table 9–2 outlines the more common inadequacies and their causes, the keys to correction.

IV. Interpretation

Radiographs are used in conjunction with clinical examination for a complete program of treatment. Periodic radiographs permit continuing evaluation. As part of the permanent record, radiographs help to document the oral condition for comparative purposes as well as legal.

The quality of the radiographs determines their usability for diagnostic interpretation. Techniques for the preparation of radiographs must be perfected in order that radiographs have maximum interpretability with minimum radiation exposure of the patient.

A. **Prerequisites for Interpretation**
1. Mounting. Mount radiographs in an opaque mount to prevent light between each radiograph from creating glare and producing a blinding effect.
2. Viewbox. Use an adequately lighted viewbox. Dimmed room light improves visibility for contrasting radiolucent and radiopaque areas. Holding the radiographs up to view by window, room, or unit light is very inadequate and only gross interpretation can be accomplished. When a viewbox is larger than the mount used, cover the edges to block out peripheral light.
3. Hand magnifying glass. Examine radiographs on a viewbox through a magnifying glass. Viewboxes are available which have a built-on magnifying glass.

B. **Systematic Examination**
1. Observe one radiographic feature at a time. Examine all of the radiographs for that feature, rather than taking each radiograph separately to find everything. It is important to note comparisons for each change over the entire survey.
2. When examining a particular tooth, compare the appearance of that tooth in each radiograph where it appears, including bite-wings. At different angulations different findings may become apparent.

C. **Coordination with Clinical Examination**

A description of radiographic examination of the teeth may be found on page 216, and of the periodontal tissues on page 202. Correlation of radiographic findings with the clinical examination, using probe and explorer, is basic to an understanding of the true oral condition of the patient.

Table 9-2. Analysis of Radiographs: Causes of Inadequacies

Inadequacy	*Cause: Factors in Correction*
Image	
Elongation	Insufficient vertical angulation
Foreshortening	Excessive vertical angulation
Superimposition (overlapping)	Incorrect horizontal angulation (central ray not directed through interproximal)
Partial Image	Cone-cut (incorrect direction of central ray or incorrect film placement)
	Incompletely immersed in processing tank
	Film touched other film or side of tank during processing
Blurred or Double Image	Patient, tube, or packet movement during exposure
	Film exposed twice
Stretched Appearance of Trabeculae or Apices	Bent film
No Image	Machine misfunction from time switch to wall plug
	Failure to turn on the machine
	Film placed in fixer before developed
Density	
Too Dark	Excessive exposure
	Excessive developing
	Developer too warm
	Unsafe safelight
	Accidental exposure to white light (may be completely black)
Too Light	Insufficient exposure
	Insufficient development or excessive fixation
	Too cool solutions
	Use of old, contaminated, or poorly mixed solutions
	Film placement: leaded side toward teeth
	Films used beyond expiration date
Fog	
Chemical Fog	Imbalance or deterioration of processing solutions
Light Fog	Unintentional exposure to light to which the emulsion is sensitive, either before or during processing.
	(1) Unsafe safelight
	(2) Darkroom leak
Radiation Fog	Improper film storage of unused film and exposed film prior to processing
Reticulation (puckered or pebbly surface)	Sudden temperature changes during processing, particularly from warm solutions to very cold water

Table 9–2, *continued*

Inadequacy	Cause: Factors in Correction
Artifacts	

Dark Lines	Bent or creased film
	Static electricity
	  (1) Film removed from wrapper with excessive force
	  (2) Wrapper sticking to film when opened with wet fingers or if there was excessive moisture from patient's mouth
	Fingernail used to grasp film during opening

Herringbone Pattern (light film)	Packet placed in mouth backwards with foil next to teeth
Stains and Spots	Unclean film hanger Splatterings of developer, fixer, dust Finger marks Insufficient rinsing after developing before fixing Splashing dry negatives with water or solutions Air bubbles adhering to surface during processing (insufficient agitation) Overlap of film on film in tanks or while drying Paper wrapper stuck to film (film not dried when removed from patient's mouth)
Discoloration at later date after storage of completed radiographs	Incomplete processing or rinsing Storage in too warm a place Storage near chemicals

TECHNICAL HINTS

I. Never Hold a Film in a Patient's Mouth During Exposure

II. Inquire If the Patient Is Receiving Radiation Treatment

It may be necessary to minimize the number of exposures. The patient's physician should be consulted.

III. Film Placement

Dot on film packet is placed toward the occlusal or incisal to prevent superimposition of the embossed dot on the negative from appearing over the image.

IV. Check State Radiation Protection Laws

Many states have regulations concerning x-ray unit registration, inspection, safety requirements, and limitations for use of x rays.[50]

V. Record in Patient's Permanent Record

When a patient refuses to have radiographs made, record this in the patient's permanent record. Obtain patient's signature to a statement indicating such refusal in the event a legal issue should arise related to an operation performed.

VI. Who Owns Dental Radiographs?

They are part of the dentist's record and remain his property the same as other parts of the case record.[51] The first rule is to never give radiographs to a patient. If they are to be loaned to another dentist, they should be sent or delivered directly, preferably with a letter indicating, if known, when they will next be needed and should be returned. Conservatism should be exercised in loaning radiographs to other dentists. As a part of valuable permanent records, it is never known when they will be needed as evidence of the careful diagnosis and treatment provided.

VII. Film Storage

Film should always be stored in a clean, dry place. Keep in lead-lined container. Watch expiration dates. Store oldest film in front for next use. Purchase as needed, not in excess quantity.

VIII. Study Informational Sheets

It is important to study the informational sheets provided in package of film. This applies particularly when a new brand of film is being used.

IX. Stain Removal from Clothes

A. Do not launder before spot removal.
B. **Commercially Prepared Spot Removers.** (Available from dental supply companies.)
C. **Removal of Spots in Nylon Materials**[52]
   1. Prepare solution containing
      Sodium hypochlorite ½ oz. 15 cc
      (5% solution)
      (household bleach)
      Acetic acid   ½ oz. 15 cc
      (5% solution)
      (household vinegar)
      Water at about 100° F 1 gal (3.8 liters)
      (38° C)
   2. Soak the stained portion in the solution for five to ten minutes, then soak in *fresh* fixer.
   3. Rinse thoroughly in plain water. Dry.

X. X-ray Film Contamination by Stannous Fluoride

Stannous fluoride can cause artifacts on the finished radiograph. When radiographs are to be made following a topical application of stannous fluoride solution, it is recommended that citric acid be used for washing the hands. Stannous fluoride contamination of the hands is impossible to remove by ordinary handwashing procedures.[53]

XI. Radiopaque Polishing Agent

Zircate residue at the gingival margin will appear as a thin (white) opaque line in radiographs taken soon after polishing, in spite of rinsing or spraying. The microfine particles of metallic oxide in Zircate are radiopaque.[54]

FACTORS TO TEACH THE PATIENT

I. When the Patient Asks About the Safety of Radiation

A. Adapt the answer to the patient. Certain patients will have more fear; others will have more knowledge about x rays. If the hygienist expresses confidence this will aid in allaying fears. Hesitation will increase the patient's doubt.
B. Radiographs are essential to diagnosis and treatment. Without the information provided, the dentist can only guess at conditions not visible to him.
C. The benefits resulting from the intelligent use of x rays outweigh any possible negative effects.
D. Modern x-ray machines are equipped for safety. For the patient who will understand, details about filtration, collimation, film speed, and short exposure times can be explained.
E. It has never been shown that any harm has resulted to a patient from the small amount of x ray from dental sources. Exposure is distributed to different areas and the amount to any one area is small.
F. When the patient understands ionizing radiation, it may be important to explain more concerning the effects.

II. Educational Features in Dental Radiographs

(Avoid diagnosis. For teaching, it may be advisable to use radiographs of someone other than the patient.)
A. Position of unerupted permanent teeth in relation to primary teeth.
B. Detection of early carious lesions not visible in clinical examination.
C. Effects of loss of teeth and the importance of having replacements.
D. Periodontal changes and other pathology appropriate to education of individual patient.

References

1. American Dental Association, Council on Dental Materials and Devices: *Guide to Dental Materials and Devices*, 7th ed. Chicago, American Dental Association, 1974–1975, pp. 142–144.
2. Statement of the American Academy of Oral Roentgenology's Stand Regarding the Use of X-rays in Dentistry, *Oral Surg., 15*, 1350, November, 1962.
3. Glenner, R. A.: 80 Years of Dental Radiography, *J. Am. Dent. Assoc., 90*, 549, March, 1975.
4. Ennis, L. M.: Resumé of Roentgenology (Henry Cline Fixott, Sr. Memorial Lecture), *Oral Surg., 15*, 680, June, 1962.
5. Wuehrmann, A. H. and Manson-Hing, L. R.: *Dental Radiology*, 3rd ed. St. Louis, Mosby, 1973, pp. 4–15.
6. Langland, O. E. and Sippy, F. H.: *Textbook of Dental Radiography*. Springfield, Charles C Thomas, 1973, pp. 11–35.
7. Stafne, E. C.: *Oral Roentgenographic Diagnosis*, 3rd ed. Philadelphia, Saunders, 1969, pp. 387–397.
8. General Electric, Technical Services X-ray Department: *X-ray Generation and Radiographic Principles in Dentistry*. Milwaukee, Pub. 13–3549B.
9. American Dental Association, Council on Dental Materials and Devices: op. cit., pp. 130–138, 237–238.
10. Wuehrmann and Manson-Hing: op. cit., pp. 35–50, 73–78.
11. National Council on Radiation Protection and Measurements: *Dental X-ray Protection*. NCRP Report No. 35, Issued March 9, 1970.
12. American Dental Association, Council on Dental Materials and Devices: American Dental Association Specification No. 22 for Intraoral Dental Radiographic Film, in *Guide to Dental Materials and Devices*, 7th ed. Chicago, American Dental Association, 1974–1975, p. 237.
13. Stafne: op. cit., pp. 411–416.
14. Langland and Sippy: op. cit., pp. 85–98.
15. Weissman, D. D. and Sobkowski, F. J.: Comparative Thermoluminescent Dosimetry of Intraoral Periapical Radiography, *Oral Surg., 29*, 376, March, 1970.
16. Winkler, K. G.: Influence of Rectangular Collimation and Intraoral Shielding on Radiation Dose in Dental Radiography, *J. Am. Dent. Assoc., 77*, 95, July, 1968.
17. Richards, A. G.; New Method for Reduction of Gonadal Irradiation of Dental Patients, *J. Am. Dent. Assoc., 65*, 1, July, 1962.
18. Ice, R. D., Updegrave, W. J., and Bogucki, E. I.: Influence of Dental Radiographic Cones on Radiation Exposure, *J. Am. Dent. Assoc., 83*, 1297, December, 1971.
19. Glaze, S. and White, S. C.; Interpatient Microbiological Cross-contamination Via Dental X-ray Machines, *I.A.D.R. Program and Abstracts of Papers*, February, 1974, p. 214.
20. Langland and Sippy: op. cit., pp. 166–169.
21. Park, J. K.: Radiographic Technique in the Contour Dental Chair, *J. Am. Dent. Hyg. Assoc., 46*, 351, September-October, 1972.
22. Venokur, P. C., Einbender, S., and Myers, B. S.: Modified X-ray Technique for Dentistry with Patients in the Supine Position, *Oral Surg., 38*, 148, July, 1974.
23. Baum, A. T. and Morgan, E.: Reduction of X-ray Dose by Variable Rectangular Collimation and Reflex Optical Direction of Dental X-ray Beams and by Supine Position of the Patient, *J. Am. Dent. Assoc., 85*, 1091, November, 1972.
24. Eastman Kodak Company: *X-rays in Dentistry*. Rochester, Eastman Kodak, 1972, pp. 42–53.
25. Stafne: op. cit., pp. 330–341.
26. Anderson, P. C.: *Dental Radiology*. Albany, Delmar, 1974, pp. 46–55.
27. American Dental Association, Council on Dental Materials and Devices: op. cit., p. 134, 274.
28. American Dental Association, Council on Dental Materials and Devices: List of Classified Dental Materials and Devices Revised to Jan. 1, 1975, *J. Am. Dent. Assoc., 90*, 181, January, 1975.
29. American Dental Association, Council on Dental Materials and Devices: Preliminary Report on Radiographic Holding, Paralleling, and Shielding Devices, *J. Am. Dent. Assoc., 77*, 884, October, 1968.
30. STABE Disposable Dental Film Holder, Greene Dental Products, Inc., 12801 Arroyo Street, San Fernando, California 91342.
31. *Utilization of the Extension Cone Paralleling, Bisecting Angle and Interproximal Techniques with Rinn Instruments*, Elgin, Illinois, Rinn Corporation, 1975, 51 pp.
32. Eastman Kodak Company: op. cit., pp. 16–29.
33. Anderson: op. cit., pp. 23–26.
34. Stafne: op. cit., pp. 352–357.
35. Eastman Kodak Company: op. cit., pp. 34–41.
36. Manson-Hing, L. R.: Evaluation of Radiographic Techniques, including Pantomography, *J. Am. Dent. Assoc., 87*, 145, July, 1973.
37. American Dental Association, Council on Dental Materials and Devices, van Aken, J.: Panoramic X-ray Equipment, *J. Am. Dent. Assoc., 86*, 1050, May, 1973.
38. Wuehrmann and Manson-Hing: op. cit., pp. 157–169.
39. Phillips, J. E.: Panoramic Radiography, *Dent. Clin. North Am.*, p. 561, November, 1968.
40. Eastman Kodak Company: op. cit., pp. 66–72.
41. Yale, S. H., Moos, W. S., and Videka, M. A.: Measurement of Gonadal Dose in Children during Intraoral Radiography, *Oral Surg., 13*, 1081, September, 1960.
42. Scandrett, F. R., Tebo, H. G., Miller, J. T., and Quigley, M. B.: Radiographic Examination of the Edentulous Patient. Part I. Review of the Literature and Preliminary Report Comparing Three Methods, *Oral Surg., 35*, 266, February, 1973.

43. Scandrett, F. R., Tebo, H. G., Quigley, M. B., and Miller, J. T.: Radiographic Examination of the Edentulous Patient, *Oral Surg.,* 35, 872, June, 1973.
44. American Dental Association, Council on Dental Materials and Devices: op. cit., pp. 137–138.
45. Wuehrmann and Manson-Hing: op. cit., pp. 173–174.
46. American Dental Association, Council on Dental Materials and Devices: op. cit., pp. 139–141.
47. Kilpatrick, H. C.: Auxiliary Equipment for Dental Practitioners, *Dent. Clin. North. Am.,* 15, 183, January, 1971.
48. Pestritto, S. T., Anderson, S. J., and Braselton, J. A.: Comparison of Diagnostic Quality of Dental Radiographs Produced by Five Rapid Processing Techniques, *J. Am. Dent. Assoc.,* 89, 353, August, 1974.
49. American Dental Association: System of Tooth Numbering and Radiograph Mounting, Approved by the American Dental Association House of Delegates, October, 1968.
50. American Dental Association, Councils on Legislation, Dental Research, and Dental Materials and Devices: Radiation Hygiene and Practice in Dentistry: State Regulation of Dental X Rays, *J. Am. Dent. Assoc.,* 76, 107, January, 1968.
51. Langland and Sippy: op. cit., p. 333.
52. Anderson: op. cit., p. 83.
53. Yamane, G. M., Meskin, L. H., and Mehaffey, P.: Stannous Ion Contamination of Radiographic Films. Etiology and Prevention, *J. Am. Dent. Hyg. Assoc.,* 42, 147, 3rd Quarter, 1968.
54. Fowler, A.: Letter to the Editor, *J. Am. Dent. Hyg. Assoc.,* 46, 412, November-December, 1972.

Suggested Readings

Alcox, R. W. and Jameson, W. R.: Patient Exposures from Intraoral Radiographic Examinations, *J. Am. Dent. Assoc.,* 88, 568, March, 1974.
American Academy of Oral Roentgenology, Radiation Protection Committee: The Effective Use of X-ray Radiation in Dentistry, *Oral Surg.,* 16, 294, March, 1963.
American Dental Association, Council on Dental Materials and Devices: New American Dental Association Specification No. 26 for Dental X-ray Equipment, *J. Am. Dent. Assoc.,* 89, 386, August, 1974.
Bean, L. R. and Devore, W. D.: Effect of Protective Aprons in Dental Roentgenography, *Oral Surg.,* 28, 505, October, 1969.
Calvert, K. and Carmichael, C.: Open-end Lead-lined Dental X-ray Cones, *Oral Surg.,* 23, 328, March, 1967.
Colon, P. G.: The Short and Long of It—X-rays, *Dent. Hyg.,* 48, 341, November-December, 1974.

Evans, M. R.: Dental Roentgenology, in Richardson, R. E., Barton, R. E., and Brauer, J. C., eds.: *The Dental Assistant,* 4th ed. New York, McGraw-Hill, 1970, pp. 376–404.
National Council on Radiation Protection and Measurements: *Basic Radiation Protection Criteria.* NCRP Report No. 39, Issued January 15, 1971. National Council on Radiation Protection and Measurements, 4201 Connecticut Avenue, N.W., Washington, D.C. 20008.
Richards, A. G.: Sources of X-Radiation in the Dental Office, *Dent. Radiogr. Photogr.,* 37, 51, No. 3, 1964.
Richards, A. G.: New Concepts in Dental X-ray Machines, *J. Am. Dent. Assoc.,* 73, 69, July, 1966.
Richards, A. G.: Questions and Answers: Radiation Exposure, *J. Am. Dent. Assoc.,* 76, 237, February, 1968.
Updegrave, W. J.: Simplified and Standardized Intraoral Radiography with Reduced Tissue Irradiation, *J. Am. Dent. Assoc.,* 85, 861, October, 1972.
Wuehrmann, A. H.: Procedure for Lining Open-end Dental X-ray Cylinders with Lead Foil, *Oral Surg.,* 30, 64, July, 1970.
Wuehrmann, A. H.: Evaluation Criteria for Intraoral Radiographic Film Quality, *J. Am. Dent. Assoc.,* 89, 345, August, 1974.

Children

Bachman, L. H.: Pedodontic Radiography, *Dent. Radiogr. Photogr.,* 44, 51, No. 3, 1971.
Bean, L. R. and Isaac, H. K.: X-ray and the Child Patient, *Dent. Clin. North Am.,* 17, 13, January, 1973.
Khanna, S. L. and Harrop, T. J.: A Five-Film Oral Radiographic Survey for Children, *J. Dent. Child.,* 40, 42, January-February, 1973.
Silha, R. E.: The Versatile Occlusal Dental X-ray Film. Part III. A New Pedodontic Survey, *Dent. Radiogr. Photogr.,* 39, 40, No. 2, 1966.
Silha, R. E.: Special Radiographic Surveys, *Dent. Radiogr. Photogr.,* 45, 23, No. 2, 1972.

Panoramic Radiography

Jerman, A. C., Kinsley, E. L., and Morris, C. R.: Absorbed Radiation from Panoramic Plus Bitewing Exposures vs Full-Mouth Periapical Plus Bitewing Exposures, *J. Am. Dent. Assoc.,* 86, 420, February, 1973.
Johnson, C. C.: Analysis of Panoramic Survey, *J. Am. Dent. Assoc.,* 81, 151, July, 1970.
Langland, O. E. and Sippy, F. H.: *Textbook of Dental Radiography.* Springfield, Charles C Thomas, 1973, pp. 306–326.
Smith, C. J. and Fleming, R. D.: A Comprehensive Review of Normal Anatomic Landmarks and Artifacts as Visualized on Panorex Radiographs, *Oral Surg.,* 37, 291, February, 1974.
Updegrave, W. J.: The Role of Panoramic Radiography in Diagnosis, *Oral Surg.,* 22, 49, July, 1966.
Weissman, D. D. and Longhurst, G. E.: Comparative Absorbed Doses in Periapical Radiography. II Panorex, *Oral Surg.,* 33, 661, April, 1972.

Chapter 10

Study Casts

As accurate reproductions of the teeth, gingiva, and adjacent structures, study casts can be useful and frequently indispensable adjuncts in the care of the patient. The study casts, radiographs, and clinical examination with recordings and chartings, together with the medical and dental histories, are utilized in the diagnosis, total treatment planning, treatment, and subsequent maintenance through recall by the dentist and the dental hygienist.

I. Purposes and Uses of Study Casts

A. To serve as a permanent record of the patient's present condition.
B. To give sharper delineation and corroboration of the observations made during the oral inspection.
C. To observe normal conditions, the variations of and departures from the normal at the outset of treatment, and, by comparison with subsequent periodic casts, to compare and evaluate certain aspects of treatment.
D. During charting of the teeth to record missing teeth, anomalies of size, shape, or number, partial eruption, tooth positions such as drifting, tilting, and open or closed spacing, and other factors.
E. During inspection of the occlusion to observe the static relations (Angle's classification, malrelations of groups of teeth, and malpositions of individual teeth; pages 225–227) and other features such as wear patterns and the effects of premature loss of teeth.
F. During periodontal charting to record anatomic features such as the position, size, and shape of the gingiva and interdental papillae, and the position of freni.
G. To be an effective visual aid to use when the oral conditions are explained and the dental and dental hygiene treatment plan is presented; to enable the patient to visualize and understand the need for the specific care outlined.
H. To serve as a guide to clinical treatment procedures.
I. To supplement clinical observations in the selection of an oral disease and plaque control program for the patient's own treatment, and to serve as a visual aid in teaching aims and procedures of the recommended measures to the patient.

II. Terms Used*

A. **Cast** (Also called a model): Positive likeness of some desired form.

B. **Study Cast or Diagnostic Cast:** Positive likeness of dental structures.

C. **Impression:** Imprint or negative likeness which becomes the mold or form in which the cast is produced.

D. **Interocclusal Record:** A record of the positional relation of the teeth to each other.

III. Steps in the Preparation of Study Casts

The steps noted here are detailed in the sections following.

A. **Clinical Procedures**
   1. Assemble materials and equipment.
   2. Prepare the patient.
   3. Select and prepare the impression trays.
   4. Make the mandibular impression.
   5. Make the maxillary impression.
   6. Make the interocclusal record for occluding the casts.

B. **Paraclinical Procedures**
   1. Assemble materials and equipment.
   2. Prepare the impressions for pouring.
   3. Pour the casts.
   4. Trim and finish the casts.
   5. Polish the casts.

CLINICAL PROCEDURES

The need for and uses of study casts are explained to the patient when the steps in diagnosis and treatment planning are outlined. As with any procedure not familiar to a patient, an explanation is in order. The reactions of patients who have

*Definitions are taken or adapted from and in accord with the *Glossary of Prosthodontic Terms*, third edition, 1968, edited by the Nomenclature Committee of the Academy of Denture Prosthetics, J. C. Hickey, C. O. Boucher, and G. A. Hughes. Additional definitions to those included in this chapter may be found in the Glossary, page 741.

had an impression made previously may range from indifference to dread, and the dental hygienist will direct the conversation and approach accordingly.

When the radiographic survey has been made for the new patient prior to the study casts, it will have been determined as to whether precautions to prevent gagging require special application. With all patients, a calm approach, an exhibition of confidence, a direct and efficient procedure, and a gentle handling of the patient's oral tissues will increase rapport and contribute to a satisfactory result.

I. Assemble Materials and Equipment

A. Coverall (plastic drape), towel, and mouthwash.

B. Impression Trays
   1. Perforated type generally used: small, medium, and large sizes are available.
   2. Care of trays: for use in the patient's mouth, trays must be clean, shiny, and sterilized.

C. Mixing bowl: clean, dry, flexible rubber or plastic with smooth, unscratched surface.

D. Spatula: clean, dry, stiff, with a smooth, rounded end that will reach every part of the bowl without scraping or cutting its surface.

E. Saliva ejector.

F. Dental materials
   1. Wax for preparation of tray rim: soft utility wax.
   2. Alginate: irreversible hydrocolloid.

G. Water thermometer.

II. Prepare the Patient

A. **Brief Explanation of Procedure**

B. **Drape the Patient**
   Drape patient with a protective coverall and towel.

C. **Inspect the Oral Cavity**
   Note labially and buccally displaced teeth, height of palate, undercut areas,

mandibular tori, and other factors which may influence the size or preparation of the impression tray and the procedures to be carried out during impression making.

D. **Free the Mouth of Debris**
1. Spray proximal areas; use dental floss.
2. When there is excess, tenacious debris, plaque control instruction should be started so that debris and plaque can be removed during brushing by the patient.
3. When impressions are made at an initial appointment, and the dentist requests that gross deposits be removed prior to making the impression, the patient's medical history must be reviewed and cleared with respect to systemic problems which may require special procedures before instrumentation such as antibiotic premedication (page 71).

E. **Request Patient to Rinse with Mouthwash.**
1. To aid in the removal of saliva and debris and lessen the numbers of surface microorganisms.
2. To lower the surface tension; aids in preventing bubbles in the impression.
3. To provide a pleasant taste and feeling for the patient.
4. To distract an anxious patient while the trays are being prepared.

F. **Dry the Teeth**
   Use a cotton roll or compressed air stream to reduce bubbles.

G. **Prevention of Gagging**
1. Approach with confidence to reassure the patient.
2. Work as quickly and efficiently as possible.
3. Use a topical anesthetic (page 511).
   a. Cold water or an ice cube held in the mouth has some anesthetic effect.
   b. Salt: a small amount (¼ teaspoon) on the tongue to swallow just before the tray is to be inserted may relieve tissue reactions.
   c. Apply topical anesthetic to posterior palatal area, or patient may rinse with a commercial topical agent. A spray topical preparation is contraindicated because of proximity to throat where coughing may be initiated.
4. Technique considerations
   a. Avoid excessive impression material in the tray.
   b. Seat the maxillary tray from posterior to anterior as described in section VI, E, 3 (page 151).
   c. Instruct patient to breathe deeply through his nose before the tray is inserted and to continue after insertion; bring head forward.

III. **Preparation of the Impression Tray**

A. **Try-in for Selection of Proper Size and Shape**
1. *Width*
   a. Objectives: to allow an adequate thickness of impression material on the facial and lingual of each tooth to provide strength and rigidity to the impression.
   b. Tray flanges may be spread to accommodate for extra width in the molar regions, particularly lingual to the mandibular molars in the mylohyoid region.
   c. When a tooth is in marked labio-, bucco-, or linguoversion, a minimum thickness of ⅛ to ¼ inch is suggested, but even then the fragility of the impression material in that area is increased.
   d. The tray that is too wide may appear in correct relation to the

facial surfaces but may impinge on the lingual cusps of molars.

2. *Length*
   a. Objective: to allow coverage of the retromolar area of the mandibular and the tuberosity of the maxilla.
   b. Anteriorly there should be at least ¼ inch clearance labial to the most protruded incisor without impingement on lingual gingiva.

3. *Maxillary Tray Try-in*
   a. Operator position: side back of patient (11:00, figure 5–5, page 53).
   b. With left index finger, retract the patient's left lip and cheek.
   c. At the same time, use the side of the tray (carried by right thumb on top of handle and fingers under) to distend the right side of the patient's mouth to gain entry (figure 10–1).
   d. With a rotary motion, insert the tray.
   e. Orient the tray beneath the arch and center it using the tray handle and the midline (usually between the central incisors and in line with the middle of the nose) as guides for positioning.

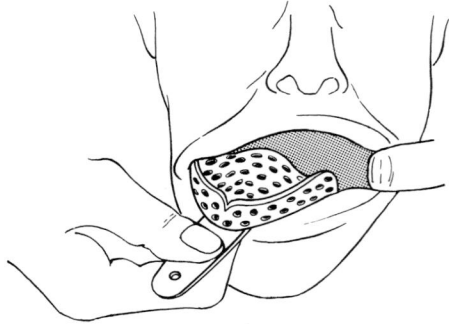

Figure 10–1. Maxillary impression tray insertion. The patient's left lip and cheek are retracted while the side of the tray is used to distend the right lip and cheek to gain entry. The tray is inserted with a rotary motion. The procedure for the mandibular tray insertion is similar.

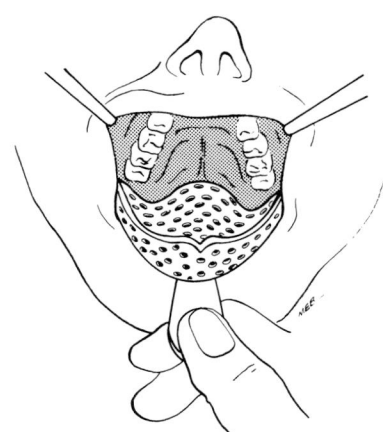

Figure 10–2. Selection of impression tray. To determine adequate coverage, the posterior border of the tray is held in position while the front of the tray is lowered to observe the relationship of the posterior border to the maxillary tuberosity areas which are to be covered by the impression. The mandibular tray position is examined similarly by lifting the tray to observe coverage of the retromolar areas.

   f. Bring the front of the tray to a position ¼ inch labial to the most labially inclined incisor.
   g. Seat the tray by bringing the posterior up before the anterior; retract the lip as the anterior is brought into place.
   h. Evaluate the size of the tray: gently lower the front of the tray while holding the posterior border in place (figure 10–2) and examine the relationship of the posterior border to the most posterior molars and the tuberosity areas to determine whether there will be ample coverage. By moving the tray up and down it is possible to observe the relation to the facial surfaces of all teeth, malaligned teeth, protuberances, and other features to assay the space allowed for the impression material.

4. *Mandibular Tray Try-in*
   a. Operator position: in front of patient (7:30 to 8:00, figure 5–5, page 53).

b. With left index and middle fingers, retract the patient's right lip and cheek.

c. At the same time, use the side of the tray (carried by right thumb and fingers) to distend the left side of the mouth to gain entry, similar to the procedure illustrated in figure 10–1 for the maxillary tray.

d. With a rotary motion insert the tray.

e. Orient the tray over the dental arch and center it using the tray handle and the midline (usually between the central incisors and in line with the center of the chin) as guides for positioning.

f. Bring the tray rim to about ¼ inch anterior to the most labially positioned incisor; instruct the patient to raise the tongue to permit the lingual flange of the tray to pass by the lateral borders of the tongue without interference.

g. As the tray is lowered, retract the cheeks in the posterior regions to make certain the buccal mucosa is not caught beneath the edge of the tray; hold the lip out to ascertain that there is clearance to the base of the vestibule.

h. Evaluate the size of the tray: lift the tray handle while keeping the posterior in position, similar to the procedure illustrated in figure 10–2 for the maxillary, to determine whether there will be ample coverage posteriorly to include the retromolar areas, and laterally to allow for ¼ inch thickness of impression material on the facial and lingual aspects of the teeth.

5. Reselect larger or smaller trays as indicated and repeat try-in; when in doubt, the larger tray is used rather than the smaller.

B. **Application of Wax Rim around Borders of Trays (Beading)**

1. *Purposes*

a. To position the loaded trays without the metal rims causing discomfort to the soft tissues.

b. To seat the vestibular periphery firmly into position with reduced pressure on the displaced tissues.

c. To prevent penetration of the incisal or occlusal surfaces through the impression material and thus prevent a defective cast.

d. To provide a slight undercut at the rim as an aid in the retention of the alginate in the tray during placement and removal.

e. To create a posterior palatal seal to aid in preventing excess material from passing into the throat.

2. *Procedure*

a. Attach a strip of soft utility wax firmly around the entire periphery of each tray (figure 10–3).

b. Mandibular tray: add extra layers from canine to canine labially and notch the wax, to fit about the labial frenum.

c. Maxillary tray

(1) Add extra layers as needed to extend the tray into the vestibule above the anterior teeth and notch the wax to fit about the labial frenum (figure 10–4).

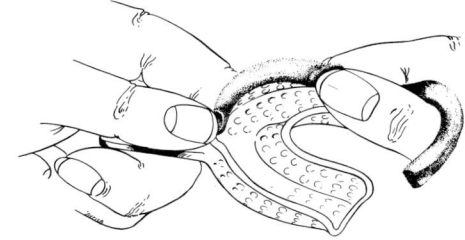

Figure 10–3. Beading the tray. A strip of soft utility wax is applied around the periphery of each tray.

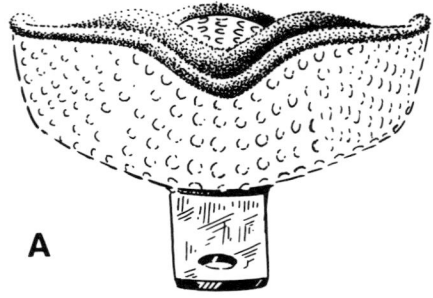

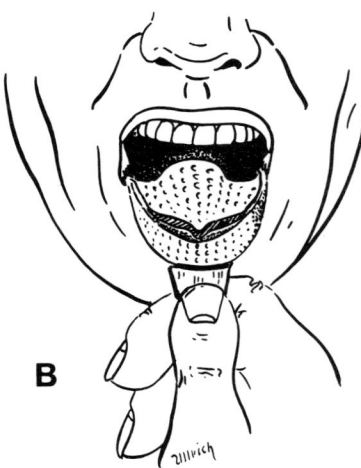

Figure 10–4. **A.** Tray with double layer of beading wax about the labial frenum. The extra wax extends the tray, protects the soft tissue from the metal rim, and provides a more complete impression of the area. **B.** Try-in after beading. The wax should contact all borders of the mucous membrane, displace the soft tissue outward, and prevent the teeth from contacting the tray.

of a mouth mirror for lingual areas; hold the tray in position.

e. Characteristics of the completed molding: when the tray is held firmly, the wax will contact all borders of the mucous membrane, will displace the soft tissue outward and upward, and the teeth will not touch the tray.

IV. The Impression Material

A. **Factors Related to the Impression Material Which Contribute to a Satisfactory Impression**

Texts on dental materials should be reviewed for complete information about the irreversible hydrocolloids.[1,2,3,4] American Dental Association Specification No. 18 applies to the requirements expected for an approved product.[5] Some of the pertinent properties related to the clinical procedures essential to making an accurate impression are listed here.

1. *Powder.* The alginate material deteriorates on standing, particularly at higher temperatures and humidity.
   a. Keep metal container tightly closed; store in a cool place.
   b. Use individually sealed packages except when large numbers of impressions are made regularly; powder is preweighed for the packages and measuring is less accurate than weighing; heat and moisture are eliminated.
   c. Individual package may be refrigerated in hot weather provided the powder is used immediately on opening. If left exposed, water condenses on the powder. The bulk container cannot be refrigerated for that reason.

2. *Water.* Temperature controls gelation time.

(2) Apply extra thickness across the posterior palatal seal area.

(3) When a patient has a high palatal vault, apply extra wax to support the impression material in that area.

d. Try the rimmed trays in the mouth and examine by retraction of the lips and cheeks and by use

a. At room temperature (68–70° F, 20–21° C), an ideal gelation time between three to four minutes provides adequate working time.

b. Temperature of the water should be measured with a thermometer at the time of mixing.

c. Control in hot humid weather: use cooler water and refrigerate the bowl and spatula.

3. *Strength and quality of the set impression* depend on:

a. Powder-water ratio accurately weighed and measured.

b. Spatulation (one minute) to allow chemical reactions to proceed uniformly.

c. Holding the impression material in position for an optimum period (two clocked minutes after the mix on the spatula has lost its stickiness). The elasticity of most alginates improves with time, therefore a superior reproduction can be obtained by waiting; distortion can result when the impression is left in the mouth too long.

4. *Surface Accuracy.* The cast must be poured immediately to prevent loss of water from the impression which will result in permanent distortion.

B. Mixing the Impression Material

1. Follow manufacturer's specifications precisely: total time lapse for mixing and insertion is approximately two minutes.

2. Place measured water (at 68–70° F, 20–21° C measured with a thermometer) in a clean dry mixing bowl.

3. Sprinkle measured powder (from individually sealed package or premeasured from large container) into the water.

4. Quickly incorporate the powder and water using a clean, dry, stiff spatula.

5. Mix for one minute (clocked) vigorously incorporating powder into the water, until a smooth, creamy mix is obtained.

C. Filling the Tray (30 seconds working time)

The mandibular impression is made first to introduce the patient to the procedure in an area where discomfort or gagging is least likely.

1. Fill the tray from one end to the other, being careful not to trap air bubbles.

2. Adapt the material to the tray thoroughly; press slightly through the perforations in the tray.

3. Do not overload; fill to a level just below the edge of the wax rim.

4. Wet index finger with cold water and pass lightly over the surface of the impression material: smooth the surface and make a slight indent where the dental arch will insert.

5. Quickly gather the excess material from the bowl and bring the material on the spatula near to patient.

V. The Mandibular Impression

A. Precoat Potential Areas of Air Entrapment

This prevents air bubbles in the finished impression.

1. Take a small amount of impression material from the spatula on the index finger.

2. Apply quickly with a positive pressure to

a. Undercut areas such as distal surfaces of teeth adjacent to edentulous areas, cervical areas of erosion or abrasion, or gingival surfaces of fixed partial dentures.

b. Vestibular areas, particularly anterior areas about the freni.

c. Occlusal surfaces.

B. Insertion of Tray

1. Follow the procedure for insertion of mandibular tray described on

page 146, III, A, 4. Briefly, from the front of the patient, retract patient's right lip and cheek with left fingers; use side of tray to distend the left lip and cheek; rotate the tray into position, center it over the teeth, introduce the tray ¼ inch anterior to the labial surface of the most anterior incisor, instruct patient to raise tongue while tray is lowered, retract cheeks and lip to clear the way for impression material to reach the base of the vestibule.

2. Seat the tray directly downward with a slight vibratory motion to aid in filling all crevices between the teeth.

3. Instruct the patient to extrude the tongue briefly to mold the lingual borders of the impression.

4. Apply equal bilateral pressure firmly, holding the middle fingers over the premolar regions and using the thumbs to support the mandible; or, if equal pressure can be maintained with one hand, place the index finger over the patient's right premolar area and the middle finger over the left with the thumb under the edge of the mandible for stabilization. Mold cheeks around buccal.

5. Saliva ejector: when the impression tray is held with one hand or when assistance is available, a saliva ejector may be slipped in over the tray and then removed before the tray is removed.

C. **Setting Time**

When the leftover material on the spatula has lost its surface stickiness (tackiness), the impression is held in position two more clocked minutes.

D. **Removal of Impression**

1. Hold tray with right thumb and fingers.

2. Retract right cheek and lip with left fingers and release the edge of the impression by depressing the buccal mucosa.

3. Do not rock the impression back and forth to release it as these movements may cause permanent distortion.

4. Remove the impression with a sudden jerk or snap.

E. **Rinse**

Rinse under cool running water to remove saliva.

F. **Inspect and Evaluate the Impression**

Observe surface detail, proper extension over retromolar area, and the peripheral roll (rounded border of the impression) generally.

G. **Repeat the Procedure**

Correct mistakes, rather than be satisfied with a substandard impression.

H. **Wrap Mandibular Impression in a Wet Towel** while making the maxillary impression.

VI. The Maxillary Impression

A. **Request Patient to Rinse**

To clear particles left from the mandibular impression, and to relax the oral muscles.

B. **Examine the Maxillary Teeth**

Teeth should be examined for particles of mandibular impression material: remove. Request patient to use mouthwash.

C. **Prepare the Alginate**

Fill the tray as described previously (IV, B and C, page 149).

D. **Precoat Undercut Areas**

Precoat undercut areas, vestibular areas, and occlusal surfaces (Procedure V, A above).

E. **Insertion of Tray**

1. Follow the procedure for insertion of maxillary tray described on page 146, III, A, 3. Briefly, from the side

back position, retract the patient's left lip with the left fingers; use side of tray (held by right hand) to distend the right lip and cheek; insert the tray with a rotary motion; center it over the teeth using the small gap in the red wax border to relate to the labial frenum.

2. Introduce the material to the teeth so that the wax rim is about ¼ inch labial to the most labially inclined incisor.

3. Seat the tray
   a. Seat the tray from posterior to anterior to direct the impression material forward and thus prevent irritation to the soft palate area.
   b. Retract the lip and bring the tray to place with a slight vibratory motion to allow the material to flow into crevices and proximal areas.
   c. The middle finger of each hand is placed over the premolar region to support and guide the tray; the index fingers and thumbs hold the lip out.
   d. Request the patient to form a tight "O" with his lips to mold the impression material.
   e. Maintain equal pressure on each side of the tray throughout the setting of the alginate. If assistance is available, or if the pressure to hold the tray can be maintained with one hand, a saliva ejector can be inserted.

F. **Setting Time**

When the material on the spatula has lost its surface stickiness, the impression is held in place for two more clocked minutes.

G. **Removal of Impression**

Hold the tray handle with the right thumb and fingers, and retract the left lip and cheek with left fingers. Elevate the cheek on the left over the edge of the impression to break the seal, and remove the impression with a sudden jerk.

H. **Rinse**

Rinse under cool running water to remove saliva.

I. **Inspect**

Examine surface detail and proper extension to include tuberosity areas and a complete reproduction of the height of the vestibule.

J. **Repeat Procedure**

Repeat procedure rather than be satisfied with a substandard impression.

K. **Wrap Impression in a Damp Towel**

This is to prevent dehydration and distortion; however, impressions should be poured promptly.

L. **Check Manufacturer's Specifications**

Check for use of a fixative.

VII. The Interocclusal Record (Wax Bite)

A. **Purposes**

1. To relate the maxillary and mandibular casts correctly.
2. To place between the casts during trimming and storage to prevent breakage of teeth.

B. **Indication for Special Need**

Many, if not most, casts will orient to each other readily in only one position, but when there are problems such as openbite, crossbite, edentulous areas, end-to-end, or edge-to-edge relations which may interfere with direct occlusion of the casts, a wax bite is generally needed.

C. **Procedure**

1. Have patient practice opening and closing on the posterior teeth to assure that the correct position can be obtained easily.

2. Ask patient to rinse with cold water.
3. Shape a double layer of soft baseplate wax in the form of the arch, warm slightly over a gas burner, and place over the maxillary occlusal surfaces.
4. Request patient to close; press the wax on the facial to shape it accurately to the arch.
5. Remove carefully to prevent distortion; chill in cold water.

PARACLINICAL PROCEDURES

Supplemental to the chairside clinical procedures is the laboratory work involved in the production of the study casts from the impressions. These duties may be the responsibility of the dental laboratory technician or the dental assistant, as directed by the dentist.

The most frequent error in the use of the alginates for impressions is in delay in pouring the cast. Undue dehydration or water loss from the alginate will cause permanent distortion, an uneven surface, and hence an inaccurate cast. Regard for the sensitive properties of the dental materials, precision and practice in laboratory procedures, and pride in the production of neat, smooth, well-proportioned study casts determine the finished product's appearance, usefulness, and accuracy.

I. Equipment and Materials

A. Mixing bowl: clean, dry flexible rubber or plastic, with smooth, unscratched surface.
B. Spatula: clean, dry, stiff, with a smooth, rounded end that will reach every part of the bowl without scraping or cutting its surface.
C. Plaster knife: sharp.
D. Vibrator.
E. Mechanical mixer.
F. Model-base formers, glass or ceramic slab, wax paper or other non-absorbent surfaced material.

G. Dental materials
  1. Baseplate wax (and wax spatula).
  2. White dental stone.
H. Model trimmer.
I. Compass or dividers.
J. Plastic ruler.
K. Waterproof sandpaper.
L. Soap solution.

II. Preparation of the Impressions

A. Rinse impressions under cool running water; shake out excess water gently, and apply gentle blast of compressed air.
B. Mandibular: create an artificial floor of the mouth in the impression to facilitate pouring and trimming of the cast.
  1. Trim the lingual impression material all around so that there is a consistent height from the occlusal and incisal surfaces to the base of the impression.
  2. Using alginate:
    a. Mix a small portion of alginate.
    b. Hold the mandibular impression upright in the left hand with the middle and ring fingers extended from under the tray into the tongue area.
    c. Apply alginate over the fingers to form a flat bridge slightly above the lingual flanges of the impression.
    d. Smooth the surface with a finger moistened with cool water; hold until the alginate sets.
    e. When assisted at the chair, the floor for the mandibular impression can be made while the maxillary impression is being held for setting. There is usually sufficient alginate mixed with that for the maxillary impression to use for this purpose.
  3. Using baseplate wax
    a. Cut a piece of baseplate wax to the shape of the lingual periphery of the impression.

b. Seal into place with a warm spatula, taking care that no heat is applied to the anatomic portions of the impression.

c. Cool under running water.

III. Pouring the Casts: Mixing the Stone

A. **Factors Related to Dental Stone Which Contribute to a Successful Cast**

Texts on dental materials should be reviewed for complete information about gypsum products.[6,7,8,9] Some pertinent properties are listed here as reference points.

1. *Dental Stone.* Sensitive to changes in the relative humidity of the atmosphere.

   a. Store in airtight container; close soon after use; do not let water enter the container.

   b. Keep the spoon or scoop used to remove the powder clean and dry.

2. *Water.* Controls the strength, rigidity, and hardness of the cast.

   a. Temperature: generally, cooler water decreases the setting time and warmer water increases it.

   b. Quantity: follow manufacturer's proportions exactly. Increasing the water over the specifications prolongs the setting time and reduces the strength.

3. *Spatulation.* Prolonged or very rapid mixing can hasten the chemical reaction and shorten the setting time.

B. **The Mix**

1. Measure the water and powder by the manufacturer's specifications.

   a. White stone is generally preferred for study casts. Plaster produces a cast more susceptible to breakage.

   b. Ratio of 30–40 ml. water to 100 Gm. stone.

2. Place measured water (room temperature) in a clean, dry, mixing bowl.

3. Sift in the powder gradually to prevent air trapping and to allow each particle to become wet.

4. Wait briefly until all powder is wet, then vibrate to release large bubbles.

5. Spatulation: with clean, stiff spatula.

   a. Hand spatulate for not less than 30 and not more than 60 seconds.

   b. Contact the entire inner surface of the bowl so no powder is left unincorporated.

   c. Do not whip or beat as this encourages bubble formation.

   d. Vibrate during and after spatulation to remove bubbles.

   e. Mechanical mixer or vacuum mixer used when available.

6 Result: smooth, homogeneous, creamy mix.

C. **Pouring the Cast**

1. Shake water out of the impression.

2. Hold the impression tray by the handle and press handle against the vibrator.

3. With a small amount of stone mix on the end of the spatula, start at one posterior corner and allow the mix to flow through the impression. Use small amounts and vibrate continually.

   a. Tip the impression so that the material will pass into the tooth indentations and flow slowly down the side, across the occlusal or incisal, and up the other side of the impression of each tooth.

   b. Air will be trapped if the process is hurried, or if too large a quantity of mix is poured in at one time without attentive control of the flow.

4. When all tooth indentations are covered, larger amounts of mix are

added to fill the impression slightly over the periphery. Vibrate.

D. One-Step Method for Forming the Base of the Cast

1. Fill rubber model-base former with the remainder of the mix, or form a mass of stone on a glass or ceramic slab or other nonabsorbable surface (wax paper on a smooth surface). Add excess stone at the heel areas.
2. Invert the poured impression onto the base.
   a. Use a slight back-and-forth motion to secure the two parts together.
   b. Common error: inverting the impression before the stone is firm enough to prevent it from flowing out of the impression.
3. Adjust tray to proper position.
   a. Occlusal plane (at premolars) should be parallel with the base of the model-base former or tabletop.
   b. Midline (anterior as judged by handle of impression tray) centered at the midline of the model-base former.
   c. Accommodate position so that a tooth in labio- or buccoversion will not protrude over the trimming line of the art portion (figure 10–6).
4. Add stone on peripheral and heel areas to provide a smooth surface; remove excess so that wax periphery of the tray is visible. When excess stone above the edge of the tray rim is permitted to set, it is difficult to separate the tray, and the use of a knife to carve the excess from the tray may damage the cast.
5. Final set occurs within one hour. Separate one hour after pouring to prevent damage to the surface of the cast.

E. Other Methods for Forming the Base of the Cast

1. *Two-step or Double-pour.* Both maxillary and mandibular impressions are poured and left upright (Steps III, C, 1 through 4, page 153). Stone is then prepared separately for the bases, and the model-base formers are filled or the mass is placed on the smooth nonabsorbent surface.

   The impression is inverted and held on the surface of the new stone while the sides and periphery are shaped and smoothed. An advantage in this method is that there is no danger of inverting the poured impression too soon so that the unset stone can fall away from the occlusal and incisal portions and leave bubbles in strategic places.

2. *Boxing Technique.* The object is to form a wall around the impression before pouring to provide a shape for the base as well as to prevent the need for inverting the poured impression. A cylinder of utility wax is attached slightly below the periphery of the impressions and completely around the entire impression. Boxing wax or baseplate is applied around the rope of utility wax and attached to it by means of a warm spatula at a height which allows for proper thickness of the final cast, about ½ inch. Care must be taken not to displace the impression dimensionally, or to touch the anatomic portions with the warm spatula. Pouring is carried out as described previously.

   Work-model formers with side walls to provide the boxing effect are available. Such a mold has a slot through the rubber where the handle of the impression tray can be inserted.

F. **Separation of the Impression and the Cast**
   1. Objective: to remove tray and impression material without breaking the teeth.
   2. When model-base former was used, remove it first.
   3. Cut away stone from the periphery to free the margin of the tray.
   4. Remove the tray by itself.
   5. Cut the impression material along the line of the occlusal surfaces and peel off the impression material (with care not to scratch the stone cast during cutting).
   6. Direct removal: when the teeth are in reasonably normal alignment, the tray and the impression material may be removed with a straight pull after first releasing the anterior portion by a slight downward and forward movement. When this method is used, do not apply lateral pressures or rock the tray back and forth, as it is easy to break the teeth by using such forces.
G. Trimming is started promptly, or if delayed, the cast should be thoroughly soaked before trimming.

IV. Trimming the Casts[10,11,12]

The exact proportions of the study casts, and the steps required to accomplish the trimming and finishing depend on several factors. These include the measurements of the patient's dental arches, the positions of the teeth, and the preferences of the dentist. Development of a routine, systematic procedure for trimming can lead to the production of consistent, attractive, and useful diagnostic casts.

The method described here is dependent on the use of a precision-type model trimmer. No specific directions are provided for the use of angulators which are available to fit on the table of the model trimmer to give average set angles for trimming the margins of the casts; when

these are available, directions are usually supplied by the manufacturer.

When a mechanical model trimmer is not available, greater skill must be developed to produce well-proportioned and smooth casts. The use of the model-base formers or a boxing method can be developed to a higher degree of precision. Trimming with a plaster knife must be started as soon as the impression is separated. Plaster files are available to aid in cutting the borders of the base.

Before the step by step description of the trimming procedure, an outline of the characteristics of the finished casts is provided as an overall guide.

A. **Objectives: Characteristics of the Finished Casts**
   1. *Overall base shape:* figure 10–5.
   2. *Proportions:* approximately ⅓ art portion and ⅔ anatomic (figure 10–6 A).
   3. *Bases:* mean occlusal plane of the related casts is parallel with both bases which are parallel with each other (figure 10–6 B).
   4. *Posterior Borders*
      a. At a right angle with the bases (figure 10–6 B).
      b. Maxillary and mandibular posterior borders are in the same plane: when standing, the casts will rest together in natural intercuspation (figure 10–6 B).
      c. Perpendicular to the median line from the incisors through the

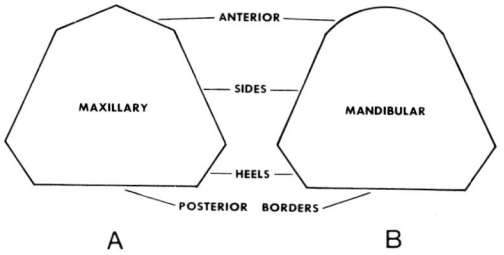

Figure 10–5. Base shapes for maxillary and mandibular study casts with designations of trimmed areas.

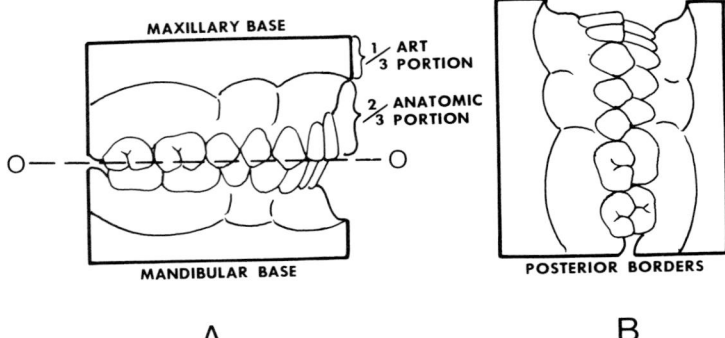

Figure 10–6. Finished study casts. **A.** Proportions and planes. The *Art* portion is ⅓ and the *anatomic* portion ⅔ of the total height of the cast. Note parallelism of the maxillary and mandibular bases with the mean occlusal plane (0–0). **B.** Posterior borders are at right angles to the bases. When the maxillary and mandibular casts are placed on their posterior borders, the teeth will intercuspate.

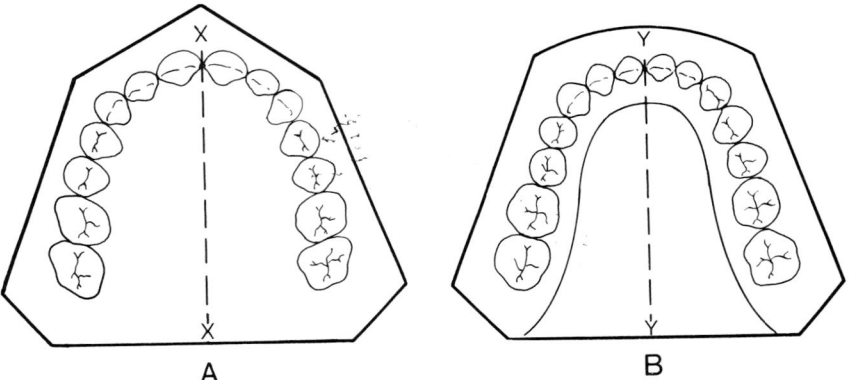

Figure 10–7. Occlusal views of finished casts, **A.** Maxillary, **B.** Mandibular. The posterior border is perpendicular to the median line from the incisors through the palate (X-X), and the middle of the tongue (Y-Y). The tuberosity areas of the maxillary arch and the retromolar areas of the mandibular arch are preserved.

palate (maxillary) and the middle of the tongue (mandibular) (figure 10–7).

5. *Sides:* symmetrical angulation with posterior border and heel cuts (figure 10–7); parallel with a line through the central grooves of the premolars of the same side.

6. *Heels:* one-half inch cuts parallel with the mesiodistal plane of the opposite canine (figure 10–7).

7. *Anterior:* mandibular is shaped in an arc, maxillary in a point, with the cuts extending from the canine area (figure 10–7).

8. *Borders:*
   a. Posterior: to include retromolar area and tuberosity (figure 10–7).
   b. Sides: ¼ to ⁵/₁₆ inch from bony protuberance over premolars and molars; anatomy of mucobuccal fold included in the cast.
   c. Anterior: ¼ to ⁵/₁₆ inch from the most protruded tooth or from the depth of the mucobuccal fold, whichever is most labial.

9. *Surfaces of the cast:* smooth and polished with air bubbles removed or filled.

B. **Preliminary Steps to Trimming the Cast**
  1. Casts must be wet: soak at least five minutes.
  2. Remove bubbles of stone on or about the teeth with a small sharp instrument: use care not to scar the cast.
  3. Level down excess stone which is distal to the retromolar area and tuberosity so that casts may be occluded. Do not shorten the cast anteriorly-posteriorly at this time.
  4. Trim casts conservatively on the sides to make a smooth surface for marking.

C. **Trimming the Bases**
  1. *Objectives*
    a. To make bases parallel with the mean occlusal plane and to each other.
    b. To make correct proportions for the height of the casts: art portion ⅓ and anatomic portion ⅔ (figure 10–6 A).
  2. *Mandibular Cast Is Trimmed First*
    a. Measure the greatest height of the anatomic portion (usually this is from the tip of the canine to the depth of the vestibule) with a plastic ruler (figure 10–8).
    b. Divide by two: this will be the height of the art portion.
    c. Add the measured height of the anatomic portion to the height of the art portion for the total height

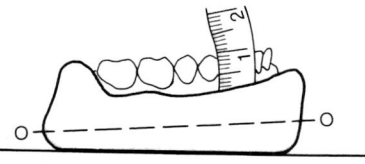

Figure 10–8. Preparation for trimming the base. The anatomic portion is measured at its greatest height which is usually from the tip of the canine to the depth of the vestibule. One-half of this measurement will be the height of the art portion. The trimming line (0–0) is parallel with the mean occlusal plane. See text for details.

of the cast. Set compass or dividers at this measurement.
    d. Place the cast teeth down on a flat surface and mark a line around the art portion at the height calculated in part 2c above. This line should be parallel with the occlusal plane (line 0–0 in figure 10–8). Trim the cast at the line.
  3. *Maxillary Cast*
    a. Measure the greatest depth of the anatomic portion (usually at the canine) and divide by two to obtain the height of the art portion.
    b. Relate the two casts (use the wax bite if necessary) and place the mandibular base on the flat surface.
    c. Measure from the base of the mandibular cast to the highest point of the maxillary anatomic portion (usually in the vestibule over the canine), and add this figure to the height of the maxillary art portion calculated in part *a* above.
    d. Set the compass at this measurement and mark a line around the maxillary cast at the total height. The line must be parallel to the base of the mandibular cast and to the occlusal plane. Trim.

D. **Posterior Borders**
  1. Select the longest cast to trim first by measuring from the incisors to points distal to the retromolar and tuberosity areas.
  2. On the longest cast, place the tip of the compass at the gingival border behind the midline anteriorly (usually this is between the central incisors) and mark an arc ¼ inch distal to the tuberosity (if the maxillary cast) or retromolar area (if the mandibular cast) on each side.

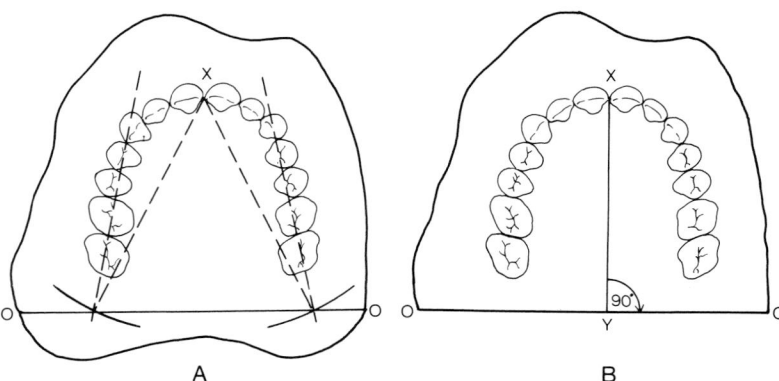

Figure 10–9. Trim line for the posterior borders. **A.** On the longest cast, use a compass to draw arcs from the anterior midline point (X) to ¼ inch distal to the tuberosity area (maxillary) or retromolar area (mandibular). Intersect the arc with a line through the central grooves of the molars and connect the two points across the cast (0–0). **B.** Check that the 0–0 line is perpendicular to the median line from the incisors through the palate or tongue (X–Y) before trimming.

3. Intersect the arc with a line through the central grooves of the molars (figure 10–9 A).
4. Connect the two points across the back of the cast (0–0 in figure 10–9 A). Check that this line is perpendicular to the median line from the incisors through the palate or the tongue (X–Y in figure 10–9 B).
5. With the base of the cast flat on the model trimmer table, trim on the line marked for the posterior border.
6. For the shorter cast: relate the two casts with the wax bite and place flat on the base of the first-trimmed cast. Bring them carefully to the cutting surface of the model trimmer, and trim until the two posterior borders are even and parallel.
7. Check by placing the casts on their posterior borders and bringing them together. They should relate in their natural intercuspation (figure 10–6 B).

E. Sides and Heels

1. Select the widest cast to trim first: casts are usually widest at the molar region.
2. Mark with ruler two symmetrical lines ¼ to ⁵/₁₆ inch buccal from the buccal bony prominence at the premolar regions and parallel with lines through the central grooves of the premolars (figure 10–10 A).
   a. Check that the lines form equal angles with the posterior border.
   b. Before trimming make certain that the lines when cut would not remove any vestibular anatomy.
   c. Trim the sides with the base flat on the model trimmer table.
3. Mark trimming lines for the heels: cuts are ½ inch wide and parallel with a line through the mesiodistal plane of the opposite canine (figure 10–10 B). Trim with base flat on the model trimmer table.
4. Relate the opposite cast with the wax bite and trim the sides and heels to match the previously trimmed cast.

F. Anterior

1. *Maxillary*
   a. With a ruler draw to shape of a point at the midline from the canine areas two lines labial to the depth of the mucobuccal fold or the most labially inclined tooth approximately ¼ to ⁵/₁₆ inch (figure 10–11 A).
   b. Before trimming check that both

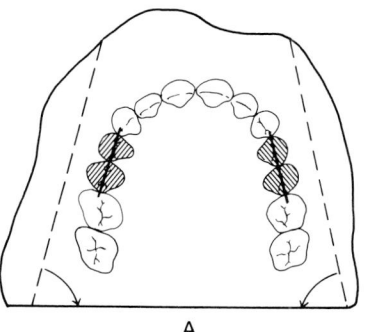
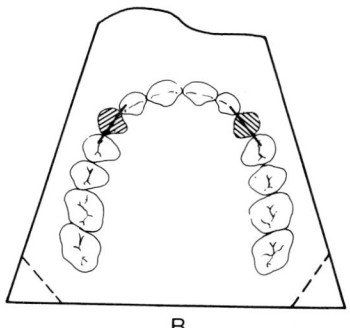

Figure 10–10. Trim lines for the sides and heels. **A.** On the widest cast, the trim lines for the sides are drawn parallel with lines through the central grooves of the premolars. The two symmetrical lines form equal angles with the posterior border of the cast. **B.** Mark trim lines for the heels ¼ inch wide and parallel with lines through the mesiodistal plane of the opposite canine. The lines are symmetrical with each other and form equal angles with the posterior border.

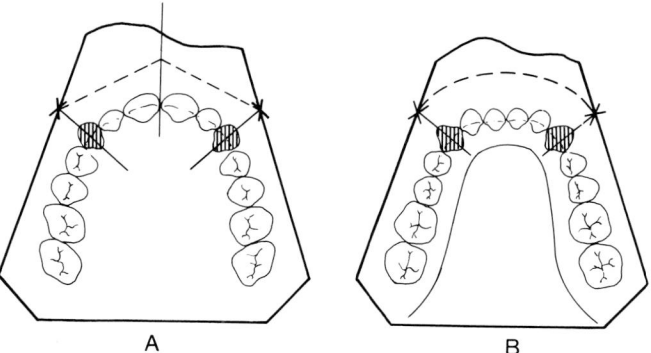

Figure 10–11. Trim lines for anterior. **A.** Maxillary lines are drawn from opposite the middle of each canine to meet in a point at the midline and approximately ¼ inch labial to the most labially positioned tooth. **B.** Mandibular line forms an arc drawn from the middle of each canine approximately ¼ inch labial to the most labially positioned tooth.

sides of the cast will be the same length from the intersection of the front cut to the heels.

2. *Mandibular*

   a. Sketch the shape of an arc from canine to canine to conform generally with the curvature of the anterior teeth and approximately ¼ to ⁵/₁₆ inch labial to the depth of the mucobuccal fold or the most labially inclined or positioned tooth (figure 10–11 B).

   b. Before trimming, check that both sides of the cast will be the same length from the intersection of the front cut to the heels.

G. **Finishing and Polishing**

   1. Trim rough edges and margins of both casts and the lingual portion of the mandibular cast to even off irregularities and make the depth of the vestibule visible. Remaining bubbles are removed.

   2. Use waterproof sandpaper and a plaster smoothing stone to remove marks left by the model trimmer on the art portion. Sandpaper is not used on the anatomic portion.

   3. Fill any holes in the wet casts with stone applied with a spatula to the flat surfaces of the art portion or a camel's hair brush to the anatomic portion. Smooth off excess.

4. Finish and polish:
   a. Allow casts to dry thoroughly for two to three days.
   b. Smooth the art portion with fine sandpaper.
   c. Soak in heated soap solution for 30 to 60 minutes. Concentrated model gloss soap is available commercially, or a super-saturated solution of Ivory flakes may be used (approximately one cup of flakes to five cups of water).
   d. Rub with chamois, cotton, or a soft cloth.
   e. Talc or baby talcum powder with olive oil may be used followed by rubbing with a chamois or soft cloth.

TECHNICAL HINTS

 I. Label each cast with the patient's name and the date. These may be inscribed into the posterior border of the cast before soaping and polishing.
 II. Boxes of an appropriate size are available commercially for the storage of one or more pairs of casts.
III. Note in the patient's permanent record the size of impression tray used. When casts are made periodically for follow-up, time is saved both in the sterilization of all sizes for try-in, and by preparing the wax rim in advance of the patient's appointment.
 IV. Make duplicate cast for the permanent record when the dentist uses the original for the design of prosthesis or fabrication of a secondary impression tray. The duplicate cast is made by taking a laboratory impression of the original and pouring it in the same manner as the original.
  V. To care for the model trimmer, following its use, allow motor to run until clear water is flowing through and all particles of stone have been washed away.
 VI. Replace scratched mixing bowls.
VII. Sterilize aluminum impression trays. Clean completely and sterilize by autoclave or dry heat.

FACTORS TO TEACH THE PATIENT

  I. Importance of having study casts and for what they are used. Reasons for comparative casts following treatment or at a later date.
 II. Use of the casts of other patients to show effects of treatment or what can happen if the prescribed treatment is not carried out.
III. Areas which present difficulty in the plaque control and oral physical therapy program: use of devices can be demonstrated on the patient's own study cast.

References

1. American Dental Association, Council on Dental Materials and Devices: *Guide to Dental Materials and Devices*, 7th ed. Chicago, American Dental Association, 1974–1975, pp. 71–73.
2. Peyton, F. A. and Craig, R. G., eds.: *Restorative Dental Materials*, 4th ed. St. Louis, Mosby, 1971, pp. 187–191.
3. Phillips, R. W.: *Elements of Dental Materials for Dental Hygienists and Assistants*, 2nd ed. Philadelphia, Saunders, 1971, pp. 74–79.
4. Phillips, R. W.: *Skinner's Science of Dental Materials*, 7th ed. Philadelphia, Saunders, 1973, pp. 114–123.
5. American Dental Association, Council on Dental Materials and Devices: op. cit., pp. 219–223.
6. Ibid., pp. 86–91.
7. Peyton and Craig: op. cit., pp. 213–234.
8. Phillips, R. W.: *Elements of Dental Materials for Dental Hygienists and Assistants*, 2nd ed. Philadelphia, Saunders, 1971, pp. 35–50.
9. Phillips, R. W.: *Skinner's Science of Dental Materials*, 7th ed. Philadelphia, Saunders, 1973, pp. 55–82.
10. Barton, R. E. and Rigsby, B. E.: Pouring Models, in Peterson, S., ed.: *The Dentist and His Assistant*, 3rd ed. St. Louis, Mosby, 1972, pp. 291–304.
11. Graber, T. M.: *Orthodontics, Principles and Practice*, 3rd ed. Philadelphia, Saunders, 1972, pp. 403–413.

12. Strang, R. H. W. and Thompson, W. M.: *A Textbook of Orthodontia*, 4th ed. Philadelphia, Lea & Febiger, 1958, pp. 786–798.

Suggested Readings

Hill, C. J. and Gellin, M. E.: Impression Making for the Young Child Who Gags, *J. Am. Dent. Assoc.*, *81*, 161, July, 1970.

McGrath, J.: Role of the Auxiliary in Orthodontics, in Castano, F. A. and Alden, B. A., eds.: *Handbook of Expanded Dental Auxiliary Practice*. Philadelphia, Lippincott, 1973, pp. 202–207.

Polan, M., Frommer, S., and Roistacher, S.: Incidence of Viable Mycobacteria Tuberculosis on Alginate Impressions in Patients with Positive Sputum, *J. Prosthet. Dent.*, *24*, 335, September, 1970.

Rudd, K. D.: Making Diagnostic Casts Is Not a Waste of Time, *J. Prosthet. Dent.*, *20*, 98, August, 1968.

Rudd, K. D. and Morrow, R. M.: A Simplified Method for Mixing Dental Stone, *J. Prosthet. Dent.*, *32*, 675, December, 1974.

Schwarzrock, S. P. and Jensen, J. R.: *Effective Dental Assisting*, 4th ed. Dubuque, Iowa, Brown, 1973, pp. 471–481.

Simon, W. J.: *Clinical Dental Assisting*. Hagerstown, Maryland, Medical Department, Harper & Row, 1973, p. 102–119.

Thompson, E. O.: Constructing and Using Diagnostic Models, *Dent. Clin. North Am.*, p., 67, March, 1963.

Chapter 11

The Gingiva

The true test of successful treatment, the real evaluation of the effects of scaling and related instrumentation, is the *health* of the gingival tissues. The objective of all treatment is to bring the diseased gingiva to a state of health which can be maintained by the patient. To do this, the first thing is to learn to recognize normal healthy tissue, to observe certain characteristics of color, texture, and form, to test for bleeding, and to apply this knowledge to the treatment and supervision of the patient's gingiva until health is attained.

An outline of the clinical features of the periodontal tissues in health and disease is included in this chapter. It is expected that complete information about the gross and microscopic anatomy of the periodontium and the periodontal pathology will have been studied or will be studied in preparation for clinical practice. Textbooks and other references are listed in *Suggested Readings* at the end of the chapter for review.

OBJECTIVES

The ultimate objective is that the dental hygienist's knowledge and skill in examination and evaluation of the periodontal tissues will be applied in patient care so that each patient will attain and maintain optimum oral health. The dental hygienist will know when the treatment provided by dental hygiene services is definitive in restoring health and when more advanced treatment is needed. The patient can be properly informed so that complete treatment can be provided.

Specific objectives for the dental hygienist are to be able to

I. Recognize normal periodontal tissues.
II. Know the features of the periodontal tissues which must be examined for a complete evaluation.
III. Recognize the basic signs of periodontal involvement of varying degrees.
IV. Identify the dental hygiene treatment and instruction needed.
V. Outline the patient's preventive periodontal program (pages 294, 386).

THE FIELD OF OPERATION

The techniques of dental hygiene are applied directly to the teeth, the gingiva, and the gingival sulcus. Detailed knowledge and understanding of the anatomy and normal clinical appearance of the field of operation are prerequisite to meaningful examination and treatment.

I. The Teeth

A. Clinical Crown

The part of the tooth which is above the junctional epithelium. It can be considered the part of the tooth where clinical techniques are applied (figure 11–1).

B. Clinical Root

The part of the tooth which is below the base of the gingival sulcus or periodontal pocket. It is the part of the root to which periodontal fibers are attached.

C. Anatomic Crown

The part of the tooth covered by enamel.

D. Anatomic Root

The part of the tooth covered by cementum.

II. Oral Mucosa

The lining of the oral cavity, the oral mucosa, is a mucous membrane composed of connective tissue covered with stratified squamous epithelium. There are three divisions or categories of oral mucosa.

A. Masticatory Mucosa

1. Covers the *gingiva* and the *hard palate*, the areas used most during the mastication of food.
2. Except for the free margin of the gingiva, the masticatory mucosa is firmly attached to underlying tissues.
3. The epithelial covering is generally keratinized.

B. Lining Mucosa

1. Covers the inner surfaces of the *lips and cheeks*, the *floor of the mouth*, the *under side of the tongue*, the *soft palate*, and the *alveolar mucosa.*
2. These tissues are not firmly attached to underlying tissue.
3. The epithelial covering is not generally keratinized.

C. Specialized Mucosa

1. Covers the *dorsum* (upper surface) *of the tongue.*
2. Anterior part is composed of many papillae, some contain the tastebuds.

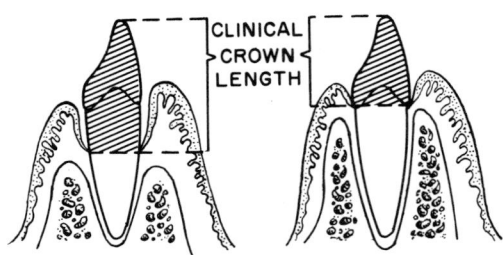

Figure 11–1. Diagram to show clinical crown. The clinical crown is the part of the tooth coronal to the junctional epithelium. *Left,* when there is increased pocket depth, the clinical crown may extend to a position where the clinical crown length is longer than the clinical root length. The clinical root is the part of the tooth with periodontal tissues attached. *Right,* when the junctional epithelium is at the cementoenamel junction, the clinical crown and anatomic crown are the same.

III. The Periodontium

The periodontium is the functional unit of tissues which surrounds and supports the tooth. There are four parts: the gingiva and the attachment apparatus made up of the periodontal ligament, cementum, and bone.

A. Gingiva

The part of the masticatory mucosa which surrounds the necks of the teeth and is attached to the teeth and the alveolar bone.

B. Periodontal Ligament

Connective tissue fibers which surround the root and connect the tooth with the bone.

C. Cementum

The calcified tissue which covers the root and attaches the fibers of the periodontal ligament to the tooth.

D. Alveolar Bone

The bone of the mandible and the maxilla which surrounds the roots of the teeth to support them. Periodontal ligament fibers are attached to the bone.

THE GINGIVA AND RELATED STRUCTURES

The gingiva is made up of the free gingiva, the attached gingiva, and the interdental gingiva or interdental papilla (figure 11–2).

I. Free Gingiva (Marginal Gingiva)

The free gingiva is closely adapted around each tooth. It connects with the attached gingiva at the free gingival groove, and attaches to the tooth at the coronal portion of the junctional epithelium.

A. Free Gingival Groove

1. A shallow linear groove which demarcates the free from the at-

tached gingiva. Generally about one-third of the teeth show a visible gingival groove when the gingiva is in health.[1]

2. In the absence of disease and pocket formation, the gingival groove runs somewhat parallel with, and about 0.5 to 1.5 millimeters from, the gingival margin[2] and is approximately at the level of the bottom of the gingival sulcus.

B. Oral Epithelium (outer gingival epithelium, figure 11–3)

1. Covers the free gingiva from the gingival groove over the gingival margin.
2. It is composed of keratinized stratified squamous epithelium.

C. Gingival Margin (gingival crest, margin of the gingiva, or free margin)

1. It is the edge of the gingiva nearest the incisal or occlusal.
2. Marks the opening of the gingival sulcus.

D. Gingival Sulcus (crevice)

1. It is the crevice or groove between the free gingiva and the tooth.

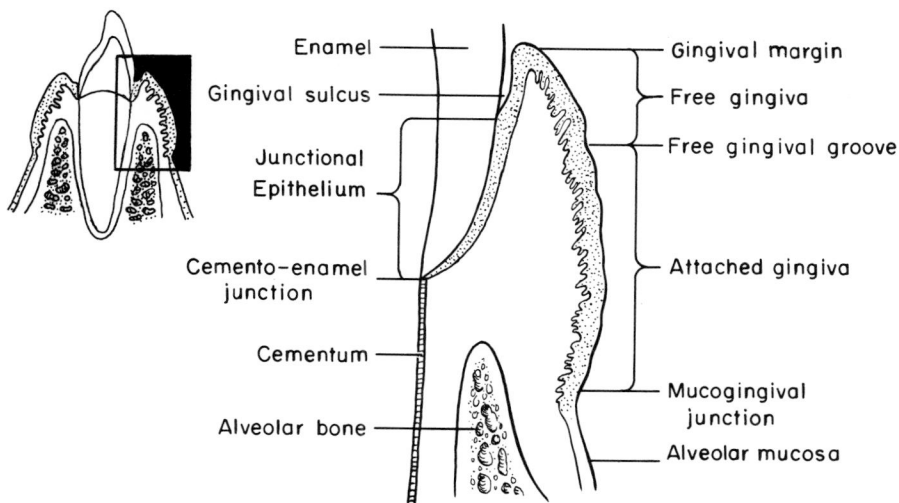

Figure 11–2.   Parts of the gingiva. Diagram to illustrate the parts of the gingiva and adjacent tissues of a partially erupted tooth. Note that the junctional epithelium is on the enamel. When fully erupted, the junctional epithelium will be on the cementum and cementoenamel junction.

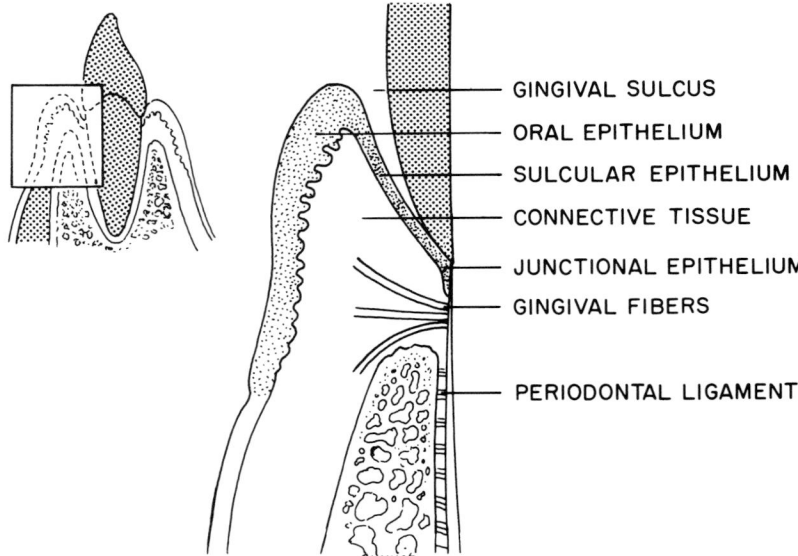

Figure 11–3.   The gingival tissues. Cross section to show the histologic relationships of the oral, sulcular, and junctional epithelium, and the connective tissue of the gingiva.

2. Boundaries (figure 11–3)
   a. Inner: tooth surface. May be the enamel, cementum or part of each, depending on the position of the junctional epithelium.
   b. Outer: sulcular epithelium.
   c. Base: coronal margin of the junctional epithelium. The base of the sulcus or pocket is also called the "depth of the sulcus" or the "bottom of the pocket."
3. Sulcular epithelium: the continuation of the oral epithelium covering the free gingiva. Sulcular epithelium is not keratinized.
4. Depth of sulcus: approximately 1 to 2 millimeters. Healthy sulci are shallowest and may be only 0.5 millimeters. The average depth of the healthy sulcus is about 1.8 millimeters.[3]
5. Gingival sulcus fluid (sulcular fluid, crevicular fluid)[4,5]
   a. A serum-like fluid secreted from the connective tissue through the epithelial lining of the sulcus or pocket.

   b. Occurrence: slight to none in a normal sulcus; increased with inflammation; and considered part of the local defense mechanism.

II. Junctional Epithelium (Epithelial Attachment, Epithelial Cuff)

A. **Description:** the junctional epithelium is a cuff-like band of stratified squamous epithelium which is continuous with the sulcular epithelium and completely encircles the tooth. The *epithelial attachment* is the inner part of the junctional epithelium which is adjacent to the tooth and which provides the actual attachment.

B. **Size:** 3 to 4 layers of cells thick in the young and up to 20 cells thick in later life. The length ranges from 0.25 to 1.35 millimeters.[6]

C. **Position**
   1. As the tooth erupts, the attachment is on the enamel; during eruption the epithelium moves toward the cementoenamel junction (figure 11–4).

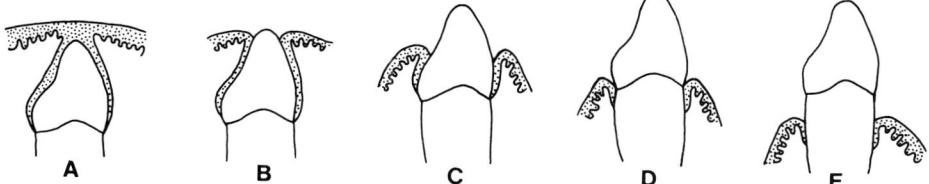

Figure 11–4.   Position of junctional epithelium. **A.** Before eruption the oral epithelium covers the tooth. **B.** As the tooth emerges, the junctional epithelium joins the oral epithelium as the gingival sulcus is formed. **C.** Partial eruption with the junctional epithelium along the enamel (see also figure 11–2). **D.** Eruption complete, with junctional epithelium at the cementoenamel junction. **E.** When there is disease or other cause, the junctional epithelium recedes along the root.

2. At full eruption the attachment is on the cementum where it becomes firmly attached. The coronal margin of the junctional epithelium is at the cementoenamel junction.
3. With wear of the tooth on the incisal or occlusal, and in disease, the attachment can recede along the root surface (figure 11–4 E).

D. **Relation of Crest of Alveolar Bone to the Junctional Epithelium:** the distance between the base of the attachment and the crest of the alveolar bone is approximately 1.0 to 1.5 millimeters. This distance is maintained in disease when the epithelium moves along the root surface during pocket formation.

E. **Attachment of the Epithelium to the Tooth Surface:** an adhesive, organic, mucopolysaccharide substance secreted by the epithelial cells provides a seal at the base of the sulcus and along the border of the junctional epithelium and the tooth surface.

III. Interdental Gingiva (Interdental Papilla)

A. **Location:** between the teeth; it occupies the interproximal space. The tip and lateral borders are continuous with the free gingiva, while other parts are attached gingiva.

B. **Shape**
1. Varies with spacing or overlapping of the teeth: a papilla may be flat or saddle-shaped when there are wide spaces between the teeth, or tapered and narrow when the teeth are crowded or overlapped.
2. Between anterior teeth: pointed, pyramidal.
3. Between posterior teeth.
   a. Flatter than anterior papillae which is caused by wider teeth, wider contact areas, and flattened interdental bone.
   b. Two papillae, one facial and one lingual, connected by a col, are found when teeth are in contact.

C. **Col**
1. A depression between the lingual and facial papillae which conforms to the proximal contact area (figure 11–5).
2. The center of the col area is not keratinized, which makes it more susceptible to disease. Most periodontal disease begins in the col area.

IV. Attached Gingiva

A. **Dimensions**
1. Continuous with the oral epithelium of the free gingiva and is covered with keratinized stratified squamous epithelium.
2. Maxillary lingual: continuous with the palatal mucosa.
3. Mandibular facial and lingual, and maxillary facial: demarcated from

the alveolar mucosa at the muco-gingival junction by the mucogin-gival lines.

B. **Attachment:** firmly bound to the un-derlying cementum and alveolar bone.

C. **Shape:** follows the depressions be-tween the eminences of the roots of the teeth.

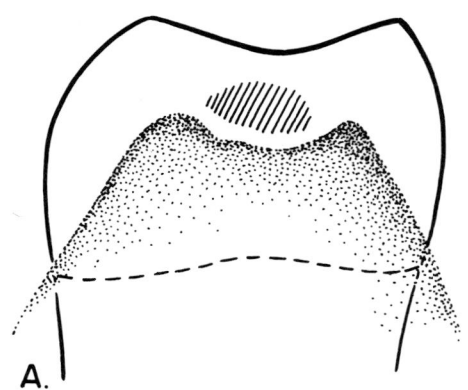

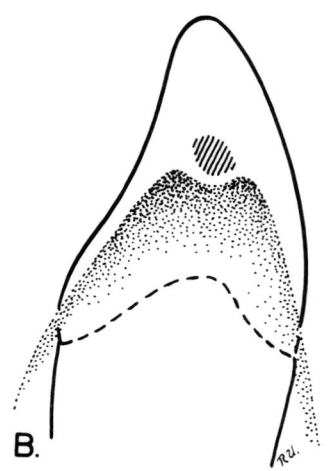

Figure 11–5. Col. The col is the depression between the lingual and facial papillae under the contact area. Contact area is represented by the striped line areas. **A.** Mesial of mandibular molar to show wide col area, and **B.** mesial of mandibular lateral incisor shows narrow anterior col. The col deepens when there is gingival enlargement.

D. **Mucogingival Junction**
1. Mucogingival lines: scalloped lines which mark the connection be-tween the attached gingiva and the alveolar mucosa. A mucogingival line is found on the facial of all quadrants, and on the lingual of the mandibular arch. There is no alveolar mucosa on the palate; the palatal tissue is firmly attached to the bone of the roof of the mouth. There are three mucogingival lines: facial and lingual mandibular, and facial maxillary. In figure 11–6 the facial maxillary and mandibular muco-gingival lines are shown in relation to the attached gingiva and the alveolar mucosa.
2. A sharp contrast can be seen be-tween the light pink of the keratinized, stippled, attached gin-giva, and the darker, alveolar mu-cosa.

V. Alveolar Mucosa

A. **Description:** movable tissue loosely attached to the underlying bone. Has a smooth, shiny surface with non-keratinized epithelium which is thin. Underlying vessels may be seen through the epithelium.

B. **Frena** (Singular: frenum or frenulum)
1. A frenum is a narrow fold of mucous membrane which passes from a more fixed to a movable part, for example, from the gingiva to the lip, cheek, or undersurface of the ton-gue. A frenum serves to check undue movement.
2. Locations
a. Maxillary and mandibular an-terior frena: at midlines between central incisors. Figure 11–6 shows diagrammatically the an-terior frena.
b. Lingual frenum: from undersur-face of the tongue.

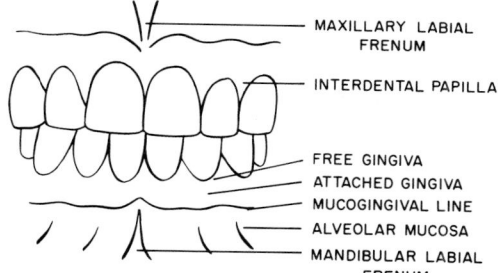

MAXILLARY LABIAL FRENUM

INTERDENTAL PAPILLA

FREE GINGIVA
ATTACHED GINGIVA
MUCOGINGIVAL LINE
ALVEOLAR MUCOSA
MANDIBULAR LABIAL FRENUM

Figure 11–6. Parts of the gingiva, labial view. Maxillary and mandibular mucogingival lines are shown in relation to the attached gingiva, alveolar mucosa, and labial frena.

    c. Buccal frena: in the canine–premolar areas, both maxillary and mandibular.
3. Attachment of frena in relation to the attached gingiva
    a. May be closely associated with the mucogingival line.
    b. When the attached gingiva is narrow or missing, the frena may tend to pull on the free gingiva.

THE RECOGNITION OF GINGIVAL AND PERIODONTAL DISEASES

The recognition of normal gingiva, gingival diseases, and deeper periodontal involvement depends on a disciplined, step-by-step examination. To recognize the signs of disease, a basic examination must include clinical observation for gingival tissue changes, bleeding, exudate, pockets, furcation involvement, mucogingival involvement, occlusion factors, tooth mobility, and a radiographic examination.

It is also necessary to know the extent of the disease. *Gingival diseases* are confined to the gingiva, whereas *periodontal diseases* include all parts of the periodontium, namely, the gingiva, periodontal ligament, bone, and cementum.

Patients may or may not have specific symptoms to report because periodontal diseases are insidious in development. Subjective symptoms, those which the patient notices himself, may include bleeding gingiva, sometimes only with brushing, sometimes with drooling at night, or sometimes spontaneously. Other possible symptoms are sensitivity to hot and cold, tenderness or discomfort while eating or some pain after eating, food retained between the teeth, unpleasant mouth odors, chronic bad taste, or a feeling that the teeth are loose. Most of these are symptoms of advanced disease.

I. Clinically Normal

The terms "clinically normal" or "clinically healthy" may be used to designate gingival tissue which is pale pink, has a knife-edge gingival margin which adapts closely around the tooth, is stippled, firm, has minimal sulcus depth, and no bleeding is elicited when probed. Although "normal" will vary with anatomic, physiologic, and other factors, general characteristics form a baseline for a contrast in the recognition of disease.

II. Causes of Tissue Changes

Disease changes which occur produce alterations in the color, size, position, shape, consistency, surface texture, bleeding readiness, and exudate production.

To understand the changes which take place in the gingival tissues during the transition from health to disease, it is necessary to have a clear picture of what plaque is, the role of plaque microorganisms in the development of disease, and the inflammatory response by the body.

When the products of the plaque microorganisms cause breakdown of the intercellular substances of the sulcular epithelium, injurious agents can pass into the connective tissue where an inflammatory response is initiated. An inflammatory response means that there is increased blood flow, increased permeability of capillaries, and increased collection of defense cells and tissue fluid. It is these changes that produce the tissue alterations such as color, size, shape, and consistency, which are described in the next section.

III. Descriptive Terminology

The degree of severity and distribution of a change should be noted when inspecting the gingiva. When a deviation from normal affects a single area, it can be designated by the number of the adjacent tooth and the surface of the tissue involved, namely, facial, lingual, mesial, or distal. Teeth numbering systems are described on page 60.

A. **Severity.** Severity is expressed as slight, moderate, or severe.

B. **Distribution.** Terms used for describing distribution are
   1. *Localized.* Localized means that the gingiva is involved only about a single tooth or a specific group of teeth.
   2. *Generalized.* Generalized means that the gingiva is involved about all or nearly all of the teeth throughout the mouth. A condition may also be generalized throughout a single arch, the maxillary or mandibular.
   3. *Marginal.* A change which involves the free or marginal gingiva. This is specified as either localized or generalized.
   4. *Papillary.* A change which involves a papilla but not the rest of the free gingiva around a tooth. A papillary change may be localized or generalized.
   5. *Diffuse.* When the attached gingiva is involved as well as the free gingiva, it is referred to as a diffuse change. A diffuse condition is most frequently localized, rarely generalized.

IV. Early Recognition of Tissue Changes

Marked changes, such as moderate to severe generalized redness, enlargement, sponginess, deep pockets, and definite mobility, are relatively easy to detect even with limited experience, provided there is good light and accessibility for vision. In contrast, when changes are subtle, localized about one or a few teeth, and of a lesser degree of severity, more skillful application of knowledge is needed.

Early recognition of gingival and periodontal disease prevents neglect of conditions which can develop into severe disease. Treatment is less complicated, and the success of treatment and recovery to healthy tissue is predictable when early recognition makes early treatment possible.

THE GINGIVAL INSPECTION

The inspection of the gingiva includes evaluation of the color, size, shape, consistency, surface texture, position, mucogingival lines, bleeding, and exudate. These are summarized in table 11–1, which is a clinical reference chart.

I. Color

A. **Normal**
   1. Pale pink; darker in people with darker complexions.
   2. Factors influencing color.
      a. Vascular supply.
      b. Thickness of epithelium.
      c. Degree of keratinization.
      d. Physiologic pigmentation: melanin pigmentation occurs frequently in Negroes, Orientals, Indians, and Caucasians of Mediterranean countries.

B. **Changes in Disease**
   1. In chronic inflammation: dark red, bluish red, magenta, or deep blue.
   2. In acute inflammation: bright red.
   3. Extent: deep involvement can be expected when color changes ex-

tend into the attached gingiva; or from the marginal gingiva to the mucogingival line; or over into alveolar mucosa.

II. Size

A. **Normal**
1. Free gingiva: flat, not enlarged, fits snugly around the tooth.
2. Attached gingiva.
   a. Width of attached gingiva varies between patients and between teeth for an individual, from 1 to 9 millimeters.[7]
   b. Wider in maxilla than mandible: broadest zone related to incisors, narrowest at the canine and premolar regions.

B. **Changes in Disease**
1. Free gingiva and papillae: become enlarged, which may be localized or limited to specific areas or generalized throughout the entire gingiva. The col deepens as the papillae increase in size.
2. Attached gingiva: decreases in amount as the pocket deepens. How to measure the amount of attached gingiva is described on page 193.

III. Position

The *actual* position of the gingiva is the level of the junctional epithelium (epithelial attachment) which is not directly visible but can be determined by probing (page 186). The *apparent* position of the gingiva is the level of the gingival margin which is seen by direct observation.

A. **Normal:** in an adult, for the fully erupted tooth, the apparent position of the gingival margin is normally at the level of, or slightly below, the enamel contour or prominence of the cervical third of a tooth.

B. **Changes in Disease**
1. Location
   a. With gingival enlargement (in-crease in size) the apparent position may be high on the enamel.
   b. With recession, the gingival margin is apical to the cementoenamel junction.
2. Recession: exposure of root surface resulting from apical movement of the gingiva.
3. To measure recession: place a probe parallel with the long axis of the tooth and measure from the cementoenamel junction to the gingival margin for apparent recession, and to the bottom of the pocket for actual recession.

IV. Shape (Form or Contour)

A. **Normal**
1. Free gingiva
   a. Follows a curved line around each tooth; may be straighter along wide molar surfaces.
   b. The margin is knife-edged or slightly rounded on facial and lingual; closely adapted to the tooth surface.
2. Papillae
   a. Teeth with contact area: facial and lingual pointed or slightly rounded papillae with col area under the contact (figure 11–5).
   b. Spaced teeth (with diastemas): interdental gingiva is flat or saddle-shaped.

B. **Changes in Disease**
1. Gingival margin
   a. Bulbous or rounded
   b. Festoon ("McCall's festoon"): an enlargement of the marginal gingiva with the formation of a life-saver–like gingival prominence.
   c. Gingival cleft ("Stillman's cleft"): straight or apostrophe–shaped indentation which extends from the gingival margin along the root surface; may extend to the alveolar mucosa.

Table 11–1. Inspection of the Gingiva. Clinical Reference Chart

	Normal Appearance	Changes in Disease Clinical Appearance	Causes for Changes
Color	Uniformly pale pink Variations in pigmentation related to complexion, race	Acute: bright red	Inflammation: capillary dilation increased blood flow
		Chronic: bluish pink, bluish red	Vessels engorged Blood flow sluggish Venous return impaired Anoxemia
		pink	Increased fibrosis
		Attached gingiva: color change may extend to the mucogingival line	Deepening of pocket, mucogingival involvement
Size	Flat, not enlarged Fits snugly around the tooth	Enlarged	Edematous: inflammatory fluid cellular exudate vascular enlargement hemorrhage Fibrotic: new collagen fibers
Shape	Marginal gingiva: Knife-edge, flat Follows a curved line about the tooth	Marginal gingiva: rounded rolled bulbous	Inflammatory changes: edema or fibrosis
	Papillae: (1) Normal contact, papilla is pointed and pyramidal; fills the interproximal area (2) Space (diastema) between teeth: gingiva is flat or saddle-shaped	Papillae: bulbous flattened blunted cratered	Bulbous with gingival enlargement Cratered in acute necrotizing ulcerative gingivitis
Consistency	Firm, resilient Attached gingiva firmly bound down	Soft, spongy, dents readily when pressed with probe. Associated with red color, smooth shiny surface, loss of stippling, bleeding on probing	Edematous: fluid between cells in connective tissue
		Firm, hard, resists probe pressure Associated with pink color, stippling, bleeding only in depth of pocket	Fibrotic: collagen fibers

	Normal Appearance	Changes in Disease Clinical Appearance	Causes for Changes
Surface texture	Free gingiva: smooth Attached gingiva: stippled	Acute condition: loss of stippling, with smooth, shiny gingiva Chronic: hard, firm, with stippling, sometimes heavier than normal	Inflammatory changes in the connective tissue; edema, cellular infiltration Fibrosis
Position of Gingival Margin	Fully erupted tooth: margin is 1–2 mm. above cementoenamel junction, at or slightly below the enamel contour.	Enlarged gingiva: margin is higher on the tooth, above normal, pocket deepened. Recession: margin is more apical; root surface is exposed.	Edematous or fibrotic (see Size, page 172) Junctional epithelium has migrated along the root; gingival margin follows.
Position of Junctional Epithelium	Fully erupted tooth: the junctional epithelium is at the cementoenamel junction During eruption: along the enamel surface	Position, determined by use of probe, is on the root surface.	Apical migration of the epithelium along the root
Mucogingival Lines	Make clear demarcation between the pink, stippled, attached gingiva and the darker alveolar mucosa with smooth shiny surface and thin keratinization.	No attached gingiva: (1) color changes may extend full height of the gingiva; mucogingival line obliterated. (2) Probing reveals that the bottom of the pocket extends into the alveolar mucosa. (3) Frenal pull may displace the gingival margin from the tooth.	Deepening of the pocket Apical migration of the junctional epithelium Attached gingiva decreases with pocket deepening Inflammation extends into alveolar mucosa.
Bleeding	No spontaneous bleeding or upon probing	Spontaneous bleeding Bleeding on probing: Bleeding near margin in acute condition; bleeding deep in pocket in chronic.	Degeneration of the sulcular epithelium with ulceration Blood vessels engorged Tissue edematous
Exudate	No exudate on pressure.	White fluid, pus, visible on digital pressure Amount not related to pocket depth	Inflammation in the connective tissue Excessive accumulation of white blood cells with serum and tissue fluid makes up the exudate (pus).

Several possible causes exist, one of which is incorrect toothbrushing.

2. Papillae: bulbous, flattened, blunted, or cratered. Figure 11–7 illustrates the shape of normal compared with enlarged, bulbous gingiva.

V. Consistency

A. **Normal**
1. Firm and resilient when palpated with the side of a blunt instrument (probe).

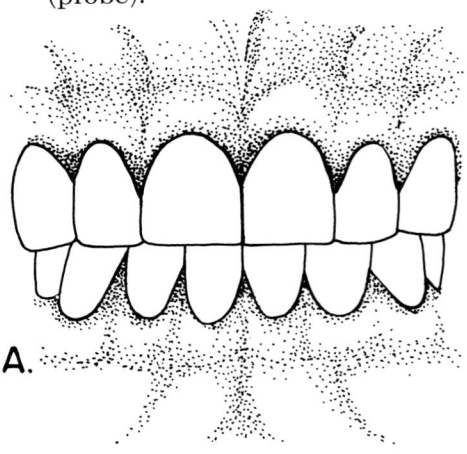

A.

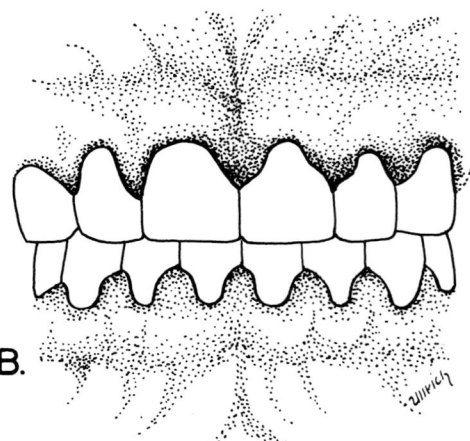

B.

Figure 11–7. Shape of the gingiva. **A.** Normal contour. **B.** Gingival enlargement with rounded marginal gingiva and bulbous papillae.

2. Attached gingiva is bound down firmly to the underlying bone.

B. **Changes in Disease**
1. To determine consistency: gently press side of probe on free gingiva. Soft, spongy gingiva will dent readily; firm hard tissue resists.
2. Soft spongy gingiva is related to acute stages of inflammation with increased infiltration of fluid and inflammatory elements. The tissue appears red, may be smooth and shiny with loss of stippling, has marginal enlargement, and bleeds readily on probing.
3. Firm, hard gingiva is related to chronic inflammation with increased fibrosis. The tissue may appear pink and well stippled. Bleeding, when probed, usually will occur only in the deeper part of a pocket, not near the margin.
4. Retraction of the margin away from the tooth: normally the free gingiva fits snugly about the tooth. When the margin tends to hang slightly away or is readily displaced with a light air blast, it means that the gingival fibers which support the margin have been destroyed.

VI. Surface Texture

A. **Normal**
1. Free gingiva: smooth.
2. Attached gingiva: stippled (minutely "pebbled" or "orange peel" surface).
3. Interdental gingiva: the free gingiva is smooth; the center portion of each papilla is stippled.

B. **Changes in Disease**
1. Early inflammatory changes: may be loss of stippling, with smooth, shiny surface.
2. Hyperkeratosis may result in a leathery, hard, or nodular surface.
3. Chronic disease: tissue may be hard

and fibrotic with a normal pink color, and have normal or deep stippling.

VII. Bleeding

A. Normal
1. No bleeding: healthy tissue does not bleed.
2. Gingival Index Score: zero (page 278).

B. Changes in Disease
1. Bleeding occurs spontaneously or when pockets are probed.
2. Changes in sulcular epithelium during the inflammatory process result in a thin, ulcerated pocket wall which bleeds readily. Development of inflammation and pocket formation are described on page 177.
3. Gingival Index Score: 2 or 3, depending on the severity of the condition.

VIII. Exudate

A. Normal: none, except slight gingival sulcus fluid (page 166).

B. Changes in Disease
1. Suppuration: Formation or secretion of pus.
2. White fluid may appear at the entrance to the pocket or may be squeezed out of the sulcus by light finger pressure on the external wall of the pocket. Pus is a semi-fluid creamy, yellow-white product of inflammation composed mainly of leukocytes and serum.
3. Amount of exudate: is related to the severity of the acute inflammation, not to the depth of the pocket.

IX. The Gingiva of Young Children[8-10]

A. Normal
1. *Primary dentition.*
   a. Color: pink or slightly red.
   b. Shape: thick, rounded, or rolled.
   c. Consistency: firm, but not tightly adapted to the teeth; it may be easily displaced with a light air jet.
   d. Surface texture: may or may not have stippling; high percentage have shiny gingiva.
   e Width of attached gingiva ages 3 to 5: between 1 and 6 millimeters.[7]
   f. Interdental gingiva.
      (1) Anterior: diastemas are frequently present and the papillae are flat or saddle-shaped; when teeth are in contact, the usual pyramid or col is present.
      (2) Posterior: col between facial and lingual papillae when teeth are in contact (figure 11–5).
2. *Mixed dentition.*
   a. Constant state of change related to exfoliation and eruption.
   b. Free gingiva may appear rolled or rounded, slightly reddened, shiny, and with a lack of firmness.
   c. Position: the gingiva covers varying portion of the anatomic crown, depending on the stage of eruption (figure 11–4).

B. Changes in Disease

Gingival disease is common in children and increases in prevalence until a high of over 90 percent can be found in the 9- to 14-year-old group. Periodontal disease can occur in the primary dentition as well as in a percentage of children of all ages. Definite periodontal disease can be observed during the teen-age years. Periodontosis is a condition involving severe bone loss particularly about incisors and first molars, which is usually first diagnosed in the 15- to 25-year-old group.

Examination of the periodontal tissues for a child is not different from that of an adult. A complete examination is necessary, including probing around each tooth.

X. The Gingiva after Periodontal Treatment

The characteristics of "normal healthy gingiva" take on different dimensions for the patient who has completed the treatment for pockets, bone loss, and other signs of periodontal disease. The junctional epithelium will be apical to the usual normal position, yet after healing the sulcus depth will be within normal range and no bleeding should occur when probed.

Depending on the exact treatment performed, examination will show changes from the initial evaluation. For example, where the initial examination showed a deficiency of attached gingiva with frenal pull, mucogingival surgery was designed and treatment satisfactorily completed to create new attached gingiva. With each recall, a thorough careful examination is necessary to control factors which may permit recurrence of disease.

GINGIVAL AND PERIODONTAL POCKETS

A pocket is a diseased sulcus. It is the presence or absence of disease that distinguishes a pocket from a sulcus, and not the depth as measured with a probe. A pocket has an *inner wall, the tooth surface*, and an *outer wall, the sulcular epithelium* of the free gingiva. The two walls meet at the base of the pocket. The base of the pocket is the coronal margin of the junctional epithelium.

The presence of a pocket is an indicator of gingival and/or periodontal diseases. The elimination of pockets is basic to all treatment. When pockets are eliminated, plaque removal in the sulcus by the patient is made possible. The control of plaque microorganisms which initiate gingival and periodontal diseases is essential for the arrest and control of disease.

Most periodontal diseases are inflammatory, inflammatory combined with trauma from occlusion, or complicated by inflammation. The inflammatory diseases are divided into *gingivitis*, when only the gingiva is involved, and *periodontitis*, which means inflammation is in the gingiva and the deeper parts of the periodontium, namely, the cementum, periodontal ligament, and alveolar bone.

I. Types of Pockets

Pockets are divided into *gingival* and *periodontal* types to clarify the degree of anatomic involvement. They are then further categorized by their position in relation to the alveolar bone, that is, whether their pocket base is suprabony or intrabony (figure 11–8).

A. **Gingival Pocket**
   1. Definition: a pocket formed by gingival enlargement without apical migration of the junctional epithelium (figure 11–8A).

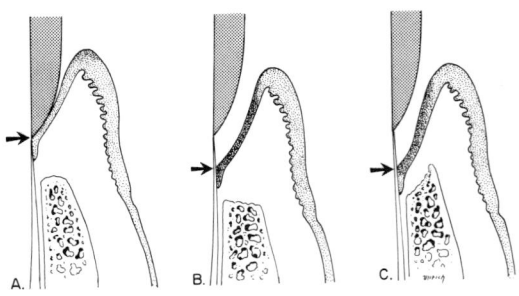

Figure 11–8. Types of pockets. Arrow indicates coronal margin of the junctional epithelium. **A.** Gingival pocket formed by gingival enlargement. Junctional epithelium has not migrated along root surface. **B.** Periodontal pocket which is suprabony. The junctional epithelium has migrated apically along the cementum. **C.** Periodontal pocket which is intrabony, in which the top of the junctional epithelium is apical to the crest of the interdental bone.

2. Other names: pseudopocket, false pocket, relative pocket.
3. The margin of the gingiva has moved toward the incisal or occlusal without the deeper periodontal structures becoming involved.
4. The tooth wall is enamel.
5. During eruption, the base of the pocket is at various levels along the enamel. The base of the pocket of the fully erupted tooth is at the cementoenamel junction (figure 11–4, page 167).
6. All gingival pockets are suprabony: that is, the base of the pocket is coronal to the crest of the alveolar bone.

B. **Periodontal Pockets**
1. Definition: a pocket formed as a result of disease or degeneration which caused the junctional epithelium to migrate apically along the cementum.
2. Other names: true pocket, absolute pocket.
3. The periodontal deeper structures (attachment apparatus) are involved, that is, the cementum, periodontal ligament, and bone.
4. The tooth wall is cementum or partly cementum and partly enamel.
5. The base of the pocket is on cementum.
6. Periodontal pockets may be suprabony or infrabony.
   a. Suprabony: pocket in which the base of the pocket (junctional epithelium) is coronal to the crest of the alveolar bone (figure 11–8B).
   b. Intrabony: pocket in which the base of the pocket (junctional epithelium) is below or apical to the crest of the alveolar bone (figure 11–8C).

II. **Pocket Formation**

A. **Steps in the Development of a Gingival Pocket**
1. Microorganisms of plaque produce harmful substances: enzymes and toxins.
   a. Plaque collects at and below the gingival margin.
   b. Bacterial products (enzymes and toxins) cause breakdown of epithelial intercellular substances which leads to ulceration of the sulcular epithelium.
   c. Widening of intercellular spaces permits injurious agents to penetrate into the connective tissue beneath the epithelium.
2. Inflammatory reaction in the connective tissue
   a. Dilation and increased permeability of capillaries with increased blood flow results in redness of tissue and bleeding when probed.
   b. Increased numbers of inflammatory cells collect for defense: primarily lymphocytes, plasma cells, polymorphonuclear leukocytes, and macrophages. An exudate may be produced in an acute stage.
   c. Edema from the leakage of fluid into the tissues results in an increase in size and alteration in shape of the gingival tissue.
3. Gingival pocket formation
   a. Junctional epithelium does not move at the base of the pocket.
   b. Increased depth is due to swelling from the enlarged gingiva.
4. Reversible: when plaque is controlled and calculus which is harboring plaque is removed, the number of microorganisms is reduced and the irritant is removed. The inflammation then subsides and the enlargement can decrease.

5. Continued exposure to plaque organisms means continued inflammatory reaction and increased pocket depth.

6. Chronic gingivitis develops.
   a. Destruction (inflammation) and healing (new collagen fibers and blood vessels produced) go on simultaneously.
   b. Fibrosis may result which leads to the formation of firm hard gingiva.

B. **Steps in the Development of a Periodontal Pocket**
   1. Extension of inflammation from the gingival pocket into the deeper structures.
      a. Plaque microorganisms collect in large numbers because plaque control procedures were ineffective in the depth of the gingival pocket.
      b. Plaque microorganisms continue to produce irritants: inflammation increases in severity and spreads.
      c. Inflammation spreads through the loose connective tissue along (beside) the blood vessels to the bone.[11]
      d. Most commonly the inflammation enters the bone through small vessel channels in the alveolar crest.
      e. Inflammation spreads through the bone marrow and out into the periodontal ligament.
   2. Progressive destruction of connective tissue fibers under the base of the sulcus at the apical border of the junctional epithelium.
      a. Undermining destruction: epithelium migrates along the root surface.
      b. Coronal portion of the junctional epithelium becomes detached.
      c. Since the epithelial cells must be living for migration, the junc-

tional epithelium usually remains intact and does not have ulcerations or other destructive changes such as the sulcular epithelium shows.

3. Exposed cementum where the fibers were attached becomes altered. There are changes chemically and physically and in permeability. Bacterial and inflammatory products from the periodontal pocket become incorporated. The diseased cementum contains endotoxin.

4. Pocket becomes progressively deepened as the migration of epithelium continues toward the apex of the tooth.
   a. Pocket retains plaque microorganisms and is not cleanable by the patient.
   b. Plaque retention leads to calculus formation.

C. **Systemic Influence on Pocket Formation**
   1. Pocket formation is not caused by or initiated by a systemic condition or disease.
   2. Systemic condition can influence the severity and rate of development and the response to healing.
      a. An altered, exaggerated response to plaque bacterial irritants can occur.
      b. Alteration of healing capacity and lowered resistance to infection can influence outcome of treatment.

III. **Identification of Pockets**

A. **Method**
   The use of a calibrated probe is the only accurate, dependable way in which pockets can be located, inspected, and measured. Detailed technique and charting procedures are described on pages 186–194.

B. **Signs and Symptoms Which Suggest the Presence of Pockets**

Although precise information about pockets is determined by the use of a probe, notice of clinical changes in the tissues can be of invaluable assistance while probing. All of the indicators of disease which were described with the gingival examination (pages 170–175) can provide clues to the presence of pockets.

Extended color changes, loss of stippling, margins that retract and do not fit snugly about a tooth, bleeding, exudate, and changes in form and size are all indicators of disease and pocket formation. It is the evidence of disease that determines the presence of a pocket, not the depth. A shallow pocket can be severely involved with inflammation and degeneration.

C. **Furcation Involvement**

Furcation involvement means that the pocket and bone loss have extended into the furcation area, or furca, the area between the roots of a multirooted tooth.

1. Significance of furcation involvement
    a. Furcation involvement, however incipient it may appear to be in a radiograph or by probing, indicates progressive periodontal disease.
    b. Causes and steps in pocket formation in a furcation are the same as for other pockets (pages 177–178).
2. Clinical observations
    a. When the gingiva over the furcation has not receded, the following may be seen:
        (1) The furcation is covered by the pocket wall.
        (2) No differences in color, size, or other tissue changes may exist to differentiate the area from adjacent gingiva; but

when color changes do exist, they provide clues to supplement probe examination.
    b. When the gingiva over a molar buccal furcation is receded, the root division may be seen directly.
3. Detection
    A suggested procedure for probing furcations is described on pages 191–192. Radiographic examination of furcation areas may be studied on page 203.

D. **Mucogingival Involvement**

When a pocket extends to or beyond the mucogingival junction and into the alveolar mucosa, there is mucogingival involvement. There is no attached gingiva in the area, and a probe can be passed through the pocket and past the mucogingival junction into the alveolar mucosa (figure 12–8, page 192).

1. Significance of attached gingiva
    a. Functions of the attached gingiva
        (1) Give support to the marginal gingiva.
        (2) Withstand the frictional stresses of mastication and toothbrushing.
        (3) Provide attachment or a solid base for the movable alveolar mucosa for the action of the cheeks, lips, and tongue.
    b. Barrier to passage of inflammation

    Without attachment, the inflammation from the pocket area can extend to the alveolar mucosa. The junctional epithelium (epithelial attachment) acts as a barrier to keep infection outside the body. With destruction of the connective tissue and periodontal ligament fibers under the junctional epithelium, the epithelium migrates along the root, thus a pocket is created. In mucogingival involvement the bottom of the pocket extends into the alveolar mucosa where unconfined inflammation can spread more rapidly in the loose tissue.

2. Clinical observations
   a. Color changes. Sometimes a bluish or bluish red area can be seen extending from the gingival margin to and/or beyond the mucogingival junction. Stippling is missing and the surface of the area is smooth and shiny. A probe is used to examine the extent of the involvement.
   b. Width of gingiva from gingival margin to mucogingival line. A narrow zone of gingiva, caused by recession or occurring naturally without recession, is more susceptible to developing mucogingival involvement because there is less attached gingiva at the start.
   c. Base of pocket at the mucogingival line. When the probe measures only 1 to 2 mm. and there is no bleeding on probing but the tip of the probe is at the mucogingival line, the area should be charted and called to the dentist's attention since surgery may be indicated. Such an area needs specific instruction in plaque control procedures for preventive maintenance.
   d. Frenal attachments. The frena were described on page 168. When a frenum attachment is high, and the width of the gingiva narrow, there may be a pull exerted on the gingiva when the cheek or lip is retracted. This can lead to injuries to the gingiva by food and trauma from brushing in the area. Plaque accumula-

tion, recession, and root exposure may result.

TOOTH SURFACE POCKET WALL

I. Tooth Structure Involved

A sulcus or a pocket has a gingival side, which is the sulcular epithelium, and a tooth side. In gingival pockets the tooth surface wall is enamel, while in periodontal pockets the tooth surface wall is cementum, or a combination of cementum and enamel.

The positions of the junctional epithelium and gingival margin determine whether the tooth surface wall will be cementum or enamel. Pockets may be of the same depth when measured with a probe, but because of the location of the junctional epithelium on the tooth surface, the tooth surface pocket wall varies.

II. Contents of a Pocket

A. Pocket Size

A pocket is narrow and the sulcular epithelial lining is adjacent to and follows closely the contour of the tooth. When there are calculus deposits, the pocket wall follows the contour of the calculus. The firmness of the free gingiva is influential in confining and shaping the submarginal calculus deposit.

Access of the opening of the pocket to the oral cavity provides an opportunity for material to collect. The deeper the pocket, the less it can be cleaned by toothbrushing or other plaque control devices, hence greater quantities of material can be expected to collect.

B. Substances Found

The following may be inside a pocket in contact with the tooth surface on one side and on the surface of the sulcular epithelium on the other.
1. Microorganisms and their products:

enzymes, endotoxins, and other metabolic products

2. Calculus deposits and other rough areas covered with dental plaque
3. Gingival sulcus fluid
4. Food remnants
5. Salivary mucin
6. Desquamated epithelial cells
7. Leukocytes
8. Purulent exudate made up of living and broken down leukocytes, living and dead microorganisms, and serum.

II. Nature of the Tooth Surface

Knowledge of the characteristics and quality of the tooth surface pocket wall is of prime importance in instrumentation. During the examination of the tooth surface with probe and explorer, differentiation needs to be made of the various irregularities that can occur. How the irregularities came into existence is important for interpretation and understanding.

A. Pocket Development Factors

1. The pocket deepens as a result of continuing action of the irritants and destructive agents from dental plaque.
2. The periodontal ligament fibers become detached and the junctional epithelium migrates apically.
3. The cementum becomes exposed to the open pocket and the oral fluids.
4. Cementum is altered and there are effects of physical and chemical changes which have been observed by electronmicroscope.
5. Surface changes occur as a result of exchange of minerals with oral fluids and exposure to plaque bacteria and their products. On different surfaces of the same teeth or different teeth in the same mouth, any of the following can occur[12]:

a. Hypermineralization of the surface cementum which increases with time
b. Decalcification
c. Calculus formation
d. Plaque and debris collection

B. Causes of Surface Irregularities

Surface irregularities are detected supramarginally by drying the surface with air, and observing under adequate direct or indirect light, followed by the use of an explorer as needed. Submarginally, examination is dependent, for the most part, on tactile and auditory sensitivity transmitted by a probe and an explorer (page 198). Causes of surface roughness include the following:

1. *Enamel surface*
   a. Structural defects: cracks, grooves
   b. Dental caries, decalcification
   c. Calculus deposits and heavy stain deposits
   d. Erosion, abrasion
   e. Pits and irregularities from hypoplasia
2. *Cementoenamel junction*
   Cementum overlaps enamel in 60 to 65 percent; cementum and enamel meet directly in 30 percent; or there may be a small zone of dentin between in 5 to 10 percent.[13] Despite the differences, the junction is usually smooth or with a slight groove except when cementum is worn away by abrasion. Abrasion may undermine the enamel.
3. *Cemental surface*
   a. Diseased cementum
   b. Cemental resorption
   c. Calculus
   d. Cemental caries
   e. Abrasion
   f. Deficient or overhanging filling
   g. Grooves from previous incomplete instrumentation

III. Examination of the Tooth Surface

Inspection of the tooth surface pocket wall is made with a probe and an explorer. The techniques are described on pages 199–200.

The distribution and amount of calculus, plaque, and other soft deposits are recorded with the periodontal charting and records (page 288).

FACTORS TO TEACH THE PATIENT

I. Characteristics of normal healthy gingiva.

II. The significance of bleeding: healthy tissue does not bleed.

III. What a pocket is and how it forms.

IV. How a pocket is measured with a probe and that until the sulci and pockets are probed, it is not possible to tell whether disease is present and how far it has progressed. Pockets and sulci must be checked regularly all around every tooth to be sure nothing is developing insidiously.

V. Relationship of gingival findings during inspection to the personal daily care procedures for the control of plaque.

VI. The need for meticulous care of an area of gingival recession close to the mucogingival line where, if inflammation developed, there could be serious involvement with loss of all of the attached gingiva.

VII. How the method of brushing, stiffness of toothbrush, and abrasiveness of a dentifrice can be factors in gingival recession.

References

1. Ainamo, J. and Löe, H.: Anatomical Characteristics of Gingiva. A Clinical and Microscopic Study of the Free and Attached Gingiva, *J. Periodont.*, 37, 5, January-February, 1966.

2. Sicher, H. and Bhaskar, S. N., eds.: *Orban's Oral Histology and Embryology*, 7th ed. St. Louis, Mosby, 1972, p. 232.

3. Ibid., p. 250.

4. Goldman, H. M. and Cohen, D. W.: *Periodontal Therapy*, 5th ed. St. Louis, Mosby, 1973, pp. 25–28.

5. Glickman, I.: *Clinical Periodontology*, 4th ed. Philadelphia, Saunders, 1972, pp. 14–15.

6. Ibid., p. 12.

7. Bowers, G. M.: A Study of the Width of Attached Gingiva, *J. Periodont.*, 34, 201, May, 1963.

8. Baer, P. N. and Benjamin, S. D.: *Periodontal Disease in Children and Adolescents.* Philadelphia, Lippincott, 1974, pp. 1–35.

9. Glickman: op. cit., pp. 259–261.

10. Kopczyk, R. A. and Lenox, J. A.: Periodontal Health and Disease in Children: Examination and Diagnosis, *Dent. Clin. North Am.*, 17, 25, January, 1973.

11. Weinmann, J. P.: Progress of Gingival Inflammation into the Supporting Structures of the Teeth, *J. Periodont.*, 12, 71, July, 1941.

12. Selvig, K. A.: Biological Changes at the Tooth-saliva Interface in Periodontal Disease, *J. Dent. Res.*, 48, 846, September–October, 1969.

13. Sicher and Bhaskar: op. cit., pp. 170–171.

Suggested Readings

Allen, D. L., McFall, W. T., and Hunter, G. C.: *Periodontics for the Dental Hygienist*, 2nd ed. Philadelphia, Lea & Febiger, 1974, pp. 7–35.

Colby, R. A., Kerr, D. A., and Robinson, H. B. G.: *Color Atlas of Oral Pathology*, 3rd ed. Philadelphia, Lippincott, 1971, pp. 76–90.

Glickman, I.: *Clinical Periodontology*, 4th ed. Philadelphia, Saunders, 1972, pp. 5–25, 185–210.

Glickman, I. and Smulow, J. B.: *Periodontal Disease: Clinical, Radiographic, and Histopathologic Features.* Philadelphia, Saunders, 1974, pp. 2–12, 38–48.

Goldman, H. M. and Cohen, D. W.: *Periodontal Therapy*, 5th ed. St. Louis, Mosby, 1973, pp. 1–44, 65–78, 94–137.

Grant, D. A., Stern, I. B., and Everett, F. G.: *Orban's Periodontics*, 4th ed. St. Louis, Mosby, 1972, pp. 3–62.

Permar, D.: *Oral Embryology and Microscopic Anatomy*, 5th ed. Philadelphia, Lea & Febiger, 1972, pp. 103–130.

Ratcliff, P. A. and Oliver, G. V.: Periodontics, in Steele, P. F., ed.: *Dimensions of Dental Hygiene*, 2nd ed. Philadelphia, Lea & Febiger, 1975, pp. 323–358.

Sicher, H. and Bhaskar, S. N., eds.: *Orban's Oral Histology and Embryology*, 7th ed. St. Louis, Mosby, 1972, pp. 218–268.

Smith, L. B., Golub, L. B., and Duperon, D. F.: An Evaluation of Crevicular Fluid and Gingival Tissue in Children, *J. Dent. Child.*, 41, 128, March-April, 1974.

Chapter 12

Examination Procedures

Parts of the gingival and dental examinations are made by direct *visual* observation, while other parts require *tactile* examination using a probe and an explorer. These two types of instruments, assisted by a mouth mirror, are key instruments in patient evaluation. Considerable skill is required for accurate and efficient probing and exploring.

General principles of instrumentation are described in Chapter 31, pages 461–469. Study of that chapter for basic descriptions of instrument parts, grasp, finger rests, and stroke, logically precedes the use of instruments in this chapter.

I. Precaution

There are several reasons why a probe or an explorer should not be applied to the teeth and gingiva until an initial review of information from the patient history and oral inspections has been made. The immediate application of information from the history was outlined on page 70. In addition, soft tissue lesions found during the intraoral and extraoral inspection may need immediate biopsy or additional diagnostic tests.

II. Basic Set-up

All tray arrangements need a basic set-up composed of a mouth mirror, probe, explorers, and cotton pliers. Wrapping these together for autoclaving increases efficiency. The packet should be labeled "basic set-up." When a complete examination tray is assembled, the basic set-up is included with other essentials (page 23).

THE MOUTH MIRROR

I. Description

A. **Parts.** There are three parts: the handle, shank, and working end which is the mounted mirror or mirror head. Instrument parts are described on page 462.

B. **Mirror Surfaces**
   1. Plane (flat): may produce a double image.
   2. Concave: magnifying.
   3. Front surface: the reflecting surface is on the front of the lens rather than the back as with plane or magnifying mirrors. The front surface eliminates "ghost" images.

C. **Diameters.** Diameters vary from ⅝ to 1¼ inches. In addition, special examination mirrors are available in 1½- to 2-inch diameters.

D. **Attachments.** Mirrors may be threaded plain stem or cone socket to be joined to a handle. Since mirrors tend to become scratched, replacement of the working end is possible without purchasing new handles.

E. **Handles**
   1. Thicker handles contribute to a more comfortable grasp and greater control.
   2. Wider mirror handles are especially useful for mobility determination (page 201).

F. **Disposable Mirrors**
   1. Plastic in one piece or a handle with replaceable head for professional use; may have front surface.
   2. Take-home mirrors for patient instruction. Patient may observe his own gingiva, or teeth with disclosing agent applied. One type has a light attachment.

II. Purposes and Uses

The mouth mirror is used to provide:

A. **Indirect Vision.** This is particularly needed for distal surfaces of posterior teeth and lingual surfaces of anterior teeth.

B. **Indirect Illumination.** Reflection of light from the dental overhead light to any area of the oral cavity is accomplished by adapting the mirror.

C. **Transillumination.** Reflection of light through the teeth.
   1. Mirror is held to reflect light from the lingual while the teeth are examined from the facial.
   2. Mirror is held for indirect vision on the lingual while light from the overhead dental light passes through the teeth. Translucency of

enamel can be seen clearly while dental caries or calculus deposits appear opaque.

D. **Retraction.** The mirror is used to protect or prevent interference by the cheeks, tongue, or lips.

III. Technique for Use

A. Use modified pen grasp with finger rest on tooth surface (pages 463–464).

B. Retraction
   1. Use petrolatum or other lubricant on dry or cracked lips and corners of mouth.
   2. Adjust the mirror position so that the angles of the mouth are protected from undue pressure of shank of the mirror.
   3. Insert and remove mirror carefully to avoid hitting the teeth since this can be very disturbing to the patient.

C. Maintain clear vision
   1. Warm mirror with water, rub along buccal mucosa to coat mirror with thin transparent film of saliva, and request patient to breathe through his nose, to prevent condensation of moisture on mirror: use a detergent or other means for keeping a clear surface.
   2. Discard scratched mirrors.

IV. Care of Mirrors

A. Dismantle mirror and handle for sterilization.

B. Examine carefully after scrubbing with brush prior to sterilization to assure removal of debris around back, shank, and rim of reflecting surface.

C. Handle carefully during sterilization procedures to prevent other instruments from scratching the reflecting surface.

D. Consult manufacturer's specifications for sterilizing or disinfecting procedures which may cloud the mirror, particularly the front surface type.

INSTRUMENTS FOR APPLICATION OF AIR

I. Purposes and Uses

With appropriate, timely application of air to clear saliva and debris and/or dry the tooth surfaces, the following can be accomplished:

A. **Improve and Facilitate Examination Procedures**
1. Make a thorough, more accurate inspection.
2. Dry supramarginal calculus, particularly small deposits which are light in color, so that it can be readily explored and removed. Dried calculus appears chalky and presents a contrast to tooth color.
3. Deflect free gingival margin for observation into the submarginal area. Submarginal calculus appears dark usually.
4. Make identification of areas of decalcification and carious lesions easier.
5. Recognize location and condition of restorations, particularly tooth-color restorations.

B. **Improve Visibility of the Field of Operation during Instrumentation**
1. Dry area for finger rest to provide stability during instrumentation.
2. Facilitate positive scaling techniques.
3. Minimize operating time.
4. Evaluate complete removal of calculus after instrumentation.

C. **Prepare Teeth and/or Gingiva for Certain Procedures**
1. Dry tooth surfaces for application of caries-preventive agents.
2. Make impression for study cast.
3. Apply topical anesthetic.

II. Compressed Air Syringe

A. **Description**
1. Air source: air compressor with tubing attachment to syringe.
2. Air tip: with angled working end which can be turned for maxillary or mandibular application. Tip is removable for sterilization.

B. **Technique for Use**
1. Use palm grasp about the handle of the syringe; place thumb on release lever or button on handle.
2. Test the air flow so that the strength of flow can be controlled.
3. Make controlled, relatively short, gentle applications of air.
4. Supplement air drying with use of saliva ejector and folded gauze sponge placed in vestibule.

C. **Precautions**
1. Avoid sharp blasts of air on sensitive cervical areas of teeth or open carious lesions. Such areas may be dried by blotting with a gauze sponge or cotton roll to avoid causing discomfort to the patient.
2. Forceful application of air may direct saliva and debris out of the oral cavity and contaminate the working area and operator, and create aerosols (pages 27–28). When air is directed toward the posterior region of the patient's mouth, it may cause coughing.
3. Avoid silicate cement or other restorations which may be harmed by excessive drying.
4. Avoid startling the patient: forewarn when air is to be applied.

D. **Care of Compressed Air Syringe**
1. Clean inside of air tip with pipe cleaner prior to sterilization.
2. Sanitize syringe by vigorous wiping with a gauze sponge moistened with disinfecting solution.

III. Manual Chip Blower

This instrument is not commonly used because of the availability and efficiency of the compressed air syringe. Consideration is given here because of its portability and therefore it may be used for home visits or wherever compressed air is not available. A main consideration is the particular attention which must be paid to sterilization.

A. **Description.** Rubber bulb attached to air tip with angled working end.

B. **Technique for Use**
1. Hold rubber bulb firmly in palm; use index finger and thumb to steady the shank of the air tip to prevent it from moving against the patient's oral tissues. The remaining fingers depress the bulb to force air out.
2. Hold away from the oral tissues when the pressure on bulb is released to prevent suction of debris and saliva into the air tip and bulb.

C. **Care.** Separate air tip and bulb. Clean inside of air tip with pipe cleaner prior to sterilization. Air tip is sterilized; bulb can only be rubbed vigorously with disinfecting solution.

PROBE

I. Description

A. **Parts**
There are three parts: the handle, the angled shank, and the working end which is the probe itself.

B. **Probe Characteristics**
1. Slender, rod-like working end; may be straight or tapered; round, flat or rectangular in cross section with a smooth, rounded end.
2. Marked in millimeters at intervals specific for each kind of probe.

C. **Examples of Probes.** In table 12–1 several probe markings are listed with examples and descriptions. Figure 12–1 shows a comparison of types of probe markings and sizes.

II. Selection

The probe chosen for use by a dentist or a dental hygienist is frequently the instrument first used when a particular technique was learned, or one that provides comfort during use because of habit. Analysis of a probe and comparison with other probes is recommended. Important features to be considered in probe selection are

A. **Adaptability.** The probe should be adaptable around the complete circumference of each tooth, both posterior and anterior, so that no millimeter of pocket depth can be neglected. Flat probes require more attention to adaptation and are useful primarily on facial and lingual surfaces.

B. **Markings.** Markings should be easy to read so that pocket depth can be readily identified and specifically measured and no disease area will be overlooked.

III. Purposes and Uses

A probe is used to

A. **Make a Sulcus and Pocket Survey**
1. Examine the shape, topography, and dimensions of sulci and pockets.
2. Measure pocket depths as a factor in the identification of severity of disease and for charting.
3. Determine relationship of the gingival margin, junctional epithelium, and the mucogingival line to detect the width of the attached gingiva (figure 12–9, page 193).

Table 12-1. Types of Probes

Probe Markings (in mm.)	Examples	Description
Marks at 3–6–8	University of Michigan O Premier O Marquis M-1	Round, fine, narrow diameter
Marks at 1, 2, 3–5–7, 8, 9, 10	Williams Goldman-Fox University of Michigan with Williams markings Glickman Merritt A and B	Round Flat (rectangular) Fine, round, narrow diameter Round, with longer shank Round, single bend in shank
Marks at 1, 2, 3–5, 6, 7, 8, 9, 10	Nabers #3N	Flat, double-ended with ends at right angles to each other
Marks at 3–6–9–12	Hu-Friedy Color-coded Marquis Color-coded	Round
No marks	Gilmore Nabers 1N and 2N	Tapered, sharper than other probes Curved, with curved shank for adaptation in a furcation

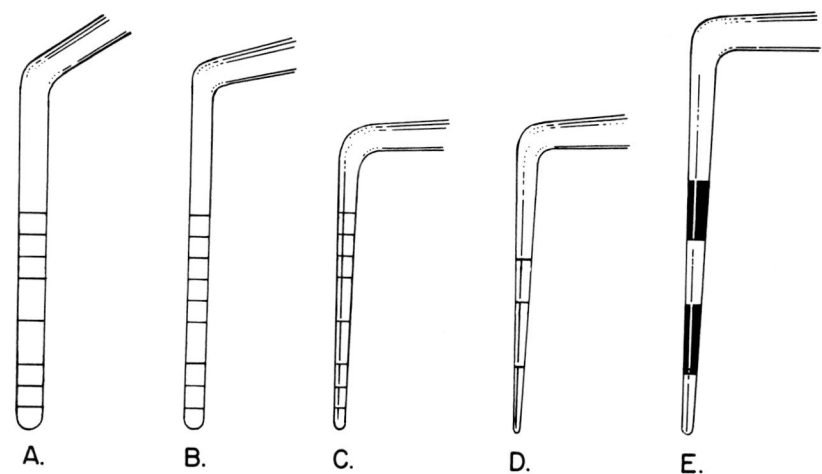

A.   B.   C.   D.   E.

Figure 12–1. Examples of probes. Names and calibrated markings for probes shown are **A.** Goldman-Fox (1-1-1-2-2-1-1-1, flat), **B.** Nabers (1-1-1-2-1-1-1-1, flat), **C.** Williams (1-1-1-2-2-1-1-1, round), **D.** Michigan O (3-3-2, round), **E.** Hu-Friedy or Marquis Color-coded (3-3-3-3, round). See Table 12–1 for additional data on probes.

B. **Make Other Gingival Determinations**
1. Evaluate gingival bleeding on probing, and prepare the gingival bleeding index (page 278).
2. Measure the extent of gingival recession.
3. Determine the consistency of the gingival tissue.

C. **Guide to Instrumentation**
1. Define depth for application of scaling, root planing, and curetting instruments, and depth for use of an explorer for evaluation of these procedures.
2. Detect anatomical configuration of roots, submarginal deposits, and root irregularities which complicate instrumentation. For this, the probe is used in conjunction with the explorer.

D. **Evaluate Success and Completeness of Treatment**
1. Evaluate tissue response to professional treatment postoperatively on an immediate, short-term basis as well as at periodic recall appointments.
2. Evaluate patient's self-treatment through plaque control procedures.
3. Signs of health revealed by probing
   a. No bleeding: healthy tissue does not bleed.
   b. Reduced pocket depth; comparison of pre- and postoperative pocket depths.
   c. Tissue is firm as shown by application of the probe to the surface of the free gingiva.

IV. Procedure for Use of Probe

The information in Chapter 11 concerning the gingival examination, the normal tissues, and the development and types of pockets, should be studied in conjunction with this outline of probing techniques.

A pocket is a diseased gingival sulcus. The use of a probe is the only accurate, dependable method to locate, inspect, and measure sulci and pockets.

Strategic use of light, retraction, a mouth mirror, and air for drying surfaces is necessary for efficiency and accuracy during the examination and measurement of sulci and pockets.

A. **Pocket Characteristics: Guide to Probing**
1. A pocket is measured from the base of the pocket (top of junctional epithelium) to the gingival margin. Figure 12–2 shows two pockets of different depths beneath gingival margins which are at the same level.
2. The pocket (or sulcus) is continuous around the entire tooth, and the entire pocket or sulcus must be measured. "Spot" probing is inadequate.
3. The depth varies around an individual tooth: it is unusual for a pocket to measure the same all around a tooth or even around one side of a tooth.
   a. The junctional epithelium assumes a varying position around the tooth.

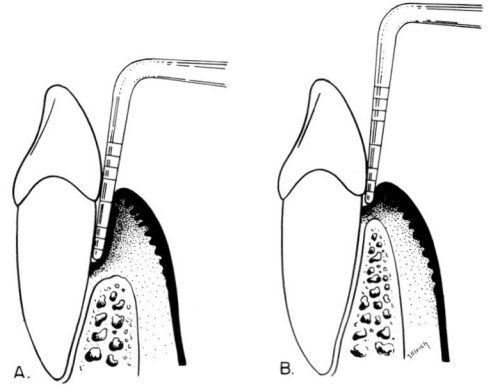

Figure 12–2. Pocket depth. A pocket is measured from the top of the junctional epithelium to the gingival margin. Contrast probe measurements of two pockets with gingival margins at the same level. **A.** Deep periodontal pocket (7 mm.). Junctional epithelium has migrated apically. **B.** Shallow pocket (2 mm.).

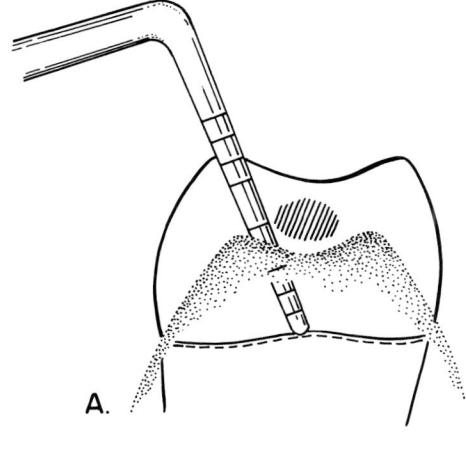

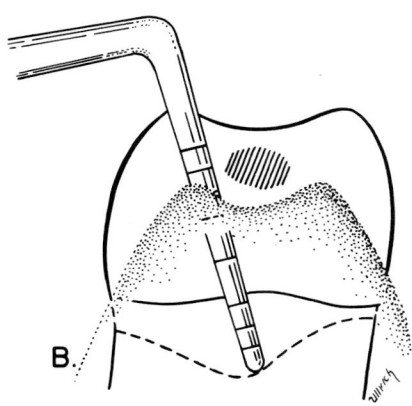

Figure 12–3. Proximal surface probing. **A.** Probe must be applied more than halfway across from the facial to overlap with probing from the lingual. **B.** Probe in area of crater formation. A pocket is usually deeper on the proximal under the contact area than on facial or lingual.

direction of probing. Examples are concave surfaces, anomalies, shape of cervical third, and position of furcations.

6. Pocket depth is not proportional to the severity of disease in the pocket. The sulcular epithelium of a shallow pocket may show more advanced degeneration and necrosis than the sulcular epithelium of a deeper pocket.

B. **Preparation for Probe Insertion**
1. Grasp probe with modified pen grasp (page 463).
2. Establish finger rest on a neighboring tooth in the same dental arch.
3. Hold side of instrument tip flat against the tooth near the gingival margin with the probe approximately parallel with the long axis of the tooth for insertion. The cervical third of a primary tooth is more convex (figure 12–4).
4. Gently insert the tip under the gingival margin.
   a. Healthy or firm fibrotic tissue: insertion is more difficult be-

   b. The gingival margin varies in its position on the tooth.
4. Proximal surface pockets
   a. Gingival and periodontal disease begin in the col area more frequently than other areas (page 167).
   b. Pocket may be deepest directly under the contact area because of crater formation in the alveolar bone (figure 12–3).
5. Anatomical features of the tooth wall of the pocket influence the

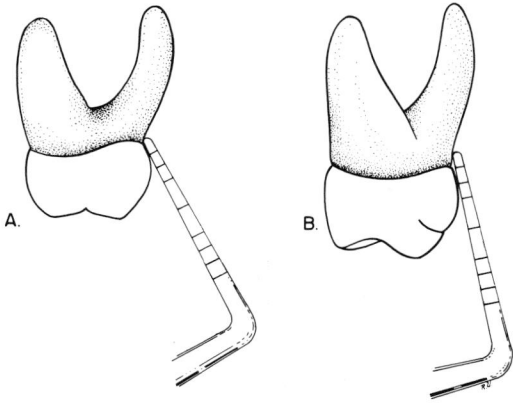

Figure 12–4. Probe placement on lingual of maxillary primary and permanent molars. **A.** Accentuated convexity of the cervical third and widespread roots of the primary tooth complicate probe placement. Probe may encounter the root. **B.** Permanent tooth with less convexity of the cervical third and roots that are less spread. Probe placement is easier than on primary tooth.

cause of the close adaptation of the tissue to the tooth surface; underlying gingival fibers are strong and tight.

b. Spongy, soft tissue: gingival margin is loose and flabby due to the destruction of underlying gingival fibers. Probe will insert readily and bleeding can be expected.

C. **Advance Probe to Base of Pocket**

1. Hold probe flat against the root surface. Widespread roots of primary molars may make this probe position difficult unless the tissue is unduly distended by the probe (figure 12–4).

2. Move the probe along the tooth surface vertically down to the base of the sulcus or pocket.

   a. Maintain contact of the side of the tip of the probe with the tooth.

   b. Interference: as the probe is passed down the side of the tooth, roughness may be felt. Possible causes of root roughness are listed on page 181. Evaluation of the topography and nature of the tooth surface is important to instrumentation.

c. Obstruction by hard bulky calculus deposit on tooth surface: lift the probe away from tooth and follow over the edge of the calculus until the probe can move vertically into the pocket again.

d. The bottom of the sulcus or pocket will feel soft and elastic (compared with tooth surface and calculus deposits) and, with slight pressure, the tension of the junctional epithelial tissue can be felt.

3. Position probe for reading.

   a. Bring the probe to position as nearly parallel with the long axis of the tooth as possible for reading the depth.

   b. Interference of the contact area does not permit placing the probe parallel for the measurement directly beneath the contact area. Hold the side of shank of the probe against the contact to minimize the angle.

D. **Read the Probe**

1. Measurement is made from the gingival margin to the base of the pocket.

2. Count the millimeters which show

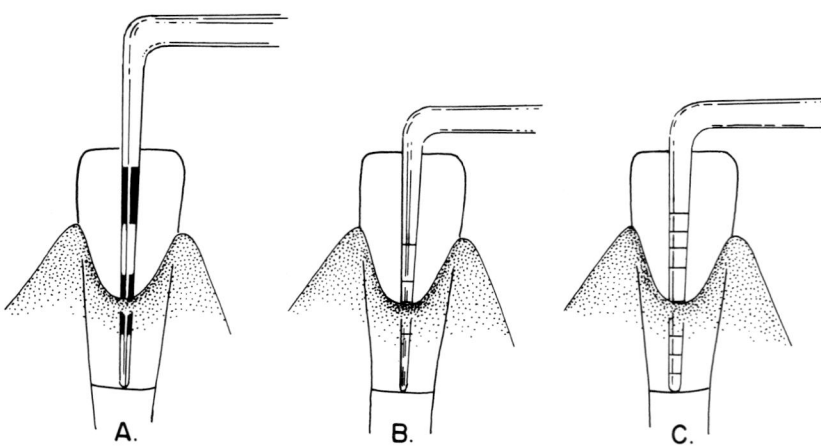

Figure 12–5. Measurement of same pocket with three different probes. **A.** Hu-Friedy or Marquis Color-coded, **B.** Michigan O. **C.** Williams.

on the probe above the gingival margin and subtract the number from the total number of millimeters marked on the particular probe being used. A comparison of pocket measurement using probes with different calibrations is shown in figure 12–5.

3. When the gingival margin appears at a level between probe marks, use the higher mark for the final reading.

4. Drying the area being probed improves visibility for specific reading.

E. **Circumferential Probing:** Probe stroke

1. Maintain the probe in the sulcus or pocket of each tooth as the probe is moved in a walking stroke to measure from distal to mesial.
   a. It is not correct to remove the probe and reinsert it to make individual readings.
   b. Repeated withdrawal and reinsertion will cause unnecessary trauma to the gingival margin and hence increase postoperative discomfort.

2. Walking stroke
   a. Hold the side of the tip against the tooth at the base of the pocket.
   b. Walking stroke: move the probe up (coronally) about 1 to 2 mm. and back to the attachment in a "touch . . . touch . . . touch . . ." rhythm (figure 12–6).
   c. Observe probe measurement at the gingival margin at each touch.
   d. Advance millimeter by millimeter along the facial into the proximal areas.

3. Horizontal stroke: To test bleeding from the sulcular epithelium, the probe is applied inside the pocket

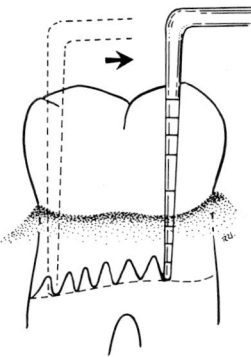

Figure 12–6. Probe walking stroke. The side of the tip of the probe is held in contact with the tooth. From the base of the pocket the probe is moved up and down in 1 to 2 mm. strokes. The junctional epithelium is contacted on each down stroke to identify the pocket depth in that area.

wall. The technique is shown for a gingival or bleeding index on page 278 and figure 19–1, page 279.

F. **Probing Proximal Surfaces**
1. Continue the walking stroke around each line angle and onto the proximal surfaces.
2. Roll the instrument handle between the fingers to keep the side of the probe tip adapted to the tooth surface as the tooth contour varies.
3. Continue stroke under the contact area. Overlap strokes from facial with strokes from lingual to assure full coverage (figure 12–3). Make sure that the col area under each contact has been thoroughly examined.

G. **Evaluation of Tooth Surface.** During the movement of the probe on the surface, irregularities can be felt and evaluated. Although the probe is not as sensitive as a fine explorer, it can be of assistance especially during the preliminary examination. Types of irregularities are described on page 181.

H. **Probing Furcation Areas**
   When a pocket extends into a furcation, special adaptation of the probe

must be made to determine the extent and topography of the furcation involvement.

1. Anatomic features related to probing
   a. Bifurcation (teeth with two roots)
      (1) Mandibular molars: the furcation area is accessible for probing from the facial and lingual.
      (2) Maxillary first premolars: the furcation area is accessible from the mesial and distal, under the contact area.
      (3) Primary mandibular molars: widespread roots.
   b. Trifurcation (teeth with three roots)
      (1) Maxillary molars: there is a palatal root and two buccal roots, the mesiobuccal and the distobuccal roots. Access for probing is from the mesial, buccal, and distal.
      (2) Maxillary primary molars: widespread roots (figure 12–4).
2. Examination methods
   a. Beginning furcation: probe to measure pocket depth, and then inspect the area by adapting the probe closely to the tooth surface and moving the end of the probe over the anatomical curvatures of the roots. Check radiograph for early signs of furcation involvement (page 203).
   b. Probe to measure pocket depths at points of access for each bifurcation or trifurcation area. Position of gingival margin will vary. Figure 12–7 shows apparent recession and 3-mm. pocket in bifurcation.
   c. Use probe in diagonal or horizontal position to examine between roots when there is gingival recession or a flexible, short,

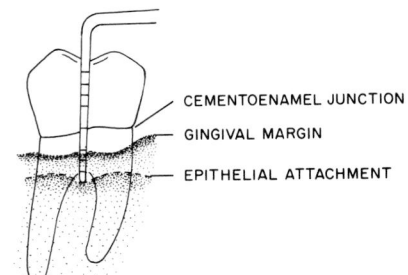

Figure 12–7. Furcation involvement. Probe inserted into bifurcation in area of gingival recession shows pocket of less than 3 mm. The probe is used to examine the topography of the furcation area.

soft pocket wall which permits access.
   d. Use a curved instrument such as a curved probe (Nabers 1N or 2N) or a curet to inspect advanced furcation.
   e. Anatomic variations which complicate furcation examination: fused roots, anomalies such as extra roots, or low or high furcations.

I. **Probing Mucogingival Involvement**

When a pocket extends to or beyond the mucogingival junction, the probe may pass through the pocket directly into the alveolar mucosa (figure 12–8). Mucogingival involvement was described on pages 179–180.

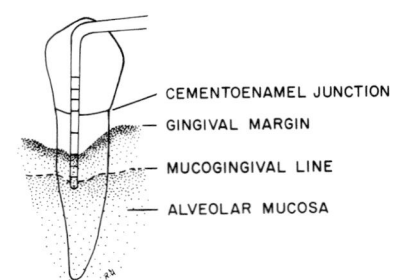

Figure 12–8. Mucogingival involvement. Probe in position for measuring pocket depth where there is no attached gingiva. Absence of attached gingiva permits probe to pass through mucogingival line into alveolar mucosa.

J. **Examine the Amount of Attached Gingiva**
1. Observe the amount of gingiva by retracting the lip and cheek from the facial. Note where the movable alveolar mucosa unites with the gingiva at the mucogingival junction. This is the mucogingival line and, when the line is drawn on a periodontal chart, the distance between the gingival margin and the mucogingival line should be clearly noted.

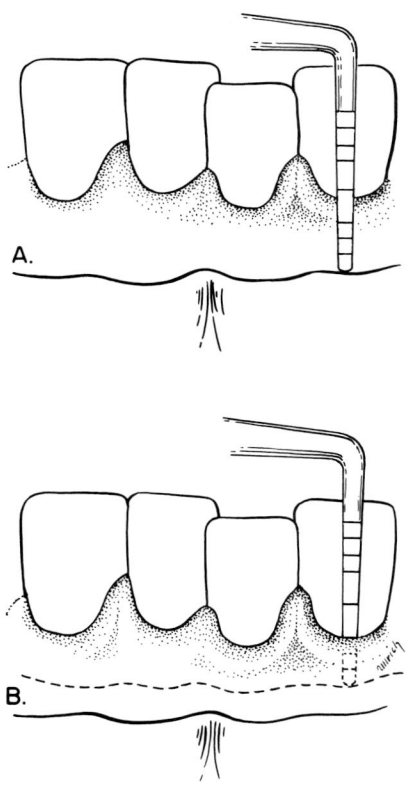

Figure 12–9. Measuring the width of the attached gingiva. **A.** Place probe on the surface of the gingiva and measure from the mucogingival line to the gingival margin to determine the total width of the gingiva. **B.** Measure the pocket. Dotted line represents the junctional epithelium at the bottom of the pocket. Subtract the pocket measurement (B) from the total width of the gingiva (A) to obtain the width of the attached gingiva.

2. To measure the amount of attached gingiva
   a. Place the probe on the external surface of the gingiva and measure from the mucogingival line to the gingival margin to determine the width of the total gingiva (figure 12–9 A).
   b. Insert the probe and measure pocket depth (figure 12–9 B).
   c. Subtract the pocket depth from the total gingival measurement to get the width of the attached gingiva.

K. **Test Frenal Attachments**
The maxillary and mandibular anterior and buccal frena and the lingual frenum were described on page 168.
1. Facial frena. To test the frena from the facial, pull out the lip or cheek gently, and lift the alveolar mucosa at the mucogingival line. If such tension moves the gingival margin away from a tooth, the high frenum attachment should be noted on the patient's record for review by the dentist.
2. Lingual frenum. To test the lingual frenum, request patient to lift the tip of the tongue to the palate. Observe the freedom of movement as well as the gingival attachment of the frenum and its relation to the free gingiva.

V. Periodontal Charting

Pocket charting is a part of the complete periodontal recordings. The summary of periodontal observations and records may be found on page 288.

The procedure described here assumes the use of a chart form with outline drawings of teeth with both facial and lingual root drawings. The exact procedure and format is entirely the choice of an individual dentist. A composite chart to include dental as well as periodontal findings is frequently used.

In the preparation of the charting, colors used should contrast with other colors on the chart. For example, when red is used to chart dental caries on a composite charting, red would not be a good color selection for drawing the gingival margin because of possible interference with a drawing of a Class V carious lesion. One procedure for a relatively simple charting system is described here.

A. **Teeth Identification.** Mark missing, unerupted, or impacted teeth. Prepare these markings in advance of the patient's appointment by reviewing and comparing the radiographs and the study casts.

B. **Draw Gingival Lines**
   1. Gingival margin
      a. Draw the outline of the position and contour of the gingival margin on the chart form as it appears in relation to the teeth both facial and lingual.
      b. Prepare in advance of the patient's appointment when study casts are ready.
   2. Mucogingival lines (page 168)
      a. Use contrasting color to that used for drawing the gingival line.
      b. Draw on the facial for all quadrants; draw lingual only on mandibular.
      c. Study casts: when parts or all of the mucogingival lines show clearly on the casts, the drawing can be made in advance of the patient's appointment.

C. **Record Pocket Measurements**
   1. Record all diseased pockets of any depth.
   2. Record deepest millimeter measurement for each of the six areas around a tooth as shown in figure 12–10. Areas numbered 1, 3, 4, 6 extend from the line angle to under the contact area.

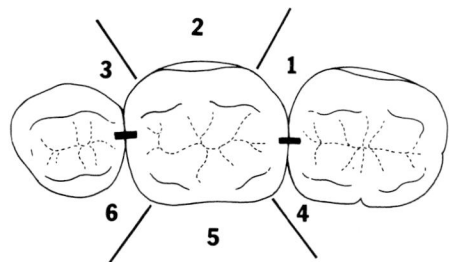

Figure 12–10. Charting pocket measurements. The pocket (sulcus) is measured completely around each tooth. Record the deepest measurement for each of the six areas around the tooth. Areas 1, 3, 4, 6 extend from the line angle to under the contact area.

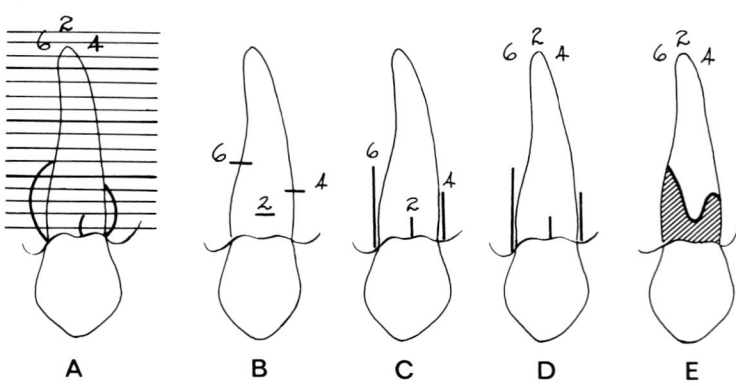

Figure 12–11. Methods for charting pocket measurements. **A.** Chart form with horizontal lines at millimeter intervals. Pocket measurements are written about the apex. Other chart forms do not have the millimeter markings, and may be used with **B.** horizontal lines, **C.** and **D.** vertical lines, or **E.** a continuous line to define the entire pocket area which can be shaded.

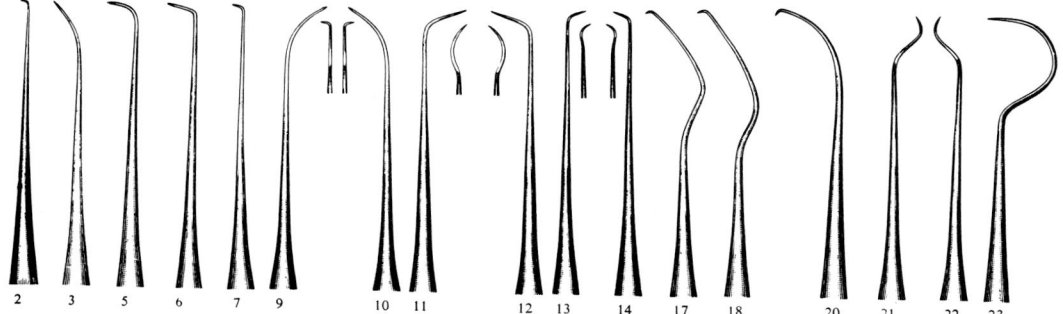

Figure 12–12. Explorers. This series from Numbers 2 through 23 shows standard shapes of explorer tips. Numbers 2 through 7, 17, 18, 20, and 23 are single instruments. Numbers 9 and 10, 11 and 12, 13 and 14, and 21 and 22 are paired instruments. (Courtesy of the S. S. White Company, Philadelphia, Pennsylvania.)

3. Supplement the six recordings with additional readings to show particular areas of unusually deep pockets, furcation involvement or mucogingival involvement.
4. Where to record on the charting form: figure 12–11 shows five possible methods for recording the millimeter depth.

D. Record Special Disease Problems

Furcation involvement, mucogingival involvement, and frenal pull must be recorded either by a conspicuous symbol, or by writing directly on the chart or in the record. See previous section for methods of examination.

EXPLORERS

I. Description

The basic parts of an instrument are described on page 462.

A. Working End

1. Slender, wire-like, metal *tip* approximately 1 to 2 mm. in length, which is circular in cross section and tapers to a fine sharp *point.*
2. Design
   a. Single: a single instrument may be universal and adaptable to any tooth surface, or it may be designed for specific groups of surfaces. In figure 12–12, Numbers 2 through 7, 17, 18, 20, and 23 are single instruments.
   b. Paired: paired instruments are mirror images of each other, curved to provide access to contralateral tooth surfaces. In figure 12–12, Numbers 9 and 10, 11 and 12, 13 and 14, and 21 and 22 are paired.
   c. Design of individual explorer: middle of working end (tip) should be centered over the long axis of the handle (figure 12–13).

B. Shank

1. Straight, curved, or angulated: whether a shank is straight, curved or angulated depends on the use and adaptation for which the explorer was designed. In figure 12–12 compare the straight shanks of Numbers 2, 5, 6, 7, 13, 14 with the others in the series which are not straight. A curved shank permits application of the instrument to proximal surfaces, particularly of posterior teeth.
2. Flexibility: the slender wire-like

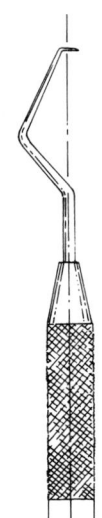

Figure 12–13. Explorer design. The middle of the tip should be centered over the long axis of the handle.

explorers have a degree of flexibility which contributes to increased sensitivity.

C. **Handle**
1. Weight: for increased acute tactile sensitivity, a lightweight handle is more effective.
2. Diameter: a wider diameter with serrations for friction while grasping can prevent finger cramping from too tight a grasp. With a lighter grasp, tactile sensitivity can be increased.

D. **Construction**
1. Single-ended: one working end, usually a single explorer (see A.2 above).
2. Double ended: a double-ended instrument has two working ends, one on each end of a common handle. Most paired instruments are available double-ended. Other double-ended instruments combine two single instruments, for example, two unpaired explorers or an explorer with a probe.

II. General Purposes and Uses

An explorer is used to

A. Detect, by tactile sense, the texture and character of the tooth surface.

B. Examine the supramarginal tooth surfaces for calculus, decalcified and carious lesions, defects or irregularities in the surfaces and margins of restorations, and other irregularities which are not apparent to direct observation. An explorer is used to confirm direct observation.

C. Examine the submarginal tooth surfaces for calculus, decalcified and carious lesions, diseased cementum and other cemental changes which can result from periodontal pocket formation.

D. Define the extent of instrumentation needed and guide techniques for
1. Scaling and root planing.
2. Polishing a restoration.
3. Removal of an overhanging filling.

E. Evaluate the completeness of treatment as shown by the smooth, glassy tooth surface or the smooth restoration.

III. Preparation of Explorers

Sharpen and retaper a dull explorer tip (page 491). With the explorer tip sharp and tapered, the following can be expected:

A. Increased tactile sensitivity with less pressure required.

B. Prevention of unnecessary trauma to the gingival tissue because with less pressure there can be greater control.

C. Decreased operating time with increased patient comfort.

IV. Specific Explorers and Their Uses

A variety of explorers are available as shown by the examples in figure 12–12. The function of each type is related to its adaptability to specific surfaces of teeth at particular angulations. For example, certain explorers can be used effectively for detection of dental caries in pits and fissures, and others are designed to be adapted to examine proximal surfaces for calculus or dental caries. By other criteria, some can be used submarginally, while others cannot be adapted submarginally without inflicting damage to the sulcular epithelium, and therefore are limited to supramarginal examination only.

A. **Submarginal Explorer (Number 17 in figure 12–12)**
   1. Other names and numbers: Orban Number 20, G-2, pocket explorer.
   2. Shape: the pocket explorer has an angulated and curved shank with a short tip at a right-angle bend (figure 12–13). The tip should be measured to make sure the tip is not over 2 millimeters, as a longer tip cannot be adapted to narrow roots, particularly because the pocket narrows near the base.
   3. Use
      a. Submarginal root examination: Number 17 is the instrument of choice.
      b. Characteristics which make Number 17 more effective for submarginal exploration than other types of explorers.
         (1) Back of tip can be applied directly to the junctional epithelium without lacerating. When a straight or sickle explorer is directed toward the base of the pocket, the sharp tip can pass into the epithelium without resistance.
         (2) The short tip can be adapted to rounded tooth surfaces and line angles. Long tips of other explorers have tangential relationship with the tooth, and cause distension and trauma to sulcular epithelium.

(3) Narrow short tip can be adapted at the base where the pocket narrows without undue displacement of the pocket soft tissue wall.
      c. Supramarginal use of Number 17: it may be adapted to all surfaces, is especially useful for proximal surface examination, and is not readily adaptable to pits and fissures.

B. **Sickle or Shepherd's Hook (Number 23 in figure 12–12)**
   1. Use: examining pits and fissures and supramarginal smooth surfaces; examining surfaces and margins of restorations.
   2. Adaptability
      a. Difficult to apply to proximal surfaces as the wide hook can contact an adjacent tooth, and the straight long section of the tip can pass over a small proximal carious lesion.
      b. Not effective for submarginal exploration because of reasons listed under A.3.b. above. When the point is directed to base of a pocket, there is danger of trauma to the junctional epithelium. In the attempt to prevent such damage, the operator may not explore to the base of the pocket, thus providing incomplete service.

C. **Pigtail or Cowhorn (Numbers 21 and 22 in figure 12–12)**
   1. Use: proximal surfaces: for calculus, dental caries, or margins of restorations.
   2. Adaptability: as paired, curved tips, they are applied to opposite tooth surfaces.

D. **Straight (Numbers 2, 6, 7 in figure 12–12)**
   1. Use: supramarginal, for pits and fissures, tooth irregularities of smooth surfaces, and surfaces and margins of restorations.

2. Adaptability
   a. For pit and fissure caries: the explorer tip is held parallel with the long axis of the tooth and applied straight into a pit.
   b. Not adaptable deep in submarginal area: straight shanked instruments or those with long tips do not adapt in the apical portion of the pocket near the junctional epithelium or on line angles.

BASIC TECHNIQUES FOR USE OF EXPLORERS

Prerequisite to the effective use of an explorer and to making interpretations of findings is knowledge of the anatomical surface features of each tooth, and the anatomy and characteristics of a sulcus and pocket. The latter were described on pages 165 and 176.

Development of ability to use an explorer and a probe is achieved first by learning the anatomy of the tooth surface and the types of irregularities which may be encountered on the surfaces. The second step is repeated practice of a careful and deliberate technique for application of the instruments.

The objective is to adapt the instruments in a consistent manner which will relay consistent comparative information about the nature of the tooth surface. Concentration, patience, attention to detail, and alertness to each irregularity, however small it may seem, are necessary.

I. Use of Sensory Stimuli

Both explorers and probes can transmit tactile stimuli from tooth surfaces to the fingers. A fine explorer usually gives a more acute reaction to small irregularities than a thicker explorer. Probes vary in diameter; the narrower types provide greater sensitivity.

A. **Tooth Surface Irregularities**

There are three basic tactile sensations which must be distinguished when probing or exploring. These may be grouped as normal tooth surface, irregularities created by excesses or elevations in the surface, and irregularities caused by depressions in the tooth surface. Examples of these are listed here.

1. *Normal*
   a. Tooth structure: the smooth surface of enamel and root surface that has been planed; anatomical configurations such as cingula, furcations.
   b. Restored surfaces: smooth surfaces of metal (gold, amalgam) and the softer feeling of plastic; smooth margin of a restoration.

2. *Irregularities: increases or elevations in tooth surface.*
   a. Deposits: calculus, and stain which is thick.
   b. Anomalies: enamel pearl; unusually pronounced cementoenamel junction.
   c. Restorations: overcontoured, irregular margins (overhang).

3. *Irregularities: depressions, grooves.*
   a. Tooth surface: decalcified or carious lesion, abrasion, erosion, pits such as those caused by enamel hypoplasia, areas of cemental resorption on the root surface.
   b. Restorations: deficient margin, rough surface.

B. **Types of Stimuli**

During exploring and probing, distinction of irregularities can be made through auditory and tactile means.

1. *Tactile.* Tactile sensations pass through the instrument to the fingers and hand and to the brain for registration and action. Tactile sensations, for example, may be the result of catching on an overcontoured restoration, dropping into a carious lesion, hooking the edge of a restoration or lesion, encounter-

ing an elevated deposit, or simply rubbing over a rough surface.

2. *Auditory.* As an explorer or probe moves over the surface of enamel, cementum, a metallic restoration, a plastic restoration, or any irregularity of tooth structure or restoration, a particular surface texture is apparent. With each contact, sound may be created. The clean smooth enamel is quiet, the rough cementum or calculus is scratchy or noisy. Sometimes a metallic restoration may "squeak" or have a metallic "ring." With experience, differentiations can be made.

II. Procedures: Supramarginal

A. Use of Vision

Supramarginal exploration for defects of the tooth surface differs from submarginal in that, when a surface is dried, much of the actual exploration is to confirm visual observation. The exceptions are the proximal areas near and around contact areas which cannot be directly observed.

Unnecessary exploring should be avoided. With adequate light and a source of air, proper retraction, and use of mouth mirror, dried supramarginal calculus can generally be seen since it is apt to be either chalky white or brownish yellow, and in contrast to tooth color. A minimum of exploration can confirm the finding.

B. Facial and Lingual Surfaces

1. Choice of explorer: almost all explorers can be adapted to the middle and incisal thirds of facial and lingual surfaces. For the cervical (gingival) third the pocket explorer, Number 17, is recommended. Application and stroke are made as described for submarginal surfaces (page 200). The tip can be directed away from the gingival margin to prevent laceration.

2. Use side of tip with the point always on the tooth surface.

3. Move the instrument in short walking strokes over the surface being examined for calculus, or direct the tip gently into a suspected carious lesion.

4. Cervical sensitivity: avoid deliberate exploration of cervical third areas where there is recession or where the patient has previously exhibited sensitivity. If necessary to dry a sensitive area, avoid an air blast, and blot with a gauze sponge or a cotton roll. Methods for desensitization are described on pages 564–566.

C. Proximal Surfaces

1. Choice of explorer: submarginal explorer Number 17 or the pigtails (Numbers 21 and 22 in figure 12–12), or other explorer with curved working end.

2. Lead with the tip onto the proximal surface, rolling the handle between the fingers to assure adaptation around the line angle.

3. Explore under the proximal contact area when there is recession of the papilla and the area is exposed. Overlap strokes from facial and lingual to assure full coverage.

III. Procedures: Submarginal

A. Choice of Explorer: Submarginal explorer Number 17.

B. Essentials for Detection of Tooth Surface Irregularities

1. Definite but light grasp.
2. Consistent finger rest with light pressure.
3. Definite contact of the instrument with the tooth.
4. Light touch as the instrument is moved over the tooth surface.

C. Steps

1. With the tip in contact with the tooth supramarginally, hold the part

of the shank which is next to the tip parallel with the long axis of the tooth, and gently slide the tip under the gingival margin into the sulcus or pocket.

2. Keep the point in contact with the tooth at all times to prevent lacerations of the sulcular epithelium. Adapt the tip closely to the tooth surface on the side of the point.

3. Slide the explorer tip over the tooth surface to the base of the pocket until, with the back of the tip, the resistance of the soft tissue of the junctional epithelium is felt (figure 12–14). Calculus deposits may obstruct direct passage of the instrument to the base of the pocket. Lift the tip slightly away from the tooth surface and follow over the deposit to proceed to the base of the pocket.

4. Stroke: use a "walking" stroke, vertical or diagonal (oblique).
   a. Lead with the tip: move it ahead as the instrument progresses (figure 12–15).

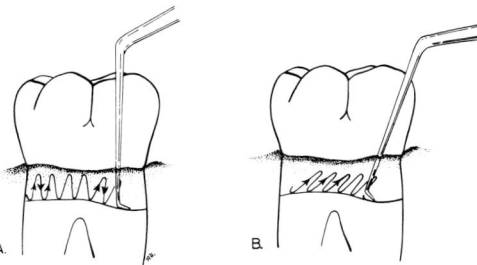

Figure 12–15. Explorer walking stroke. With the side of the tip of the explorer in contact with the tooth surface at all times, the explorer is moved over the surface in A. vertical walking stroke, or B. diagonal or oblique walking stroke. Complete exploration of the tooth surface is needed; therefore groups of strokes are overlapped.

b. Length of stroke depends on the depth of a pocket, for example,
   (1) Shallow pocket: the stroke may extend the entire depth, from the base of the pocket to just beneath the gingival margin.
   (2) Deep pocket: controlled strokes of 2 to 3 mm. long can provide more acute sensitivity to the surface and allow improved adaptation of the instrument. It is advisable to divide a deep pocket and first explore all of the apical section next to the base of the pocket, and then move up to explore another section, overlapping to assure full coverage.

c. Do not remove the explorer from the pocket for each stroke on a particular surface because
   (1) Trauma to the gingival margin caused by repeated withdrawal and reinsertion can cause the patient postoperative discomfort.
   (2) Concentration on the texture of the tooth surface is interrupted.
   (3) More time is consumed.

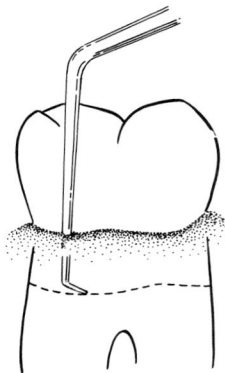

Figure 12–14. Use of submarginal explorer. The section of the shank next to the working tip is held parallel with the long axis of the tooth. The sharp explorer tip is held in contact with the tooth surface at all times. The explorer is passed into the pocket and over the surface until the back of the working end meets resistance from the junctional epithelium at the base of the pocket.

5. Proximal surface
   a. Lead with tip of instrument: do not "back into" an area.
   b. Continue the stroke around the line angle: roll the instrument handle between the fingers to keep the tip closely adapted as the tooth contour changes.
   c. Continue stroke under the contact area. Overlap strokes from facial and lingual to assure full coverage.

IV. Record Findings

A. Supramarginal Calculus
1. Distribution. Supramarginal calculus is generally localized. It is most commonly confined to the lingual of the mandibular anterior teeth, and the buccal of the maxillary first and second molars, opposite the openings to the salivary ducts (page 249)
2. Amount: slight, moderate, heavy

B. Submarginal Calculus
1. Distribution. Submarginal calculus can be either localized or generalized.
2. Amount: slight, moderate, heavy

C. Other Irregularities of the Tooth Surface: Note on the chart or in the record any other deviation from normal detected while using the explorer.

MOBILITY EXAMINATION

Because of the nature and function of the periodontal ligament, teeth have a slight normal mobility. Mobility can be considered abnormal or pathologic when it exceeds normal. Increased mobility can be an important clinical sign of disease.

I. Causes of Mobility

A. *Inflammation* in the periodontal ligament which leads to degeneration or destruction of the fibers.

B. *Loss of sufficient support* by alveolar bone and periodontal ligament (destroyed in periodontal disease).

C. *Trauma from occlusion:* injury to the periodontal tissues which results from occlusal forces (page 229).

II. Procedure for Determination of Mobility

A. Position the patient for clear visibility with maximum light and ready accessibility through convenient retraction.

B. Stabilize the head. Motion of the head, lips, or cheek can interfere with a true evaluation of tooth movement.

C. Use two single-ended metal instruments with wide blunt ends, held with a modified pen grasp. Using wooden tongue depressors or plastic mirror handles is not recommended because of their flexibility. Testing with the fingers without the metal instruments can be misleading since the soft tissue of the finger tips can be moved and give an illusion of tooth movement.

D. Apply specific, firm finger rests (fulcrums). A standardized finger rest pressure contributes increased consistency to the determinations. The teeth may be dried with air or sponge to prevent slipping of the instruments or the finger on the finger rest.

E. Apply the blunt ends of the instruments to opposite sides of a tooth, and rock the tooth to test horizontal mobility. Keep both instrument ends on the tooth as pressure is applied first from one side and then the other.

F. Test vertical mobility (depression of the tooth into its socket) by applying, on the occlusal or incisal surface, pressure with one of the mirror handles.

G. Test each primary abutment tooth of a fixed partial denture.

H. Move from tooth to tooth in a systematic order.

III. Record Degree of Movement

A. *Scale:* N, 1, 2, 3 or I, II, III are frequently used, sometimes with a + to indicate mobility between numbers.

B. *Recording:* although subjective, interpretation may be considered as follows:
N = Normal, physiologic
1 = slight mobility, greater than normal
2 = moderate mobility, greater than 1 mm. displacement
3 = severe mobility, may move in all directions, vertical as well as horizontal.

C. The letter N means *normal* mobility. All teeth that have a periodontal ligament have normal mobility. No tooth has zero mobility except in a condition such as ankylosis when there is no periodontal ligament.

D. Chart Form: a chart form used should provide for a place to record mobility, and preferably more than one place so that comparative readings may be recorded at successive recall appointments.

RADIOGRAPHIC EXAMINATION

Radiographs provide essential information to aid and supplement clinical findings. During other phases of the examination, and especially during probing, the mounted radiographs should be on a viewbox for viewing in conjunction with examination. When the radiographs have not been processed at the time of probing, areas for special confirmation can be marked on the record for review at the next appointment.

For observing evidence of periodontal involvement, periapical radiographs are needed. Bite-wing radiographs do not show the complete periodontal tissues which extend around the roots. When there is moderate to severe bone loss, the crest of the bone cannot be seen in a bite-wing survey.

Principles for use of radiographs were described on pages 136–137. The need for mounted radiographs which are free from errors of technique, and viewed on an adequately lighted viewbox, cannot be overemphasized. A magnifying reading glass is of special assistance when studying periodontal findings.

I. Radiographic Changes in Periodontal Diseases

A. **Bone Level**
   1. Normal bone level: the crest of the interdental bone appears from 1.0 to 1.5 mm. from the cementoenamel junction (figure 12–16).
   2. Bone level in periodontal disease: the height of the bone is lowered progressively as the inflammation is extended and bone is resorbed.

B. **Shape of Remaining Bone**
   1. *Horizontal*
      a. When the crest of the bone is parallel with a line between the cementoenamel junctions of two adjacent teeth, it is called "horizontal bone loss" (figures 12–17 and 12–18).
      b. When inflammation is the sole destructive factor, the bone loss usually appears horizontal.
      c. Generalized: when the amount of remaining bone is fairly evenly distributed throughout the dentition, it is described as generalized horizontal bone loss. It may be designated either by millimeters from the position of the normal bone level or by percentage. When making estimates, referral to the table of average root lengths can be helpful (Appendix, tables A–3 and A–4).

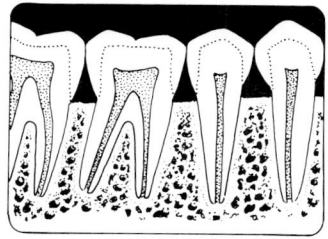

Figure 12–16. Drawing of a radiograph to show normal bone level, 1 to 1.5 mm. from the cementoenamel junction.

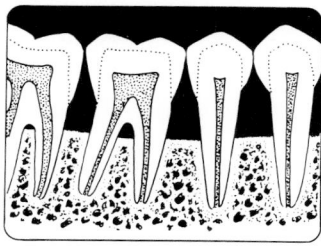

Figure 12–17. Horizontal bone loss. Bone level in periodontal disease is more than 1 to 1.5 mm. from the cementoenamel junction. When bone loss is horizontal the crest of the alveolar bone is parallel with a line between the cementoenamel junctions of adjacent teeth. Note early furcation involvement in the second molar and moderate furcation involvement in the first molar.

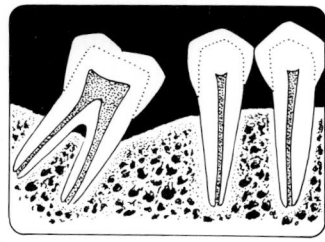

Figure 12–18. Horizontal bone loss. Second molar has drifted mesially into the space created when the first molar was removed. Note that the level of the crestal bone is parallel with a line between the cementoenamel junctions of the second premolar and the tipped second molar.

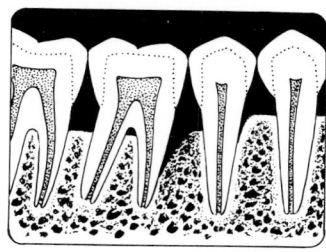

Figure 12–19. Angular or vertical bone loss, mesial of the first molar. The level of the crestal bone between the second premolar and the first molar is not parallel with a line between the cementoenamel junctions of the same teeth.

  d. Localized: when bone loss is confined to specific areas.
  2. *Angular or Vertical*
  a. Reduction in height of crestal bone which is irregular; the bone level is not parallel with a line joining the adjacent cementoenamel junctions (figure 12–19); and there is greater bone loss on the proximal surface of one tooth than on the adjacent tooth.
  b. Angular bone loss is more commonly localized than generalized.
  c. When inflammation and trauma from occlusion are combined in causing the destruction and irregular shape of the bone, the bone appears with "angular defects" or with "vertical bone loss."

C. **Crestal Lamina Dura**
  1. *Normal:* white, radiopaque; continuous with and connects the lamina dura about the roots of two adjacent teeth; covers the interdental bone.
  2. *Evidence of disease:* the crestal lamina dura is indistinct, irregular, radiolucent, fuzzy.

D. **Furcation Involvement**
  1. *Normal:* bone fills the area between the roots (figure 12–16).
  2. *Evidence of disease:* radiolucent area in the furcation.
  a. Early: beginning furcation involvement may appear as a small radiolucent black dot or as a slight thickening of the periodontal ligament space. It can be confirmed by probing. Early furcation involvement is shown in the second molar in figure 12–17.
  b. Furcation involvement of maxillary molars may become advanced before radiographic evi-

dence can be seen. Superimposition of the palatal root may mask a small area of involvement. When the proximal bone level in the radiograph appears at the level where the furcation is normally located, furcation involvement should be suspected and probed for confirmation.

c. Maxillary first premolar furcation: furcation involvement cannot be seen in a radiograph except at an unusual angulation or unusual position of the tooth. With correct vertical and horizontal angulation the roots are superimposed.

d. Furcations may show at one angulation but not at another; variations in technique can obscure a furcation involvement. All furcations must be carefully probed.

E. **Periodontal Ligament Space**

1. *Normal:* the periodontal ligament is connective tissue, hence appears radiolucent in a radiograph. It appears as a fine black radiolucent line next to the root surface. On its outer side is the lamina dura, the bone lining the tooth socket, which appears radiopaque (figure 12–20).

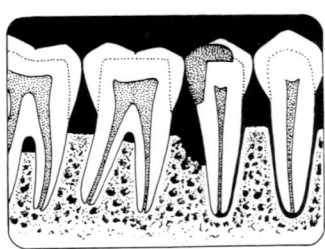

Figure 12–20. Periodontal ligament space. First and second molars have a normal periodontal ligament space which appears as a fine black line about the roots. The first premolar shows thickening of the ligament space about the entire root, and the second premolar has thickening about the mesial only.

2. *Evidence of disease:* widening or thickening

a. Angular thickening or triangulation: the space is widened only near the coronal third, near the crest of the interdental bone.

b. Complete periodontal ligament thickened along an entire side of a root to the apex, or around the root (figure 12–20). When viewed at different angulations (in the various radiographs of a complete survey), the ligament space may appear of varying thicknesses, which can show that the disease involvement is not consistent around the entire root or that other structures are superimposed.

II. Early Periodontal Disease

The real service which a dental hygienist can perform is to recognize *early signs* of periodontal involvement so that treatment can be initiated to arrest the disease and prevent more severe involvement which could lead to tooth loss. To recognize severe bone loss, advanced furcation involvement, and marked thickening of the periodontal ligament space is not difficult after a basic understanding is gained. The difficult part is to watch carefully for incipient, often isolated indications of early periodontal disease. These changes can be seen in all age groups, from small children to the elderly.

A. **Earliest Signs**

The early signs of periodontal involvement do not show in a radiograph. Only after the inflammation has extended from the soft tissue (gingivitis) to the supporting periodontal tissues, and there is sufficient bone resorption, will there be radiographic evidence.

B. **Initial Bone Destruction**
  1. Pathway of inflammation: the usual interproximal pathway of inflammation from gingivitis to periodontitis is directly from the inflamed gingival connective tissue into the crest of the interdental bone (page 178).
  2. Initial bone destruction takes place at the crest of the interdental bone in the crestal lamina dura.

C. **Radiographic Evidence**
  1. Crestal lamina dura will appear slightly irregular, fuzzy, and radiolucent. At this stage it is best examined with a hand magnifying glass.
  2. Angular thickening of the periodontal ligament space (triangulation) may also be apparent.

III. Other Radiographic Findings

Any other radiographic findings which may be directly or indirectly related to periodontal involvement and its contributing factors should be noted in the record for the attention of the dentist. Certain findings have a direct relation to dental hygiene care and instruction, particularly local factors which contribute to food impaction or plaque retention.

A. **Calculus**
  Gross deposits, primarily those on proximal surfaces, may be seen in radiographs. Observing these may be helpful, but the probe and explorer are needed to define the exact location and extent.
  The density and contrast of the radiograph influence whether or not calculus is seen. Since all deposits are not visible, the use of radiographs has limited value for specific calculus detection.

B. **Overhanging Restorations**
  Some proximal overhanging margins may be seen in radiographs. The use of an explorer is necessary to detect irregular margins and to examine all proximal margins which do not reveal irregularities in the radiographs. Superimposition can mask an overhanging margin.

C. **Dental Caries**
  Clinical and radiographic identification of carious lesions is described on pages 215–216. Certain findings should be noted for their relationship to the periodontal tissues.
  1. Large carious lesions may leave open contact areas which permit food impaction and hence damage to the periodontal tissues.
  2. Carious lesions, either enamel or cemental caries, hold plaque and provide a rough surface for retention of food debris and materia alba.
  3. Cemental caries and decalcification interfere with accomplishing the objectives of root planing (pages 181, 504).

D. **Relationship to Pockets**
  Radiographs do not show pockets; soft tissue does not show in a radiograph. Since a pocket is measured from the gingival margin to the base of the pocket, both of which are soft tissue, pockets cannot be seen in a radiograph. Probing is necessary to identify pockets.

TECHNICAL HINTS

  I. Use topical anesthetic to help alleviate discomfort from probing.
  II. The most common errors in probing are
  A. Not passing the probe to the full pocket depth.
  B. Not holding the probe as parallel with the long axis of a tooth as possible, and therefore obtaining a false reading.
  C. Not measuring around the entire

tooth and therefore missing pockets. This most commonly applies to proximal pockets. The probe must be passed more than halfway across from the facial to overlap with the probe used on the lingual which should also be passed more than halfway across.

III. Check the calibrations on a new probe by measuring on a standard millimeter ruler.

IV. When bleeding is readily elicited on probing or exploring and tooth surfaces are obscured so that examination is complicated, initiate tooth-brushing and other appropriate plaque control methods. Explain the problem to the patient, and outline a specific home care routine designed to reduce gingival inflammation. Postpone the complete examination for one week when it would be expected that the gingival condition would be improved.

V. Replace mirror head frequently. Scratched mirrors obscure vision and delay procedures.

VI. Handle explorers and probes carefully. Because the tips are pliable and relatively fragile, precautions must be taken against breakage, bending, or catching in a perforated tray of a sterilizing unit.

FACTORS TO TEACH THE PATIENT

I. The need for a careful, thorough examination if treatment is to be complete and effective.

II. Information about the materials and techniques of examination and how their use makes the examination complete. Examples are the complete radiographic survey, probing 360 degrees around every tooth, and exploring each submarginal tooth surface.

III. Why bleeding can occur when probing. Healthy tissue does not bleed.

IV. Relation of pocket measurements to normal sulci.

V. Significance of mobility.

VI. Signs of periodontal disease in radiographs.

Suggested Readings

Allen, D. L., McFall, W. T., and Hunter, G. C.: *Periodontics for the Dental Hygienist*, 2nd ed. Philadelphia, Lea & Febiger, 1974, pp. 92–104.

Grant, D. A., Stern, I. B., and Everett, F. G.: *Orban's Periodontics*, 4th ed. St. Louis, Mosby, 1972, pp. 313–321, 365–366, 530–533.

Pattison, A. M. and Behrens, J.: *Dental Hygiene: the Detection and Removal of Calculus*. Reston, Virginia, Reston Publishing, 1973, pp. 10, 78–148.

Parr, R. W.: *Examination and Diagnosis of Periodontal Disease*. DHEW Publication No. (HRA) 74–36, Washington, U.S. Government Printing Office, pp. 31–54, 70–76.

Quong, T. L.: Types and Use of Periodontal Probe, *J. Hawaii Dent. Assoc.*, 5, 8, February, 1972.

Tibbetts L. S.: Use of Diagnostic Probes for Detection of Periodontal Disease, *J. Am. Dent. Assoc.*, 78, 549, March, 1969.

Mobility

Glickman, I.: *Clinical Periodontology*, 4th ed. Philadelphia, Saunders, 1972, pp. 215, 257, 492.

O'Leary, T. J.: Tooth Mobility, *Dent. Clin. North Am.*, 13, 567, July, 1969.

Pameijer, C. H. and Stallard, R. E.: A Method for Quantitative Measurements of Toothmobility, *J. Periodont.*, 44, 339, June, 1973.

Wasserman, B. H., Geiger, A. M., and Turgeon, L. R.: Relationship of Occlusion and Periodontal Disease. Part VII—Mobility, *J. Periodont.*, 44, 572, September, 1973.

Radiographs

Glickman, I.: *Clinical Periodontology*, 4th ed. Philadelphia, Saunders, 1972, pp. 499–509.

Goldman, H. M. and Cohen, D. W.: *Periodontal Therapy*, 5th ed. St. Louis, Mosby, 1973, pp. 84–89, 319–321.

Wuehrmann, A. H. and Manson-Hing, L. R.: *Dental Radiology*, 3rd ed. St. Louis, Mosby, 1973, pp. 300–310.

Chapter 13

The Teeth

Clinical examination of the teeth is essential prior to treatment to provide guidelines for treatment planning, instrumentation, instruction, and follow-up evaluation. In general, patients tend to be more concerned about their teeth than about their gingiva. The reasons may be related to personal appearance, degree of information which is usually greater about teeth than gingiva, and the sensitivity and pain associated with ailments of the teeth.

Background study of histology, dental anatomy, and oral pathology is important to this phase of clinical practice. *Suggested Readings* at the end of this chapter have been selected for additional information, reference, and review.

I. Objectives

With information from the patient's personal dental history (table 6–3, page 77) and a thorough clinical and radiographic examination, the dental hygienist will be able to

A. Prepare a charting and provide a record of deviations from the normal teeth for the diagnostic work-up.

B. Identify the dental hygiene treatment and instruction needed in relation to the teeth for the particular patient.

C. Outline the patient's preventive dental program (pages 294, 386).

D. Utilize the specific data needed during treatment for instrument selection and adaptation.

II. Clinical Examination of the Teeth

Following is a list of major factors to observe when examining the teeth. A number of these are described in other chapters, for which page references are noted. Information about hypoplasia, attrition, erosion, abrasion, dental caries, and tooth vitality will be described in this chapter. Table 13–1 lists factors to observe during the examination of the teeth and suggests relationships to appointment procedures.

A. **General Characteristics**
  1. Number of teeth; eruption pattern (Appendix, tables A–1 and A–2).
  2. Anomalies of size, form, number.
  3. Replacements: restorations for individual teeth and groups of teeth (fixed and removable).

Table 13-1.   Examination of the Teeth

Feature	To Observe	Suggested Relationship to Appointment Procedures
Morphology	Number of teeth (missing teeth verified by radiographic examination) Size, shape Arch form Position of individual teeth	Selection and adaptation of instruments Areas prone to dental caries initiation, particularly the difficult-to-reach areas during plaque control
	Injuries; fractures of the crown (root fractures observed in radiographs)	Pulp test for vitality may be indicated
Development	Anomalies and developmental defects Pits and white spots	Distinguish hypoplasia and dental fluorosis from decalcification
Eruption	Sequence of eruption: normal, irregular Unerupted teeth observed in radiographs	Care in using floss in the col area where the epithelium is usually less mature Procedures for preservation of primary teeth
Deposits Food debris Plaque Calculus Supramarginal Submarginal	Overall evaluation of self-care and plaque control measures Relation of appearance of teeth to gingival health Extent and location of plaque, debris and calculus Calculus and the tooth surface pocket wall	Need for instruction and guidance Frequency of follow-up and recall
Stains Extrinsic Intrinsic	Extrinsic: colors relate to causes Intrinsic: dark, grayish Tobacco stain	Need for test for pulp vitality Stain removal procedures; selection of polishing agent Dentifrice recommendation Plaque control emphasis for plaque-related stains Provide information concerning the oral effects of smoking (page 103)
Regressive Changes	Attrition: primary and permanent Abrasion: physical agents which may be a cause Erosion	Evaluate causes and treat or counsel for prevention Dietary analysis: for finding foods that may be related Selection of non-abrasive dentifrice Habit evaluation
Exposed Cementum	Relation to gingival recession, pocket formation Hypersensitivity	Special care areas where only slight attached gingiva remains (pages 179–180) Non-abrasive dentifrice advised Caries preventive measures to prevent cemental caries Care during instrumentation Indication for application of desensitizing agent (page 563)

Feature	To Observe	Suggested Relationship to Appointment Procedures
Dental Caries	Areas of decalcification Carious lesions (proximal lesions observed in radiographs) Arrested caries	Charting Treatment plan Preventive program for caries control, fluoride, dietary factors Follow-up and frequency of recall
Restorations	Contour of restorations Proximal contact (see separate heading later in this table) Surface smoothness Staining	Check for inadequate margins. Chart and correct inadequate margins. Selection of instruments and polishing agents Dentifrice selection to prevent discoloration
Factors Related to Occlusion Tooth Wear	Facets; worn-down cusp tips Health of supporting structures; observation of radiographs for signs of trauma from occlusion	Need for study of bruxism and other parafunctional habits
Proximal Contacts	Use of floss to find open contact areas Areas of food retention	Correction of inadequate contacts; chart Use of floss by patient
Mobility	Degree; comparison of chartings Possible causes	Need for reduction of inflammatory factors which may be related Dentist will identify and treat factors related to trauma from occlusion
Classification	Angle's classification (pages 225–227)	Relationship to orthodontic treatment needs
Habits	Nail or objects biting; lip or cheek biting Observe effects on lip, cheek, teeth. Tongue thrust; reverse swallow	Guidance for habit correction when indicated
Edentulous Areas	Radiographic evaluation for impacted, unerupted teeth, retained root tips, other deviations from normal	Supplemental fulcrum selection during instrumentation Applied plaque control procedures for abutment teeth
Replacements for Missing Teeth Dentures Partial dentures	Teeth and tissue which support an appliance Cleanliness of an appliance Factors which contribute to food and debris retention	Preventive measures for harm to supporting teeth and soft tissues Instruction in personal care of fixed and removable dentures; use of floss under fixed partial denture; other appropriate care
Saliva	Amount and consistency Dryness of mouth	Relation to instruction for prevention of dental caries: more caries can be expected in a dry mouth. Fluoride: plan preventive program.

B. **Deposits:** calculus, plaque, materia alba (pages 235, 249)

C. **Color**
1. Intrinsic stains (page 263)
2. Extrinsic stains (page 260)

D. **Developmental Defects**
1. Enamel hypoplasia
2. Amelogenesis Imperfecta; Dentinogenesis Imperfecta (page 264)

E. **Physical Injuries:** fractures

F. **Regressive changes**
1. Attrition
2. Erosion
3. Abrasion

G. **Occlusion** (pages 221–231)
1. Proximal contact relation: areas of food impaction
2. Mobility (page 201)

H. **Dental Caries and Decalcification**

I. **Vitality of Pulp**

ENAMEL HYPOPLASIA

I. Definition: Enamel hypoplasia is a defect which occurs as a result of a disturbance in the formation of the organic enamel matrix.

II. Types and Etiology

A. **Hereditary:** enamel is partly or wholly missing; an anomaly.

B. **Systemic** (environmental): factors which may contribute include severe nutritional deficiency particularly rickets, fever-producing diseases such as measles, chicken pox, and scarlet fever, congenital syphilis, hypoparathyroidism, birth injury, prematurity, Rh hemolytic disease, idiopathic.

C. **Local:** affecting a single tooth; caused by trauma or periapical inflammation about a primary tooth which can injure the adjacent developing permanent tooth.

III. Appearance

A. **Hereditary:** may appear brown (page 264).

B. **Systemic:** is also called "chronologic hypoplasia" because the lesions are found in areas of those teeth where the enamel was formed during the systemic disturbance.
1. Single narrow zone, smooth or pitted, means the disturbance was for a short period of time (figure 13–1).
2. Multiple: disturbance to the ameloblast occurred over a period of time, or several times.
3. Teeth most frequently affected: first molars, incisors, canines, because the disturbances generally occur during the first year when those teeth are calcifying. A table of tooth development is available for reference in Appendix, tables A–1 and A–2.

C. **Local:** a single tooth with a yellow or brown intrinsic stain.

ATTRITION

I. Definition: Attrition is the physiologic wearing away of a tooth as a result of tooth-to-tooth contact, as in mastication.[1]

II. Occurrence

A. **Location:** may be found on occlusal, incisal, and proximal surfaces.

B. **Age Factor:** increases with age, and more attrition is seen in men than women of comparable age.

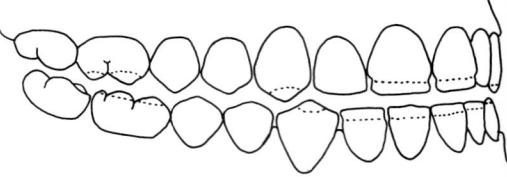

Figure 13–1. Enamel hypoplasia. Chronologic hypoplasia, usually in the form of grooves or pits, appears in the enamel at a level corresponding to the stage of development of the teeth. For this patient the disturbance in enamel development occurred at approximately 10 months of age.

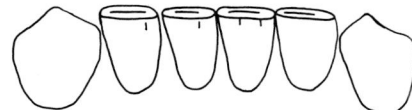

Figure 13–2. Attrition. Attrition of the incisal surfaces of mandibular anterior teeth which has extended to expose the dentin. Dentin usually appears as a brown line or ring.

III. Etiology

A. **Usage:** wear of surfaces on each other.

B. **Predisposing Factors:** coarse foods, chewing tobacco, heavy chewing habits, or abrasive dusts associated with certain occupations.

IV. Appearance

A. **Initial lesion:** small polished facet on a cusp tip or ridge, or slight flattening of an incisal edge.

B. **Advanced:** gradual reduction in cusp height, flattening of occlusal plane (figure 13–2).

C. **Staining of Exposed Dentin May Occur:** usually brown.

D. **Radiographic:** the pulp chamber and canals may be narrowed and sometimes obliterated due to formation of secondary dentin.

EROSION

I. Definition: Erosion is the loss of tooth substance by a chemical process that does not involve known bacterial action.[1] Enamel is usually involved before the root surface.

II. Occurrence

A. **Location:** facial surfaces of any teeth; most frequently cervical third of anterior teeth.

B. **Usually Involves Several Teeth.**

III. Etiology

The lesion is apparently due to some form of chemical dissolution. Microorganisms are not involved.

A. **May Be Idiopathic** (unknown).

B. **Acid of Chronic Vomiting:** affects lingual surfaces, particularly anterior teeth.

C. **Dietary Acid.** Labial surfaces are more commonly affected.
1. Carbonated beverages or lemon juice used frequently.
2. Lemons or other citrus fruit sucked frequently.

D. **Occupational:** workers in industries using acids.

IV. Appearance

A. Smooth, shallow, hard, shiny (in contrast to dental caries, in which appearance is soft and discolored).

B. Shape: varies from shallow saucer-like depressions to deep wedge-shaped grooves; margins are not sharply demarcated.

C. May progress to involve the dentin and stimulate secondary dentin.

D. May occur in combination with dental caries, calculus, or dental restorations.[2]

ABRASION

I. Definition: Abrasion is the pathologic wearing away of tooth substance through some abnormal mechanical process.[1]

II. Occurrence

A. **Location:** exposed root surfaces generally.

B. **Other types:** at incisal edge.

III. Etiology

The lesion originates from a mechanical abrasive activity. The action of microorganisms is not essential for the development of abrasion. Dental caries may occur in the abraded area as a secondary lesion.

A. **Abrasive Agent.** The most common cause is an abrasive dentifrice applied with vigorous horizontal toothbrushing (figure 13–3).

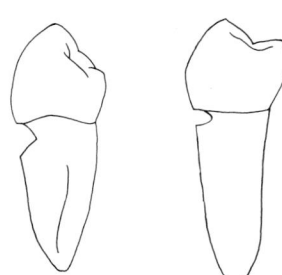

Figure 13–3. Abrasion. Profile view of facial surface of mandibular premolars to show shape of areas of abrasion on the cementum. Note that the area of abrasion undermines the enamel.

B. **Other Types.** Abrasion may occur at the incisal or occlusal surfaces.
  1. Opening bobby pins may leave a small notch in one incisal edge. People with this habit usually utilize the same tooth each time.
  2. Occupations: tacks held by carpenters, pins by dressmakers.
  3. Pipe held between teeth; usually held in the same place over many years.

IV. Appearance

A. Saucer-shaped or wedge-shaped with hard, smooth, shiny surface and clearly defined margins.
B. Except for incisal biting habits, the lesions occur initially on exposed cementum, then extend into the dentin.

DENTAL CARIES

Dental caries is a disease of the calcified structures of the teeth which is characterized by decalcification of the mineral components and dissolution of the organic matrix. As defined by the World Health Organization, dental caries is a "localized, post-eruptive, pathological process of external origin involving softening of the hard tooth tissue and proceeding to the formation of a cavity."[3]

I. Development of Dental Caries

Required for a carious lesion to develop are microorganisms, carbohydrate, primarily sucrose, and the susceptible tooth surface. Dental plaque contains numerous types of acid-forming bacteria, and *Streptococcus mutans* has been specifically implicated. The role of plaque, and the factors in the initiation of caries are described in Chapter 15, pages 235–247.

A. **Enamel Caries**
  1. Steps in the formation of a cavity
    a. Starts in pits or fissures, or smooth surfaces which are not accessible for cleaning.
    b. Follows the general direction of the enamel rods.
    c. Spreads at the dentinoenamel junction.
    d. Continues along the dentinal tubules (figure 13–4).
  2. Types of dental caries: described by location.
    a. *Pit and Fissure.* Caries begins in a minute fault in the enamel.
      (1) Occurs where three or more lobes of the developing tooth join; there is imperfect closure of the enamel plates. *Examples:* occlusal pits of molars and premolars.

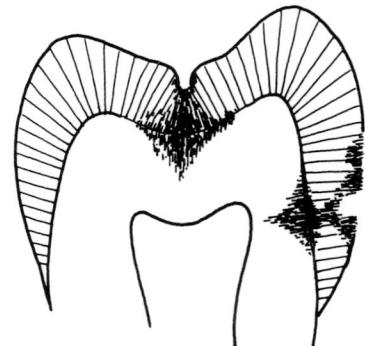

Figure 13–4. Cones of dental caries in a pit and fissure and on a smooth tooth surface. Dental caries follows the general direction of the enamel rods, spreads at the dentinoenamel junction, then continues along the dentinal tubules.

(2) Occurs at the endings of grooves of the teeth. *Example:* the buccal groove of a mandibular molar.

b. *Smooth Surface.* Caries begins in smooth surfaces where there is no pit, groove, or other fault. It occurs in areas where dental plaque collects, such as proximal tooth surfaces, cervical thirds of teeth, and other difficult-to-clean areas.

B. Cemental Caries (Root Caries)

1. Steps in the formation of a cavity in the cementum
   a. Rough root surfaces are conducive to the collection of plaque.
   b. Microorganisms essential to root caries have been shown to differ from those responsible for enamel caries.[4]
   c. Invasion of the cementum takes place either along Sharpey's fibers or between bundles of fibers.
   d. Microorganisms tend to spread laterally between the concentric layers of cementum.[5]
2. Incidence
   Cemental caries increases with age and with increased exposure of cementum. Therefore the population with periodontal involvement can show a high incidence of cemental caries. A high percentage of teeth with root surface caries have not had previous enamel caries.[6]
3. Location
   a. Above the junctional epithelium (epithelial attachment) in the exposed cementum.
   b. May undermine the cervical enamel.
4. Description
   a. Soft, shallow lesions, ill defined. They may have a broad or a narrow base.

b. Color: dark brown or deep yellowish brown.

II. Classification of Cavities

A. G. V. Black's Classification[7]

The standard method for classifying dental caries was developed by Dr. G. V. Black, a noted dental educator who divided the categories into five classes, according to surfaces of the teeth; each class is represented by a Roman numeral. These categories are customarily used for carious lesions, cavity preparations, and finished restorations. See table 13–2 for definitions and examples.

B. Nomenclature by Surfaces

1. *Simple Cavity.* Involves one tooth surface. *Example:* occlusal cavity.
2. *Compound Cavity.* Involves two tooth surfaces. *Example:* mesio-occlusal cavity, referred to as an "M-O" cavity.
3. *Complex Cavity.* Involves more than two tooth surfaces. *Example:* mesio-occlusal-distal, referred to as an "M-O-D" cavity.

III. Other Descriptive Terminology

A. **Primary Dental Caries.** On a surface not previously affected; sometimes called initial or incipient dental caries.

B. **Secondary.** On surface which previously has been affected and has been restored.

C. **Recurrent** (generally referred to as secondary). On tooth surface adjacent to a restoration when the lesion is believed to be a continuation of the previous carious lesion.

D. **Rampant.** Widespread formation of chalky areas and incipient cavities in numerous teeth over a comparatively short time lapse. Most characteristically found in teen-age patients.

Table 13–2. Dental Caries Charting: Classification of Cavities

Classification: Location	Appearance	Method of Examination
Class I. **Cavities in Pits or Fissures** a. Occlusal surfaces of premolars and molars. b. Occlusal two-thirds of facial and lingual surfaces of molars. c. Lingual surfaces of maxillary incisors.		Direct or indirect visual Exploration Radiographs not useful
Class II. **Cavities in Proximal Surfaces of Premolars and Molars**		Early caries: by radiographs only Moderate caries not broken through from proximal to occlusal: (1) Visual by color changes in tooth and loss of translucency (2) Exploration from proximal. Extensive caries involving occlusal: direct visual.
Class III. **Cavities in Proximal Surfaces of Incisors and Canines Which Do Not Involve the Incisal Angle**		Early caries: by radiographs or transillumination. Moderate caries not broken through to lingual or facial: (1) Visual by tooth color change (2) Exploration (3) Radiograph Extensive caries: direct visual.
Class IV. **Cavities in Proximal Surfaces of Incisors or Canines Which Involve the Incisal Angle**		Visual Transillumination
Class V. **Cavities in the Cervical ⅓ of Facial or Lingual Surfaces** (not Pit or Fissure)		Direct visual: dry surface for vision Exploration to distinguish decalcification: whether rough or hard and unbroken. Area may be sensitive to touch.

214

E. **Arrested Caries.** Caries which becomes stationary and does not show a tendency to progress further is called arrested. It frequently takes on a dark brown or reddish brown color.[8]

F. **Nursing Bottle Caries.** Nursing bottle caries is a form of rampant caries found in very young children who routinely have been given a nursing bottle at times when they are going to sleep. The nursing bottle may contain sweetened milk or other fluid sweetened with sucrose. Maxillary anterior teeth are most severely affected. The position of the tongue during sucking is under the nipple and extended out over the mandibular anterior teeth which are usually found to have less caries than the other primary teeth.

RECOGNITION OF CARIOUS LESIONS

Both visual and exploratory means are used to recognize dental caries.

I. Preparation

Dry each tooth or group of teeth with compressed air and carefully inspect each surface, first visually, and then with an explorer as necessary to confirm visual findings.

II. Visual Inspection

Characteristic changes in the color and translucency of tooth structure may be observed which are either definite signs of dental caries progress, or lead the examiner to suspect dental caries which can then be followed by the use of an explorer. Variations in color and translucency include the following:

A. Chalky white areas of decalcification.
B. Grayish white discoloration of marginal ridges due to dental caries of the proximal surface underneath.
C. Grayish white color spreading from margins of restorations due to lesions of secondary dental caries.

D. In relation to an amalgam restoration: dental caries appears translucent in outer portion and white and opaque adjacent to the amalgam.
E. Open carious lesions may vary in color from yellowish brown to a dark brown.
F. Less discoloration is generally present when dental caries progresses rapidly than when it progresses slowly.
G. Dull, flat white, opaque areas under direct light show loss of translucency particularly of the enamel.
H. Dark shadow on a proximal surface may be shown by transillumination; this type of observation is especially useful for anterior teeth and unrestored posterior teeth.

III. Exploratory Inspection

A. **Choice of Explorer**

Explorers and their specific uses were described on pages 195–198. For detection of tooth irregularities the following recommendations are made:
1. Occlusal surfaces: straight explorer.
2. Middle and incisal thirds of facial and lingual surfaces: All explorers can be adapted to these surfaces. A straight explorer usually can be applied more easily to the pits such as the buccal pit of a molar or the cingulum pit of an incisor.
3. Gingival or cervical third, facial and lingual: Number 17, the submarginal explorer can be adapted best to prevent laceration of the gingival margin.
4. Proximal: either the Number 17 or the pigtail paired explorers.
5. Cemental caries on root surfaces submarginally: Number 17.

B. **Smooth Surface Caries**
1. Technique. Adapt the side of the tip of the explorer closely to the tooth surface as described on page 200. Examine for hardness versus softness, roughness versus smoothness,

and continuity of tooth surface versus breaks in continuity.

2. Restorations. Follow the margins of all restorations around with an explorer. Overhanging margins may or may not appear in the radiographs depending on superimposition. Chart all irregularities of existing restorations.

C. **Pit and Fissure Caries**

When a pit or fissure is discolored, it is not possible to determine whether dental caries is present except when a large obvious cavity can be seen. When a cavity is obvious, it should not be explored.

1. Choice of explorer. Of those pictured in figure 12–12, page 195, numbers 6 and 23 have the best adaptability for occlusal pits and fissures.

2. Technique
   a. Direct the explorer tip so that it can pass directly into the pit or fissure. When it is not positioned correctly, caries in a small narrow pit can be undetected.
   b. Explorer will catch when dental caries is present and there will be evidence of softening of tooth structure.

RADIOGRAPHIC EXAMINATION

During the clinical examination, information revealed by radiographs is utilized for supplementation and confirmation. Neither clinical nor radiographic examination is complete without the other. A few principal items to be seen in a radiographic examination of the teeth are:

Anomalies
Impactions
Fractures
Internal or root resorption
Dental caries
Periapical radiolucencies

I. Technique Principles

Periapical radiographs usually provide sufficient information concerning the teeth, but panoramic, extraoral, or occlusal radiographs may be needed for detecting or defining anomalies and pathologic lesions outside the scope of periapical radiographs. Bite-wing radiographs or periapical radiographs made by a paralleling technique with no overlapping are most satisfactory for dental caries detection.

Principles for examination were described on page 136. Mounted radiographs on an adequately lighted viewbox are a necessity during charting and treatment procedures. For the detection of early carious lesions a hand magnifying glass can be of invaluable assistance.

II. Detection of Dental Caries

Radiographs are not needed for facial, lingual, or occlusal carious lesions because they are accessible and best observed by exploration and direct vision. Because of superimposition of other parts of the tooth, facial, lingual, and occlusal carious lesions need to be fairly well advanced before they are definitely discernible in a radiograph.

A. **Proximal Caries**

It has been shown by research that many proximal surface lesions are missed if radiographs are not used. In one study 75 percent of the proximal surface lesions were not found without radiographs.[9]

1. Small proximal lesions. Properly angulated radiographs with no overlapping are required for the detection of small lesions that involve the enamel or extend slightly into the dentin.

2. Proximal overhanging restorations. Because of superimposition it is not necessarily true that there is no overhanging filling, or dental caries

under that filling, if none can be seen in the radiograph. An explorer must be passed around the complete margin to confirm the condition.

B. **Cemental Caries**
1. Location. Although most cemental carious lesions occur in the vicinity of and just beneath the cementoenamel junction, the lesions may also be found more apically located on the root. The use of an explorer submarginally can sometimes locate a cavity which appeared indefinite in the radiograph.
2. Appearance. Cemental caries appears as a saucer-shaped lesion in a radiograph. It sometimes appears to undermine the enamel or it may appear beneath an overhanging filling.

TESTING FOR PULPAL VITALITY

Any tooth suspected of being devital must be tested for pulpal vitality or degree of vitality. This is particularly significant prior to treatment involving periodontal surgery, any restorative procedures, and orthodontic appliance placement. Diagnosis of vitality cannot be made on a pulp test alone, but on consideration of all data from the patient history and clinical and radiographic examinations.

A tooth may become devital from bacterial causes particularly invasion of the pulp from dental caries or periodontal disease. Physical causes may be mechanical or thermal injuries. Examples of mechanical injuries are trauma, such as a blow, or iatrogenic dental procedures such as cavity preparation or too-rapid orthodontic movement.[10,11]

I. Observations Which Suggest Loss of Vitality

A. **Clinical**
1. Discoloration of a tooth crown (intrinsic stains, page 263–264).

2. Fractured: part of the crown may be missing.
3. Large carious lesion or large restoration.
4. Fistula with opening into the oral cavity over the apical region of a tooth.

B. **Radiographic**
1. Apical radiolucency which may indicate a granuloma, cyst, or abscess.
2. Bone loss with a thickened periodontal ligament space extending to the apex.
3. Fractured root.
4. Large carious lesion or restoration which appears closely related to the pulp chamber.

II. Response to Pulp Testing

A. **Rationale**
Electrical pulp testing is based on the knowledge that an electrical stimulus can create pain to which a patient can react. The pulp tester, therefore, determines the conduction of stimuli to the sensory receptors. The vitality of the pulp is dependent upon its blood supply and not on its nerve supply. For that reason a positive or negative pulp test may not always show the true condition of the pulp.

B. **Factors Which Influence the Response**
1. Degree of pulpal degeneration or inflammation: a necrotic pulp will give no response at all, while an acutely or chronically inflamed pulp will respond at varying degrees between no response and full normal response.
2. Pain perception threshold: the lowest perceptible intensity of pain caused by a threshold stimulus. A threshold stimulus is the minimum stimulus necessary to induce patient response.

3. Reaction to pain may vary with a patient's attitude, age, sex, emotional security, fatigue, drugs used, as well as the size of the pulp and thickness of the dentin, particularly the amount of secondary dentin.
4. Nerve transmission blocks: injuries or lesions of nerves, and anesthetics.
5. Adjacent metal restorations or continuous bridgework.

III. Electrical Pulp Testers

Although thermal tests using hot or cold applications have been used, the electrical pulp testers are considered more consistent and reliable.

A. **Types**
   1. Battery-operated
      a. Advantages: hand held so operator can work alone; portability.
      b. Disadvantage: battery can run down. Some types have a light to indicate current in circuit.
      c. Examples: Vitapulp (Pelton and Crane); Dentotest (Parkell).
   2. Plug-in
      a. Advantage: more dependable than battery-operated.
      b. Examples: Burton Vitalometer; Ritter Sensitron Model A; S. S. White Pulp Tester No. 2 A.

B. **Precaution**
   The application of an electrical current to a patient with an artificial pacemaker by the use of a device such as an ultrasonic scaler, pulp tester, desensitizing equipment, or electrosurgical instrument can interfere with pacemaker function and may constitute a serious health hazard.[12,13] A review of the patient history is necessary prior to application of a pulp tester.

C. **Technique for Preparation and Use of Equipment**
   Manufacturer's instructions are provided for each tester and should be followed carefully. When the tester rheostat is separate from the applicator tip, an assistant is needed.

D. **General Procedures**[14]
   1. Assemble equipment and pretest current on the skin of finger of the operator to determine that current is passing through.
   2. Explain briefly to the patient what is to be done, but avoid detailed description which could create anxiety or apprehension.
   3. Dry the teeth to be tested to prevent the current from passing to the gingiva: isolate with cotton rolls and insert a saliva ejector, or use rubber dam.
   4. Moisten the end of the tip of the tester with a small amount of toothpaste. Another electrolyte (conductor) may be used if the consistency allows it to remain where placed and not flow over the tooth surface.
   5. Instruct the patient to signal when a sensation is felt: suggest raising a hand or making a sound.
   6. Application of tester tip
      a. Apply first to at least one tooth other than the one in question, preferably an adjacent tooth and the same tooth on the contralateral side, in order to determine a normal response for the patient.
      b. Place without pressure but with definite contact on sound tooth structure within the middle third of the crown of single rooted tooth and the middle third of each cusp of a multirooted tooth (figure 13–5).
      c. Avoid contact with the gingiva or other soft tissues or restorations as a false reading could result.

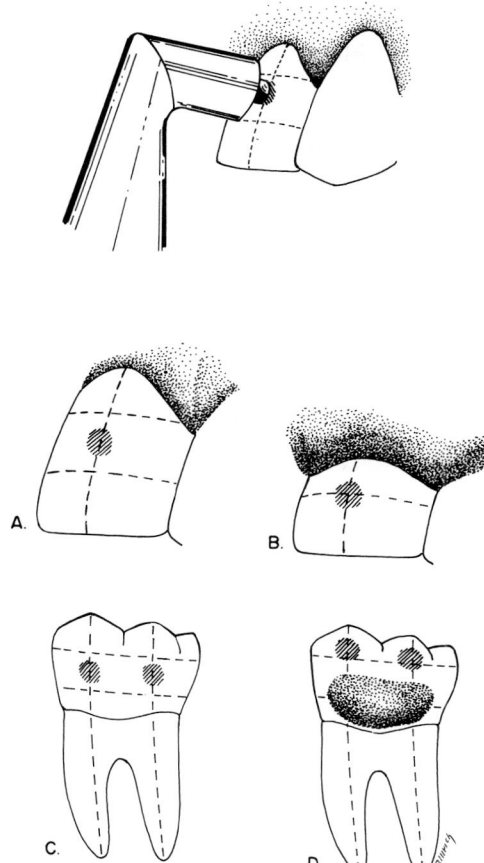

Figure 13-5. Pulp tester in position. **A.** Correct contact point for tip of pulp tester is within the middle third of the crown. Avoid contact with gingiva or restorations. **B.** Adjustment of position of the contact point because of gingival enlargement. **C.** Contact points on multirooted tooth. Place tip of pulp tester in middle third over each root. **D.** Adjustment of position of the contact points because of large Class V restoration.

7. Start with the rheostat at zero, advance slowly but steadily, stopping only momentarily after each number. Do not proceed with such regularity that the patient can count and anticipate.
8. Test each tooth at least twice. Average the readings.
9. Record on patient's record: the lowest number (average number) at which minimal stimulus induced

response. Record for all teeth tested, not only the tooth in question.

FACTORS TO TEACH THE PATIENT

I. The cause and process of dental caries formation and development and the route of attack through the enamel into the dentin.
II. About the hardness of the enamel and why a cavity is usually larger in the dentin before there is evidence from the external surface.
III. Why radiographs are necessary to detect incipient caries.
IV. Reasons for preservation of primary teeth.
V. Frequency of complete oral examination in relation to a continuing preventive program.
VI. Methods for dental caries prevention: fluorides, dietary sugar control, plaque prevention and control.
VII. Preventive measures for control and prevention of tooth abrasion: dentifrice selection and correction of brush selection and use.
VIII. Dietary factors related to erosion.
IX. When the patient asks specific questions about oral findings, explain why it is necessary for the dentist to observe and check before explanations can be made.

References

1. Shafer, W. G., Hine, M. K., and Levy, B. M.: *A Textbook of Oral Pathology*, 3rd ed. Philadelphia, Saunders, 1974, pp. 285–290.
2. Sognnaes, R. F., Wolcott, R. B., and Xhonga, F. A.: Dental Erosion. 1. Erosion-like Patterns Occurring in Association with Other Dental Conditions, *J. Am. Dent. Assoc.*, 84, 571, March, 1972.
3. World Health Organization : *Standardization of Reporting of Dental Diseases and Conditions.* Geneva, World Health Organization, Technical Report Series, Number 242, 1962.
4. Sumney, D. L. and Jordan, H. V.: Characterization of Bacteria Isolated from Human Root Surface Carious Lesions, *J. Dent. Res.*, 53, 343, March-April, 1974.

5. Shafer, Hine, and Levy: op. cit., pp. 404–405.
6. Sumney, D. L., Jordan, H. V., and Englander, H. R.: The Prevalence of Root Surface Caries in Selected Populations, *J. Periodont.*, *44*, 500, August, 1973.
7. Blackwell, R. E.: *G. V. Black's Operative Dentistry* Vol. II, 9th ed. Milwaukee, Medico-Dental Publishing Company, 1955, pp. 1–4.
8. Shafer, Hine, and Levy: op. cit., p. 394.
9. Hennon, D. K., Stookey, G. K., and Muhler, J. C.: Prevalence and Distribution of Dental Caries in Preschool Children, *J. Am. Dent. Assoc.*, *79*, 1405, December, 1969.
10. Grossman, L. I.: *Endodontic Practice*, 7th ed. Philadelphia, Lea & Febiger, 1970, pp. 13–23, 34.
11. Ingle, J. I.: *Endodontics*. Philadelphia, Lea & Febiger, 1965, pp. 270–292, 416–419.
12. Wooley, L. H., Woodworth, J., and Dobbs, J. L.: A Preliminary Evaluation of the Effects of Electrical Pulp Testers on Dogs with Artificial Pacemakers, *J. Am. Dent. Assoc.*, *89*, 1099, November, 1974.
13. Ore, D. E. and Shriner, W. A.: Doctor: Don't Shut Off That Pacemaker, *Chicago Dent. Soc. Rev.*, pp. 22–23, August, 1974.
14. American Dental Association, Council on Dental Materials and Devices, Millard, H. D.: Electric Pulp Testers, *J. Am. Dent. Assoc.*, *86*, 872, April, 1973.

Suggested Readings

Burkett, L. W.: *Oral Medicine*, 6th ed. Philadelphia, Lippincott, 1971, pp. 186–202.
Colby, R. A., Kerr, D. A., and Robinson, H. B. G.: *Color Atlas of Oral Pathology*, 3rd ed. Philadelphia, Lippincott, 1971, pp. 55–69.
Kerr, D. A. and Ash, M. M.: *Oral Pathology*, 3rd ed. Philadelphia, Lea & Febiger, 1971, pp. 51–66, 133–136, 167–178.
Kerr, D. A., Ash, M. M., and Millard, H. D.: *Oral Diagnosis*, 4th ed. St. Louis, Mosby, 1974, pp. 193–213.
Massler, M. and Schour, I.: *Atlas of the Mouth*, 2nd ed. Chicago, American Dental Association, Plates 7–16.
Mitchell, D. F., Standish, S. M., and Fast, T. B.: *Oral Diagnosis/Oral Medicine*, 2nd ed. Philadelphia, Lea & Febiger, 1971, pp. 126–135.
Rowe, N. H.: Dental Caries, in Steele, P. F., ed.: *Dimensions of Dental Hygiene*, 2nd ed. Philadelphia, Lea & Febiger, 1975, pp. 198–222.
Shafer, W. G., Hine, M. K., and Levy, B. M.: A *Textbook of Oral Pathology*, 3rd ed. Philadelphia, Saunders, 1974, pp. 34–66, 366–432, 490–493.
Winter, G. B. and Brook, A. H.: Enamel Hypoplasia and Anomalies of the Enamel, *Dent. Clin. North Am.*, *19*, 3, January, 1975.

World Health Organization: *The Etiology and Prevention of Dental Caries*. Report of a WHO Scientific Group, Geneva, World Health Organization, 1972, Technical Report Series, No. 494.
Wuehrmann, A. H. and Manson-Hing, L. R.: *Dental Radiology*, 3rd ed. St. Louis, Mosby, 1973, pp. 274–330.

Cemental Caries

Glickman, I. and Smulow, J. B.: *Periodontal Disease: Clinical, Radiographic, and Histopathologic Features*, Philadelphia, Saunders, 1974, p. 102.
Hazen, S. P., Chilton, N. W., and Mumma, R. D.: The Problem of Root Caries. I. Literature Review and Clinical Description, *J. Am. Dent. Assoc.*, *86*, 137, January, 1973.
Jordan, H. V. and Sumney, D. L.: Root Surface Caries: Review of the Literature and Significance of the Problem, *J. Periodont.*, *44*, 158, March, 1973.

Nursing Bottle Caries

Katz, S., McDonald, J. L., and Stookey, G. K.: *Preventive Dentistry in Action*. Upper Montclair, N. J., D. C. P. Publishing, 1972, pp. 55–57.
Kroll, R. G. and Stone, J. H.: Nocturnal Bottle-Feeding as a Contributory Cause of Rampant Dental Caries in the Infant and Young Child, *J. Dent. Child.*, *34*, 454, November, 1967.
Silver, D. H.: The Prevalence of Dental Caries in 3-Year-Old Children, *Brit. Dent. J.*, *137*, 123, August 20, 1974.
Snawder, K. D.: The Nursing-Bottle Syndrome and Related Problems, in Goldman, H. M., Gilmore, H. W., Irby, W. B., and Olsen, N. H.: *Current Therapy in Dentistry*, Volume 5. St. Louis, Mosby, 1974, p. 473.

Pulp Vitality

Bhaskar, S. N. and Rappaport, H. M.: Dental Vitality Tests and Pulp Status, *J. Am. Dent. Assoc.*, *86*, 409, February, 1973.
Johnson, R. H., Dachi, S. F., and Haley, J. V.: Pulpal Hyperemia—A Correlation of Clinical and Histologic Data from 706 Teeth, *J. Am. Dent. Assoc.*, *81*, 108, July, 1970.
Kerr, D. A., Ash, M. M., and Millard, H. D.: *Oral Diagnosis*, 4th ed. St. Louis, Mosby, 1974, pp. 328–336.
Mitchell, D. F., Standish, S. M., and Fast, T. B.: *Oral Diagnosis/Oral Medicine*, 2nd ed. Philadelphia, Lea & Febiger, 1971, pp. 100–104.
Mumford, J. M. and Björn, H.: Problems in Electrical Pulp-testing and Dental Algesimetry, *Int. Dent. J.*, *12*, 161, June, 1962.
Sommer, R. F., Ostrander, F. D., and Crowley, M.: *Clinical Endodontics, A Manual of Scientific Endodontics*. Philadelphia, Saunders, 1966, pp. 86–92.
Sturdevant, C. M., Barton, R. E., and Brauer, J. C.: *The Art and Science of Operative Dentistry*. New York, McGraw-Hill, 1968, pp. 53–56.

Chapter 14

The Occlusion

The occlusion is examined and recorded as part of the oral inspection. The dental hygienist, by studying the occlusion of each patient, can contribute significantly to the complete dental care and instruction. Recognition of malocclusion assists the dentist in his referral of patients to the orthodontist, gives many valuable points of reference for patient instruction, and determines necessary adaptations in techniques.

I. Objectives for Observing Occlusion

Recognition of the patient's occlusion and understanding the oral health problems of malocclusion can aid in accomplishing the following:

A. Provide information for the diagnostic work-up and planning dental hygiene care.

B. Plan personalized instruction in relation to such factors as oral habits, masticatory efficiency, personal oral care procedures, and predisposing factors to dental and periodontal disease.

C. Adapt techniques of instrumentation to malpositioned teeth or groups of teeth.

D. Plan the frequency of recall appointments for professional care on the basis of deposit retention areas, particularly those which are difficult to reach in routine personal care.

E. Assist by recording the general features of malocclusion for special consideration by the dentist who may wish to refer the patient to an orthodontist.

II. Definitions

A. **Occlusion**

The contact of the teeth in the mandibular arch with those in the maxillary arch.

B. **Static Occlusion**

The relationships of the teeth when the jaws are closed in centric occlusion is called static occlusion.

C. **Functional Occlusion**

Functional or dynamic occlusion refers to tooth contacts while the mandible is in action such as during mastication and swallowing.

D. **Centric Occlusion**

The centric occlusion is the relation of opposing occlusal surfaces which provides the maximum planned contact and/or intercuspation.

E. **Centric Relation**

Centric relation is the most unstrained, retruded anatomical and functional position of the heads of the condyles of the mandible in the glenoid fossae of the temporomandibular joints.

STATIC OCCLUSION

Static occlusion relationships may be efficiently observed in occluded study casts, although they can be seen directly in the oral cavity when there is adequate retraction of lips and cheeks. Classification of malocclusion and the variations which occur with each category are described here.

I. Normal (Ideal) Occlusion

The ideal mechanical relationship between the teeth of the maxillary arch and the teeth of the mandibular arch.

A. All teeth in maxillary arch in maximum contact with all teeth in mandibular arch in a definite pattern.

B. Maxillary teeth slightly overlapping the mandibular teeth on the facial surfaces.

II. Malocclusion

Any deviation from the ideal relationship of the maxillary arch and/or teeth to the mandibular arch and/or teeth.

III. Types of Facial Profile (figure 14–1)

A. **Mesognathic.** Having slightly protruded jaws which give the facial outline a relatively flat appearance (straight profile).

B. **Retrognathic.** Having a prominent maxilla and a deficient, retruded mandible (convex profile).

C. **Prognathic.** Having a prominent, protruded mandible and normal (usually) maxilla (concave profile).

IV. Malrelations of Groups of Teeth

A. **Crossbites**
   1. Anterior: maxillary incisors are lingual to the mandibular incisors (figure 14–10).
   2. Posterior: maxillary or mandibular posterior teeth are either buccal or lingual to their normal position: this may occur bilaterally or unilaterally (figure 14–2).

B. **Edge-to-Edge Bite.** Incisal surfaces of maxillary teeth occlude with incisal surfaces of mandibular teeth instead of overlapping as in ideal occlusion (figure 14–3).

C. **End-to-End Bite.** Molars and premolars occlude cusp-to-cusp as viewed mesiodistally (figure 14–4).

D. **Openbite.** Lack of occlusal or incisal contact between maxillary and mandibular teeth because either or both have failed to reach the line of occlusion. The teeth cannot be brought

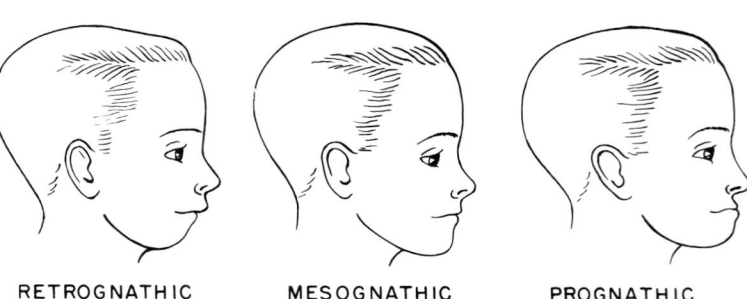

RETROGNATHIC   MESOGNATHIC   PROGNATHIC

Figure 14–1.   Types of facial profiles.

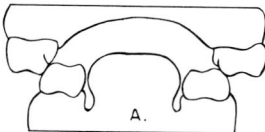 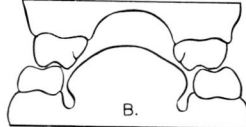 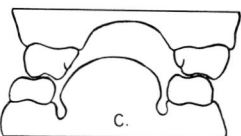

Figure 14–2. Posterior crossbite. **A.** Mandibular teeth lingual to normal position. **B.** Mandibular teeth buccal to normal position. **C.** Unilateral crossbite: right side normal; left side, mandibular teeth buccal to normal position.

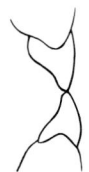

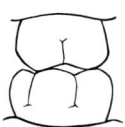

Figure 14–3. Edge-to-edge bite. Incisal surfaces occlude.

Figure 14–4. End-to-end bite. Molars in cusp-to-cusp occlusion as viewed from the buccal.

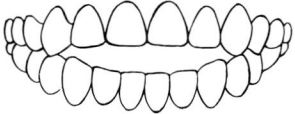

Figure 14–5. Openbite. Lack of incisal contact. Posterior teeth in their normal occlusion.

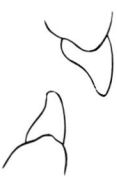 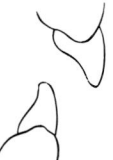

Figure 14–6. Overjet. Maxillary incisors are labial to the mandibular incisors. There is a measurable horizontal distance between the incisal edge of the maxillary incisors and the incisal edge of the mandibular incisors.

Figure 14–7. Underjet. Maxillary incisors are lingual to the mandibular incisors. There is a measurable horizontal distance between the incisal edges of the maxillary incisors and the incisal edges of the mandibular incisors.

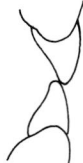 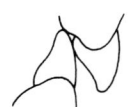 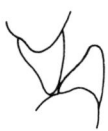

Figure 14–8. Normal overbite. Profile view to show position of incisal edge of maxillary tooth within the incisal third of the facial surface of the mandibular incisor.

Figure 14–9. Severe anterior overbite. Incisal edge of maxillary tooth is at the level of the cervical third of the facial surface of the mandibular anterior tooth. See facial view in 14–11 C.

Figure 14–10. Anterior crossbite. Maxillary anterior teeth are lingual to the mandibular anterior teeth. This occurs in Angle's Class III malocclusion.

together and a space remains due to the arching of the line of occlusion (figure 14–5).

E. **Overjet.** The horizontal distance between the labioincisal surfaces of the mandibular incisors and the linguoincisal surfaces of the maxillary incisors (figure 14–6). One way to measure the amount of overjet is to place the tip of a probe on the labial surface of the mandibular incisor and, holding it horizontally against the incisal edge of the maxillary tooth, read the millimeters distance.

F. **Underjet** (maxillary teeth are lingual to mandibular teeth). The horizontal distance between the labioincisal surfaces of the maxillary incisors and the linguoincisal surfaces of the mandibular incisors (figure 14–7).

G. **Overbite (Vertical Overlap).** Overbite is the vertical distance by which the maxillary incisors overlap the mandibular incisors.
1. *Normal overbite.* An overbite is considered normal when the incisal edges of the maxillary teeth are within the incisal third of the mandibular teeth as shown in figure 14–8 in side view and in figure 14–11 viewed from the anterior.
2. *Moderate overbite.* When the incisal edges of the maxillary teeth appear within the middle third of the mandibular teeth, it is called moderate overbite (figure 14–11B).
3. *Severe overbite.* When the incisal edges of the maxillary teeth are within the cervical third of the mandibular teeth, it is called severe overbite, and when in addition the incisal edges of the mandibular teeth are in contact with the maxillary lingual gingival tissue, it is called very severe. A side view of very severe overbite is shown in figure 14–9.

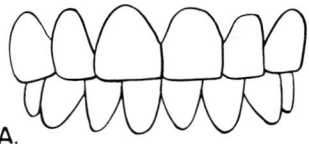

A.

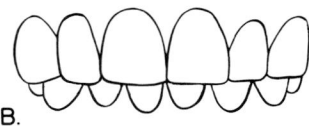

B.

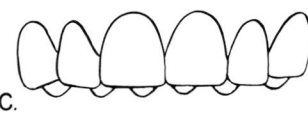

C.

Figure 14–11. Overbite, anterior view. **A.** Normal overbite; the incisal edges of the maxillary teeth are within the incisal third of the facial surfaces of the mandibular teeth. **B.** Moderate overbite: the incisal edges of the maxillary teeth are within the middle third of the facial surfaces of the mandibular teeth. **C.** Severe overbite: the incisal edges of the maxillary teeth are within the cervical third of the facial of the mandibular teeth. When the incisal edges of the mandibular teeth are in contact with the maxillary lingual gingival tissue, it is considered very severe overbite. See profile view figure 14–9.

4. *Anterior crossbite.* The opposite situation occurs in anterior crossbite when the maxillary anterior teeth are lingual to the mandibular anterior teeth (figure 14–10).
5. *Clinical examination of overbite.* Normal, moderate, and severe anterior overbite are observed directly when the teeth are closed in occlusion. With the posterior teeth closed together, the lips can be retracted and the teeth observed as in figure 14–11. The degree of anterior overbite is judged by the position of the incisal edge of the

maxillary teeth: normal (slight) within the incisal third of the mandibular incisors; moderate overbite within the middle third; and severe overbite within the cervical third. By placing a mouth mirror under the incisal edge of the maxillary teeth it is sometimes possible to see the mandibular teeth contact with the maxillary lingual gingiva. When this is not possible, an examination of the lingual gingiva may reveal teeth prints, or at least enlargement and tenderness from the contact.

V. Malpositions of Individual Teeth

A. **Labioversion.** A tooth which has assumed a position labial to normal.

B. **Linguoversion.** Position lingual to normal.

C. **Buccoversion.** Position buccal to normal.

D. **Supraversion.** Elongated above the line of occlusion.

E. **Torsoversion.** Turned or rotated.

F. **Infraversion.** Depressed below the line of occlusion. (Example: primary tooth that is submerged or ankylosed.)

DETERMINATION OF THE CLASSIFICATION OF OCCLUSION

The determination of the classification of occlusion is based upon the principles of Edward H. Angle, which he presented in the early 1900s. He defined normal occlusion as "the normal relations of the occlusal inclined planes of the teeth when the jaws are closed"[1] and based his system of classification upon the relationship of the maxillary first permanent molars.

Although authorities have since agreed that the maxillary first permanent molars do not occupy a fixed position in the dental arch, Angle's system serves to provide an acceptable basis for a useful classification. A more comprehensive picture of malocclusion is made by the orthodontist who studies the relationships of the position of the teeth to the jaws, the face, and the skull.

Four general classes of malocclusion are described below. These are designated by Roman numerals. Since the mandible is movable and the maxilla is stationary, the classes describe the relationship of the mandible to the maxilla. For example, in Distoclusion (Class II) the mandible is distal, whereas in Mesioclusion (Class III) the mandible is mesial to the maxilla, as compared to the normal position.

Relative to the incidence of malocclusion, various surveys have been made which cannot be compared directly because of differences in methodology. Only between two and four percent of the population has normal or ideal occlusion. More than two-thirds of the population have been found to have malocclusion severe enough to require orthodontic treatment.

The prevalence of malocclusion is significantly less in communities where there is fluoride in the drinking water. Since there is less dental caries and fewer teeth are extracted, one factor which contributes to malocclusion is reduced or missing, namely, tooth loss with shifting of the positions of remaining teeth. A list of suggested readings is supplied at the end of the chapter for readers interested in studying surveys of the prevalence of malocclusion.

I. Normal (Ideal) Occlusion (figure 14–12)

A. **Facial Profile**
   Mesognathic (figure 14–1).

B. **Molar Relation**
   The mesiobuccal cusp of the maxillary first permanent molar occludes with the buccal groove of the mandibular first permanent molar.

Normal (Ideal) Occlusion.

Molar relationship: mesiobuccal cusp of maxillary first permanent molar occludes with the buccal groove of the mandibular first permanent molar.

Malocclusion

Class I: Neutroclusion. Molar relationship same as Normal, with malposition of individual teeth or groups of teeth.

Class II: Distoclusion.

Molar relationship: buccal groove of the mandibular first permanent molar is distal to the mesiobuccal cusp of the maxillary first permanent molar by at least the width of a premolar.

Division 1: mandible is retruded and all maxillary incisors are protruded.

Division 2: mandible is retruded and one or more maxillary incisors are retruded.

Class III: Mesioclusion.

Molar relationship: buccal groove of the mandibular first permanent molar is mesial to the mesiobuccal cusp of the maxillary first permanent molar by at least the width of a premolar.

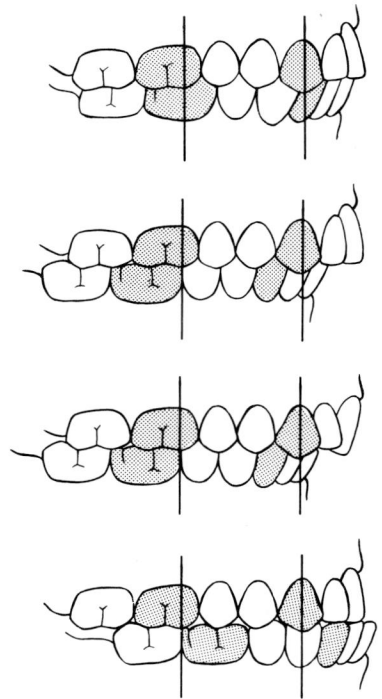

Figure 14–12.   Normal occlusion and classification of malocclusions.

C. **Canine Relation**

The maxillary permanent canine occludes with the distal half of the mandibular canine and the mesial half of the mandibular first premolar.

II. Malocclusion

A. **Class I or Neutroclusion** (figure 14–12)
1. *Facial Profile.* Same as Normal Occlusion (I, A, above).
2. *Molar Relation.* Same as Normal Occlusion (I, B, above).
3. *Canine Relation.* Same as Normal Occlusion (I, C, above).
4. *Malposition* of individual teeth or groups of teeth.
5. *General Types of Conditions Which Frequently Occur in Class I.*
   a. Crowded maxillary or mandibular anterior teeth.
   b. Protruded or retruded maxillary incisors.

c. Anterior crossbite.
d. Posterior crossbite.
e. Mesial drift of molars resulting from premature loss of teeth.

B. **Class II or Distoclusion** (figure 14–12)
1. *Description.* Mandibular teeth posterior to normal position in their relation to the maxillary teeth.
2. *Facial Profile.* Retrognathic; maxilla protrudes; lower lip is full and often rests between the maxillary and mandibular incisors; the mandible appears retruded or weak (figure 14–1, Retrognathic).
3. *Molar Relation*
   a. The buccal groove of the mandibular first permanent molar is distal to the mesiobuccal cusp of the maxillary first permanent molar by at least the width of a premolar.

b. When the distance is less than the width of a premolar the relation should be classified as "tendency toward Class II."

4. *Canine Relation*
   a. The distal surface of the mandibular canine is distal to the mesial surface of the maxillary canine by at least the width of a premolar.
   b. When the distance is less than the width of a premolar the relation should be classified as "tendency toward Class II."

5. *Class II, Division 1*
   a. Description: the mandible is retruded and all maxillary incisors are protruded.
   b. General types of conditions which frequently occur in Class II, Division 1 malocclusion: deep overbite, excessive overjet, abnormal muscle function (lips), short mandible, or short upper lip.

6. *Class II, Division 2*
   a. Description: the mandible is retruded, and one or more maxillary incisors are retruded.
   b. General types of conditions which frequently occur in Class II, Division 2 malocclusion: maxillary lateral incisors protrude while both central incisors retrude, crowded maxillary anterior teeth, or deep overbite.

7. *Subdivision.* One side is Class I, the other side is Class II (may be Division 1 or 2).

C. **Class III or Mesioclusion** (figure 14–12)
   1. *Description.* Mandibular teeth are anterior to normal position in relation to maxillary teeth.
   2. *Facial Profile.* Prognathic; lower lip and mandible are prominent (figure 14–1).

3. *Molar Relation*
   a. The buccal groove of the mandibular first permanent molar is mesial to the mesiobuccal cusp of the maxillary first permanent molar by at least the width of a premolar.
   b. When the distance is less than the width of a premolar the relation should be classified as "tendency toward Class III."

4. *Canine Relation*
   a. The distal surface of the mandibular canine is mesial to the mesial surface of the maxillary canine by at least the width of a premolar.
   b. When the distance is less than the width of a premolar the relation should be classified as "tendency toward Class III."

5. *General Types of Conditions Which Frequently Occur in Class III Malocclusion*
   a. True Class III: maxillary incisors are lingual to mandibular incisors in an anterior crossbite (figure 14–10).
   b. Maxillary and mandibular incisors are in edge-to-edge occlusion.
   c. Mandibular incisors very crowded, but lingual to maxillary incisors.

OCCLUSION OF THE PRIMARY TEETH[2]

I. **Normal** (Ideal)

A. **Canine Relation**
   Same as permanent dentition.
   1. *With primate spaces* (page 752 for definition).
      a. Mandibular: between mandibular canine and first molar (figure 14–13A).
      b. Maxillary: between maxillary lateral incisor and canine (figure 14–13B).

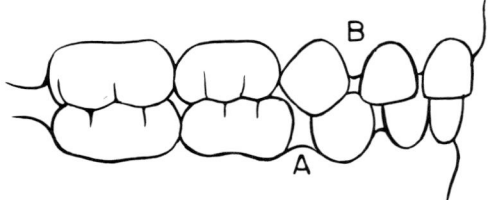

Figure 14–13. Primary teeth showing primate space. **A.** Mandibular primate space between canine and first molar. **B.** Maxillary primate space between lateral incisor and canine.

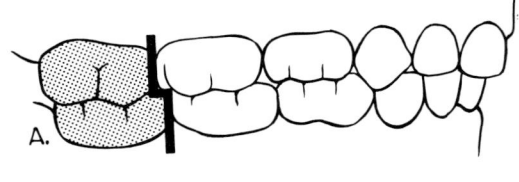

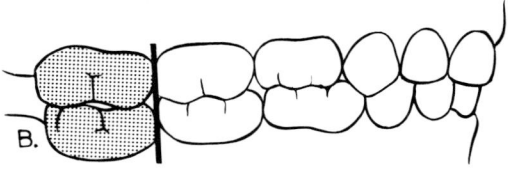

Figure 14–14. Eruption patterns of first permanent molars. **A.** Terminal step. Distal surface of mandibular second primary molar is mesial to the distal surface of the maxillary primary molar. **B.** Terminal plane. Distal surfaces of mandibular and maxillary second primary molars are on the same vertical plane. Permanent molars erupt in end-to-end occlusion.

2. *Without primate spaces:* closed arches.

B. **Second Molar Relation**

The mesiobuccal cusp of the maxillary second primary molar occludes with the buccal groove of the mandibular second primary molar.

1. Variations in distal surfaces relationships: terminal step.
   a. The distal surface of the mandibular molar is mesial to that of the maxillary, thereby forming a mesial step (figure 14–14A).
   b. Morphological variation in molar size: maxillary and mandibular molars have approximately the same mesiodistal width.
2. Variation: terminal plane
   a. The distal surfaces of the maxillary and mandibular molars are on same vertical plane (figure 14–14B).
   b. The maxillary molar is narrower mesiodistally than the mandibular molar (occurs in high percentage of cases).
3. Effects on occlusion of first permanent molars
   a. Terminal step: first permanent molar erupts directly into proper occlusion (figure 14–14A).
   b. Terminal plane: first permanent molars erupt end-to-end. With mandibular primate space there is early mesial shift of primary molars into the primate space and the permanent mandibular molar shifts into proper occlusion. Without primate spaces there is late mesial shift of permanent mandibular molar into proper occlusion following exfoliation of second primary molar (figure 14–14B).

II. **Malocclusion of the Primary Teeth:** Same as permanent dentition.

FUNCTIONAL OCCLUSION

In contrast to the static occlusion which pertains to the relationship of the teeth when the jaws are closed, the functional occlusion consists of all contacts during chewing, swallowing, or other normal action. Functional occlusion is associated with performance.

The pressures or forces created by the muscles of mastication are transmitted from the teeth, after contact, to the periodontium. Such forces are necessary to maintain the occlusal relationship of the teeth and guide the teeth during eruption. The forces are also necessary to provide functional stimulation for the preservation of the health of the attachment apparatus, namely the periodontal ligament, the cementum, and the alveolar bone.

I. Types of Occlusal Contacts

A. **Functional Contacts.** Functional contacts are the normal contacts that are made between the maxillary teeth and the mandibular teeth during chewing and swallowing. Each contact is momentary, so the total contact time is only a few minutes each day.

B. **Parafunctional Contacts.** Parafunctional contacts are those made outside the normal range of function. They result from occlusal habits and neuroses, and are potentially injurious to the periodontal supporting structures. Parafunctional contacts can be divided into the following:
   1. Tooth-to-tooth contacts: bruxism, clenching, tapping, doodling.
   2. Tooth-to-hard object contacts: nail biting, occupationally utilized objects such as tacks or pins, smoking equipment such as a pipe stem or hard cigarette holder.
   3. Tooth-and-oral tissues: lip or cheek biting.

II. Proximal Contacts

Proximal contacts serve to stabilize the position of teeth in the dental arches and to prevent food impaction between the teeth. Attrition or wear of the teeth occurs at the proximal contacts.

A. **Drifting.** When proximal contact is lost, teeth can drift into spaces created by unreplaced missing teeth. There is also a natural tendency for mesial migration of teeth toward the midline.

In the absence of disease, the surrounding periodontal tissues adapt to repositioned teeth (figure 12–18, page 203).

B. **Pathologic Migration.** With destruction of the supporting structures of a tooth due to periodontal disease, and a force to move a tooth weakened by disease and bone loss, migration of the tooth can result. Pathologic migration occurs when disease is present, in contrast to drifting which is migration with a healthy periodontium.

TRAUMA FROM OCCLUSION

Periodontal tissue injury caused by repeated occlusal forces which exceed the physiologic limits of tissue tolerance is called trauma from occlusion. Other names are periodontal traumatism, occlusal traumatism, and periodontal trauma.

I. Types of Trauma from Occlusion

A. **Primary.** When the excessive occlusal force is exerted on a tooth with normal bone support, it is called *primary trauma from occlusion*. An example is the effect of a restoration placed above the line of occlusion.

B. **Secondary.** When the excessive occlusal force is exerted on a tooth with bone loss and inadequate alveolar bone support, and the ability of the tooth to withstand occlusal forces is impaired, it is called *secondary trauma from occlusion*. It is likely that when a tooth has lost the support of the surrounding bone, even the pressures of what are usually considered normal occlusal forces can create lesions of trauma from occlusion.

II. Effects of Trauma from Occlusion

The attachment apparatus (periodontal ligament, cementum, and alveolar bone) has as its main purpose the maintenance of the tooth in the socket in a functional state. In a healthy situation, occlusal pressures and forces during chewing and swallowing are readily dispersed or absorbed, and no unusual effects are produced.

A. **Excess Forces**

   When the forces of occlusion are greater than can be taken care of by the attachment apparatus, damage can result. Circulatory disturbances, tissue destruction from crushing under pressure, bone resorption, and other pathologic processes are initiated.

B. **Relation to Inflammatory Factors**
   1. *Trauma from occlusion does not cause gingivitis, periodontitis, or pocket formation.* The steps in the development of inflammatory disease and pockets were outlined on pages 177–178.
   2. In the presence of inflammatory disease, the existing periodontal destruction may be aggravated or promoted by trauma from occlusion.

III. Methods of Application of Excess Pressure

To understand the nature of the occlusal forces that can cause periodontal trauma from occlusion, it is helpful to recognize types of tooth contacts that can overburden a tooth or group of teeth.[3]

A. *Individual teeth that touch before full closure.* The contact is premature and may put excessive force on an individual tooth.

B. *Two or a few teeth in contact during movement of the jaw.* The teeth involved receive a disproportionate amount of force.

C. *Initial contacts on inclined planes of cusps.* Following the initial contact, when the teeth are brought together in a closed position, there may be excess pressure on the teeth where initial contact was made.

D. *Heavy forces not in a vertical or axial direction.* Normal occlusal relationships imply a direct cusp-to-fossa position during closure, with the force of occlusion in a vertical direction toward the tooth apex and parallel with the long axis. When pressures are exerted laterally or horizontally, there is excess force placed on the periodontal attachment apparatus.

E. *Increased frequency, intensity, and duration of contacts.* When there are parafunctional habits such as bruxism, clenching, tapping, or biting objects, many more than usual tooth contacts are made each day, and the intensity and duration are altered.

IV. Recognition of Signs of Trauma from Occlusion

No one clinical or radiographic finding will clearly define the presence of trauma from occlusion. Diagnosis of the condition is complex. The possible observations listed below should be looked for specifically and recorded for evaluation and correlation with the patient history and all other clinical determinations.

A. **Clinical Findings Which May Occur in Trauma from Occlusion**
   1. Tooth mobility
   2. Fremitus*
   3. Sensitivity of teeth to pressure and/or percussion.
   4. Pathologic migration.
   5. Wear facets or atypical occlusal wear.
   6. Open contacts related to food impaction.
   7. Neuromuscular disturbances in the

*Fremitus is a palpable vibration or movement. To determine whether a tooth has fremitus, place an index finger on each maxillary tooth in succession around the arch as the patient taps the teeth together.

muscles of mastication. In severe cases muscle spasm can occur.

8. Temporomandibular joint symptoms.

B. **Radiographic Findings**

Characteristics which may occur in trauma from occlusion include:

1. Widened periodontal ligament spaces, particularly angular thickening (triangulation). This finding frequently occurs in conjunction with tooth mobility.

2. Angular (vertical) bone loss in localized areas (figure 12–19, page 203).

3. Root resorption.

4. Furcation involvement.

5. Thickened lamina dura. Although related to occlusal forces, thickened lamina dura should not necessarily be considered a detrimental or destructive effect of trauma from occlusion. It may be a defense reaction to strengthen tooth support against occlusal forces. Thickened lamina dura is frequently associated with teeth which have undergone orthodontic treatment.

TECHNICAL HINTS

I. Observe the facial profile as the patient enters and is seated in the dental chair to estimate the classification of occlusion before examination of the teeth.

II. Avoid mention of a dentofacial deformity which would make the patient feel self-conscious.

III. Avoid suggesting to the patient or a parent the possible procedures which the orthodontist may use in the treatment of the case, as complications of the case become known only after the complete diagnosis.

IV. To aid in closing to centric relation: Instruct the patient to curl the tongue and try to hold the tip of tongue as far back as possible while closing.

V. When a small child has difficulty in occluding, the operator may firmly but gently press the cushions of the thumbs on the mucous membrane over the pterygomandibular raphe, holding the thumbs between the cheek and buccal surfaces of the teeth, as the patient is requested to close.

VI. Study the occlusion of the patient with removable dentures with the dentures in place in the mouth.

FACTORS TO TEACH THE PATIENT

I. Interpretation of the *general* purposes of orthodontic care (function and esthetics) to patients whom the dentist has referred to an orthodontist.

A. Dependence of masticatory efficiency on the occlusion of the teeth.

B. Influence of masticatory efficiency on food selection in the diet.

C. Influence of masticatory efficiency and diet on the nutritional status of the body and oral health.

II. Interpretation of the dentist's suggestions for the correction of oral habits.

III. The space maintaining function of the primary teeth in prevention of malocclusion of permanent teeth.

IV. The role of malocclusion as a predisposing factor in the formation of dental caries and periodontal diseases.

V. Plaque removal methods for reducing dental calculus and soft deposit retention in areas where teeth are crowded, displaced, or otherwise not in normal occlusion.

VI. The relation of the occlusion and the position of the teeth to the patient's personal oral care procedures.

A. Selection of the proper type of toothbrush.
B. Application of thorough tooth-brushing method or methods.
C. Use of dental floss.
VII. Specific reasons for frequency of recall when related to malocclusion.

References

1. Angle, E. H.: *Malocclusion of the Teeth,* 7th ed. Philadelphia, S. S. White, 1907.
2. Baume, L. J.: Physiological Tooth Migration and Its Significance for the Development of the Occlusion.
    I. The Biogenetic Course of the Deciduous Dentition, *J. Dent. Res.,* 29, 123, April, 1950.
    II. The Biogenesis of the Accessional Dentition, *J. Dent. Res.,* 29, 331, June, 1950.
    III. The Biogenesis of the Successional Dentition, *J. Dent. Res.,* 29, 338, June, 1950.
    IV. The Biogenesis of Overbite, *J. Dent. Res.,* 29, 440, August, 1950.
3. Allen, D. L., McFall, W. T., and Hunter, G. C.: *Periodontics for the Dental Hygienist,* 2nd ed. Philadelphia, Lea & Febiger, 1974, pp. 74–76.

Suggested Readings

Baer, P. N. and Benjamin, S. D.: *Periodontal Disease in Children and Adolescents.* Philadelphia, Lippincott, 1974, pp. 109–127.
Gianelly, A. A.: Diagnosis of Incipient Malocclusions, *J. Am. Dent. Assoc.,* 79, 658, September, 1969.
Graber, T. M.: *Orthodontics,* 3rd ed. Philadelphia, Saunders, 1972, pp. 204–254.
Herman, E.: Dental Considerations in the Playing of Musical Instruments, *J. Am. Dent. Assoc.,* 89, 611, September, 1974.
Hitchcock, H. P.: Face Development and Tooth Eruption, in Finn, S. B.: *Clinical Pedodontics,* 4th ed. Philadelphia, Saunders, 1973, pp. 309–331.
Kerr, D. A., Ash, M. M., and Millard, H. D.: *Oral Diagnosis,* 4th ed. St. Louis, Mosby, 1974, pp. 214–245.
Lieberman, M. A. and Gazit, E.: Guides to Orthodontic Treatment Timing, *J. Am. Dent. Assoc.,* 88, 555, March, 1974.
Proffit, W. R. and Norton, L. A.: Orthodontics in General Practice, in Morris, A. L. and Bohannan, H. M., eds.: *The Dental Specialties in General Practice.* Philadelphia, Saunders, 1969, pp. 197–210.
van der Linden, F. P. G. M.: Theoretical and Practical Aspects of Crowding in the Human Dentition, *J. Am. Dent. Assoc.,* 89, 139, July, 1974.
Wheeler, R. C.: *Dental Anatomy, Physiology, and Occlusion,* 5th ed. Philadelphia, Saunders, 1974, pp. 405–505.

Habits

Ayer, W. A. and Gale, E. N.: Psychology and Thumbsucking, *J. Am. Dent. Assoc.,* 80, 1335, June, 1970.
Barber, T. K. and Bonus, H. W.: Dental Relationships in Tongue-thrusting Children as Affected by Circumoral Myofunctional Exercise, *J. Am Dent. Assoc.,* 90, 979, May, 1975.
Graber, T. M.: *Orthodontics,* 3rd ed. Philadelphia, Saunders, 1972, pp. 292–328.
Lundeen, D. J., Kurtz, D. D., and Stanley, E. O.: Clinical Study of Dental Caries and Tongue Thrust, *J. Am. Dent. Assoc.,* 88, 1019, May, 1974.
Mason, R. M. and Proffit, W. R.: The Tongue Thrust Controversy: Background and Recommendations, *J. Speech and Hearing Disorders,* 39, 115, May, 1974.
Proffit, W. R. and Mason, R. M.: Myofunctional Therapy for Tongue-thrusting: Background and Recommendations, *J. Am. Dent. Assoc.,* 90, 403, February, 1975.
Sim, J. M. and Finn, S. B.: Oral Habits in Children, in Finn, S. B.: *Clinical Pedodontics,* 4th ed. Philadelphia, Saunders, 1973, pp. 370–385.
Subtelny, J. D. and Subtelny, J. D.: Oral Habits—Studies in Form, Function, and Therapy, *Angle Orthodont.,* 43, 347, October, 1973.

Trauma from Occlusion

Glickman, I.: *Clinical Periodontology,* 4th ed. Philadelphia, Saunders, 1972, pp. 250–254, 328–342, 355–356, 827–849.
Glickman, I. and Smulow, J. B.: *Periodontal Disease Clinical, Radiographic, and Histopathologic Features.* Philadelphia, Saunders, 1974, pp. 136–146.
Goldman, H. M. and Cohen, D. W.: *Periodontal Therapy,* 5th ed. St. Louis, Mosby, 1973, pp. 217–223, 315–317, 547–555.
Grant, D. A., Stern, I. B., and Everett, F. G.: *Orban's Periodontics,* 4th ed. St. Louis, Mosby, 1972, pp. 563–639.
Posselt, U.: Occlusion Related to Periodontics—Review of Literature, in Ramfjord, S. P., Kerr, D. A., and Ash, M. M., eds.: *World Workshop in Periodontics,* Ann Arbor, University of Michigan 1966, pp. 225–264.
Ratcliff, P. A. and Oliver, G. V.: Periodontics, in Steele, P. F., ed.: *Dimensions of Dental Hygiene,* 2nd ed. Philadelphia, Lea & Febiger, 1975, pp. 337–338, 363–365.

Prevalence of Malocclusion

Ast, D. B., Allaway, N., and Draker, H. L.: The Prevalence of Malocclusion, Related to Dental Caries and Lost First Permanent Molars, in a Fluoridated City and a Fluoride-deficient City, *Amer. J. Orthodont.,* 48, 106, February, 1962.
Ast, D. B., Carlos, J. P., and Cons, N. C.: The Prevalence and Characteristics of Malocclusion Among Senior High School Students in Upstate New York, *Am. J. Orthodont.,* 51, 437, June, 1965.

Emrich, R. E., Brodie, A. G., and Blayney, J. R.: Prevalence of Class I, Class II, and Class III Malocclusions (Angle) in an Urban Population. An Epidemiological Study, *J. Dent. Res.*, *44*, 947, September–October, 1965.

Erickson, D. M. and Graziano, F. W.: Prevalence of Malocclusion in Seventh Grade Children in Two North Carolina Cities, *J. Am. Dent. Assoc.*, *73*, 124, July, 1966.

Horowitz, H. S.: A Study of Occlusal Relations in 10 to 12 Year Old Caucasian and Negro Children—Summary Report, *Int. Dent. J.*, *20*, 593, December, 1970.

Mills, L. F.: Epidemiological Studies of Occlusion. IV. The Prevalence of Malocclusion in a Population of 1455 School Children, *J. Dent. Res.*, *45*, 322, March-April, 1966.

Salzmann, J. A.: The Effects of Fluoride on the Prevalence of Malocclusion, *J. Am. Coll. Dent.*, *35*, 82, January, 1968.

Chapter 15

Dental Plaque and Other Soft Deposits

During the inspection of the teeth it is necessary to recognize and assess the soft and hard deposits which accumulate on tooth surfaces. The soft deposits are acquired pellicle or cuticle, dental plaque, materia alba, and food debris, each of which is an entity, and the terms should not be interchanged. The hard, calcified deposit on teeth is dental calculus which is described in Chapter 16. A classification with definitions of the dental deposits is presented in table 15–1.[1]

ACQUIRED PELLICLE

The acquired pellicle is an amorphous, organic, tenacious membranous layer which forms over exposed tooth surfaces as well as restorations and dental calculus. Its thickness varies from 0.1 to several micra, usually thicker near the gingiva. Pellicles are acellular, that is, they are free from bacteria or other cell forms.

I. Development

A. Formation

Within minutes after all external material is removed by polishing with an abrasive, the acquired pellicle begins to form. It is composed primarily of glycoproteins which are selectively adsorbed to the tooth surface. The adsorbed material becomes a highly insoluble coating over the teeth, calculus deposits, restorations, and complete and partial dentures.

B. Source of Materials

Supramarginal pellicle is derived from the saliva, and submarginal pellicle is from the gingival sulcus fluid.

II. Types of Pellicles[2]

A. Surface Pellicle, unstained

The unstained pellicle is clear, translucent, insoluble, and not readily visible until disclosing agent is applied. When stained with a disclosing agent, it appears thin, with a pale staining which contrasts with the thicker, darker staining of dental plaque.

B. Surface Pellicle, stained

Unstained pellicle can take on extrinsic stain and become brown or grayish (page 262). The stain may be derived from dentifrices, particularly stannous fluoride-containing dentifrices, tobacco, or foods.[3,4]

Table 15–1. Tooth Deposits

Category	Tooth Deposit	Description	Derivation
Nonmineralized	Acquired Pellicle	Translucent, homogeneous, thin, unstructured film covering and adherent to the surfaces of the teeth, restorations, calculus, and other firm surfaces in the oral cavity.	Supramarginal: saliva Submarginal: gingival sulcus fluid
	Dental Plaque	Dense, organized bacterial system embedded in an intermicrobial matrix which adheres closely to the teeth, calculus, and other firm surfaces in the oral cavity Water irrigation removes only the outer layer of loose organisms.	Colonization of oral micro-organisms
	Materia Alba	Loosely adherent, unstructured, white or grayish white mass of oral debris and bacteria which lies over dental plaque Vigorous rinsing and water irrigation can remove materia alba.	Incidental mechanical accumulation
	Food Debris	Unstructured, loosely attached particulate matter Self-cleansing activity of tongue and saliva, and rinsing vigorously will remove debris.	Food retention following eating
Mineralized	Calculus	Calcified dental plaque; hard, tenacious mass which forms on the clinical crowns of the natural teeth and on dentures and other appliances	Plaque mineralization
	a. Supramarginal	Occurs coronal to the margin of the gingiva; is covered with dental plaque	Supramarginal: source of the minerals is saliva
	b. Submarginal	Occurs between the junctional epithelium and the opening of the sulcus or pocket at the margin of the gingiva; below the margin of the gingiva; is covered with dental plaque.	Submarginal: source of minerals is the gingival sulcus fluid

(Adapted from Schroeder, H. E.: *Formation and Inhibition of Dental Calculus*. Vienna, Hans Huber, 1969, pp. 14–15.)

C. **Subsurface Pellicle**

Surface pellicle is continuous with pellicle which is embedded in tooth structure, particularly where the tooth surface is partially decalcified.[5]

III. Significance of Pellicle

A. **Protective.** Pellicle appears to provide a barrier against acids, thus it may aid in reducing dental caries attack.[5]

B. **Nidus for Bacteria.** Pellicle participates in plaque formation by serving as a nidus for the colonization of microorganisms.

C. **Attachment of Calculus.** One mode of calculus attachment is by the acquired pellicle (page 252).

DENTAL PLAQUE

Dental plaque is a dense, noncalcified mass of bacterial colonies in a gel-like intermicrobial matrix. It adheres firmly to the acquired pellicle and hence to the teeth, calculus, and fixed and removable restorations. Plaque can be removed by mechanical methods such as toothbrushing and flossing, but not by irrigation or rinsing.

The microorganisms of dental plaque play an important part in the development of dental caries and inflammatory periodontal diseases. For that reason, the prevention and control or removal of plaque has special significance in patient counseling and care. Instruction and supervision in plaque control methods are important parts of each patient's treatment plan.

I. Classification

A. **By Location on Tooth**

Plaque may be divided into three parts, namely, *coronal* plaque, which is on tooth surfaces not in contact with the gingiva; *gingival* plaque, with reference to plaque in contact with the gingival margin; and *submarginal* plaque which is found within the sulcus or pocket.[6]

It is more in general use to divide plaque into two categories demarcated by the gingival margin. Dental calculus is defined in the same manner (page 249).

1. Supramarginal plaque, coronal to the gingival margin.
2. Submarginal plaque, located between the junctional epithelium and the gingival margin, within the sulcus or pocket.

B. **By Pathogenic Effects**

The role of plaque in the initiation and perpetuation of both dental caries and periodontal diseases has led to a realization that all dental plaque is not the same, but that the content and effects vary. The principal differences between plaques are brought about by chemical and microbial components. On the basis of their pathogenic effects, the three main categories of plaques are as follows:

1. Cariogenic plaque: associated with the initiation of dental caries.
2. Periodontal-disease-producing plaque: directly involved in promoting the inflammatory responses demonstrated by the gingival and periodontal tissues.
3. Calculus plaque or calculogenic plaque: invites mineralization of the plaque, leading to calculus formation.

II. Clinical Characteristics

Examination for dental plaque constitutes a specific part of the inspection of the teeth and gingiva for patient evaluation and treatment planning. The evaluation of plaque goes hand in hand with examination for signs of gingival inflammation (page 170) because of the close relation between plaque and the occurrence of gingivitis.

Table 15–2. Characteristics of Dental Plaque and Materia Alba

Characteristic	Dental Plaque	Materia Alba
Clinical Appearance	Tooth: dull, dingy, slimy Thin, freshly deposited plaque: transparent (seen by application of disclosing agent) or stained light brown or gray from foods, tobacco, or chromogenic bacteria Heavy, older plaque: matted, fur-like surface, usually stained	Soft, cheese-like, mealy White or cream-colored Opaque May extend over the gingival margin Adjacent gingival margin frequently shows signs of irritation with redness and enlargement
Distribution	Initially on proximal surfaces and cervical areas from which it creeps over the tooth surfaces Heaviest deposits on: Areas protected from cleaning Proximal surfaces Cervical third, particularly facial surfaces Lingual mandibular molars	Surfaces not exposed to cleansing by brushing and flossing May cover entire crown of a tooth out of occlusion Collects in open interdental areas. Heaviest deposits on: Facial cervical third Lingual mandibular molars Facial maxillary molars
Occurrence	All teeth and on removable appliances Aways present before mineralization of calculus; occurs over the surface of calculus deposits	Associated with unclean areas of the mouth, and teeth out of occlusion
Method of Removal	Toothbrushing, flossing Not removed by rinsing or water spray	Toothbrushing Vigorous rinsing and water spray can remove
Recurrence	Pellicle forms within minutes Disclosable plaque forms within 12 to 24 hours after complete removal	Readily when teeth are not cleaned regularly by toothbrushing
Composition and Structure	Gel-like mat of masses of microorganisms and intermicrobial matrix Early plaque: coccoid forms predominate, then filaments Older plaque: vibrios and spirochetes primarily Structured: filamentous organisms are arranged at right angles to the tooth surface	Nonstructured accumulation of: masses of living and dead microorganisms (similar to types found in dental plaque); food debris particles; desquamated epithelial cells; disintegrated leukocytes
Source	Product of bacterial growth	Product of accumulation and bacterial growth
Attachment	Firm: adheres closely to the acquired pellicle over the tooth surface and removable appliances Attaches to irregularities in the tooth surface	Loosely attached Adheres to dental plaque, teeth, restorations, and gingiva
Significance to Oral Health	Cariogenic plaque: harbors the strains of streptococci which form acid to decalcify tooth structure leading to dental caries Calculogenic plaque: provides matrix for mineralization of calculus. Periodontal-disease-producing plaque: direct relation to the initiation of periodontal disease	Contributes to initiation and progress of dental caries, dental calculus, and gingivitis and periodontal diseases Unesthetic Contributes to halitosis: contains decomposing food debris

A. **Distribution of Plaque**
   1. During formation
       Plaque formation begins at the gingival margin, particularly on proximal surfaces, and increases rapidly when left undisturbed. It spreads over the gingival third and on towards the middle third of the crown.
   2. Tooth surfaces involved
       a. Most frequent plaque occurs on proximal surfaces and around the gingival third, associated with protected areas (table 15–2).
       b. Least amounts occur on the palatal surfaces of maxillary teeth because of the activity of the tongue.
       c. Mandibular teeth accumulate more plaque than maxillary teeth.
       d. More rapid collection occurs on rough surfaces of teeth, restorations, and calculus.
       e. Thick dense deposits usually collect in difficult-to-clean areas such as under overhanging margins of crowns or fillings, under ledges of calculus, and associated with carious lesions.
       f. Deposits may extend over an entire crown of a tooth which is unopposed, out of occlusion, or not used during mastication.

B. **Detection**
   1. *Direct vision*
       a. Thin plaque: may be translucent and therefore not visible.
       b. Stained plaque: may acquire stains which make it visible, for example, yellow, green, tobacco, as described on pages 260–262.
       c. Thick plaque: the tooth may appear dull, dingy, with a matted fur-like surface. Materia alba or food debris may collect over the plaque.

   2. *Use of explorer*
       a. Tactile examination. When calcification has started, plaque may feel slightly rough; otherwise the surface may feel only somewhat slippery due to the coating of soft, slimy plaque.
       b. Removal of plaque. When no plaque is visible, an explorer can be passed over the tooth surface and, when plaque is present, it will adhere to the explorer tip. This technique is used when evaluating for a Plaque Index (page 279).
   3. *Use of disclosing agent.* When a disclosing agent is applied, plaque takes on the color and becomes readily visible (page 381). Disclosing agent should not be applied until after the evaluation of the oral mucosa and gingival color has been recorded.

C. **Clinical Record**
   1. Record plaque by location and extent (slight, moderate, or heavy). An index may be used.
   2. Plaque recordings and indices are kept for comparison in conjunction with the instructional plan for plaque control by the patient, both current and for recall appointments.
   3. Inspection records are included with the complete charting and oral examination (page 288).

III. Formation of Plaque

A. **Steps**
    Plaque is formed in three basic steps, namely, pellicle formation, bacterial colonization, and plaque maturation. Plaque formation does not occur randomly but involves a series of complex interactions, all of which are not completely researched.
   1. *Formation of a pellicle.* The pellicle forms on the tooth surface by

rapid and selective adsorption of components from the saliva (page 235).

2. *Bacteria attach to the pellicle.* There is prompt initial attachment of bacteria to the pellicle by rapid and selective adsorption of specific bacteria from the oral environment. Innate characteristics of the bacteria and the pellicle determine the adhesive interactions which make a particular organism adsorb to a particular pellicle.

3. *Bacterial multiplication.* Microcolonies form in layers as the bacteria multiply and grow. With increased size of colonies, they meet and coalesce to form a continuous bacterial mass.

4. *Plaque growth and maturation.* The increase in the mass and thickness of plaque results from
   a. Continued bacterial growth and multiplication.
   b. Continuous adsorption of bacteria to the plaque surface.

5. *Matrix formation.* The carbohydrate–protein–lipid matrix material is derived mainly from saliva for supramarginal plaque and from gingival sulcus fluid for submarginal plaque. Other materials are from the bacteria themselves.

B. **Plaque Adhesion Interactions**[7]
   1. If plaque is to develop and adhere to the teeth, mechanisms for adhesive interaction must be effective. The following interactions occur:
      a. Between cells and the pellicle and tooth.
      b. Cell-to-cell of the same species.
      c. Cell-to-cell between different species.
   2. Agents or substances which provide adhesion
      a. Surface components of the cells adsorb to the surface compo-

nents of pellicle or other organisms.
      b. Extracellular polysaccharide synthesized by the microorganisms are sticky and aid in the aggregation of bacteria. The most profuse of these is dextran produced by *Streptococcus mutans* from sucrose in the diet.
      c. Salivary constituents can interact. For example, *Streptococcus sanguis* interacts with components from the saliva which facilitate bacterial accumulation.
      d. Matrix–mediated interaction by the fibrillar structure of the matrix occurs.

IV. Composition

Plaque is composed of microorganisms and intermicrobial matrix. Organic and inorganic solids constitute approximately 20 percent, and water 80 percent. Microorganisms make up at least 70 percent of the solid matter, which is higher in submarginal plaque than in supramarginal.

Composition differs between individuals and between different tooth surfaces of an individual. As plaque ages, it changes.

A. **Inorganic Elements**[8,9]
   1. *Calcium and phosphorus.* The concentration of calcium, phosphorus, magnesium, and fluoride are higher in plaque than in saliva, which illustrates the ability of plaque to concentrate inorganic minerals.

   Plaque on the lingual surfaces of the mandibular anterior teeth contains a higher concentration of calcium and phosphate than on the other teeth, and the amount is even higher on those same surfaces in heavy calculus formers.

   2. *Fluoride.* Fluoride in plaque is higher when fluoridated water is used and is increased following

topical applications of fluoride or the use of dentifrices.[9-11] It has also been shown that the amount of plaque was decreased following the use of an 0.2 percent sodium fluoride mouth rinse.[12]

B. **Organic Components**

In addition to the organic matrix and the microorganisms, plaque (particularly submarginal plaque) may have a few epithelial cells and leukocytes which contribute to the organic content. Materials contained within the matrix vary. Diet influences the available fermentable carbohydrate. Constituents of the matrix may include, or are derived from, the following:

1. Products of bacterial metabolism: acids, antigens, enzymes, toxins, and endotoxins.
2. Salivary constituents: proteins, carbohydrates, lipids.
3. Soluble food components, particularly fermentable carbohydrates.
4. Broken down cells of microorganisms.
5. Shed leukocytes and epithelial cells.
6. Extracellular polysaccharides synthesized from sucrose by bacteria. Dextran is the major carbohydrate component.
7. Submarginal plaque: contains components from the gingival sulcus fluid.

C. **Plaque Microorganisms**

Dental plaque consists of a complex mixture of microorganisms which occur primarily as microcolonies. The population density is very high and increases as plaque ages. The probability of the development of dental caries and gingivitis increases as the number of microorganisms increases.

Changes in the types of organisms occur within plaque as the plaque matures. When oral hygiene practices are discontinued, the numbers of bacteria increase rapidly. The changes in oral flora follow a pattern such as the following:[13,14]

1. Days 1–2. Early plaque consists primarily of cocci. Streptococci, which dominate the bacterial population, include *Streptococcus mutans* and *Streptococcus sanguis*.
2. Days 2–4. The cocci still dominate and increasing numbers of filamentous forms may be seen on the surface of the cocci colonies. Gradually the filamentous forms grow into the cocci layer and replace them. Slow plaque formers continue to form plaque comprised primarily of cocci for a longer time than fast plaque formers.
3. Days 6–10. Filaments increase in numbers, and a more mixed flora begins to appear with rods, spirilla, and fusobacteria. Plaque near the gingival margin is thicker and develops a more mature flora earlier, with spirochetes and vibrios. As plaque spreads coronally, the new plaque has the characteristic coccal forms.

As plaque matures and thickens, more gram-negative and anaerobic organisms appear. During the period when this is happening, signs of inflammation are beginning to be observable in the gingiva.

4. Older plaque. Vibrios and spirochetes are prevalent, along with cocci and filamentous forms. The densely packed filamentous microorganisms arrange themselves perpendicular to the tooth surface in a palisade.

D. **Comparison of Supramarginal and Submarginal Plaque**

The sulcus or pocket provides a different environment for plaque than the supramarginal areas. Many more microorganisms are found in the sulcus, and especially in a pocket. In fact, almost the entire volume of pocket contents is microorganisms.

1. *Effect of anatomic form*[15]
    a. Shape. Plaque in a pocket is molded to the outline of the pocket wall. The shape of the pocket favors deposit retention.
    b. Cleaning limitations. A shallow sulcus can be cleaned by toothbrushing and other devices, but a deep pocket has a protected, deep, narrow base which cannot be reached by mechanical devices or by the saliva or tongue for self-cleansing.
2. *Microorganisms*[14,16]
    a. Types of organisms. Deep, closed pockets create an environment favorable to the general growth of microorganisms and specifically to anaerobic growth.
    b. Flora. A more complex flora can be found in submarginal plaque earlier in development than is typical of supramarginal plaque. Spirochetes, fusiforms, and *Bacteroides melaninogenicus* occur in greater numbers than in supramarginal plaque. These are organisms especially related to periodontal diseases.
    c. Arrangement of microorganisms
        (1) External surface (the part next to the sulcular and junctional epithelia) has leukocytes, desquamated epithelial cells, and many spirochetes. Spirochetes tend to grow preferentially next to the gingival tissues.
        (2) Deep part of the pocket: the flora varies with the type of periodontal disease.
    d. Source of nutrients. Plaque matrix materials and nutrients for the bacteria are obtained from the gingival sulcus fluid.

V. Effect of Diet on Plaque

A. **Content**
    1. Dental plaque is a product o bacterial growth and is not com posed of food.
    2. Sucrose
        a. Dental caries. The relationshi of the sucrose content of the die and its frequency of use to th development of dental caries i well defined in research an clinical application. Denta caries initiation is outlined i figure 15–1.
        b. Effect of sucrose on amount an pH of plaque. When a hig sucrose diet is used, plaqu forms and grows more pro fusely.[17] Patients fed sucrose b stomach tube had a les acidogenic plaque than patien who were fed by mouth.[18]

B. **Food Intake**
    Food particles are not needed in th mouth for plaque to form. In one stud neither varying the number of meal nor feeding by stomach tube affecte the development of plaque.[19] I another study less plaque develope in a group of stomach-fed patient when compared with those fed b mouth.[18]

C. **Texture of Diet**
    1. *Mechanical removal of plaque.* Th friction of mastication has bee shown to affect only the occlusa and incisal thirds of the crowns o teeth. Plaque on the gingival thir collected in spite of a normal die with coarse bread and fresh fruit, or chewing raw carrots three time daily as the only methods for per sonal care.[20] Chewing apples di not affect moderate amounts o plaque, but did tend to remove foo debris in a group of 12-year-olds.
    2. *Soft Diet.* A soft diet tends to favo plaque accumulation. Although no

CARBOHYDRATE + ORAL MICROBIAL ENZYMES = ACID FORMATION
FOODSTUFF   (Dextran-Forming
(Sucrose)   Streptococci)

ACID +   TOOTH SURFACE   = DECALCIFICATION
(Initial Dental Caries)

Figure 15–1.   Dental caries initiation.

well documented in the literature, clinical experience has shown the soft diet, especially one with excess fermentable carbohydrates, to lead to excess plaque formation. In one experiment using dogs, it was shown that more plaque developed when a soft diet was used.[22]

IGNIFICANCE OF DENTAL PLAQUE

Dental Plaque and Dental Caries

Dental caries is a disease of the dental lcified structures (enamel, dentin, and mentum) which is characterized by calcification of the mineral components d dissolution of the organic matrix. linical characteristics and types of vities were described on pages 212–215.

Essentials for Dental Caries

1. *Susceptible Tooth Surface.* A tooth with optimum fluoride content resists the process of dental caries (pages 421–423).
2. *Specific Microorganisms.*[23] Dental plaque contains many acidogenic microorganisms, especially streptococci, which have been shown to be involved in the etiology of dental caries. *Streptococcus mutans* has particular cariogenic potential in the development of smooth surface caries.
3. *Carbohydrate Source: Sucrose*
   a. Cariogenic microorganisms have the ability to synthesize carbohydrates into extracellular polysaccharides (dextrans, levans, and other glucans and fructans) and intracellular polysaccharides which are stored. *Streptococcus mutans, Streptococcus sanguis,* and *Streptococcus mitis* are involved in enamel caries.

   Other organisms, *Actinomyces viscosus* and *Actinomyces naeslundii,* are involved in root surface caries. They do not produce glucans, but synthesize other surface constituents for aggregation and plaque formation.[24]
   b. Dextran and other substances contribute to plaque formation and plaque adherence to the tooth; they may also serve as a barrier to the diffusion of buffers which might be available to neutralize the acids formed in plaque.
   c. Acid is formed by the breakdown of the sucrose. The acid acts to dissolve the tooth surface. With sufficient exposures (use of sucrose frequently) tooth structure breaks down. At first an area of decalcification (soft white spot) appears and then a definite carious lesion results.
   d. When there is no available sucrose in the diet, stored intracellular polysaccharides can be converted into acid. There are many more polysaccharide-storing organisms in the plaque of the caries-active than in the plaque of the caries-free person.
   e. The dental caries process within the plaque and on the tooth surface is outlined in figure 15–1.

B. **Contributing Factors**
   1. *Time.* Acid formation begins *immediately* when the sucrose from food is taken into the plaque.
   2. *The pH of the Plaque.* The plaque's pH is lowered promptly and it takes from one to two hours for the pH to return to a normal level, assuming the plaque is left undisturbed.
      a. Plaque pH before eating ranges from 6.2 to 7.0; it is lower in the caries-susceptible person and higher in the caries-resistant.
      b. Immediately following sucrose intake into plaque, a rapid drop in the pH of the plaque occurs.[25,26]
      c. Critical pH for enamel decalcification averages about 5.0, below which the enamel will decalcify.
      d. The amount of decalcification depends on the length of time and the frequency with which the acid with a pH below 5.0 is in contact with the tooth surface.
   3. *Frequency of Carbohydrate Intake.* With each meal or snack, when sucrose is used, the pH of the plaque is lowered provided the specific streptococci are present. Large amounts of sucrose eaten at mealtimes can be expected to be less cariogenic than small amounts eaten at frequent intervals during the day.[27] These and other related facts can be presented to the patient when the diet is discussed as a part of the basic instruction or as part of a total dental caries control program with dietary analysis (pages 410–414).

II. Dental Plaque and Periodontal Diseases

Dental plaque is unquestionably the single most important etiological factor in most periodontal diseases.[28] The variations in clinical manifestations in different individuals can be accounted for by the differences in the bacterial activi within the plaque as well as the tiss response and resistance to the microc ganisms and their products.

A. **Initiation of Gingival Disease**
   Experiments have been conduct in which the teeth of humans we completely cleaned of plaque, and tl subjects were instructed to withho all personal plaque remov techniques (toothbrushing, flossir etc.). Samples of plaque which d veloped over 22 days were examine and the types of microorganisms corded. The findings were describe earlier in this chapter under IV. C. page 241. In these patients, clinic signs of gingivitis appeared as early the tenth day, while in a majority subjects it was between 15 and days. When plaque removal proc dures were reinstated, the gingi returned to normal in approximate one week.[13]

   Microorganisms of the dent plaque at the gingival margin multip and extend beneath the margin; tl area of contact between the plaqu and the soft tissue increases; and the is a high concentration of microc ganisms in contact with the sulcu epithelium. The irritation from tl bacteria and their products leads degeneration of the sulcul epithelium and inflammation in tl adjacent connective tissue. The ste in the development of gingivitis an pocket formation are described pages 177–178.

B. **Calculus Formation**
   Dental plaque may form a matrix calculus formation (page 253). Tl significance of calculus is describe on page 256.

C. **Tooth Deposits and Incidence of Gi gival and Periodontal Diseases**
   A positive association betwee amounts of plaque, oral debris, ar

calculus and the severity of periodontal diseases has been shown.[29,30]

MATERIA ALBA

Materia alba ("white material") distinguishes itself clinically by being a bulky, loosely connected, soft deposit which is clearly visible without application of a disclosing agent. It is white, or grayish-white, and characteristically may resemble cottage cheese. Other properties are compared with dental plaque in table 15–2.

Materia alba forms over dental plaque. It is a product of informal accumulation of living and dead bacteria, desquamated epithelial cells, disintegrating leukocytes, salivary proteins, and particles of food debris. Although the bacterial count is high, it has been shown that the bacterial counts of materia alba are significantly lower than for dental plaque, and there are fewer living organisms in materia alba.[31]

Surface bacteria in contact with the gingiva can contribute to gingival inflammation, but the degree of inflammation is less than from dental plaque.[32] Although clinically, tooth surface decalcification and dental caries are frequently seen under materia alba, the direct effect of the dental plaque under the materia alba is the significant action, and materia alba bacteria are not the specific etiologic agents.

Clinical distinction between materia alba, food debris, and dental plaque is necessary, but patient instruction for the removal of all three involves the same basic plaque control procedures. Materia alba can be removed with a water spray or oral irrigator whereas dental plaque cannot.

FOOD DEBRIS

Loose food particles following eating collect about the cervical third and proximal embrasures of the teeth. Many of the factors related to deposit retention (pages 268–271) apply to food debris as well as materia alba and dental plaque.

When there are open contact areas, mobility of teeth or irregularities of occlusion such as plunger cusps, food may be forced between the teeth during mastication and vertical food impaction result. Horizontal or lateral food impaction occurs in facial and lingual embrasures, particularly when the interdental papillae are reduced or missing.

The role of food in the oral cavity during plaque formation was described briefly on page 242. Food debris adds to a general unsanitary condition of the mouth. Food with sucrose contributes to dental caries as the liquified sugar diffuses rapidly into the plaque and hence to the acid-forming bacteria.

Some self-cleansing through the action of the tongue, lips, saliva, and related factors takes place as described on page 267. Debris removal by toothbrushing, flossing, and water irrigation is a specific part of the total plaque control program. Cleansing of debris from about fixed prosthetic and orthodontic appliances is important to the plan for oral sanitation.

TECHNICAL HINTS

I. Check all surfaces of restorations and prosthetic appliances and remove rough areas. Soft deposits accumulate on rough or irregular surfaces more rapidly and in greater quantity than on smooth surfaces.

II. Withhold the use of a disclosing agent until the intraoral mucosal and gingival examinations have been made. Coloring agents can disguise soft tissue changes and deviations from normal.

FACTORS TO TEACH THE PATIENT

I.   Location, composition, and properties of dental plaque with emphasis on its role in dental caries and periodontal disease initiation.

II. The cause and prevention of dental caries.

III. Effects of personal oral care procedures in the prevention of dental plaque and materia alba.

IV. Plaque control procedures with special adaptations for individual needs.

V. Sources of sucrose in the diet with suggestions for control.

VI. Relationship of frequency of eating sucrose-sweetened foods to dental caries.

References

1. Schroeder, H. E.: *Formation and Inhibition of Dental Calculus.* Vienna, Hans Huber, 1969, pp. 14–15.
2. Meckel, A. H.: Formation and Properties of Organic Films on Teeth, *Arch. Oral Biol., 10,* 585, July-August, 1965.
3. Manly, R. S.: A Structureless Recurrent Deposit on Teeth, *J. Dent. Res., 22,* 479, December, 1943.
4. Vallotton, C. F.: An Acquired Pigmented Pellicle of the Enamel Surface. II. Clinical and Histologic Studies, *J. Dent. Res., 24,* 171, June-August, 1945.
5. Meckel, A. H.: The Nature and Importance of Organic Deposits on Dental Enamel, *Caries Res., 2,* 104, No. 2, 1968.
6. Goldman, H. M. and Cohen, D. W.: *Periodontal Therapy,* 5th ed. St. Louis, Mosby, 1973, pp. 181–184.
7. Gibbons, R. J. and van Houte, J.: On the Formation of Dental Plaques, *J. Periodont., 44,* 347, June, 1973.
8. Mandel, I. D.: Relation of Saliva and Plaque to Caries, *J. Dent. Res., 53,* 246, March-April, 1974, Supplement.
9. Grøn, P., Yao, K., and Spinelli, M.: A Study of Inorganic Constituents in Dental Plaque, *J. Dent. Res., 48,* 799, September-October, 1969.
10. Jenkins, G. N., Edgar, W. M., and Ferguson, D. B.: The Distribution and Metabolic Effects of Human Plaque Fluorine, *Arch. Oral Biol., 14,* 105, January, 1969.
11. Birkeland, J. M.: Fluoride Content of Dental Plaque after Brushing with a Fluoride Dentifrice, *Scand. J. Dent. Res., 80,* 80, No. 1, 1972.
12. Birkeland, J. M.: Effect of Fluoride on the Amount of Dental Plaque in Children, *Scand. J. Dent. Res., 80,* 82, No. 1, 1972.
13. Löe, H., Theilade, E., and Jensen, S. B.: Experimental Gingivitis in Man, *J. Periodont., 36,* 177, May-June, 1965.
14. Listgarten, M. A., Mayo, H. E., and Tremblay, R.: Development of Dental Plaque on Epoxy Resin Crowns in Man, *J. Periodont., 46,* 10, January, 1975.
15. Kelstrup, J. and Theilade, E.: Microbes and Periodontal Disease, *J. Clin. Periodont., 1,* 15, No. 1, 1974.
16. Socransky, S. S.: Relationship of Bacteria to th Etiology of Periodontal Disease, *J. Dent. Re 49,* 203, March-April, 1970 (Part 1).
17. Carlsson, J. and Egelberg, J.: Effect of Diet Early Plaque Formation in Man, *Odont. Rev 16,* 112, No. 1, 1965.
18. Littleton, N. W., Carter, C. H., and Kelley, R. Studies of Oral Health in Persons Nourishe by Stomach Tube. I. Changes in pH of Plaq Material after the Addition of Sucrose, *J. A Dent. Assoc., 74,* 119, January, 1967.
19. Egelberg, J.: Local Effect of Diet on Plaq Formation and Development of Gingivitis Dogs. III. Effect of Frequency of Meals a Tube Feeding, *Odont. Revy, 16,* 50, No. 1965.
20. Lindhe, J. and Wicén, P-O.: The Effects on th Gingivae of Chewing Fibrous Foods, *Periodont. Res., 4,* 193, No. 3, 1969.
21. Birkeland, J. M. and Jorkjend, L.: The Effect Chewing Apples on Dental Plaque and Foc Debris, *Comm. Dent. Oral Epidemiol., 2,* 16 No. 4, 1974.
22. Egelberg, J.: Local Effect of Diet on Plaq Formation and Development of Gingivitis Dogs. I. Effect of Hard and Soft Diets, *Odon Revy, 16,* 31, No. 1, 1965.
23. Fitzgerald, R. J.: Plaque Microbiology a Caries, *Alabama J. Med. Sci., 5,* 239, Jul 1968.
24. Jordan, H. V. and Hammond, B. F.: Filamento Bacteria Isolated from Human Root Surfac Caries, *Arch. Oral Biol., 17,* 1333, Septembe 1972.
25. Stephan, R. M.: Intra-oral Hydrogen-Ion Co centrations Associated with Dental Cari Activity, *J. Dent. Res., 23,* 257, August, 194
26. Rosen, S. and Weisenstein, P. R.: The Effect Sugar Solutions on pH of Dental Plaques fro Caries-Susceptible and Caries-Free Ind viduals, *J. Dent. Res., 44,* 845, Septembe October, 1965.
27. Gustafsson, B. E., Quensel, C. E., Lanke, L. Lundquist, C., Grahnén, H., Bonow, B. E and Krasse, B.: The Vipeholm Dental Cari Study. The Effect of Different Levels Carbohydrate Intake on Caries Activity in 4 Individuals Observed for Five Years, *Act Odont. Scand., 11,* 232, No. 3–4, 1954.
28. World Health Organization: *Periodontal Di ease.* Technical Report Series, No. 20 Geneva, World Health Organization, 1961, 4 pp.
29. Ash, M. M., Jr., Gitlin, B. M., and Smith, W. A Correlation Between Plaque and Gingivitis, *Periodont., 35,* 424, September-Octobe 1964.
30. Russell, A. L.: Epidemiology of Periodont Disease, *Int. Dent. J., 17,* 282, June, 1967.
31. Salkind, A., Oshrain, H. I., and Mandel, I. D Materia Alba and Dental Plaque, *J. Peric dont., 45,* 489, July, 1974.

32. Schwartz, R. S., Massler, M., and LeBeau, L. J.: Gingival Reactions to Different Types of Tooth Accumulated Materials, *J. Periodont.*, 42, 144, March, 1971.

Suggested Readings

Bahn, A. N.: Microbial Potential in the Etiology of Periodontal Disease, *J. Periodont.*, 41, 603, November, 1970.

Dawes, C., Jenkins, G. N., and Tonge, C. H.: The Nomenclature of the Integuments of the Enamel Surface of Teeth, *Brit. Dent. J.*, 115, 65, July 16, 1963.

Eastcott, A. D. and Stallard, R. E.: Sequential Changes in Developing Human Dental Plaque as Visualized by Scanning Electron Microscopy, *J. Periodont.*, 44, 218, April, 1973.

Fundak, C. P. and Ash, M. M.: Pilot Investigation of Correlations between Supragingival Plaque, Subgingival Plaque and Gingival Crevice Depth, *J. Periodont.*, 40, 636, November, 1969.

Galil, K. A. and Gwinnett, A. J.: Scanning Electron Microscopy: Observations on Occlusal Human Dental Plaque, *J. Can. Dent. Assoc.*, 39, 472, July, 1973.

Genco, R. J., Evans, R. T., and Ellison, S. A.: Dental Research in Microbiology with Emphasis on Periodontal Disease, *J. Am. Dent. Assoc.*, 78, 1016, May, 1969.

Gibbons, R. J., Socransky, S. S., De Araujo, W. C., and van Houte, J.: Studies of the Predominant Cultivable Microbiota of Dental Plaque, *Arch. Oral Biol.*, 9, 365, May-June, 1964.

Gildenhuys, R. R. and Stallard, R. E.: Comparison of Plaque Accumulation on Metal Restorative Surfaces, *Dent. Surv.*, 51, 56, January, 1975.

Glickman, I.: *Clinical Periodontology*, 4th ed. Philadelphia, Saunders, 1972, pp. 291–300.

Hiep, N., Stallard, R. E., and Shapiro, L.: Dental Plaque, *J. Periodont.*, 45, 117, February, 1974.

Hutchins, D. W. and Parker, W. A.: A Study of Plaque Distribution in the Gingival Crevice, *Oral Surg.*, 35, 385, April, 1973.

Katz, S., McDonald, J. L., and Stookey, G. K.: *Preventive Dentistry in Action.* Upper Montclair, N.J., D. C. P. Publishing, 1972, pp. 45, 115–118.

Keyes, P. H.: Research in Dental Caries, *J. Am. Dent. Assoc.*, 76, 1357, June, 1968.

Leach, S. A.: The Acquired Integuments of the Teeth: A Biochemical Review, *Brit. Dent. J.*, 122, 537, June 20, 1967.

Leach, S. A.: A Review of the Biochemistry of Dental Plaque, in McHugh, W. D., ed.: *Dental Plaque.* Edinburgh, E. & S. Livingstone, 1970, pp. 143–156.

Listgarten, M. A.: Dental Plaque: Its Structure and Prevention, *J. Dent. Child.*, 39, 347, September-October, 1972.

Mackler, S. B. and Crawford, J. J.: Plaque Development and Gingivitis in the Primary Dentition, *J. Periodont.*, 44, 18, January, 1973.

Mandel, I. D.: Dental Plaque: Nature, Formation and Effects, *J. Periodont.*, 37, 357, September-October, 1966.

Mandel, I. D., Levy, B. M., and Wasserman, B. H.: Histochemistry of Calculus Formation, *J. Periodont.*, 28, 132, April, 1957.

Nizel, A. E.: *Nutrition in Preventive Dentistry: Science and Practice.* Philadelphia, Saunders, 1972, pp. 3–47.

Nolte, W. A., ed.: *Oral Microbiology*, 2nd ed. St. Louis, Mosby, 1973, pp. 21–26, 233–240, 251–267.

Permar, D.: Our Old Friend, Nasmyth's Membrane, *J. Am. Dent. Hyg. Assoc.*, 44, 31, 1st Quarter, 1970.

Schroeder, H. E. and de Boever, J.: The Structure of Microbial Dental Plaque, in McHugh, W. D., ed.: *Dental Plaque.* London, E. & S. Livingstone, 1970, pp. 49-72.

Schwartz, R. S. and Massler, M.: Tooth Accumulated Materials: A Review and Classification, *J. Periodont.*, 40, 407, July, 1969.

Socransky, S. S. and Manganiello, S. D.: The Oral Microbiota of Man from Birth to Senility, *J. Periodont.*, 42, 485, August, 1971.

Plaque Prevention

Carlson, H. C. and Porter, C. K.: Inhibitory Effect of a Synthetic Antibiotic Mouthwash (QR-711) on Dental Plaque and Gingivitis in Young Adults, *J. Periodont.*, 44, 225, April, 1973.

Esposito, E. J.: Effect of Daily Rinsing with Alexidine on Supragingival Plaque pH, *J. Periodont.*, 45, 833, November, 1974.

Kaslick, R. S., Shapiro, W. B., and Chasens, A. I.: Studies on the Effects of a Urea Peroxide Gel on Plaque Formation and Gingivitis, *J. Periodont.*, 46, 230, April, 1975.

Keyes, P. H. and McCabe, R. M.: The Potential of Various Compounds to Suppress Microorganisms in Plaques Produced *in vitro* by a Streptococcus or an Actinomycete, *J. Am. Dent. Assoc.*, 86, 396, February, 1973.

Keyes, P. H. and Shern, R. J.: Chemical Adjuvants for Control and Prevention of Dental Plaque Disease, *J. Am. Soc. Prev. Dent.*, 1, 18, January-February, 1971.

Löe, H., ed.: Symposium on Chlorhexidine in the Prophylaxis of Dental Diseases, *J. Periodont Res.*, Supplement No. 12, 1973.

Löe, H.: A Review of the Prevention and Control of Plaque, in McHugh, W. D., ed.: *Dental Plaque.* Edinburgh, E & S Livingstone, 1970, pp. 259–270.

Loesche W. J., Green, E., Kenney, E. B., and Nafe, D.: Effect of Topical Kanamycin Sulfate on Plaque Accumulation, *J. Am. Dent. Assoc.*, 83, 1063, November, 1971.

Lusk, S. S., Bowers, G. M., Tow, H. D., Watson, W. J., and Moffitt, W. C.: Effects of an Oral Rinse on Experimental Gingivitis, Plaque Formation, and Formed Plaque, *J. Am. Soc. Prev. Dent.*, 4, 31, July-August, 1974.

Mandell, I. D.: New Approaches to Plaque Prevention, *Dent. Clin. North Am.*, *16*, 661, October, 1972.

Parker, R. B.: Our Common Enemy, *J. Am. Soc. Prev. Dent.*, *1*, 15, January-February, 1971.

Parsons, J. C.: Chemotherapy of Dental Plaque—A Review, *J. Periodont.*, *45*, 177, March, 1974.

Turesky, S., Glickman, I., and Sandberg, R.: *In vit* Chemical Inhibition of Plaque Formation, *Periodont.*, *43*, 263, May, 1973.

Weinstein, L.: Antimicrobial Chemoprophylaxis Dentistry, *Dent. Clin. North. Am.*, *16*, 75 October, 1972.

Chapter 16

Dental Calculus

Dental calculus, which is calcified dental plaque, is a hard, tenacious mass which forms on the clinical crowns of the natural teeth and on dentures and other dental appliances. Calculus is significant in the progression of inflammatory periodontal disease. The control of plaque deposits by the patient, supplemented by complete calculus removal by the dental hygienist, can reduce or eliminate gingival inflammation. There is a close relationship between the amount of plaque and calculus on the teeth and the severity of most gingival and periodontal diseases.

Comprehensive understanding of the characteristics, origin, development, and methods of prevention of calculus is essential to patient examination, evaluation, treatment, and instruction. For successful treatment and prevention the patient needs to know the interrelationship between plaque, calculus, and oral health, the need for complete removal of calculus, and the reasons for the painstaking manner in which scaling procedures must be carried out.

Classification and Distribution

Dental calculus is classified by its location on a tooth surface as related to the adjacent free gingival margin, that is, supramarginal and submarginal (figure 16–1).

A. **Supramarginal Calculus**
1. Location: on the clinical crown above the margin of the gingiva.
2. Distribution
   a. Most frequent sites: lingual of mandibular anterior teeth and buccal of maxillary first and second molars, opposite the openings of the ducts of the salivary glands.
   b. Crowns of teeth out of occlusion; nonfunctioning teeth; or teeth that are neglected during plaque removal (toothbrushing, flossing, or other personal care).
   c. Surfaces of dentures and dental appliances.
3. Other names for supramarginal calculus
   a. Supragingival*
   b. Extragingival

*The terms supra- and subgingival are at present probably the most widely used. Supra- and submarginal are more specific in their definition since the margin of the free gingiva is the dividing line between the two categories. The gingiva includes free, interdental, and attached. Hence, the terms supra- and subgingival are not as accurate.

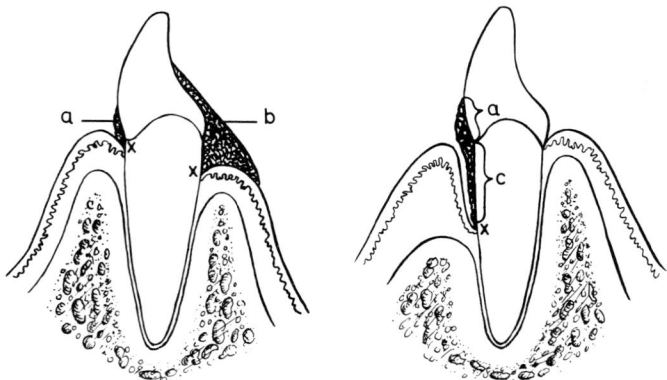

Figure 16–1.   Location of dental calculus. **a.** Supramarginal calculus. **b.** Extensive accumulation supramarginal calculus over crown, exposed root surface, and margin of the free gingiva. **c.** Submargin calculus along root surface to bottom of periodontal pocket. **x.** Bottom of pocket. Note level of crest alveolar bone in relation to bottom of the pocket.

      c. Coronal: indicating that the calculus is on the anatomic crown.
      d. Salivary: a term which indicates that the source of the calculus is the saliva.

B. **Submarginal Calculus**
    1. Location: on the clinical crown beneath the margin of the gingiva. It extends to the bottom of the pocket. As the pocket is deepened by disease, calculus formation results.
    2. Distribution
      a. May be generalized or localized on single teeth or a group of teeth.
      b. Facial surfaces have least; proximal surfaces have heaviest deposits.
      c. Relation to supramarginal: submarginal deposits may follow closely the location of the supramarginal deposits. Increased amounts of supramarginal calculus provide greater surface for plaque collection and hence periodontal inflammatory reaction may be increased, which in turn encourages submarginal deposits.
    3. Other names for submarginal calculus

      a. Subgingival
      b. Serumal: term which indicate the source of the calculus mate rials is the blood serum.

II. Occurrence

A. Calculus occurs at all ages and on bot permanent and primary teeth. In survey of children ages 9 to 14, 56 to 8 percent had supramarginal and 30 t 67 percent had submarginal calculu in the various age, sex, and racial ethnic groups measured.[1] In anothe study, in normal children 9 percent c ages 4 to 6, 18 percent of ages 7 to 9 and 43 percent of ages 10 to 15 ha calculus. In a group of children wit cystic fibrosis ages 10 to 15, 90 percen had calculus, and in a group of th same age with asthma, 100 percent ha calculus.[2]

B. Incidence increases with age, and i some populations 100 percent of th people over 30 have calculus, usuall due to continuing accumulation, no an increased tendency to form nev deposits as age advances.

III. Clinical Characteristics

A. **Appearance and Consistency**
    Identification of calculus prior t removal depends on knowledge of th

Table 16–1.   Clinical Characteristics of Dental Calculus

Characteristic	Supramarginal Calculus	Submarginal Calculus
Color	White, creamy-yellow, or gray May be stained by tobacco, food, or other pigments Slight deposits may be invisible until dried with compressed air	Light to dark brown, dark green, or black Stains derived from blood pigments from diseased pocket
Shape	Amorphous, bulky Gross deposits may: (1) Form interproximal bridge between adjacent teeth (2) Extend over the margin of the gingiva Shape of calculus mass is determined by the anatomy of the teeth, contour of gingival margin, and pressure of the tongue, lips, cheeks	Flattened to conform with pressure from the gingival pocket wall Combinations of the following calculus formations occur[3] (1) Crusty, spiny, or nodular (2) Ledge or ring-like formations (3) Thin, smooth veneers (4) Finger and fern-like formations (5) Individual calculus islands
Consistency and Texture	Moderately hard Newer deposits less dense and hard Porous Surface covered with plaque	Brittle, flint-like Harder and more dense than supramarginal calculus Newest deposits near bottom of pocket are less dense and hard. Surface covered with plaque
Size and Quantity	Quantity has direct relationship to: (1) Personal oral care procedures and plaque control measures (2) Physical character of diet (3) Individual tendencies (4) Function and use Increased amount in tobacco smokers	Related to pocket depth Increased amount with age because of accumulation Quantity is related to personal care, diet, and individual tendency as it is with supramarginal. Submarginal is primarily related to the development and progression of periodontal disease
Distribution on Individual Tooth	Above margin of gingiva May cover a large portion of the visible clinical crown, or may form fine thin line near gingival margin	Below margin of gingiva Extends to bottom of the pocket and follows contour of junctional epithelium With gingival recession, submarginal calculus may become supramarginal and become covered with typical supramarginal calculus
Distribution on Teeth	Symmetrical arrangement on teeth except when influenced by (1) Malpositioned teeth (2) Unilateral hypofunction (3) Inconsistent personal care (4) Abrasion from food Occurs with or without associated submarginal deposits Location related to openings of the salivary gland ducts: (1) Buccal of maxillary molars (2) Lingual mandibular anterior teeth	May be generalized or localized on a few teeth Heaviest on proximal surfaces, lightest on facials Occurs with or without associated supramarginal deposits

appearance, consistency, and distribution. Selection of instruments and techniques depends on understanding the texture, morphology, and mode of attachment of calculus. Table 16–1 provides a summary of clinical characteristics.

B. **Supramarginal Examination**
1. Direct inspection. Supramarginal deposits may be seen directly, or indirectly using a mouth mirror.
2. Use of compressed air. Small amounts of calculus which have not been stained are frequently invisible when they are wet with saliva. With a combination of retraction, light, and drying with air, small deposits usually can be seen. An explorer may be used when visual examination is not definite (page 199).

C. **Submarginal Examination**
1. *Visual examination* of calculus within a pocket
   a. Dark edge of calculus may be seen at or just beneath the margin.
   b. Diseased gingival margin does not adapt closely to a tooth surface, thus permitting a view into the pocket where calculus can be seen.
   c. Gentle air blast can deflect the margin from the tooth for observation into the pocket.
   d. Transillumination: when light shines through anterior teeth, a dark opaque shadow-like area seen on a proximal tooth surface could be submarginal calculus. Supramarginal calculus may also be found by this method. Without calculus, stain, or thick soft deposit, the tooth is translucent.
2. *Gingival tissue color change.* Dark calculus may reflect through a thin margin and suggest the presence of submarginal calculus.

3. *Tactile examination*
   a. Probe. While probing for sulcus/pocket depth, a rough submarginal tooth surface can be felt when calculus is present. Although there are other causes for roughness, submarginal calculus is the most frequent (page 198).
   b. Explorer. The use of the submarginal explorer Number 1 was described on page 199. Each submarginal area must be examined carefully to the bottom of the pocket, completely around each tooth.

D. **Clinical Record**
Calculus deposits are described in the examination record. The location of supra- and submarginal deposits and their extent (light, moderate, or heavy) need to be designated. A calculus index may be useful (page 275).

The calculus inspection record is included with the complete charting and oral examination, page 288.

CALCULUS FORMATION

Calculus has its origin from the deposition of minerals into an organic matrix. Calculus formation occurs in three basic steps: pellicle formation, plaque formation, and mineralization. Formation of supra- and submarginal calculus is essentially the same, although the source of the elements for mineralization is not the same.

I. Pellicle Formation

The formation and characteristics of pellicle were described on page 235. The pellicle, or cuticle, is composed of mucoproteins from the saliva, and is an acellular material. Its thickness and contour vary on the tooth surface. It begins to form within minutes after a tooth is cleaned.

II. Plaque Maturation

A. Microorganisms settle in the pellicle layer.

B. Colonies are formed which originally consist primarily of cocci and rod-shaped organisms in a homogeneous ground substance (page 241).

C. Colonies grow together to form a cohesive plaque layer.

D. Mineralization centers or foci form. Within 24 to 72 hours, more and more mineralization centers develop close to the underlying tooth surface. Eventually the centers grow large enough to touch and unite.

III. Mineralization

Mineralization of dental plaque and its transformation into calculus proceeds rapidly, coincident with its growth. Mineralization may start as early as a few hours after plaque maturation.

A. **Mineral Concentrations.** Concentrations of calcium and phosphate increase daily. The mineral concentration varies in plaque of different areas. The amount of minerals is greatest on the lingual surfaces of the mandibular anterior teeth.[4]

B. **Microorganisms.** The microbial flora shifts from cocci and rods to primarily filamentous forms as mineralization continues beyond the initial stages.

C. **Organic Matrix.** The microorganisms serve as the matrix for the deposition of minerals. A calculus-like deposit has been observed on the teeth of germ-free animals,[5-7] which may indicate that other organic substances may also serve as the matrix. However, as developed on human teeth, the bacteria do have a necessary function.

D. **Source of Minerals.** Saliva is the source of elements for supramarginal calculus, and the gingival sulcus fluid supplies the material for the submarginal deposits.[8,9] Gingival sulcus fluid was described on page 166. Since the amount of gingival sulcus fluid increases in diseased pockets, more minerals are available for the deposition of more calculus.

E. **Crystal Formation.** Mineralization consists of crystal formation, namely, hydroxyapatite, octocalcium phosphate, whitlockite, and brushite, each with a characteristic developmental pattern. The crystals form in the intercellular matrix and on the surface of bacteria, and finally within the bacteria.[10-12]

F. **Mechanism of Mineralization.** The process by which minerals, mainly calcium and phosphate, become incorporated from the saliva or gingival sulcus fluid into the plaque matrix is still not completely understood. Current research studies point to the probability that calcification of calculus may involve the same phenomena as other ectopic calcifications (such as urinary or renal calculi) and with similarities to normal calcification of bone, cartilage, enamel, or dentin. For those wishing to read about this complex subject, a list of references is provided in the *Suggested Readings* at the end of this chapter.

IV. Formation Time

Formation time means the average number of days required for the primary soft deposit to change to the mature mineralized stage. The average time is about 12 days, with a range from 10 days for rapid calculus formers to 20 days for slow calculus formers.[13] Calcification can begin as early as 24 to 48 hours.

Formation time depends on individual tendency, but it is strongly influenced by the roughness of the tooth surface, and the care and character of personal plaque control measures. Determination of the approximate formation time for an individual is important to instruction and counseling, as well as treatment planning for professional care.

V. Structure of Calculus

A. **Layers.** Calculus forms in layers which are more or less parallel with the tooth surface. The layers are separated by a line which appears to be a pellicle which was deposited over the previously formed calculus, and, as mineralization progressed, the pellicle became imbedded.

The lines between the layers of calculus can be called incremental lines. They form around the tooth in supramarginal calculus, but irregularly from crown to apex on the root surface in submarginal calculus. The lines are evidence that calculus grows or increases by apposition of new layers.

B. **Surface.** The surface of a calculus mass is rough and can be detected by use of an explorer. As observed by electron microscope, the surface roughness appears as peaks, valleys, and pits. When a section of a calculus mass was fractured off and the inner fractured surface examined by the electron microscope, the surface appeared granular, and the fracture followed through the intermicrobial matrix, leaving the calcified organisms visible.[14]

C. **Outer Layer.** The outer layer is partly calcified. On the surface there is a thick, mat-like soft layer of plaque and/or materia alba. It is the outer surface of the plaque on the submarginal calculus that is in contact with the sulcular epithelium.

VI. Attachment of Calculus

Calculus is more easily removed from some tooth surfaces than others. The ease or difficulty of removal can be related to the manner of attachment of the calculus to the tooth surface.

Several modes of attachment have been observed by conventional histologic techniques and by electronmicroscopy.[15-21] On any one tooth and in any one area, more than one mode of attachment may be found. When studying the attachment types, the character of the hard smooth enamel surface, and the rough porous, cemental surface should be considered. Four general modes of attachment have been described from research.

A. *Attachment by Means of an Acquired Pellicle or Cuticle*
   1. The pellicle is a thin, acellular homogeneous layer positioned between the calculus and the tooth surface.
   2. Calculus attachment is superficial since there is no interlocking or penetration.
   3. Occurs most frequently on enamel and newly scaled root surface.
   4. Calculus may be removed readily because of the smooth attachment.

B. *Attachment to Minute Irregularities in the Tooth Surface*
   1. Enamel irregularities include cracks, lamellae, and carious defects.
   2. Cemental irregularities include tiny spaces left at previous locations of Sharpey's fibers, resorption lacunae, scaling grooves, cemental tears or fragmentation.
   3. Difficult to be certain all calculus is removed when it is attached by this method.

C. *Attachment by Direct Penetration of Microorganisms into the Cementum*
   1. Bacteria from plaque penetrate into the cementum to various depths.
   2. A calculus matrix forms within the substance of the cementum.
   3. Removal of cementum with calculus is necessary to assure complete calculus removal.

D. *Attachment by Direct Contact Between Calcified Intercellular Matrix and the Tooth Surface*
   1. Remnants of microorganisms observed by electron microscope were near the root surface in the calculus but separated from it by the calcified intercellular matrix.[21]
   2. Cementum would be removed to assure calculus removal which was attached by this method.

VII. Composition

Calculus is made up of inorganic and organic components and water. Although the percentage will vary depending on the age and hardness of a deposit, and the location from which the sample for analysis is taken, mature calculus usually contains between 75 and 85 percent inorganic components, and the rest is organic components and water. The chemical content of supra- and submarginal calculus is similar.[4,22,23]

A. Inorganic
   1. *Inorganic components.* The components are mainly salts of calcium, calcium phosphate primarily, with small amounts of magnesium phosphate and calcium carbonate.
   2. *Trace elements.* Various trace elements have been identified including Na, Cl, Zn, Sr, Br, Cu, Mn, W, Au, Al, Si, Fe, and F.[24]
   3. *Fluoride in calculus*
      a. Concentration. The concentration of fluoride in calculus varies and is influenced by the amount of fluoride received from fluoride in the drinking water, topical application,[25] dentifrices,[26,27] or any form which is received by contact with the external surface of the calculus.
      b. Uptake. Fluoride uptake has been shown to be greater in calculus and silicate restorations than in intact enamel.[28] The surface of the cementum which is more permeable has a much higher content of fluoride than the enamel surface. Supramarginal calculus has a much higher concentration than submarginal calculus, and supramarginal calculus can have a higher fluoride content than the enamel surface,[29] since the calculus would be more porous than the enamel. The importance of the complete removal of calculus prior to a topical fluoride application is explained by these facts related to the uptake of fluoride by calculus.
   4. *Crystalline salts.* At least two-thirds of the inorganic matter of calculus is crystalline, principally apatite. Predominating is hydroxyapatite, which is the same crystal present in other calcified tooth parts and bone. Calculus also contains varying amounts of the crystalline salts brushite, whitlockite, and octocalcium phosphate.[30]
   5. *Calculus compared with teeth and bone.* Dental enamel is the most highly calcified tissue in the body and contains 96 percent inorganic salts as compared with dentin 70 percent, and cementum and bone at 45 to 50 percent.[31] Mature calculus has approximately 75 to 85 percent inorganic content. A comparison of calculus with the tooth parts provides insight into the effects of instrumentation, the difficulty of distinguishing calculus from cementum or dentin when scaling submarginally, and the modes of attachment of calculus to the tooth surface.

B. Organic
The organic portion of calculus consists of microorganisms, desquamated epithelial cells, leukocytes, and

mucin from the saliva. Supra- and submarginal calculus, as well as calculus formed on artificial dentures, are all comparable in composition and similar to duct calculi.[32] Substances identified in the organic matrix include cholesterol, cholesterol esters, phospholipids, and fatty acids in the lipid fraction; reducing sugars and carbohydrate-protein complexes in the carbohydrate fraction; and keratins, nucleoproteins, amino acids in the protein portion.[33,34] Mucoprotein is the principal constituent.[32]

The microorganisms are predominantly filamentous. In early calculus, during the first five days, cocci are found with some rods.[33,35] Most of the organisms within calculus are considered nonviable. The plaque on the calculus surface contains viable organisms.

SIGNIFICANCE OF DENTAL CALCULUS

Calculus has long been considered to have an important role in the development, promotion, and recurrence of gingival and periodontal conditions. With the newer knowledge of the role of dental plaque, and with understanding that dental calculus is mineralized plaque, the actual contribution of calculus to the disease process can be recognized.

Significant to the rationale for calculus removal and the production of a smooth tooth surface are the points listed here concerning the relationship of calculus to periodontal and gingival diseases.

I. Relation to Plaque

A. Calculus is mineralized plaque. Therefore calculus prevention depends on plaque prevention.
B. Calculus has a rough surface and provides a haven for plaque collection on its surface. Calculus increases the rate of plaque formation.

II. Relation to Pocket

A. Submarginal calculus is always covered by active plaque which is in direct contact with the sulcular epithelium. Plaque bacteria initiate gingivitis and periodontitis.
B. Submarginal calculus forms as a result of the calcification of the plaque on the submarginal tooth surface. Therefore submarginal calculus is secondary to plaque, and its formation is secondary to pocket formation. Submarginal calculus is a *result* of pocket formation, not a cause.
C. With the perpetuation of inflammation in the pocket wall by the plaque on the calculus surface, the secretion of gingival sulcus fluid is promoted and increased. With more fluid come more minerals for calculus formation.

III. Limitation of Self-Cleansing Activity

With calculus deposits the shape of the teeth is changed by the mass of calculus and the pocket wall is stretched out over the bulky calculus. Calculus may fill the interproximal area. When recession occurs, the gingival margin may be beneath the bulk of the calculus. Alteration of the natural contours interferes with normal self-cleansing. The self-cleansing mechanism is described on pages 267–268.

IV. Relation to Plaque Control Techniques and Scaling

A. Plaque over a rough calculus surface is much more difficult to remove by toothbrushing than from a smooth surface. The proximal surface calculus tears and shreds dental floss as it is passed over and under the deposit.
B. Removal and prevention of calculus leaves a smooth tooth surface which is possible to keep clean by toothbrushing and flossing, and which is resistant to plaque retention.

V. Permeability of Calculus

With its rough surface and permeable structure, calculus can act as a reservoir for toxic microbial and tissue breakdown products.

VI. Drainage From Diseased Pocket

Calculus can reduce drainage from the pocket by trapping bacteria and debris. Healing is prevented and the advancement of disease encouraged.

FACTORS TO TEACH THE PATIENT

   I. What calculus is and how it forms on the teeth.
  II. The effect of calculus on the health of the periodontal tissues and therefore on the general health of the oral cavity.
III. Properties of calculus which will explain the need for detailed, meticulous scaling procedures.
IV. Reasons for producing a smooth tooth surface during scaling and planing submarginally.
  V. Plaque control measures which the patient may carry out to prevent calculus formation.

References

1. Suomi, J. D., Smith, L. W., McClendon, B. J., Spolsky, V. W., and Horowitz, H. S.: Oral Calculus in Children, *J. Periodont.*, 42, 341, June, 1971.
2. Wotman, S., Mercadante, J., Mandel, I. D., Goldman, R. S., and Denning, C.: The Occurrence of Calculus in Normal Children, Children with Cystic Fibrosis, and Children with Asthma, *J. Periodont.*, 44, 278, May, 1973.
3. Everett, F. G. and Potter, G. R.: Morphology of Submarginal Calculus, *J. Periodont.*, 30, 27, January, 1959.
4. Mandel, I. D.: Biochemical Aspects of Calculus Formation, *J. Periodont. Res.*, 9, 10, No. 1, 1974.
5. Fitzgerald, R. J. and McDaniel, E. G.: Dental Calculus in the Germ-free Rat, *Arch. Oral Biol.*, 2, 239, August, 1960.
6. Gustafsson, B. E. and Krasse, B.: Dental Calculus in Germfree Rats, *Acta Odont. Scand.*, 20, 135, No. 2, 1962.
7. Theilade, J., Fitzgerald, R. J., Scott, D. B., and Nylen, M. U.: Electron Microscopic Observations of Dental Calculus in Germfree and Conventional Rats, *Arch. Oral Biol.*, 9, 97, January-February, 1964.
8. Waerhaug, J.: The Source of Mineral Salts in Subgingival Calculus, *J. Dent. Res.*, 34, 563, August, 1955.
9. Stewart, R. T. and Ratcliff, P. A.: The Source of Components of Subgingival Plaque and Calculus, *Periodont. Abstr.*, 14, 102, September, 1966.
10. Gonzales, F. and Sognnaes, R. F.: Electron Microscopy of Dental Calculus, *Science*, 131, 156, January 15, 1960.
11. Zander, H. A., Hazen, S. P., and Scott, D. B.: Mineralization of Dental Calculus, *Proc. Soc. Exp. Biol. and Med.*, 103, 257, February, 1960.
12. McMillan, L., Hutchinson, A. C. W., and Fosdick, L. S.: Electron Microscopic Study of Dental Calculus, *Dental Prog.*, 1, 188, April, 1961.
13. Schroeder, H. E.: *Formation and Inhibition of Dental Calculus*. Vienna, Hans Huber Publishers, 1969, pp. 73–74.
14. Baumhammers, A., Conway, J. C., Saltsberg, D., and Matta, R. K.: Scanning Electron Microscopy of Supragingival Calculus, *J. Periodont.*, 44, 92, February, 1973.
15. Zander, H. A.: Attachment of Calculus to Root Surfaces, *J. Periodont.*, 24, 16, January, 1953.
16. Shroff, F. R.: An Observation on the Attachment of Calculus, *Oral Surg.*, 8, 154, February, 1955.
17. Voreadis, E. G. and Zander, H. A.: Cuticular Calculus Attachment, *Oral Surg.*, 11, 1120, October, 1958.
18. Theilade, J.: Electron Microscopic Study of Calculus Attachment to Smooth Surfaces, *Acta Odont. Scand.*, 22, 379, No. 3, 1964.
19. Kopczyk, R. A. and Conroy, C. W.: The Attachment of Calculus to Root Planed Surfaces, *Periodontics*, 6, 78, April, 1968.
20. Moskow, B. S.: Calculus Attachment in Cemental Separations, *J. Periodont.*, 40, 125, March, 1969.
21. Selvig, K. A.: Attachment of Plaque and Calculus to Tooth Surfaces, *J. Periodont. Res.*, 5, 8, No. 1, 1970.
22. Glock, G. E. and Murray, M. M.: Chemical Investigation of Salivary Calculus, *J. Dent. Res.*, 17, 257, August, 1938.
23. Mandel, I. D. and Levy, B. M.: Studies on Salivary Calculus. I. Histochemical and Chemical Investigations of Supra- and Subgingival Calculus, *Oral Surg.*, 10, 874, August, 1957.
24. Mukherjee, S.: Formation and Prevention of Supra-Gingival Calculus, *J. Periodont. Res.*, Supplementum 2, 1968, pp. 1–35.
25. Schait, A. and Mühlemann, H. R.: Fluoride Uptake by Calculus Following Topical Application of Fluorides, *Helv. Odont. Acta*, 15, 132, October, 1971.

26. Kinoshita, S., Schait, A., Schroeder, H. E., and Mühlemann, H. R.: Origin of Fluoride in Early Dental Calculus, *Helv. Odont. Acta, 9,* 141, October, 1965.

27. Mühlemann, H. R., Schait, A., and Schroeder, H. E.: Salivary Origin of Fluorine in Calcified Dental Plaques, *Helv. Odont. Acta, 8,* 128, October, 1964.

28. Hellström, I.: Fluoride Uptake in Intact Enamel, Calculus Deposits, and Silicate Fillings, *Caries Res., 4,* 168, No. 2, 1970.

29. Yardini, J., Gedalia, I., and Kohn, M.: Fluoride Concentration of Dental Calculus, Surface Enamel, and Cementum, *Arch. Oral Biol., 8,* 697, November-December, 1963.

30. Grøn, P., van Campen, G. J., and Lindstrom, I.: Human Dental Calculus. Inorganic Chemical and Crystallographic Composition, *Arch. Oral Biol., 12,* 829, July, 1967.

31. Sicher, H. and Bhaskar, S. N., eds.: *Orban's Oral Histology and Embryology,* 7th ed. St. Louis, Mosby, 1972, pp. 39, 97, 160.

32. Stanford, J. W.: Analysis of the Organic Portion of Dental Calculus, *J. Dent. Res., 45,* 128, January-February, 1966.

33. Mandel, I. D., Levy, B. M., and Wasserman, B. H.: Histochemistry of Calculus Formation, *J. Periodont., 28,* 132, April, 1957.

34. Mandel, I. D.: Histochemical and Biochemical Aspects of Calculus Formation, *Periodontics, 1,* 43, March-April, 1963.

35. Turesky, S., Renstrup, G., and Glickman, I.: Histologic and Histochemical Observations Regarding Early Calculus Formation in Children and Adults, *J. Periodont., 32,* 7, January, 1961.

Suggested Readings

Alexander, A. G.: Calculus—An Historical Review of its Association with Periodontal Disease, *Dent. Health, 7,* 39, July-September, 1968.

Alexander, A. G.: Crevicular Fluid as a Source of the Constituents of Subgingival Calculus, *Dent. Health, 8,* 1, January-March, 1969.

Alexander, A. G.: The Relationship between Tobacco Smoking, Calculus, and Plaque Accumulation and Gingivitis, *Dent. Health, 9,* 6, January-March, 1970.

Grant, D. A., Stern, I. B., and Everett, F. G.: *Orban's Periodontics,* 4th ed. St. Louis, Mosby, 1972, pp. 123–138.

Leung, S. W.: Relation of Calculus, Plaque, and Food Impaction to Periodontal Disease, *J. Dent. Res., 41,* 306, January-February, 1962.

Listgarten, M. A. and Ellegaard, B.: Electron Microscopic Evidence of a Cellular Attachment Between Junctional Epithelium and Dental Calculus, *J. Periodont. Res., 8,* 143, No. 3, 1973.

Löe, H.: A Discussion of the Possible Significance of Gingival Pocket Fluid in Periodontal Disease, *Periodont. Abstr., 16,* 52, June, 1968.

Mislowsky, W. J. and Mazzella, W. J.: Supragingival and Subgingival Plaque and Calculus Formation in Humans, *J. Periodont., 45,* 822, November, 1974.

Oshrain, H. I., Salkind, A., and Mandel, I. D.: An Histologic Comparison of Supra and Subgingival Plaque and Calculus, *J. Periodont., 42,* 31, January, 1971.

Rizzo, A. A., Scott, D. B., and Bladen, H. A.: Calcification of Oral Bacteria, *Ann. New York Acad. Sci., 109,* 14, May 31, 1963.

Mineralization Theories

Ennever, J., Vogel, J. J., and Benson, L. A.: Lipid and Calculus Matrix Calcification in Vitro, *J. Dent. Res., 52,* 1056, September-October, 1973.

Everett, F. G.: Calculus, *J. Am. Dent. Hyg. Assoc., 30,* 121, July, 1956.

Glimcher, M. J.: Specificity of the Molecular Structure of Organic Matrices in Mineralization, in Sognnaes, R. F., ed.: *Calcification in Biological Systems.* Washington, D.C., Amer. Asso. Adv. Sci., 1960, p. 421 ff.

Gressly, F.: Experimental Calculus Formation, *Periodontics, 1,* 53, March-April, 1963.

Leung, S. W.: Calculus Formation. Salivary Factors, *Dent. Clin. North Am.,* p. 723, November, 1960.

Leung, S. W. and Jensen, A. T.: Factors Controlling the Deposition of Calculus, *Int. Dent. J., 8,* 613, December, 1958.

Mandel, I. D.: Calculus Formation. The Role of Bacteria and Mucoprotein, *Dent. Clin. North Am.,* p. 731, November, 1960.

Mukherjee, S.: Formation and Prevention of Supragingival Calculus, *J. Periodont. Res.,* Supplementum 2, 1968, pp. 14–21.

Schroeder, H. E.: *Formation and Inhibition of Dental Calculus.* Vienna, Hans Huber, 1969, pp 37–44, 94–108.

Sobel, A. E.: Local Factors in the Mechanism of Calcification, *Ann. New York Acad. Sci., 60,* 713, April 27, 1955.

Weidmann, S. M.: Review of Modern Concepts on Calcification, *Arch. Oral Biol., 1,* 259, No. 3, 1960.

Chapter 17

Tooth Stains and Discolorations

Discolorations of the teeth occur in three ways: (1) stain adhering directly to the surfaces of the teeth, (2) stain contained within calculus and soft deposits on the teeth, and (3) stain incorporated within the tooth structure. The dental hygienist is mainly concerned during instructional and clinical techniques with the first two, since these may be removed by scaling and polishing, and certain stains may be prevented by the patient's routine personal care.

The significance of stains is related to the effect on the appearance of the teeth. In general, any detrimental effect on the teeth or gingival tissues is related to the soft deposit or calculus in which the stain occurs. Thick, bulky deposits of stain can conceivably be a source of irritation if they occur adjacent to the gingival crest. Certain stains provide a means for evaluating oral cleanliness and the patient's habits of personal care.

I. Definitions for the Classification of Stains

A. Extrinsic

Extrinsic stains occur on the external surface of the tooth and may be removed by techniques of scaling and polishing.

B. Intrinsic

Intrinsic stains occur within the tooth substance and cannot be removed by techniques of scaling and polishing.

C. Exogenous

Exogenous stains develop or originate from sources outside the tooth. Exogenous stains may be extrinsic and stay on the outer surface of the tooth or intrinsic and become incorporated within the tooth structure.

D. Endogenous

Endogenous stains develop or originate from within the tooth. Endogenous stains are always intrinsic and usually are discolorations of the dentin which are reflected through the enamel.

II. Application of Techniques to Stain Removal

A. Stains Occurring Directly on the Tooth Surface

1. Stains which are directly associated with the surface of the enamel or

exposed cementum are removed as much as possible during tooth-brushing by the patient. Some stains are removed by scaling while others will require polishing.

2. When stains are tenacious, excessive polishing should be avoided: precaution should be taken to prevent abrasion of the tooth surface or gingival margin, or overheating with a motor-driven polisher.

B. **Stains Incorporated within Tooth Deposits**

When stain is included within the substance of a soft deposit or calculus, it is removed with the deposit.

EXTRINSIC STAINS

Many stains are both described and classified by their colors, which is confusing for clinical designation. For example, there is a wide variety of green stains which occur on rather specifically different tooth surfaces. Green stains may result from chlorophyll preparations, from the metallic dust of certain minerals in industry, or from drugs. The most common green stain is not one of those listed above but is a clinical entity with a specific occurrence pattern and no scientific name other than "green stain." The term green stain is applied to this particular stain, whereas green stains from other causes need to be clinically designated by their etiology.

The most frequently observed stains, yellow, green, black line and tobacco will be described first; the less common orange, red, and metallic stains will follow.

I. **Yellow Stain**

A. **Clinical Appearance**

Dull, yellowish discoloration of dental plaque appears.

B. **Distribution on Tooth Surfaces**

Yellow stain is associated with presence of dental plaque. (Note distribu-tion of dental plaque, table 15–2, page 238.)

C. **Occurrence**
   1. Common to all ages.
   2. More evident when personal oral care procedures are neglected.

D. **Etiology**
   Usually food pigments.

II. Green Stain

A. **Clinical Appearance**
   1. Light or yellowish green to very dark green
   2. Embedded in dental plaque.
   3. Shape: occurs in three general forms.
      a. Small curved line following contour of labial gingival crest.
      b. Smeared irregularly, may even cover entire facial surface.
      c. Streaked, following grooves or lines in enamel.
   4. Lighter stain is frequently superimposed by soft, yellow, or gray debris.
   5. Dark green more frequently associated with adequate personal toothbrushing habits; light green stain with inadequate (unclean teeth).[1,2]
   6. Dark green occasionally becomes imbedded in surface enamel and may be observed as an intrinsic stain when superficial layers of deposit are removed.
   7. Enamel under stain: sometimes decalcified as a result of cariogenic plaque or materia alba (pages 243–244). The rough decalcified surface encourages plaque retention and recurrence of green stain.

B. **Distribution on Tooth Surfaces**
   1. Primarily labial and buccal; may extend to proximal.
   2. Most frequent: labial cervical third of maxillary anterior teeth.

C. **Composition**
1. Chromogenic bacteria and fungi.
2. Decomposed hemoglobin.
3. Inorganic elements: calcium, potassium, sodium, silicon, magnesium, phosphorus, and others in small amounts.[3]

D. **Occurrence**
1. May occur at any age; primarily found in childhood.
2. Sex: statistics vary.
   a. Males more frequently.[1,4]
   b. Females more frequently.[2]
3. Green stain tends to occur without other stains (except yellow) in the same mouth in nearly one-half the cases.[2,4]

E. **Recurrence**
Recurrence tends to depend on fastidiousness of personal care procedures.

F. **Etiology**
The etiology of green stain has not been established. It is possible that causes may vary in different mouths. Differences of opinion exist as to the effects of oral uncleanliness, chromogenic bacteria, and gingival hemorrhage. The theories and predisposing factors have been reviewed in the literature.[1-3] A summary is given below.
1. Chromogenic or fluorescent bacteria or fungi.
   a. Retained and nourished in dental plaque.
   b. Produce coloring substances.
2. Blood pigments from hemoglobin are decomposed by bacteria.
3. Predisposing factors
   a. Means for retention and proliferation of chromogenic bacteria: dental plaque, materia alba, and food debris.
   b. Gingiva with bleeding tendencies in gingivitis.
4. Role of primary enamel cuticle or Nasmyth's membrane: although in the literature the primary cuticle has been associated with green stain, current evidence shows that the cuticle or membrane is lost soon after the eruption of the teeth.[5]

III. **Black Line Stain**

A. **Other Names**
Mesenteric line,[6] pigmented dental plaque,[7] brown stain,[4] black stain.[10]

B. **Clinical Appearance**
1. Black or dark brown.
2. Continuous or interrupted fine line, one mm. wide (average), no appreciable thickness.
3. May be a wider band or even occupy entire gingival third in severe cases (rare).
4. Follows contour of gingival crest about one mm. above crest.
5. Usually demarcated from gingival crest by clear white line of unstained enamel.
6. Appears black at bases of pits and fissures.
7. Heavy deposits slightly elevated from the tooth surface, may be detected with an explorer.
8. Gingiva: firm, resilient, with little or no tendency to hemorrhage.
9. Teeth: frequently clean and shiny with a tendency to lower incidence of dental caries.

C. **Distribution on Tooth Surface**
1. Labial, buccal, and lingual; follows contour of gingival crest onto proximal surfaces.
2. Rarely on labial of maxillary anterior.
3. Most frequently: lingual and proximal surfaces of maxillary posterior teeth.

D. **Composition and Formation**[9,10]
1. The composition is like plaque in that it is composed of microor-

ganisms imbedded in an intermicrobial substance.

2. The microorganisms are primarily Gram positive rods and actinomycetes, with other bacteria in smaller percentages.

3. Calcification occurs which is similar to the regular formation of calculus.

E. **Occurrence**
   1. All ages; more common in childhood.
   2. More common in females.
   3. Frequently in clean mouths.

F. **Recurrence**
   Black line stain tends to reform despite regular personal care, but quantity may be less when plaque control procedures are meticulous.

G. **Predisposing factors:** none apparent except a natural tendency.

IV. Tobacco Stain

A. **Clinical Appearance**
   1. Light brown to dark leathery brown or black.
   2. Shape
      a. Diffuse staining of dental plaque.
      b. Narrow band which follows contour of gingival crest, slightly above the crest.
      c. Wide, firm, tar-like band may cover cervical third and extend to central third of crown.
   3. May be incorporated in calculus deposit.
   4. Heavy deposits (particularly from chewing tobacco) may penetrate the enamel and become intrinsic.

B. **Distribution on Tooth Surfaces**
   1. Cervical third, primarily.
   2. Any surface, as well as pits and fissures.
   3. Most frequent: lingual surfaces.

C. **Composition**
   1. Tar products of combustion.
   2. Brown pigment from chewing tobacco.

D. **Predisposing Factors**
   1. Natural tendencies: quantity of stain not proportional to amount of tobacco used, which may indicate individual differences.
   2. Personal oral care procedures: increased deposits occur with neglect.
   3. Extent of dental plaque and calculus available for adherence.

V. Other Brown Stains

A. **Brown Pellicle**
   1. The acquired pellicle (page 235) can take on various tones of brown or gray stain.
   2. It is smooth and structureless and recurs readily after removal.[5]
   3. It has been associated with the use of a nonabrasive-containing dentifrice or plain brush with water.[11,12]

B. **Stannous Fluoride Dentifrice**
   1. An extrinsic diffuse light brown staining occurs in some individuals who use stannous fluoride dentifrice regularly. It may resemble brown pellicle.
   2. The stain takes various forms: when it stains primarily at the cervical third and on plaque or calculus, it appears similar to a light brown tobacco stain.

VI. Orange and Red Stains

A. **Clinical Appearance**
   Orange or red stains appear at the cervical third.

B. **Distribution on Tooth Surfaces**
   1. More frequently on anterior than posterior teeth.
   2. Both labial and lingual of anterior teeth.

C. **Occurrence**
Rare (red more rare than orange).

D. **Etiology**
Chromogenic bacteria.

VII. Metallic Stains

A. **Metals or Metallic Salts from Metal-Containing Dust of Industry**
1. Clinical appearance: examples of colors on teeth.
   a. Copper or brass: green or bluish-green.
   b. Iron: brown to greenish-brown.
   c. Nickel: green.
   d. Cadmium: yellow or golden brown.
2. Distribution on tooth surfaces.
   a. Primarily anterior; may occur on any teeth.
   b. Cervical third more commonly.
3. Manner of formation.
   a. Industrial worker inhales dust through mouth, bringing metallic substance in contact with teeth.
   b. Metal imparts color to dental plaque.
   c. Occasionally stain may penetrate tooth substance and become exogenous intrinsic stain.

B. **Metallic Substances Contained in Drugs**
1. Clinical appearance: examples of colors on teeth.
   a. Iron: black (iron sulfide) or brown.
   b. Manganese (from potassium permanganate): black.
2. Distribution on tooth surfaces: general, may occur on all.
3. Manner of formation.
   a. Drug enters plaque substance, imparts color to plaque.
   b. Pigment from drug may attach directly to tooth substance.

INTRINSIC STAINS

Stains incorporated within the tooth structure may be related to the period of tooth development or may be acquired after eruption. They present no problems in that they do not weaken the tooth or make it more susceptible to disease. An occasional patient, desiring an improvement in the appearance of the anterior teeth, may request removal of a discoloration. The dentist may employ one of two alternatives in the treatment of these teeth. Improvement in tooth color can be produced by bleaching in certain instances. In other cases it is necessary to prepare a jacket crown to cover the discoloration.

I. Pulpless Teeth

It should be realized that all pulpless teeth do not discolor. Improved endodontic procedures have contributed to the prevention of many discolorations formerly associated with that cause.

A. **Clinical Appearance**
A wide range of colors exists; they may be light yellow-brown, slate gray, reddish-brown, dark brown, bluish-black, or black. Others have an orange or greenish tinge.

B. **Manner of Formation**
1. Blood and other pulp tissue elements may be made available for breakdown as a result of hemorrhages in the pulp chamber, root canal operations, or necrosis and decomposition of the pulp tissue.
2. Pigments from the decomposed hemoglobin and pulp tissue penetrate into the dentinal tubules.

II. Drugs and Metals

A. **Restorative Materials**
1. Dental amalgam: silver amalgam can impart a gray to black discolora-

tion to the tooth structure around a restoration.

   a. Due to migration of metallic ions from the amalgam restoration into the enamel and dentin.

   b. The silver, tin, and mercury ions eventually contact debris at the junction of the tooth and the restoration and form sulfides, which are products of corrosion.[13]

2. Copper amalgam used for filling primary teeth may impart a bluish-green color.

3. Silver nitrate used in a cavity base under a restoration can produce black discoloration.

B. **Endodontic Therapy and Restorative Materials**

1. Silver nitrate: bluish-black.
2. Volatile oils: yellowish-brown.
3. Strong iodine: brown.
4. Aureomycin: yellow.
5. Silver-containing root canal sealer: black.

III. Imperfect Tooth Development

A. **Enamel Hypoplasia**[14,15]

1. *Systemic Hypoplasia* (chronologic hypoplasia resulting from ameloblastic disturbance of short duration). Teeth erupt with white spots or with pits. Over a long period of time the white spots may become discolored from food pigments or other substances taken into the mouth. Figure 13–1 (page 210) shows an example of chronologic hyperplasia.

2. *Local Hypoplasia* (affects single tooth). White spots may become stained as in systemic hypoplasia.

3. *Hereditary Amelogenesis Imperfecta.* The enamel is partially or completely missing due to a generalized disturbance of the ameloblasts. Teeth are yellowish-brown or gray-brown.

B. **Dental Fluorosis**

1. Manner of formation[15]

   a. Enamel hypocalcification resulting from ingestion of excessive fluoride ion content of the drinking water (more than two parts per million) during the period of calcification.

   b. When the teeth erupt there are white spots or areas which later become discolored from oral pigments and appear light or dark brown.

   c. Severe effects produce cracks or pitting; the discoloration concentrates in these.

2. Classification[16]

   a. *Very mild:* enamel shows irregularly scattered, small, opaque, white areas; frequently only a few teeth are affected.

   b. *Mild:* enamel shows white opaque areas which involve up to one-half of the tooth surface.

   c. *Moderate:* entire enamel is affected and brown staining occurs in varying degrees.

   d. *Severe:* entire enamel is affected and discrete or confluent pitting is present.

C. **Hereditary Dentinogenesis Imperfecta ("Opalescent Dentin")**[15]

The dentin is abnormal as a result of disturbances in the odontoblastic layer during development. The teeth appear translucent or opalescent, and vary in color from gray to bluish-brown.

D. **Tetracycline**[17]

1. Tetracycline antibiotics, used widely for combatting many types of infections, are absorbed by the bones and teeth and can be transferred through the placenta and enter fetal circulation.

2. Discoloration of the teeth of a child can result when the drug is administered during the third trimes-

ter of pregnancy or in infancy and early childhood.

3. Color of teeth: may be light green to dark yellow tones, or a gray-brown. The discoloration depends on the dosage, length of time the drug was used, and the type of tetracycline.

4. Teeth involved: may be generalized or limited to specific parts of individual teeth that were developing at the time of administration of the antibiotic; enamel hypoplasia also may occur. Reference to the Table of Tooth Development can assist the identification of the source of an intrinsic stain (Appendix, tables A–1 and A–2).

IV. Other Systemic Causes

Pigments circulating in the blood are transmitted to the dentin from the capillaries of the pulp. *Example:* prolonged jaundice early in life can impart yellow or greenish discoloration to the teeth.[12]

Erythroblastosis fetalis may leave a green, brown, or blue hue to the teeth.[18] A kidney disease patient who had uremia during tooth development may have hypoplasia with a brownish discoloration.[19]

V. Exogenous Intrinsic Stains

When intrinsic stains come from an outside source, not from within the tooth, the stain is called exogenous intrinsic. Extrinsic stains can provide stain which becomes intrinsic. Tobacco and green stains are examples of this.

A. **Drugs**

1. Stannous fluoride topical application[20]

   a. Light to dark brown staining from the formation of tin sulfide.

   b. Location: most frequently in occlusal pits and grooves of posterior teeth and cervical third facial surfaces of anterior; in carious and pre-carious lesions

and margins of silicate and amalgam restorations.

   c. Has been suggested that the staining is evidence of dental caries arrestment.[21]

2. Ammoniacal silver nitrate, used in treatment of sensitive areas such as exposed cementum or for inhibition of decalcification in dental caries prevention, imparts a dark brown to black discoloration.

B. **Stain in Dentin**

Example: discoloration resulting from a carious lesion.

TECHNICAL HINTS

I. Record color, type, extent, and location of stains with the patient's examination.

II. Make additions to the Dental History as information is gained concerning the origin of stains such as those related to tooth development, systemic disease, occupations, or medications.

III. Avoid making patient feel self-conscious by overemphasizing the appearance of stains which may occur in spite of conscientious toothbrushing habits.

IV. Use tact when questioning patients with brown stain since nonsmokers do not appreciate having an assumption made concerning the etiology of the stain on the teeth.

V. Refer patient's questions concerning the removal of intrinsic stains to the dentist. Avoid expressing an opinion in terms of diagnosis or prognosis of treatment until the dentist has recommended a procedure.

FACTORS TO TEACH THE PATIENT

I. Factors which contribute to stain accumulation.

II. Personal care procedures which can aid in the prevention or reduction of stains.

III. Reasons for not using an excessively abrasive dentifrice to lessen or remove stain accumulation.

IV. Reasons for the difficulty in removal of certain extrinsic stains during scaling and polishing.

References

1. Ayers, P.: Green Stain, *J. Am. Dent. Assoc.*, 26, 2, January, 1939.
2. Springer, J.: A Clinical Study of Green Stain, *Tufts Dental Outlook*, 18, 30, December, 1944.
3. Shay, D. E., Haddox, J. H., and Richmond, J. L.: An Inorganic Qualitative and Quantitative Analysis of Green Stain, *J. Am. Dent. Assoc.*, 50, 156, February, 1955.
4. Leung, S. W.: Naturally Occurring Stains on the Teeth of Children, *J. Am. Dent. Assoc.*, 41, 191, August, 1950.
5. Meckel, A. H.: The Formation and Properties of Organic Films on Teeth, *Arch. Oral Biol.*, 10, 585, July-August, 1965.
6. Pickerill, H. P.: A Sign of Immunity, *Brit. Dent. J.*, 44, 967, September 1, 1923.
7. Bibby, B. G.: A Study of Pigmented Dental Plaque, *J. Dent. Res.*, 11, 855, December, 1931.
8. Shourie, K. L.: Mesenteric Line or Pigmented Plaque: A Sign of Comparative Freedom from Dental Caries, *J. Am. Dent. Assoc.*, 35, 805, December, 1947.
9. Theilade, J., Slots, J., and Fejerskov, O.: The Ultrastructure of Black Stain on Human Primary Teeth, *Scand. J. Dent. Res.*, 81, 528, No. 7, 1973.
10. Slots, J.: The Microflora of Black Stain on Human Primary Teeth, *Scand. J. Dent. Res.*, 82, 484, No. 7, 1974.
11. Manly, R. S.: A Structureless Recurrent Deposit on Teeth, *J. Dent. Res.*, 22, 479, December, 1943.
12. Robinson, H. B. G.: Lesions of the Teeth: Stains, *Dent. Surv.*, 44, 54, November, 1968.
13. Phillips, R. W., Swartz, M. L., and Norman, R. D.: *Materials for the Practicing Dentist.* St. Louis, Mosby, 1969, pp. 19–20.
14. Sicher, H. and Bhaskar, S. N., eds.: *Orban's Oral Histology and Embryology*, 7th ed. St. Louis, Mosby, 1972, pp. 89–90.
15. Shafer, W. G., Hine, M. K., and Levy, B. M.: *A Textbook of Oral Pathology*, 3rd ed. Philadelphia, Saunders, 1974, pp. 52–57.
16. Dean, H. T.: Investigation of Physiological Effects by Epidemiological Method, in Moulton, F. R., ed.: *Fluorine and Dental Health*. Washington, American Association for the Advancement of Science, No. 19, 1942.
17. American Dental Association, Council on Dental Therapeutics: *Accepted Dental Therapeutics*, 36th ed. Chicago, American Dental Association, 1975, pp. 178–179.
18. Shafer, Hine, and Levy: op. cit., pp. 674.
19. Bottomley, W. K., Cioffi, R. F., and Martin, A. J.: Dental Management of the Patient Treated by Renal Transplantation: Preoperative and Postoperative Considerations, *J. Am. Dent. Assoc.*, 85, 1330, December, 1972.
20. Horowitz, H. S. and Chamberlin, S. R.: Pigmentation of Teeth Following Topical Applications of Stannous Fluoride in a Nonfluoridated Area, *J. Pub. Health Dent.*, 31, 32, Winter, 1971.
21. Muhler, J. C.: Stannous Fluoride Enamel Pigmentation—Evidence of Caries Arrestment, *J. Dent. Child.*, 27, 157, 3rd Quarter, 1960.

Suggested Readings

Burke, S. W.: Oral Physiology and Oral Physiotherapy, in Steele, P. F., ed.: *Dimensions of Dental Hygiene*, 2nd ed. Philadelphia, Lea & Febiger, 1975, pp. 98–102.

Colby, R. A., Kerr, D. A., and Robinson, H. B. G.: *Color Atlas of Oral Pathology*, 3rd ed. Philadelphia, Lippincott, 1971, pp. 53, 59.

Dahl, L. O. and Shumate, J.: The Tetracyclines and Their Side Effects, *J. Am. Dent. Hyg. Assoc.*, 40, 29, 1st Quarter, 1966.

Frankel, M. A.: Tetracycline Antibiotics and Tooth Discoloration, *J. Dent. Child.*, 37, 117, March-April, 1970.

Giansanti, J. S. and Budnick, S. D.: Six Generations of Hereditary Opalescent Dentin: Report of Case, *J. Am. Dent. Assoc.*, 90, 439, February, 1975.

Kerr, D. A. and Ash, M. M.: *Oral Pathology*, 3rd ed. Philadelphia, Lea & Febiger, 1971, pp. 196–200.

Massler, M. and Schour, I.: *Atlas of the Mouth.* Chicago, American Dental Association, Plate 12.

Moffitt, J. M., Cooley, R. O., Olsen, N. H., and Hefferren, J. J.: Prediction of Tetracycline-induced Tooth Discoloration, *J. Am. Dent. Assoc.*, 88, 547, March, 1974.

Muhler, J. C.: Effect on Gingiva and Occurrence of Pigmentation on Teeth following the Topical Application of Stannous Fluoride or Stannous Chlorofluoride, *J. Periodont.*, 28, 281, October, 1957.

Richards, L. F., Westmoreland, W. W., Tashiro, M., and Morrison, J. T.: Nonfluoride Enamel Hypoplasia in Varying Fluoride-Temperature Zones, *J. Am. Dent. Assoc.*, 75, 1412, December, 1967.

Witkop, C. J.: Hereditary Defects of Dentin, *Dent. Clin. North Am.*, 19, 25, January, 1975.

Zadik, D. and Eidelman, E.: Tetracycline-Stained Teeth in Jerusalem Preschool Children, *Comm. Dent. Oral Epidemiol.*, 3, 69, March, 1975.

Chapter 18

Deposit Retention Factors

A variety of factors is responsible for the retention of soft deposits, calculus, and extrinsic stains on the teeth. Some of the retention factors were mentioned in the previous three chapters when the deposits and stains were described. In this chapter a summary is provided to serve as a check list for observation and recording during the patient examination.

Deposit retention contributes to the onset and progression of dental caries and periodontal diseases. Since dental plaque is the prime source of microorganisms involved in the etiology of both dental caries and inflammatory periodontal diseases, the retention of dental plaque is of particular significance. Calculus retention is also important. The significance and influence of calculus were outlined on page 256.

While the materials for the diagnostic work-up are being prepared, and the detailed examinations are being made, observation of predisposing and potentially disease-producing factors must be included. When the treatment plan is outlined, these factors are considered carefully in order that corrective procedures can be included in the total treatment plan.

Retention factors may be etiologic, predisposing, or contributing. These are delineated as follows:

1. *Etiologic Factor:* a factor that is the actual cause of a disease or condition.
2. *Predisposing Factor:* a factor that renders a person susceptible to a disease or condition.
3. *Contributing Factor:* that which lends assistance to, supplements, or adds to a condition or disease.

Etiologic, predisposing, and contributing factors may be local or systemic defined as follows:

1. *Local Factor:* a factor in the immediate environment of the oral cavity, or specifically in the environment of the teeth or periodontium.
2. *Systemic Factor:* a factor which results from the general physical or mental condition of a person.

SELF-CLEANSING MECHANISMS

The teeth by their anatomy, alignment, and occlusion, and the gingiva, tongue, cheeks, and saliva, function in a relationship called the self-cleansing mechanism of the oral cavity. A review of the self-cleansing mechanisms during and following mastication is included for relating the natural processes to the deviating influences.

The steps below are described for food particles, but the same processes apply to many materials which enter into or influence the formation of the deposits. These materials include mineral and organic components of the saliva, microorganisms, and foreign substances introduced into the oral cavity.

I. Food Enters the Mouth

It is carried by the tongue, assisted by the lips and cheeks, to the occlusal surfaces for grinding.

A. Salivary flow increases due to sensory reflex stimulation.
B. Saliva begins lubrication of food and oral tissues.

II. The Teeth Are Brought Together for Chewing

The food moves over the occlusal surfaces.

A. Marginal ridges: tend to force particles toward occlusal, away from proximal region.
B. Contact areas: prevent entrance to interproximal area.

III. Food Is Forced Out by Pressure of Bite

Food passes over the smooth facial and lingual surfaces.

A. Embrasures: provide spillways for the escape of particles.
B. Cervical enamel ridges: deflect particles away from free gingiva onto attached gingiva.
C. Gingival crest: prevents retention of particles by being positioned at a point below the height of contour of the cervical enamel ridge and by its close adherence to the tooth surface.

D. Interdental papilla: fills the interproximal area and prevents particles from entering.

IV. Food Particles Are Brought Back by the Tongue to Occlusal Surfaces for Additional Chewing

Process is repeated until food is ready for swallowing.

A. Salivary flow: continues to be stimulated with repeated masticatory movements.
B. Saliva: moistens food and thus reduces its adhering capacity.

V. Food Particles Remaining on the Teeth Are Removed

A. Tip of tongue: explores and attempts to dislodge remaining particles.
B. Lips and cheeks in conjunction with tongue: aid in natural rinsing process by forcing saliva over and between the teeth.
C. Saliva: continues to flow in increased amounts during rinsing and swallowing of particles, then gradually returns to its normal flow.

ANATOMIC AND PHYSIOLOGIC RETENTION FACTORS

Self-cleansing mechanisms function to a degree in nearly all mouths except when a patient has a paralysis, muscular defect, or other individual handicap. Although debris can be cleared away by self-cleansing, dental plaque adheres firmly to the tooth surface and cannot be removed by self-cleansing.

Retentive areas relate to rough surfaces of teeth and restorations, tooth contour and position, and gingival size, shape and position. Iatrogenic causes, that is, factors created by professionals during patient treatment or neglect of treatment, are significant. Factors of mastication, saliva, the tongue, cheeks, lips, and oral habits contribute as well as external factors such as diet, smoking, and personal plaque control techniques.

The patient's study casts can be especially useful for study of the physical factors. Irregularities, contour, position, malocclusion, and contact areas of the teeth, as well as the features of the gingiva, may be partially or wholly observed. Other factors can be derived from the patient history. Problem areas can be explained to the patient by demonstration with the study casts to assist in obtaining effective application of plaque control measures.

I. Teeth

A. Tooth Surface Irregularities[1]

Pellicle and plaque microorganisms attach to defective or rough surfaces including the following:

1. Pits, grooves, cracks.
2. Calculus.
3. Exposed cementum: diseased, resorbed, and other irregularities.
4. Dental caries and decalcification.
5. Iatrogenic
   a. Rough or grooved surfaces left after scaling.
   b. Inadequately polished dental restorations.

B. Tooth Contour

Altered shape may interfere with self-cleansing mechanisms and make personal care procedures difficult.

1. Congenital abnormalities
   a. Extra or missing cusps.
   b. Bell-shaped crown with prominent buccal and lingual contours tends to provide deeper retentive area in cervical third.
2. Teeth with flattened proximal surfaces have faulty contact with adjacent teeth, permitting deposits to wedge between.
3. Occlusal and incisal surfaces altered by attrition interrupt normal excursion of food during chewing.

4. Areas of erosion and abrasion (figures 13–2 and 13–3, pages 211, 212).
5. Large carious lesions.
6. Large deposits of calculus.

C. Restorations

1. Undercontoured, overcontoured, and restorations with faulty margins.
2. Dental restorations inadequately contoured allow food to enter interproximal area.
   a. Marginal ridge missing.
   b. Contact area: missing, improperly located, or of unnatural width.
3. Dental appliances
   a. Orthodontic appliances.
   b. Fixed partial denture with deficient gingival margin of an abutment tooth or an unusually shaped pontic.
   c. Removable partial denture: inadequately adapted clasps.

D. Position of Teeth

1. Malocclusion. Irregular alignment of single tooth or groups of teeth leave areas conducive to collection of microorganisms for plaque.
   a. Crowded or overlapped.
   b. Rotated.
   c. Deep anterior overbite.
      (1) Mandibular teeth force food particles against maxillary lingual gingiva.
      (2) Lingual inclination of mandibular teeth allows maxillary teeth to force food particles against mandibular labial gingiva.
2. Related to missing or extracted teeth.
   a. Inclined or migrated; contact area usually missing.
   b. Extrusion beyond line of occlusion when tooth in opposing arch is missing or ineffective.

3. Related to eruption.
   a. Incomplete eruption: below line of occlusion.
   b. Partially erupted impacted third molar.
4. Lack of function or use of teeth eliminates or decreases effectiveness of cleansing.
   a. Lack of opposing teeth.
   b. Openbite.
   c. Severe maxillary anterior protrusion.
   d. Severe crossbite with limited lateral excursion of mandible.

II. Gingiva

A. **Deviations from normal position:** provide retentive areas.
   1. Receded, leaving normal depressed area of tooth at cementoenamel junction uncovered.
   2. Extended to height of contour of teeth.
   3. Reduced height of interdental papilla leaves open interdental areas.
   4. Tissue flap over occlusal of erupting tooth.
   5. Periodontal pocket prevents free gingiva from adhering closely which increases retentive capacity of the pocket.
      a. Shape of pocket is conducive to plaque collection.
      b. Submarginal calculus provides rough retentive area.

B. **Deviation in size and contour:** enlarged or cratered gingiva creates retentive area at gingival crest.

C. **Deviation in surface texture:** poor tone and inadequate keratinization make gingiva susceptible to laceration and subsequent bleeding which releases blood elements for deposition on tooth surface.

III. Tongue, Lips, Cheeks

Limitations of normal activity prevent cleansing and rinsing functions.

A. **Congenital Malformations**
   1. Tongue: tonguetie, macroglossia.
   2. Lips: short upper lip, unusually small mouth opening.

B. **Muscle Tone and Elasticity Diminished**

C. **Muscular Coordination**
   1. Undeveloped in young child.
   2. Impaired in patients with a neuromuscular disease.

IV. Saliva

A. **Decreased quantity** limits lubricating and cleansing effects.

B. **Stagnation** of saliva permitted.
   1. Decreased activity of tongue, lips, and cheeks.
   2. Properties and quantity of saliva: thick viscid saliva in smaller amounts stagnates more readily.

V. Mastication

A. Unilateral chewing.
B. Food can be forced into interproximal areas when there are plunger cusps, inadequate contact areas, or irregular marginal ridge relationships.

VI. Mouth Breathing

Dehydration of oral tissues results in insufficient lubrication.

VII. Dietary and Eating Habits

A. **Physical Character of Diet**
   1. Soft, moist foods.
      a. Adhere to tooth surface and encourage plaque formation (page 242).
      b. Not returned readily to occlusal surface for continued chewing during mastication.
   2. Firm, crispy, fibrous foods.

a. Require more chewing, hence stimulate increased flow of saliva.

b. Are effective in mechanical cleansing of middle and incisal or occlusal thirds of crowns but do not remove dental plaque from the cervical third.

B. **Diet Selection**
1. Masticatory deficiencies limit selection of firm abrasive foods.
2. Tasteless, bland foods may fail to stimulate sufficient salivary flow.
3. Sucrose in diet increases amount of plaque and its bacterial content.

VIII. Drugs, Tobacco

A. **Drugs.** Certain drugs alter quantity of saliva.[2]

B. **Tobacco**
1. Increased plaque and calculus.[3,4]
2. Increases salivary flow.
3. Contains tar products which stain teeth.

IX. Personal Oral Care Habits

A. **Neglect**
1. The natural self-cleansing mechanisms are inadequate and must be supplemented by meticulous personal care.
2. Incomplete or inadequate brushing of less accessible areas encourages plaque and debris retention in those areas.

B. **Effects of Faulty Plaque Control Techniques in Creating Retentive Areas**
1. Alteration of position or contour of gingiva.
   a. Receded, possibly from vigorous brushing against free gingiva.
   b. Chronic horizontal or circular brushing may change shape of gingival crest.
2. Vigorous repeated horizontal brushing with an abrasive dentifrice may abrade the tooth structure and create a groove.
3. Incorrect use of toothbrush, interdental stimulator, dental floss, or tape may result in reduction in height of interdental papillae.

X. Individual Characteristics

A. **Awareness of Oral Cleanliness**
1. Self-cleansing efficiency depends in part on the individual's perception of debris by oral sensation (taste and touch).
2. Tongue activity in cleansing decreased with lack of awareness.

B. **Emotional Factors**[5]
1. Changes in salivary flow: fear and anxiety decrease flow.
2. Neglected oral care habits frequently accompany poor mental hygiene.
3. Poor diet selection, including excessive carbohydrates and other soft foods, is characteristic of the emotionally disturbed.

FACTORS TO TEACH THE PATIENT

I. The interrelationship of the natural self-cleansing mechanisms, personal oral care habits, and the professionally administered techniques in preventing deposit retention.
II. Types of foods which aid in debris removal and encourage plaque formation.
III. Information and techniques which will help to develop an awareness of oral cleanliness.
IV. Specific oral care procedures related to the individual's problem of deposit and stain retention.

References

1. Swartz, M. L. and Phillips, R. W.: Comparison of Bacterial Accumulations on Rough and Smooth Enamel Surfaces, *J. Periodont.*, 28, 304, October, 1957.

2. Lyons, D. C.: The Dry Mouth Adverse Reaction Syndrome in the Geriatric Patient, *J. Oral Med.*, 27, 110, October-December, 1972.
3. Kowalski, C. J.: Relationship Between Smoking and Calculus Deposition, *J. Dent. Res.*, 50, 101, January-February, 1971.
4. Sheiham, A.: Periodontal Disease and Oral Cleanliness in Tobacco Smokers, *J. Periodont.*, 42, 259, May, 1971.
5. Grant, D. A., Stern, I. B., and Everett, F. G.: *Orban's Periodontics*, 4th ed. St. Louis, Mosby, 1972, pp. 291–296.

Suggested Readings

Ainamo, J.: Relationship between Malalignment of the Teeth and Periodontal Disease, *Scand. J. Dent. Res.*, 80, 104, No. 2, 1972.
Alexander, A. G.: The Effect of Lack of Function of Teeth on Gingival Health, Plaque and Calculus Accumulation, *J. Periodont.*, 41, 438, August, 1970.
Alexander, A. G., Morganstein, S. I., and Ribbons, J. W.: A Study of the Growth of Plaque and the Efficiency of Self-Cleansing Mechanisms, *Dent. Pract. Dent. Rec.*, 19, 293, May, 1969.
Alexander, A. G. and Tipnis, A. K.: The Effect of Irregularity of Teeth and the Degree of Overbite and Overjet on the Gingival Health, *Brit. Dent. J.*, 128, 539, June 2, 1970.
Allen, D. L., McFall, W. T., and Hunter, G. C.: *Periodontics for the Dental Hygienist*, 2nd ed. Philadelphia, Lea & Febiger, 1974, pp. 60–77.
Buchanan, B. J.: Emotional Stress as an Etiological Factor in Periodontal Disease, *J. Am. Dent. Hyg. Assoc.*, 40, 21, First Quarter, 1966.
Glickman, I.: *Clinical Periodontology*, 4th ed. Philadelphia, Saunders, 1972, pp. 344–361.
Goldman, H. M. and Cohen, D. W.: *Periodontal Therapy*, 5th ed. St. Louis, Mosby, 1973, pp. 197–214.
Kerr, D. A. and Ash, M. M.: *Oral Pathology*, 3rd ed. Philadelphia, Lea & Febiger, 1971, pp. 193–195.
U.S. Department of Health, Education, and Welfare: *Examination and Diagnosis of Periodontal Disease*, DHEW Publication No. (HRA) 74–36. Bethesda, Maryland, 20014, 1974, pp. 58–68.
Wheeler, R. C.: *Dental Anatomy, Physiology and Occlusion*, 5th ed. Philadelphia, Saunders, 1974, pp. 98–133.

Chapter 19

Periodontal and Dental Indices

An index is an expression of clinical observations in numerical values. It is used to describe the status of the individual or group with respect to a condition being measured. By defining the number scale used and standardizing the interpretation of the observations, an index value can have consistency and reduced subjectivity when compared with a word description of a condition.

Indices using various criteria have been developed to compare the relative extent and severity of disease. For example, dental caries is indexed by the number of teeth or surfaces with carious lesions and fillings. An index for dental fluorosis identifies slight, moderate, or severe involvement of the enamel ranging respectively from white spots visible only when a tooth is dry to marked brown stains with pitting. Malocclusion indices define specific degrees of malalignment of teeth from their normal positions.

Various factors associated with disease changes in gingivitis and periodontal diseases have been used in the development of periodontal indices. Measurement criteria in current use include recession, bone loss, pocket formation,

mobility of teeth, gingival inflammation, gingival bleeding as well as plaque, calculus, and the state of oral hygiene.

An index may be used both for individuals and groups. Certain indices which were designed originally for large groups in epidemiological studies may have limited application on an individual basis. In clinical practice, an index may have significant value for patient instruction and motivation.

I. Purposes and Uses

A. For Individual Patients

An index can

1. Provide individual assessment to help a patient recognize an oral problem.
2. Reveal the degree of effectiveness of present oral hygiene practices.
3. Motivate the person in preventive or professional care for the elimination and control of oral disease.
4. Evaluate the success of individual and professional treatment over a period of time by comparing index scores.

B. **In Research**

An index is used to

1. Measure the effectiveness of specific agents for the prevention, control, or treatment of oral conditions.
2. Measure the effectiveness of mechanical devices for personal care, such as toothbrushes, interdental cleaning devices, or water irrigators.

C. **In Community Health**

An index can

1. Show the prevalence and trends of incidence of a particular condition.
2. Provide base-line data to show existing dental health practices and the needs of a community.
3. Compare the effects of a community program and evaluate the results.

II. Characteristics of an Index

A useful and effective index will

A. Be simple to use and calculate.
B. Require minimal equipment.
C. Have clear-cut criteria which are readily understandable.
D. Be as free as possible from subjective interpretation.
E. Be reproducible by the same examiner or different examiners.
F. Be amenable to statistical analysis; have validity and reliability.
G. Not require an excessive amount of time to complete.

GINGIVAL, PERIODONTAL, PLAQUE, AND CALCULUS INDICES

Several indices will be described in this chapter. The ones included have been selected because they are well known and widely used, and because they can be applied on an individual patient basis to describe the status of health. The objective of patient instruction and treatment, including all instrumentation, is the attainment of oral health by the patient; hence a means for evaluation of health status is necessary. Comparison of indices made on a continuing basis can provide practical health evaluation.

The indices to be described in the sections following are:

1. Periodontal Disease Index (PDI) by Ramfjord.[1] This is a group of indices including a Gingivitis Index, Calculus Index, Plaque Index, and the PDI itself, which is based on measurement of crevice or pocket depth related to the cementoenamel junction.
2. Simplified Oral Hygiene Index (OHI-S) by Green and Vermillion.[2] It is composed of a Debris Index and a Calculus Index, both based on tooth surface area covered by debris or calculus respectively and, added together, they make up the OHI-S.
3. Gingival Index (GI) by Löe and Silness.[3] Severity of inflammation is evaluated.
4. Plaque Index (Pl I) by Silness and Löe.[4] The thickness of plaque in the cervical third of each tooth is scored.
5. Patient Hygiene Performance (PHP) by Podshadley and Haley.[5] The tooth surface area covered by oral debris is assessed.

It should be realized that plaque indices can be applied to preventive instruction related to plaque control for dental caries as well as for gingival and periodontal disease. The *Suggested Readings* at the end of the chapter contain references to other indices. Familiarity with the various types may prove helpful when different evaluation criteria are needed.

THE PERIODONTAL DISEASE INDEX (PDI)

I. Purpose: To assess the prevalence and severity of gingivitis and periodontitis of an individual or a group, as shown by the level of the attachment of the junctional epithelium. Four indices are included in this group, namely the Gingivitis Index, Calculus Index, Plaque Index, and the Periodontal Disease Index.[1,6]

II. Selection of Teeth and Surfaces

A. Areas Measured: Six teeth are used to represent the six segments of the dentition.

Maxillary	Mandibular
#3 right first molar	#19 left first molar
#9 left central incisor	#25 right central incisor
#12 left first premolar	#28 right first premolar

B. Only fully erupted teeth are used.
C. Substitutions are not made for missing teeth; scores are derived from the teeth present.

III. Gingivitis Index

The gingiva are assessed by their color, form, consistency (density), and bleeding tendency.

A. **Procedure**
   1. Under consistent standardized light, dry the gingiva with cotton to observe color and form.
   2. Apply gentle pressure with the probe (Michigan #0) to determine consistency (density). When the color change definitely indicates the presence of inflammation, the consistency is not checked.

B. **Criteria**
   0 = Absence of signs of inflammation
   1 = Mild to moderate inflammatory gingival changes, not extending around the tooth
   2 = Mild to moderately severe gingivitis extending all around the tooth
   3 = Severe gingivitis characterized by marked redness, swelling, tendency to bleed and ulceration, not necessarily extending around the tooth

C. **Scoring**
   1. Individual teeth: add the scores for each area and divide by the number of areas examined.
   2. Gingivitis Index: add the scores for all of the examined teeth and divide

by the total number of teeth examined. The Gingivitis Index ranges from 0 to 3.

IV. Calculus Index

Because the calculus may have to be removed to determine the location of the cementoenamel junction for crevice or pocket measurements, calculus may need to be scored first.

A. **Instruments:** a #17 explorer (figure 12–12, page 195) may be used to locate submarginal calculus, although the probe (Michigan #0) used for other determinations may be sufficient for evaluation.

B. **Surface Examined:** each of the four surfaces (buccal, lingual, mesial, and distal) is given a score from 0 to 3.

C. **Criteria**
   0 = No calculus
   1 = Supramarginal calculus extending only slightly below the free gingival margin (not more than 1 mm.).
   2 = Moderate amount of supra- and submarginal calculus, or submarginal calculus only
   3 = Abundance of supra- and submarginal calculus

D. **Scoring**
   1. Individual teeth: add scores for each surface and divide by number of surfaces examined.
   2. Calculus Index for the patient: add the scores for the individual teeth and divide by the number of teeth. The Calculus Index ranges from 0 to 3.

V. Crevice (Sulcus) Depth

The crevice or sulcus depth is measured as it relates to the cementoenamel junction.

A. **Instrument:** Michigan probe #0 (figure 12–1, page 187).

B. **Locations of Measurements**
   1. Two measurements. When two measurements are made, they are at

the middle of the buccal, and at the buccal aspect of the mesial contact area with the side of the probe held touching both teeth.

2. Original PDI. Four measurements were made for each tooth, on the buccal, mesial, distal, and lingual.[1] It was later found that no significant loss in accuracy resulted from using only two measurements. The four measurements are still made for certain types of research evaluations.

C. **Measurements**
1. Measure the distance to the cementoenamel junction from the gingival margin.
   a. Scale to remove calculus when deposits interfere with detecting the location of the cementoenamel junction.
   b. Determine the location of the cementoenamel junction
      (1) By the difference in inclination of the enamel and cementum as detected by the change in direction of the probe as it is moved apically.
      (2) By the change in surface texture from the smooth enamel surface to the rougher cemental surface.
2. Measure from the gingival margin to the bottom of the crevice or pocket.
3. Subtract the distance (mm.) to the cementoenamel junction from the distance (mm.) to the bottom of the crevice or pocket.
4. Variations
   a. Junctional epithelium on the enamel: when the cementoenamel junction cannot be felt because it is not exposed, record the depth of the gingival crevice.
   b. Gingival margin on the cementum
      (1) Record the distance from the cementoenamel junction to the gingival margin as a negative score.
      (2) Record from the cementoenamel junction to the bottom of the crevice to determine loss of attachment.

D. **PDI Computation**
1. Individual teeth

0 to 3 = When the gingival crevice or pocket in none of the measured areas extends apical to the cementoenamel junction.

(Gingivitis Index)

4 = When the pockets of any two (or four) recorded areas extend apically to the cementoenamel junction not more than, but including, 3 mm. (The gingivitis score is then disregarded.)

5 = When the pocket of any of the two (or four) recorded areas extend apically to the cementoenamel junction from 3 mm. to and including, 6 mm. (The gingivitis score is disregarded.)

6 = When the pockets are more than 6 mm. apically to the cementoenamel junction in any of the two (or four) measured areas (The gingivitis score is disregarded.)

2. Total PDI
   a. Add scores for individual teeth and divide by the number of scored teeth.
   b. The PDI will range from 0 to 6. Numbers through 3 indicate gingival involvement only; numbers 4 through 6 mean there is periodontal involvement.

VI. **Dental Plaque Index**
A. **Procedure**
1. Apply Bismarck Brown disclosing agent using two saturated pellets, one for the maxillary and one for the mandibular. Bismarck Brown disclosing agent is described on page 383.
2. Patient is asked to expectorate, then rinse twice with water.
3. Direct vision or indirect with

mouth mirror is used for observing the specified surfaces.

B. **Criteria**

0 = No plaque present.

1 = Plaque present on some but not all interproximal buccal and lingual surfaces of the tooth.

2 = Plaque present on all interproximal, buccal and lingual surfaces, but covering less than one-half of these surfaces.

3 = Plaque extending over all interproximal, buccal and lingual surfaces, and covering more than one-half of these surfaces.

C. **Scoring:** Add plaque scores for each tooth and divide by the number of teeth examined. The Plaque Index ranges from 0 to 3.

SIMPLIFIED ORAL HYGIENE INDEX (OHI-S)

I. Purpose: to classify oral hygiene status by evaluation of the extent of debris and calculus on representative tooth surfaces.[2,7]

II. Selection of Teeth and Surfaces

A. Posterior. The first fully erupted tooth distal to each second premolar is examined. Buccal surfaces of the two maxillary molars and lingual surfaces of the mandibular are used. Although usually a first molar, it may be a second or third.

B. Anterior. The labial surfaces of the maxillary right and the mandibular left central incisor are scored. When either is missing, the opposite central incisor is used.

C. A tooth is considered fully erupted when it has reached the occlusal plane.

D. Examination includes the proximal surfaces to the contact area, and therefore the score is considered to represent half the circumference of each tooth examined.

III. Simplified Debris Index (DI-S)

A. **Definition of Oral Debris.** Oral debris is the soft foreign matter loosely attached to the teeth. It consists of mucin, bacteria, and food, and varies in color from grayish-white to green or orange.

B. **Examination.** The surface area covered by debris is estimated by running the side of a Number 5 explorer (or a Number 23, figure 12–12, page 195) along the tooth surface. The occlusal or incisal extent of the debris is noted as it is removed.

C. **Criteria**

0 = No debris or stain present.

1 = Soft debris covering not more than one-third of the tooth surface being examined or the presence of extrinsic stains without debris regardless of surface area covered.

2 = Soft debris covering more than one-third but not more than two-thirds of the exposed tooth surface.

3 = Soft debris covering more than two-thirds of the exposed tooth surface.

D. **Scoring**

1. At least two of the six possible surfaces must have been examined for an individual score to be calculated.

2. Simplified Debris Index (DI-S): Add the scores for the individual teeth together and divide by the number of teeth examined.

3. The DI-S ranges from 0 to 3.

IV. Simplified Calculus Index (CI-S)

A. **Examination.** An explorer is used similarly to the procedure for the DI-S previously described. The surface area covered by calculus is detected supramarginally, and submarginal calculus is explored.

B. **Criteria**

0 = No calculus present.

1 = Supramarginal calculus covering not more than one-third of the exposed tooth surface being examined.

2 = Supramarginal calculus covering more than one-third but not more than two-thirds of the exposed tooth surface, or the presence of individual flecks of submarginal calculus around the cervical portion of the tooth.

3 = Supramarginal calculus covering more than two-thirds of the exposed tooth surface or a continuous heavy band of submarginal calculus around the cervical portion of the tooth.

C. **Scoring**
1. At least two of the six possible surfaces must have been examined for an individual score to be calculated.
2. Simplified Calculus Index (CI-S): Add the scores for the individual teeth and divide by the number of teeth examined.
3. The CI-S ranges from 0 to 3.

V. Simplified Oral Hygiene Index (OHI-S)

Add together the DI-S and the CI-S. The OHI-S value ranges from 0 to 6.

VI. Comparison of OHI and OHI-S

Originally the OHI (Oral Hygiene Index) was developed.[8] After experience with the Oral Hygiene Index, the need for simplification was recognized because of the length of time required to arrive at an evaluation of the debris and calculus, as well as the need for subjective decisions for tooth selection. The basic differences between the OHI and the OHI-S are as follows:

A. **Number of Surfaces Evaluated.** In the OHI there were 12 surfaces, both lingual and facial, whereas only six are used in the OHI-S.

B. **Tooth Selection.** In the OHI the examiner had to select the tooth with the most debris or calculus in the segment. The lingual surface selected did not have to be of the same tooth as the buccal surface.

C. **Scoring.** The OHI had a possible range from 0 to 12, whereas the OHI-S may range from 0 to 6.

GINGIVAL INDEX (GI)

I. **Purpose:** To assess the gingival condition to distinguish clearly between the severity of the inflammatory lesion and the location related to the marginal gingiva completely around each tooth.[3,9]

II. **Selection of Areas for Examination**

A. **Areas Examined.** Four gingival areas (distal, buccal, mesial, lingual) are examined systematically for each tooth.

B. **Modified Procedure:** omit the distal examination for each tooth. Scoring is also modified so that the score for the mesial is doubled and the total score for each tooth is divided by 4.

III. **Procedure**

A. The teeth and gingiva are dried and, under adequate light, a mouth mirror and probe are used.

B. The probe is used to press on the gingiva to determine the degree of firmness.

C. The probe is used to run along the soft tissue wall near the entrance to the gingival sulcus to evaluate bleeding (figure 19–1).

IV. **Criteria**

0 = Normal gingiva.
1 = Mild inflammation—slight change in color, slight edema. *No bleeding on probing.*
2 = Moderate inflammation—redness, edema and glazing. *Bleeding on probing.*
3 = Severe inflammation—marked redness and edema. Ulceration. *Tendency to spontaneous bleeding.*

V. **Scoring**

A. **GI for Area.** Each of the four gingival areas (distal, buccal, mesial, lingual) is given a score of 0 to 3.

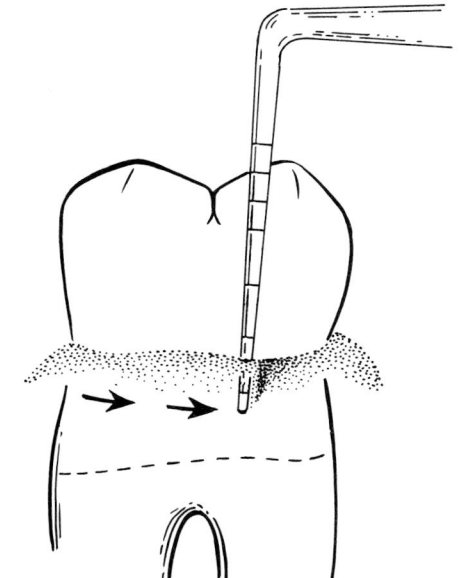

Figure 19–1. Probe stroke for bleeding evaluation. A part of the Gingival Index (GI) is to evaluate bleeding. The broken line represents the junctional epithelium at the bottom of the pocket. Insert the probe a few millimeters and move it along the soft tissue wall with slight pressure in a circumferential direction. The probe stroke for this purpose is in contrast to the walking stroke used for pocket measurement and described on page 191.

B. **GI for a Tooth.** Scores for each area are totalled and divided by four.

C. **GI for Groups of Teeth.** Scores for individual teeth may be grouped and totalled, and divided by the number of teeth. A Gingival Index may be determined for specific teeth, group of teeth, quadrant, or side of the mouth.

D. **GI for the Individual.** By totalling scores for all teeth and dividing by the number of teeth examined, the Gingival Index is determined. Indices range from 0 to 3.

PLAQUE INDEX (PL I)

I. **Purpose:** to distinguish clearly between the severity (quantity) and the location of the soft debris collections. This index was designed to match the Gingival Index (GI).[4,9]

II. Selection of Areas for Examination

A. Four gingival areas (distal, buccal, mesial, lingual) are examined systematically for each tooth.

B. Only plaque of the cervical third is evaluated with no attention to plaque which has extended to the middle or incisal thirds.

III. Instrumentation

A. The tooth is dried and examined visually for scores of 2 or 3 (see Criteria below).

B. When no plaque is visible, an explorer is used to test the surface. The explorer is passed across the tooth surface in the cervical third and near the entrance to the sulcus. When no plaque adheres to the point of the explorer, the area is considered to have a 0 score. When plaque adheres, a score of 1 is assigned.

C. Plaque, which is on the surface of calculus deposits and on dental restorations of all types in the cervical third, is evaluated and included.

D. Modified Procedures
   1. Examine only the buccal, mesial, and lingual. Assign double score to the proximal surface score, and divide the total by 4.
   2. Use a disclosing agent to assist evaluation for the 0 to 1 scores.[9]

IV. Criteria

0 = No plaque.
1 = A film of plaque adhering to the free gingival margin and adjacent area of the tooth. The plaque may be seen *in situ* only after application of disclosing solution or by using the probe on the tooth surface.
2 = Moderate accumulation of soft deposits within the gingival pocket, or on the tooth and gingival margin which can be seen with the naked eye.
3 = Abundance of soft matter within the gingival pocket and/or on the tooth and gingival margin.

V. Scoring

A. **Pl I for Area.** Each area (mesial, distal, buccal, lingual) is assigned a score from 0 to 3.

B. **Pl I for a Tooth.** Scores for each area are totalled and divided by 4.

C. **Pl I for Groups of Teeth.** Scores for individual teeth may be grouped and totalled and divided by the number of teeth. For instance a Plaque Index may be determined for specific teeth or groups of teeth. The right side may be compared with the left.

D. **Pl I for the Individual.** Add the indices for each of the teeth and divide by the number of teeth examined. The Pl I ranges from 0 to 3.

PATIENT HYGIENE PERFORMANCE (PHP)

I. Purpose. To assess location of oral debris. Debris is defined for the PHP as the soft foreign material, consisting of mucin, bacteria, and food, that is loosely attached to tooth surfaces.[5]

II. Selection of Teeth and Surfaces

A. **Teeth Examined**

Maxillary	*Mandibular*
#3 Right first molar	#19 Left first molar
#8 Right central incisor	#24 Left central incisor
#14 Left first molar	#30 Right first molar

B. **Substitutions.** When a first molar i missing or broken down, the secon molar is used, or the third when th second is missing; the adjacent centra incisor is used for a missing incisor.

C. **Surfaces.** Buccal of maxillary molar: lingual of mandibular molars, an facial of incisors are examined.

III. Procedure

A. Patient is given an erythrosin disclos ing wafer to chew and swish for 3(seconds. He may expectorate but no rinse.

B. Examination is made using a mouth mirror.

C. Each tooth surface to be evaluated i subdivided (mentally) into five sec tions (figure 19–2A) as follows:
   1. Vertically: three divisions, mesia middle, and distal.
   2. Horizontally: the middle third i subdivided into gingival, middle and occlusal or incisal thirds.

IV. Scoring

A. **Debris Score for Each Subdivision** Each of the five subdivisions is scorec for the presence of stained debris a follows:
   0 = No debris (or questionable).
   1 = Debris definitely present.
   Identify by M when all three molars or both incisors are missing.
   Identify by S when a substitute tooth i used.

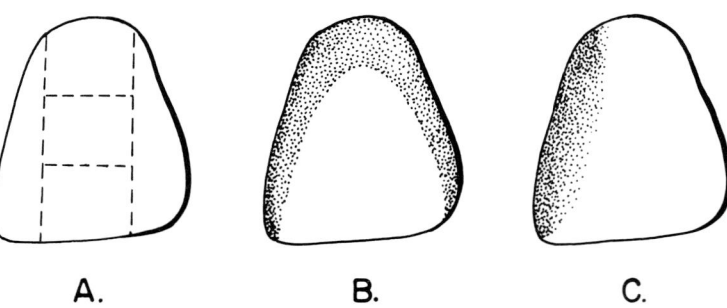

A.   **B.**   **C.**

Figure 19–2. Patient Hygiene Performance (PHP). **A.** To assess oral debris, a tooth is divided into fiv subdivisions each of which is scored one (1) if debris is shown to be present after use of a disclosing agen **B.** Example of Debris Score of 3. Shaded portion represents debris stained by disclosing agen **C.** Example of Debris Score of 1. (Podshadley and Haley, Public Health Reports, 83, 259, 1968.)

B. **Debris Score for Individual Tooth:** Add the scores for each of the five subdivisions. The scores range from 0 to 5.

C. **PHP for the Individual:** Total the scores for the individual teeth and divide by the number of teeth examined. The PHP ranges from 0 to 5.

DENTAL CARIES INDICES

I. DMFT: Decayed, Missing, Filled Teeth

A. **Purpose:** to determine total caries experience, past and present, in the permanent teeth.

B. **Procedures**
1. Standardize techniques
   When a large group is being surveyed by more than one examiner, coordination of procedures for the identification of carious lesions, particularly pits and fissures, is necessary. This can be accomplished by having all of the examiners examine a sample group of people independently. Their chartings are then compared, differences discussed, and specific criteria established.
2. Inspection. Each tooth is examined with mouth mirror and explorer under adequate light.

C. **Recordings**
1. Form for recording. For group surveys a dental inspection form should be used for efficient and convenient calculations. For individuals, the rates can be calculated directly from a dental chart.
2. Missing teeth (M) are usually divided into Me (already extracted) and Mi (indicated for extraction because of extensive breakdown). Unerupted teeth are not missing.
3. Teeth extracted for orthodontic purposes should be identified but

not counted as missing in the DMF. Identification is made by questioning the patient.
4. Only restorable teeth should be counted as the D component.
5. Each tooth is counted only once. The DMF is based on a possible total of 32 teeth. When both dental caries and a restoration appear in the same tooth, only the caries is recorded.

D. **Calculations**
1. Individual DMFT
   a. Total each component separately
   b. Total $D + M + F = DMF$

   Example:
   (1) $D = 3$, $M = 2$, $F = 5$.
   $DMF = 3 + 2 + 5 = 10$
   (2) A DMF of 10 may have different derivations. A person who had regular dental care may have a distribution : $D = 0$, $M = 0$, $F = 10$.

2. Group Average
   a. Total the DMFs for each individual examined.
   b. Divide the total DMFs by the number of individuals in the group.

   Example:
   30 people with a total DMF of 210.
   $\frac{210}{30} = 7.0$ average DMF for the group.

3. Specific Calculations
   a. Treatment needs of a group. To calculate the percent of DMF teeth needing restorations, divide the total D component by the total DMFT.

   Example: $D = 175$, $M = 55$, $F = 18$.
   Total DMFT = 248
   $\frac{D}{DMF} = \frac{175}{248} = .70$ or 70% of the teeth need restorations.

   b. Tooth mortality in a group of 20 people.

(1) To calculate the percent of DMF teeth lost by extraction, divide the total M component by the total DMFT.

Example: D = 175, M = 55, F = 18. Total DMFT = 248

$$\frac{M}{DMF} = \frac{55}{248} = .22 \text{ or } 22\% \text{ of the DMF}$$

teeth are accounted for by extraction.

(2) To calculate the percent of *all* teeth lost by extraction because of dental caries. Twenty people have $32 \times 20 = 640$ permanent teeth.

$$\frac{M}{\text{total teeth}} = \frac{55}{640} = .08 \text{ or } 8\% \text{ of all of}$$

their teeth lost because of dental caries.

c. The same type of calculation can be used to determine the percent of filled teeth.

II. DMFS: *Decayed, Missing, Filled Surfaces*

The DMFS is recorded and calculated in the same manner as the DMFT except that surfaces are counted instead of one score for each tooth.

III. deft AND defs

For primary teeth, lower case letters are used to designate the index *deft* (*d*ecayed, *e*xtracted, *f*illed *t*eeth) and the index *defs* (*d*ecayed, *e*xtracted, *f*illed *s*urfaces).

As with the DMF, the *e* component is scored to include teeth indicated for extraction or have been extracted due to breakdown from dental caries. Naturally exfoliated missing teeth are not recorded in the deft or defs.

IV. Mixed Dentition.

DMF and def are never added together. Each child is given a separate DMF and separate def.

TECHNICAL HINTS

I. Permit the patient to graph or chart the plaque or gingival index used

and correlate the numerical values with the oral findings which may be seen.

II. Keep a continuing record, graph, or chart for index recording in the patient's permanent file for observation and review at each recall appointment.

FACTORS TO TEACH THE PATIENT

I. How an index is used and calculated and what the scores mean.

II. Correlation of index scores with current oral health practices and procedures.

III. Procedures to follow to improve index scores and bring the oral tissues to health.

References

1. Ramfjord, S. P.: Indices for Prevalence and Incidence of Periodontal Disease, *J. Periodont.*, 30, 51, January, 1959.
2. Greene, J. C. and Vermillion, J. R.: The Simplified Oral Hygiene Index, *J. Am. Dent. Assoc.*, 68, 7, January, 1964.
3. Löe, H. and Silness, J.: Periodontal Disease in Pregnancy. I. Prevalence and Severity, *Acta Odont. Scand.*, 21, 533, No. 6, 1963.
4. Silness, J. and Löe, H.: Periodontal Disease in Pregnancy. II. Correlation between Oral Hygiene and Periodontal Condition, *Acta Odont. Scand.*, 22, 121, No. 1, 1964.
5. Podshadley, A. G. and Haley, J. V.: A Method for Evaluating Oral Hygiene Performance, *Pub. Health Repts.*, 83, 259, March, 1968.
6. Ramfjord, S. P.: The Periodontal Disease Index (PDI), *J. Periodont.*, 38, 602, November-December, 1967, (Part II).
7. Greene, J. C.: The Oral Hygiene Index—Development and Uses, *J. Periodont.*, 38, 625, November-December, 1967, (Part II).
8. Greene, J. C. and Vermillion, J. R.: Oral Hygiene Index: A Method for Classifying Oral Hygiene Status, *J. Am. Dent. Assoc.*, 61, 172, August, 1960.
9. Löe, H.: The Gingival Index, the Plaque Index and the Retention Index Systems, *J. Periodont.*, 38, 610, November-December, 1967, (Part II).

Suggested Readings
Other Indices

Björby, A. and Löe, H.: The Relative Significance of Different Local Factors in the Initiation and Development of Periodontal Inflammation, Scand. Symp. Periodontology, 1966. Abstr. No. 20, *J. Periodont. Res.*, 2, 76, No. 1, 1967.

Carter, H. G. and Barnes, G. P.: The Gingival Bleeding Index, *J. Periodont.*, 45, 801, November, 1974.

Dunning, J. M. and Leach, L. B.: Gingival-Bone Count: A Method for Epidemiological Study of Periodontal Disease, *J. Dent. Res.*, 39, 506, May-June, 1960.

Elliott, J. R., Bowers, G. M., Clemmer, B. A., and Rovelstad, G. H.: III. Evaluation of an Oral Physiotherapy Center in the Reduction of Bacterial Plaque and Periodontal Disease, *J. Periodont.*, 43, 221, April, 1972.

Ennever, J., Sturzenberger, O. P., and Radike, A. W.: The Calculus Surface Index Method for Scoring Clinical Calculus Studies, *J. Periodont.*, 32, 54, January, 1961.

Grossman, F. D. and Fedi, P. F.: Navy Periodontal Screening Examination, *J. Am. Soc. Prev. Dent.*, 3, 41, November-December, 1973.

Ingervall, B. and Rönnerman, A.: Index for Need of Orthodontic Treatment, *Odontol. Revy*, 26, 59, No. 1, 1975.

Massler, M.: The P-M-A Index for the Assessment of Gingivitis, *J. Periodont.*, 38, 592, November-December, 1967, (Part II).

Mühlemann, H. R. and Son, S.: Gingival Sulcus Bleeding—a Leading Symptom in Initial Gingivitis, *Helv. Odontol. Acta*, 15, 107, October, 1971.

O'Leary, T.: The Periodontal Screening Examination, *J. Periodont.*, 38, 617, November-December, 1967, (Part II).

Quigley, G. A. and Hein, J. W.: Comparative Cleansing Efficiency of Manual and Power Brushing, *J. Am. Dent. Assoc.*, 65, 26, July, 1962.

Russell, A. L.: A System of Classification and Scoring for Prevalence Surveys of Periodontal Disease, *J. Dent. Res.*, 35, 350, June, 1956.

Russell, A. L.: The Periodontal Index, *J. Periodont.*, 38, 585, November-December, 1967, (Part II).

Sandler, H. C. and Stahl, S. S.: Measurement of Periodontal Disease Prevalence, *J. Am. Dent. Assoc.*, 58, 93, March, 1959.

Shick, R. A. and Ash, M. M.: Evaluation of the Vertical Method of Toothbrushing, *J. Periodont.*, 32, 346, October, 1961.

Stahl, S. S. and Morris, A. L.: Oral Health Conditions Among Army Personnel at the Army Engineering Center, *J. Periodont.*, 26, 180, July, 1955.

Volpe, A. R., Manhold, J. H., and Hazen, S. P.: *In Vivo* Calculus Assessment: Part I. A Method and Its Examiner Reproducibility, *J. Periodont.*, 36, 292, July-August, 1965.

Uses and Applications

Alexander, A. G.: Indices for Measuring Periodontal Disease, *Dent. Health*, 9, 30, April-June, 1970.

Alexander, A. G.: Indices Used for Measuring Plaque, Calculus and Other Potential Gingival Irritants, *Dent. Health*, 10, 34, Summer, 1971.

Barnes G. P., Carter, H. G., and Fletcher, T. V.: Distribution of Bacterial Plaque by Tooth Surfaces, *J. Am. Soc. Prev. Dent.*, 2, 21, November-December, 1972.

Barrickman, R. W. and Penhall, O. J.: Graphing Indexes Reduces Plaque, *J. Am. Dent. Assoc.*, 87, 1404, December, 1973.

Chambers, D. W. and Allen, D. L.: Computer Analysis of Oral Hygiene Habits, *J. Periodont.*, 44, 505, August, 1973.

Davies, G. N.: The Different Requirements of Periodontal Indices for Prevalence Studies and Clinical Trials, *Int. Dent. J.*, 18, 560, September, 1968.

Dunning, J. M.: *Principles of Dental Public Health*, 2nd ed. Cambridge, Harvard University Press, 1970, pp. 301–307.

Fischman, S. L. and Picozzi, A.: Review of the Literature: The Methodology of Clinical Calculus Evaluation, *J. Periodont.*, 40, 607, October, 1969.

Friedman, L. A., Evans, R. I., Paver, R. C., Bridges, J. T., and Burdine, J. T.: Bacterial Plaque Disclosure Survey, *J. Periodont.*, 45, 439, June, 1974.

Garnick, J. J.: Use of Indexes for Plaque Control, *J. Am. Dent. Assoc.*, 86, 1325, June, 1973.

Lenox, J. A. and Kopczyk, R. A.: A Clinical System for Scoring a Patient's Oral Hygiene Performance, *J. Am. Dent. Assoc.*, 86, 849, April, 1973.

Mandel, I. D.: Indices for Measurement of Soft Accumulations in Clinical Studies of Oral Hygiene and Periodontal Disease, *J. Periodont. Res.*, 9, 7, Suppl. 14, 1974.

Martens, L. V. and Meskin, L. H.: An Innovative Technique for Assessing Oral Hygiene, *J. Dent. Child.*, 39, 12, January-February, 1972.

O'Leary, T. J., Drake, R. B., and Naylor, J. E.: The Plaque Control Record, *J. Periodont.*, 43, 38, January, 1972.

Orban, J. E., Stallard, R. E., and Bandt, C. L.: An Evaluation of Indexes for Periodontal Health, *J. Am. Dent. Assoc.*, 81, 683, September, 1970.

Ramfjord, S. P., Emslie, R. D., Greene, J. C., Held, A.-J., and Waerhaug, J.: Epidemiological Studies of Periodontal Diseases, *Amer. J. Public Health*, 58, 1713, September, 1968.

Ship, I. I., Cohen, D. W., and Laster, L.: A Study of Gingival, Periodontal, and Oral Hygiene Examination Methods in a Single Population, *J. Periodont.*, 38, 638, November-December, 1967, (Part II).

Waggener, E. W.: Community Dentistry, in Steele, P. F., ed.: *Dimensions of Dental Hygiene*, 2nd ed. Philadelphia, Lea & Febiger, 1975, pp. 1–24.

Young, W. O. and Striffler, D. F.: *The Dentist, His Practice, and His Community*, 2nd ed. Philadelphia, Saunders, 1969, pp. 43–56.

Chapter 20

Records and Charting

Complete and accurate examinations with proper documentation by records and chartings are basic to all patient care. All findings of the diagnostic work-up are recorded. Some systems of recording involve the completion of forms with topics and spaces to check or fill in the information, while others call for a prose-style summary.

Radiographs, study casts, photographs, and all other materials collected during the initial examination and during the continuing patient appointments, are official parts of the permanent records. A filing system which makes these records readily accessible is needed.

I. Purposes for Charting

The purpose of each type of charting is defined by its title: the dental charting includes diagrammatic representation of existing conditions of the teeth, whereas the periodontal charting indicates clinical features of the periodontium. Separate types of chart forms may be used to record the special features of each, or the two may be combined on one chart. Neatness in the marking of symbols, drawings, and labels goes hand in hand with the accuracy of the inspection itself.

A sense of responsibility to the patient and an earnest desire to be of the greatest possible assistance to the dentist are prerequisite. The dental hygienist does not diagnose: when the charting is prepared, a picture or diagram of observations made during the inspection is recorded. The charting would not be described specifically to a patient unless the dentist instructed the dental hygienist to present certain aspects of the diagnosis and treatment plan to the patient.

An accurate, detailed, and carefully recorded charting is used as follows:

A. **For Treatment Planning.** The charting is a graphic representation of the existing condition of the patient's teeth and periodontium from which needed dental procedures can be organized into a treatment plan.

B. **For Treatment.** During dental and dental hygiene appointments, the charting is useful for guiding specific techniques.

C. **For Evaluation.** Comparison can be made of existing conditions with future examinations and charting in order to evaluate the outcome of treatment.

D. **For Protection.** In the event of misunderstanding by a patient or if legal questions should arise, the records and chartings are realistic evidence.

E. **For Identification.** In the event of emergency, accident, or disaster, a patient may be identified by the teeth for which a record has been maintained.

II. Materials for Charting

A. **Instruments**
   1. Probe.
   2. Sharp explorers.
   3. Mouth mirror: clear and unscratched.
   4. Dental floss.
   5. Gauze sponges.
   6. Airtip and saliva ejector.
   7. Topical anesthetic if probing proves discomforting to the patient.

B. **Study Casts**

C. **Radiographs**
   1. Advanced preparation: to facilitate coordination between clinical and radiographic inspections, the completely processed and dried radiographs provide greater assurance of a thorough analysis.
   2. Bite-wing survey may be sufficient for the charting of dental caries, but a periapical survey is essential for periodontal evaluation.

D. **Chart Form**
   There are many variations of chart forms in current use, some available commercially, some designed by the dentist to meet his particular needs. Specifications for an adequate form include ample space to chart neatly, accurately, and completely; to label as needed for clarity; and to record in a manner that will be interpretable by all who use it.
   1. Types of forms:
      a. Anatomic tooth drawings of the complete teeth: such a chart form lends itself to combine dental and periodontal charting. Figure 20–2 is an example of this type of chart form (page 290).
      b. Anatomic with the crowns of teeth only: difficult to chart adequately the periodontal findings; designed primarily for charting dental caries.
      c. Geometric: a diagrammatic representation for each tooth with space for each surface: generally does not include the roots. Description: two circles, the inner circle representing the occlusal surface and the outer circle divided into four parts to represent the mesial, facial, distal, and lingual (figure 20–1).

E. **Marking Pencils**
   1. Pens and pencils of various colors in keeping with the system of charting selected by the dentist are needed.
   2. Sanitization. Sanitize pencils or pens to be used by rubbing vigorously with gauze sponge moistened in a chemical disinfectant.[1]
   3. Instrument arrangement. Particular care must be exercised when charting without an assistant to keep sterile dental instruments apart from materials which cannot be sterilized. Transmission of oral microorganisms to chart form, pencils, eraser, or radiographs presents a real problem in the maintenance of a clinically clean environment.

III. Clinical Procedures

A. **Patient Position.** Position for optimum visibility of and accessibility to the field of operation.

B. **Illumination.** Maximum illumination is important. Use direct or indirect (mirror) light or transillumination.

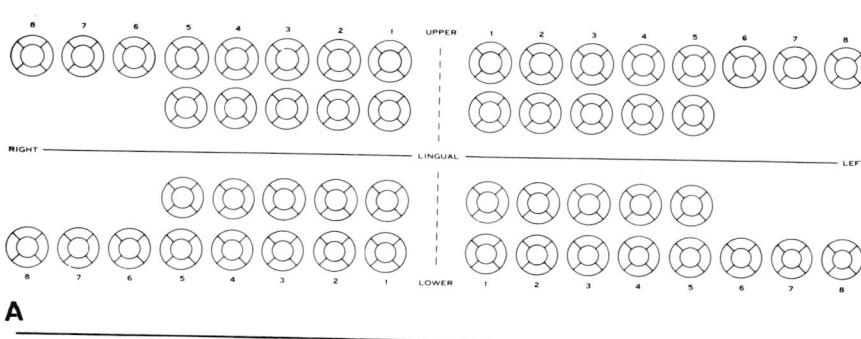

A

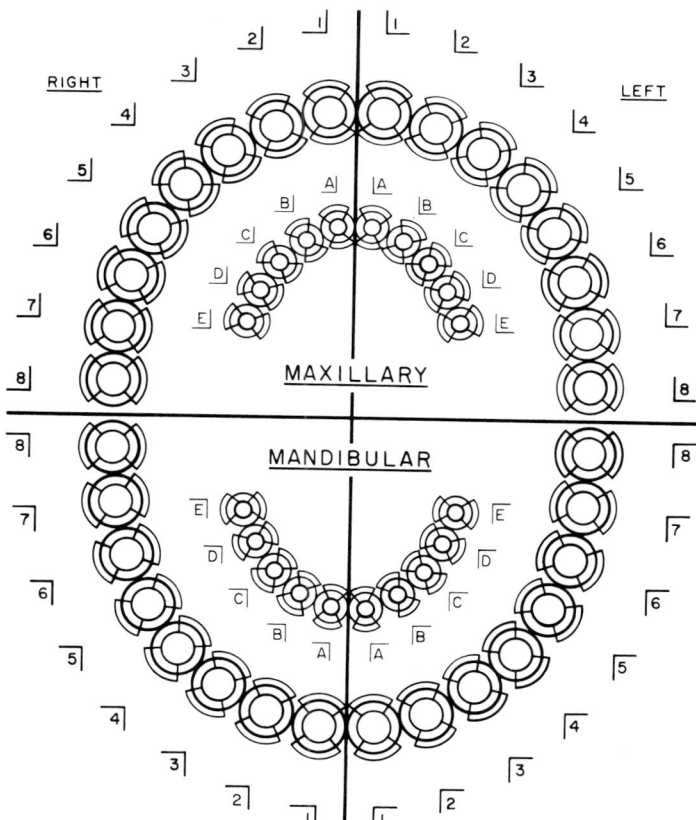

B

Figure 20–1. Geometric or graphic forms for charting. Type **A.** Linear format with primary teeth between permanent teeth. Type **B.** Permanent teeth in arch form with primary teeth inside. Teeth are numbered by Quadrant Numbers 1 through 8 (page 62).

C. **Sequence for Charting**

The use of a set routine is a prerequisite to accomplishing a complete and accurate charting. This is true not only for the tooth surface-to-surface pattern, but also for the parts of the charting itself.

It is suggested that to chart all of one kind of item for the entire mouth, rather than completely charting one tooth, helps in obtaining accuracy since only one train of thought is required at a time. For example, in the dental charting, record all of the restorations and then start again at the first tooth inspected and chart all of the deviations from normal rather than chart all restorations and deviations for each tooth separately.

PERIODONTAL RECORDS AND CHARTING

The patient's permanent records include the itemized findings of all the clinical and radiographic examinations. Material for the periodontal charting has been described on pages 193–195. Entries should be clear and easily understood by all who will read them and use them in continuing treatment.

Additions to the records are made to show the progress of treatment and comparative observations throughout the series of treatment appointments. After the mouth has been brought to a state of health which the patient can maintain, a recall plan is outlined. At each recall appointment, new and comparative records and chartings are made.

Basic periodontal recordings are listed here. Frequently the dentist prefers to do parts of the examination and assign other parts to the dental hygienist.

I. Clinical Observations of the Gingiva

A. Describe changes in color, size, position, shape, consistency, and surface texture; extent of bleeding when

probed, and areas where exudate may be pressed from the pockets (page 175 and table 11–1, page 173).

B. Describe distribution: localized or generalized, and specify the areas of severest involvement. Use tooth numbers to identify adjacent gingival tissue. Tooth numbering systems are described on pages 60–62.

C. Describe degree of severity: slight, moderate, severe.

II. Items to be Charted (pages 194–195)

A. Gingival Line and Mucogingival Lines.
B. Pocket Measurements.
C. Areas of Suspected Mucogingival Involvement.
D. Furcation Involvement.
E. Abnormal Frenal Attachments.
F. Mobility of Teeth.

III. Deposits

A. **Stains**
  1. Extrinsic: record type of stain, color, distribution, specific location by tooth number, whether slight, moderate, severe.
  2. Intrinsic: record separately from extrinsic and identify by type when known.

B. **Calculus:** record distribution and amount of supramarginal and submarginal calculus separately for treatment planning purposes.

C. **Soft Deposits**
  1. Materia alba and food debris: distribution and amount. Record location by teeth when the plaque control instruction will require special area emphasis.
  2. Dental plaque
    a. Record direct observations with or without disclosing agent: distribution and degree or amount.
    b. Plaque index recorded.

IV. Factors Related to Occlusion

Clinical signs of trauma from occlusion were described on page 230. The following list is for consideration with other records for the treatment planning.

A. **Mobility of Teeth:** record degree for each tooth (page 201). In figure 20–2, an example of a method for recording mobility is shown. The small box associated with each root apex and tooth number is to record mobility.

B. **Fremitus (page 230 footnote)**

C. **Possible Food Impaction Areas**
   1. Inquire of patient where fibrous foods usually catch between the teeth.
   2. Use dental floss to identify inadequate contact areas which may contribute to food impaction. An example of one method for recording an open contact is shown by the vertical parallel lines between teeth numbered 21 and 22 in figure 20–2.

D. **Occlusion-related Habits**
   1. Observe for evidence of, and question patient concerning, bruxism, clenching, or other oral habits.
   2. Note wear patterns and facets on study cast.
   3. Note attrition.

E. **Tooth Migration (page 229).**

F. **Sensitivity to Percussion (page 59).**

G. **Radiographic Evidences:** related to trauma from occlusion (page 231).

V. Radiographic Findings

Specific notes should be made to correlate the radiographic findings with the clinical observations listed above. The detailed description of radiographic findings in periodontal disease were described on pages 202–205. The following should be noted in particular:

A. **Bone Level:** height as related to the cementoenamel junction.

B. **Shape of Remaining Bone:** horizontal, angular.

C. **Crestal Lamina Dura:** intact, broken, or missing.

D. **Furcation Involvement**

E. **Periodontal Ligament Space:** thickening.

F. **Overhanging Fillings and Large Carious Lesions Which Are Retention Factors in Deposit Retention.**

DENTAL RECORDS AND CHARTING

The patient's permanent records include the itemized findings of the clinical and radiographic examinations along with subjective symptoms reported by the patient. Material for the dental records has been included in Chapter 13, and occlusion in Chapter 14. Mobility of teeth has been charted with the periodontal examination because the causes of mobility are periodontally oriented. The outline here is for summary in anticipation of treatment planning.

After initial entries into the record, additions are made to show the progress of treatment. At each periodic recall, new and comparative records and chartings must be prepared.

The need for meticulous examination and recording cannot be overemphasized. Finding and recording a carious lesion may mean saving a tooth for the patient's lifetime; inadvertently neglecting a tooth may eventually lead to a need for endodontic therapy or even extraction.

I. Prior to Patient Appointment

When the radiographs and study casts have been prepared at an initial appointment prior to clinical examination for charting, they are useful for the preliminary charting. Conservation of patient chair time is important.

Supplemental and confirming observations and checks are made during the clinical examination with the patient. For example, when an overhanging restoration is noted but dental caries is not visible in the radiograph, examination by exploration is required since the restoration can be superimposed over the carious lesion.

Figure 20–2 is an example of dental charting using anatomic tooth drawings. Dental findings can also be charted on a geometric form such as is shown in figure 20–1.

A. **Radiographic Charting**

The following may be charted: missing, unerupted, impacted teeth, endodontic restorations, overhanging margins of existing restorations, proximal surface carious lesions, and any other deviation from normal evident from the radiographs.

B. **Study Casts.** Record the Classification of Occlusion (pages 225–227).

II. Patient Appointment

A. Chart existing restorations, including fixed and removable prostheses.

B. Chart apparent carious lesions and other deviations from normal.

C. Coordinate clinical and radiographic findings.

D. Use dental floss. Chart inadequate contact areas and observe proximal surface roughness. Fraying of dental floss when passing over a rough proximal surface may mean the defective margin of a restoration, a sharp cavity margin, or dental calculus.

E. Pulp vitality. Record numbers in the

CODE FOR CHART

Missing tooth   **I**

Caries — red

Restorations — blue

Encircle defective restorations in red

Fixed bridge   =

Partial denture   :::

Apparent gingival position

Bone line

Periodontal pocket   ( )

Suppuration   **S**

Drift and pathological migration

Food impaction   ↓

Mobility — N-1-2-3

Overhanging margins   ▼

NV = non-vital

RCF = root filling

PT = Pulp treatment

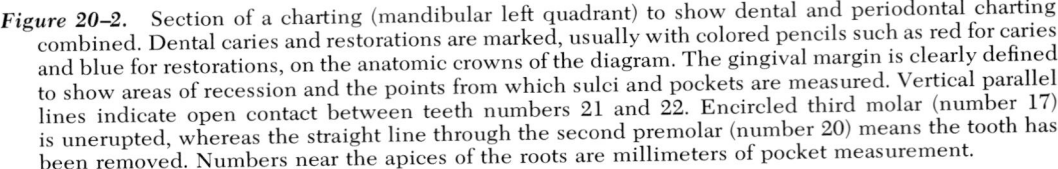

Figure 20–2. Section of a charting (mandibular left quadrant) to show dental and periodontal charting combined. Dental caries and restorations are marked, usually with colored pencils such as red for caries and blue for restorations, on the anatomic crowns of the diagram. The gingival margin is clearly defined to show areas of recession and the points from which sulci and pockets are measured. Vertical parallel lines indicate open contact between teeth numbers 21 and 22. Encircled third molar (number 17) is unerupted, whereas the straight line through the second premolar (number 20) means the tooth has been removed. Numbers near the apices of the roots are millimeters of pocket measurement.

permanent record. Chart forms are sometimes prepared with a specific place for such data to be filled in. Procedures were described on page 218.

F. Tooth sensitivity. The patient may report hypersensitive areas, or they may be discovered during instrumentation. Record the tooth number and surface for reference during the treatment phase.

TECHNICAL HINTS

A. Use a record form with adequate space for recording details.

B. Prepare permanent records in ink.

C. Use abbreviations and symbols only when their meaning will be clear to all who read them.

D. All records should be complete, accurate, clearly stated, readable, and neat.

E. Plan appointments when possible in order that radiographs and study casts will be available prior to and at the time of clinical charting. By having an initial appointment when the history and oral inspection for extraoral and intraoral mucosal examinations can be completed, time can be saved. Necessary consultations with a patient's physician, preparation with premedication when indicated for the patient susceptible to bacteremia, or other special adaptation can be made (pages 70–71).

F. When a patient asks specific questions about the charting or other recordings, explain why it is necessary for the dentist to observe and check before explanations can be made.

FACTORS TO TEACH THE PATIENT

I. The importance of making a complete study of the patient's oral problems before beginning treatment.

II. Advantages of cooperation and patience in furnishing information which will help dental personnel to interpret observations accurately in order that the correct diagnosis and appropriate treatment plan can be made.

III. All information received is completely confidential and the records are locked when the office is closed.

Reference

1. Crawford, J. J.: *Clinical Asepsis in Dentistry.* Chapel Hill, University of North Carolina, 1974, pp. 18–20.

Suggested Readings

Allen, D. L., McFall, W. T., and Hunter, G. C.: *Periodontics for the Dental Hygienist,* 2nd ed. Philadelphia, Lea & Febiger, 1974, pp. 92–107.

Castano, F. A. and Alden, B. A., eds.: *Handbook of Expanded Dental Auxiliary Practice.* Philadelphia, Lippincott, 1973, pp. 137–139.

Glickman, I.: *Clinical Periodontology,* 4th ed. Philadelphia, Saunders, 1972, pp. 490–499.

Grant, D. A., Stern, I. B., and Everett, F. G.: *Orban's Periodontics,* 4th ed. St. Louis, Mosby, 1972, pp. 313–321.

McElroy, D. L. and Malone, W. F.: *Handbook of Oral Diagnosis and Treatment Planning.* Baltimore, Williams and Wilkins, 1969, pp. 23–26.

Schwarzrock, S. P. and Jensen, J. R.: *Effective Dental Assisting,* 4th ed. Dubuque, Iowa, Wm. G. Brown, 1973, pp. 179–188.

Simon, W. J.: *Clinical Dental Assisting.* Hagerstown, Maryland, Harper & Row, 1973, pp. 79–82.

Chapter 21

The Dental Hygiene Treatment Plan

All of the information about the patient, collected as parts of the diagnostic work-up, is organized for evaluation. From the evaluation, before treatment is started, the dentist makes the diagnosis, and the treatment plan is prepared.

The *total treatment plan* is a sequential outline of the essential services and procedures which must be carried out by the dentist, the dental hygienist, and the patient to eliminate disease and restore the oral cavity to health and normal function. The *dental hygiene treatment plan*, which consists of those services to be performed by the dental hygienist with the patient, is formulated within the framework of the total treatment plan and is an integral part of it.

I. Objectives

The objectives of a treatment sequence as conducted by the dentist, patient, and the auxiliaries are:

A. To Eliminate and Control Etiologic and Predisposing Disease Factors

The principal etiologic agent in both dental caries and periodontal and gingival diseases is dental plaque. The goal should be to control the etiologic agent and thus prevent future recurrences of the same conditions.

B. To Eliminate the Signs and Symptoms of Disease

Treatment planning includes the measures to eliminate signs of disease such as carious lesions, inflammation, and pockets.

C. To Restore Normal Function

This includes occlusal adjustment, restoration of teeth, replacement of missing teeth, orthodontic tooth movement, and recontouring of gingival form (gingivoplasty).

D. To Maintain Health and Prevent the Recurrence of Disease

Methods used are to counsel and supervise the patient in daily self-care and to provide regular follow-up professional supervision and care.

II. Preparation for the Treatment Plan

A. Diagnostic Work-up

The parts of a diagnostic work-up were listed on page 57 and described in Chapters 6 through 20. The histories, dental and periodontal chartings, radiographs, study casts, recorded information from the extraoral and intraoral inspections, indices, and all other available information are studied by the dentist. The key pertinent findings which point to the disease problems are selected and the diagnosis is made.

B. **Diagnosis**

The *diagnosis* is the identification of the disease condition by recognition of characteristic signs and symptoms. A *differential diagnosis* means distinguishing the disease from other diseases which have similar manifestations.

Patients frequently have more than one disease condition. For example, dental caries and periodontal or gingival diseases commonly occur simultaneously. When the treatment plan is made, the treatment for each disease condition is outlined, and a coordinated treatment sequence is determined.

III. Parts of a Total Treatment Plan

A total treatment plan usually involves several interdependent areas of oral care based on an individual patient's diagnosis and disease symptoms. Divisions for a treatment plan are listed below with examples of services included in each.

A. **Priority Treatment**
   1. Emergency care for pain or other acute condition.
   2. Procedures such as biopsy of a lesion found during the extraoral and intraoral examination, or a laboratory test for a suspected systemic condition.

B. **Preventive Phase**
   1. Procedures for the patient's daily self-care, including plaque control.
   2. Clinical services such as topical fluoride or sealant application.

C. **Preparatory Phase**
   1. Dental caries: excavation of large carious lesions; placement of seda-

tive temporary fillings; pulp treatment as indicated.
   2. Endodontic therapy.
   3. Preparation for oral surgery: plaque control and scaling to reduce bacterial count and inflammation.
   4. Removal of hopeless teeth which cannot be successfully treated.
   5. Preparation for periodontal therapy: plaque control, complete scaling and planing, gingival curettage, tooth movement, and/or stabilization, occlusal adjustment.

D. **Treatment Phase**
   1. Gingival and periodontal treatment: elimination of inflammation and pockets; surgical procedures; occlusal adjustment.
   2. Restorative treatment.
   3. Prosthetic treatment.
   4. Orthodontic treatment.
   5. Tissue maintenance during therapy (page 296).

E. **Maintenance Phase**
   1. Patient: specific daily plaque control and other preventive measures.
   2. Professional recall at designated intervals.
      a. Complete reevaluation and updating of records, radiographs, and all parts of the diagnostic work-up.
      b. Recall treatment plan: may include any service as a continuation, supplement, or addition to previous preventive, educational, or therapeutic measures. The recall appointment is described on page 574.

PLANNING THE DENTAL HYGIENE TREATMENT PLAN

The dental hygienist's objective is to prepare a flexible, realistic, dental hygiene plan and sequence of procedures based on the plan for total care of the patient. As described on page 9, a dental hygienist's services may be divided into preventive, educational, and therapeutic, all of which are applicable at various levels in the total treatment plan. Services to be performed are dependent on state practice acts, and any examples cited here are not intended to represent a specific state.

The treatment plan is recorded in the patient's record. The patient or parent of a young or mentally disabled patient needs to understand the treatment plan and be aware of the expected outcome of each appointment as well as the total series. The role of the patient in treatment through self-care on a daily basis must be written into the treatment plan and explained to the patient.

An objective in planning dental hygiene care is to ensure the best possible sequence of procedures which will contribute to the restoration of the patient's oral health in the shortest possible time and pave the way to the long-range preventive program which will continue throughout the patient's lifetime. To achieve the goals of planned care, the dental hygienist must see the dental hygiene aspects within the total plan for the patient and contribute to the overall continuity of the corrective and maintenance phases.

I. Characteristics of a Well-planned Treatment Plan

An effective plan will be

A. Adapted to the needs of the patient's oral condition.

B. Orderly in sequence to allow for thoroughness in each procedure, and to prevent duplication or repetition of efforts.

C. Composed of purposefully selected procedures which are
1. Planned with a reasonable degree of predictability of outcome.
2. Expected to resolve the condition

and reach an optimum result in a minimum of time.
3. Projected toward a state of health which the patient can maintain with self-care procedures.

II. Steps in Planning

A. Review the patient's oral problems as described in the diagnosis and total treatment plan.

B. Identify objectives which may be attained.
1. Overall objectives of the total treatment plan: anticipated outcome of treatment and anticipated state of oral health after treatment.
2. Dental hygiene goals: short-term and long-term.

C. Select the preventive, preparatory, and treatment procedures which can be expected to meet the objectives.

D. List in sequence for the appointment series of services to be performed for each phase of the total treatment plan.

No attempt is made here to list all possible dental hygiene services, but examples are listed below for each treatment plan phase.
1. *Preventive.* A typical program includes plaque control measures, self-applied and professionally applied fluorides, and diet counseling.
2. *Preparatory.* Complete scaling, planing, and gingival curettage are major services in the preparation of a patient for periodontal surgery. *Preparatory* treatment is in contrast to *definitive* treatment. By definitive is meant the complete treatment needed by a patient to bring the oral tissues to a state of health at that time.
3. *Treatment*
   a. Periodontal: scaling, planing, and gingival curettage which were preparatory for one patient may be the definitive and cura-

tive treatment for another patient.

b. Periodontal post-surgical procedures: suture removal, removal and placement of periodontal dressings, and other postoperative care and instruction are parts of the patient's treatment plan which are performed by the dental hygienist.

c. Restorative. Finishing and polishing of restorations may best be scheduled with polishing of the teeth prior to topical fluoride application. After polishing restorations it is recommended that a topical fluoride application be made in order to protect the enamel just highly polished adjacent to the restoration.

d. Tissue maintenance during long-term therapy: when restorative, prosthetic, orthodontic, or other treatment continues over a long period, appointments are needed for gingival evaluation, supervision of plaque control measures, calculus removal, topical fluoride applications, and other procedures specific for the patient.

E. Estimate and allot time requirements for each preventive, educational, and therapeutic service.

III. Criteria for Determination of Sequence

Sequence planning involves first an outline of a series of appointments with the services to be performed. Secondly, sequence refers to the order in which the parts of an individual appointment are carried out. The sequence is influenced by numerous factors, including urgency of treatment, need for treating etiologic factors first, the severity and extent of the

case, and certain special patient requirements. These are described here with examples.

A. **Urgency**

When discomfort or pain is present the area involved would require first attention. In the dental hygiene treatment plan, this could apply to an area of the gingiva where the patient has particular difficulty, and either specially adapted plaque control instruction or scaling may be needed.

B. **Etiologic Factors Should Be Treated First**

It is necessary to arrest and control the factors which caused or contributed to the development of the existing disease. In patients with gingival or periodontal involvement, the continued success of treatment is dependent on the removal of plaque.

Disease will recur when daily control measures for the removal of the etiologic agent, plaque, are not carried out. New dental caries also can develop unless continued attention is paid to preventive measures. Because pellicle forms within minutes after a tooth surface has been completely cleaned and disclosable plaque will be present within 24 hours or less, it is necessary that plaque control measures be introduced in the treatment plan before scaling or polishing.

C. **Special Patient Requirements:** Items from the Patient History

1. Antibiotic premedication. A list of conditions which require antibiotic coverage may be found on page 71. For patients who need antibiotics, all instrumentation, including the examination procedures when instruments are used (probing, exploring) as well as tooth movement for mobility determination must be done under antibiotic coverage.

Because bacteremias have been demonstrated during brushing, flossing, and other plaque control measures, instruction and practice of these procedures must be carried out while the patient is premedicated. Appointments must be planned and conducted efficiently to prevent the need for unnecessary premedication. When a patient's physical health and strength do not contraindicate, appointments which are longer than customary may be reserved in order that more can be accomplished.

2. Chronic disease or physical handicap may influence the content or length of appointments.
3. Disease transmission problems for patients with a history of a communicable disease may require postponement of all except urgent needs.

D. **Severity and Extent of the Case**

Findings which indicate the severity of gingival or periodontal involvement include the changes in color, size, shape, consistency, and bleeding of the gingiva, pocket measurements, mobility of teeth, and radiographic signs. To determine the length of appointments and sequence of procedures, consideration is given necessarily to the depth of pockets in relation to the distribution and hardness of dental calculus. The number of appointments and the length of appointments increase with severity.

A suggested division of cases graded by severity of disease involvement follows.

1. Moderate to severe periodontal disease. For the patient who requires complicated periodontal, restorative, and prosthetic treatment, the dental hygiene treatment plan will include preventive and preparatory procedures as well as maintenance during therapy, post-surgical care, and follow-up.
2. Moderate or slight periodontal disease. The dental hygiene treatment plan will include the preventive phase, complete scaling, planing, and gingival curettage as indicated. This treatment may be definitive, or the follow-up evaluation may show the need for surgical or other additional treatment.
3. Gingivitis with supra- and submarginal calculus. The preventive phase and complete scaling are indicated and gingival pockets may require curettage. The treatment may be definitive or, upon reevaluation, gingivoplasty or other treatment may be needed.
4. Gingivitis with slight supramarginal calculus, or no calculus. Dental hygiene services usually constitute the definitive treatment. To eliminate gingival inflammation, plaque control measures may be the total treatment, which is supplemented by scaling when there is calculus, or polishing only when stain is unsightly.

E. **Individual Appointment Sequence**

1. *Evaluation.* Each appointment starts with an evaluation of the gingival tissues.
   a. Previously treated area. The area is examined for progress towards health, the signs of inflammation which may still be present, and indications for additional treatment which is needed.
   b. Effects of plaque control measures. The self-treatment by the patient is evaluated. After the color, size, shape, consistency, and other characteristics of the gingiva are observed, a disclosing agent is used to evaluate the degree of plaque present on the teeth. This in turn evaluates the

patient's techniques and thoroughness in plaque removal.

2. *Instruction.* Instruction begins when evaluation starts, and continues throughout. Specific instruction of techniques for the use of plaque removal devices, such as toothbrush, floss, or other aid, is presented before instrumentation or other professional clinical services are performed. The reasons for this sequence are presented on pages 388, 496.

3. *Clinical services.* The question of which area or quadrant should be scaled first, and in which order the other areas and quadrants should follow, can be answered for most patients by considering the following order of choices:

   a. Patient selection: when the patient indicates an area of discomfort, that area may be taken first.

   b. Apprehensive patient: to make the first scaling less complicated and help orient the patient to the procedures to be followed, the dental hygienist can select either the quadrant with the fewest teeth or the quadrant with the least deep periodontal involvement.

   c. When there is no other major reason for selection of a specific area, the quadrant that needs treatment most, that may take the longest to heal, that may have the deepest pockets, the most calculus, should be treated first.

   d. When two quadrants are to be treated at the same appointment: select a maxillary and mandibular of the same side.

SAMPLE DENTAL HYGIENE TREATMENT PLAN

It would be impossible to present sample treatment plans for each of the wide variety of patient problems or combinations of problems encountered in practice. Each case must be handled individually.

Examples of treatment sequences and plans are found in special areas of this book. An outline of a dental caries control study program may be found on page 412, a recall appointment on page 574, and a treatment sequence for a patient with acute necrotizing ulcerative gingivitis on pages 601–603.

For the patient whose dental hygiene treatment plan is sketched below, the diagnostic work-up was completed by the dental hygienist. The dentist indicated a diagnosis of generalized moderate periodontal disease. The preliminary total treatment plan includes occlusal adjustment, restorative procedures, and the prosthetic replacement of two missing teeth. There are no emergency measures required. None of the periodontal surgery or dental treatment will be started until the dental hygiene preventive and preparatory appointments have been completed and the patient's mouth has been reevaluated.

The examinations revealed slight localized supramarginal calculus and generalized moderate-to-heavy submarginal calculus. Because the patient has enlarged, spongy marginal gingiva with generalized bleeding on probing and plaque on the cervical thirds of most teeth, scaling is not started on the first appointment. The rationale for introducing plaque control before scaling is described on page 388.

More detail is included in the treatment plan recorded below than probably would be written in practice. Abbreviations would be used which could be recognized by all personnel involved in using the patient's record. For example, "Plaque I," "Plaque II," "Plaque III" would be sufficient notation for the plaque control instruction series.

APPOINTMENT I

1. Record Gingival Index (GI) and Plaque Index (Pl I).
2. Give plaque control instruction: *First Lesson*, page 388.
3. Introduce fluoride program.
   a. Dentifrice recommendation: reasons for frequent brushing to gain most benefit from fluoride in dentifrice.
   b. Mouthrinse. Demonstrate.

APPOINTMENT II

1. Plaque control evaluation
   a. Gingival tissue inspection (table 11–1, pages 172–173).
   b. Record indices.
2. Instruction: *Second Lesson*, page 390.
3. Scaling
   a. First quadrant scaling with anesthesia.
   b. Curettage as directed; dressing placed when needed.
   c. Postoperative instructions.

APPOINTMENT III

1. Remove dressing.
2. Evaluation
   a. Gingival tissue inspection; record Gingival Index.
   b. Specific examination for first quadrant scaled: note healing. Explore to check for residual calculus.
   c. Plaque evaluation: disclose and record Plaque Index.
3. Instruction: *Third Lesson*, page 391.
4. Scaling
   a. Complete first quadrant when residual calculus is found.
   b. Second quadrant scaling with anesthesia.
   c. Gingival curettage as directed; dressing when needed.

APPOINTMENT IV

1. Remove dressing.
2. Evaluation
   a. Gingival tissue inspection: record Gingival Index.
   b. Specific examination for previously scaled quadrants; explore for residual calculus.
   c. Plaque evaluation: disclose and record Plaque Index.
3. Instruction: continue as needed.
4. Scaling
   a Complete first and second quadrants.
   b. Third quadrant scaling with anesthesia.
   c. Gingival curettage as directed; dressing when needed.

APPOINTMENT V

The same basic structure is followed as outlined for Appointments III and IV. Each time the previously treated quadrants must be checked and completed. Each time the instruction is continued if the patient is still not accomplishing plaque control. The fourth quadrant is scaled under anesthesia and curettage performed as needed.

APPOINTMENT VI

1. Evaluation of four quadrants; additional scaling when indicated.
2. Reevaluation by the dentist; planning for the next phase of appointments when patient is ready as shown by the health of the gingival tissue.

APPOINTMENT VII: Maintenance During Therapy

When the restorative and prosthetic treatment extends over a period of time, periodic appointments are needed for monitoring the continued success of the patient's self-care. A gingival tissue evaluation, checks with a probe to determine bleeding, plaque checks with disclosing agents, additional instruction particularly for the care of newly fixed or removable prosthetic appliances, and motivational encouragement are essential.

APPOINTMENT VIII: Recall

The recall frequency is determined. Components of the recall appointments are described on page 574.

TECHNICAL HINTS

I. Treatment plans for minors or mentally disabled patients should be discussed with the parent or guardian. Permission should be obtained by signature, particularly when anesthesia will be used or prescriptions issued.

II. Complete records are essential. Misunderstandings can lead to legal involvements.

FACTORS TO TEACH THE PATIENT

I. Why a treatment plan is made.
II. Explanation of unclear parts of the total treatment plan.
III. Parts of the treatment plan carried out by the patient. Interrelation of roles of patient, dentist, and auxiliary personnel in eliminating disease from the patient's oral cavity.
IV. The long-term effects of comprehensive continuing care.
V. Why plaque control measures must

be learned before scaling and polishing are done.
VI. Significance of the indices as a guide to evaluating the health of the gingiva.
VII. What presurgical preparation means, consists of, and what the expected advantages are.

Suggested Readings

American Association of Dental Schools, Section on Community and Preventive Dentistry: Preventive Dentistry Curriculum: Minimal Preventive Action Guidelines for Dental Practice, *J. Dent. Educ.*, 39, 53, January, 1975.

Glickman, I.: *Clinical Periodontology*, 4th ed. Philadelphia, Saunders, 1972, pp. 531–532.

Goldman, H. M. and Cohen, D. W.: *Periodontal Therapy*, 5th ed. St. Louis, Mosby, 1973, pp. 354–371, 998–1000.

Grant, D. A., Stern, I. B., and Everett, F. G.: *Orban's Periodontics*, 4th ed. St. Louis, Mosby, 1972, pp. 328–331.

Howe, R., Morganstein, W., and Barr, C.: A New Role for the Hygienist: The Preventive Prescription, *J. Dent. Educ.*, 38, 403, July, 1974.

Kerr, D. A., Ash, M. M., and Millard, H. O.: *Oral Diagnosis*, 4th ed. St. Louis, Mosby, 1974, pp. 382–391.

McElroy, D. L. and Malone, W. F.: *Handbook of Oral Diagnosis and Treatment Planning*. Baltimore, Williams & Wilkins, 1969, pp. 69–77, 109–117.

Mitchell, D. F., Standish, S. M., and Fast, T. B.: *Oral Diagnosis/Oral Medicine*, 2nd ed. Philadelphia, Lea & Febiger, 1971, pp. 38–39, 393–394.

Stibbs, G. D.: Treatment—Clinical Procedures, in Morrey, L. W. and Nelson, R. J., eds.: *Dental Science Handbook*. Washington, Superintendent of Documents, U.S. Government Printing Office, pp. 170–174.

IV
Prevention

INTRODUCTION

This section, *Prevention*, includes procedures for plaque control, diet counseling, fluorides, sealants, and related preventive measures. In the sequence of treatment planning for the patient, initiation of preventive measures precedes dental and dental hygiene clinical services except for an emergency. The long-range success of treatment procedures is limited unless the causes of the condition being treated are removed.

Primary prevention, involving measures to prevent disease completely, is essential to continuing benefits of dental and dental hygiene treatment. The fluoridation of water supplies, and plaque and sucrose control for the prevention of dental caries, are examples of primary prevention.

Secondary preventive measures are those related to the early recognition and treatment of incipient disease before extensive lesions develop. The restoration of small carious lesions and the recognition and biopsy of a suspected lesion of the mucous membrane are examples of secondary prevention. The relationship of primary and secondary prevention to dental hygiene practice was introduced on page 9. Tertiary preventive measures are represented in more complex and involved dental and periodontal therapy, and even to the extent of the replacement of missing teeth. Prevention is still involved as long as complete breakdown and loss of function are prevented.

Preventive dentistry is the sum total of the efforts to promote, restore, and maintain the oral health of the individual. A *program for prevention* is composed of the cooperative steps taken by the patient, dentist, and dental auxiliary personnel to preserve the natural dentition and the supporting structures by preventing the onset, progress, and recurrence of oral diseases and other destructive or disfiguring conditions.

STEPS IN A PREVENTIVE PROGRAM

The dental hygienist prepares a preventive treatment plan for each patient. Planning and carrying out the preventive program may be divided into the six basic steps below. Details to describe each step are not included here, because the details were either part of the diagnostic work-up

301

described in previous chapters or will be parts of the preventive section chapters to follow.

I. Assess Patient's Needs

A. Review all information from the diagnostic work-up; history, examinations, radiographs, chartings, pages 63–300.

B. Identify the presence and severity of disease, predisposing factors, and deposit retention factors.

C. Utilize indices to rate the severity of the needs (pages 273–283).

II. Select Applicable Preventive Methods

A. Apply information about the patient: educational level, occupation, socioeconomic background, and attitudes toward oral health.

B. Recognize the influence of physical or mental handicaps.

C. Determine the current personal oral care procedures carried out by the patient, and the frequency.

D. Outline the instruction recommended for the patient.

III. Provide Instruction for Self-Care

A. Present information and demonstration for specific daily care techniques and self-applied fluoride.

B. Show methods for self-evaluation.

IV. Perform Clinical Preventive Services

A. Complete scaling.

B. Apply topical caries-prevention agents.

V. Evaluate Changes in the Patient's Oral Health

A. Evaluate gingival tissue, bleeding, plaque, and techniques performed by the patient.

B. Use successive indices to compare progress.

VI. Plan Long-Term Maintenance

A. Reevaluate periodically to monitor continuance of preventive practices.

B. Provide additional preventive measures when indicated.

PATIENT INSTRUCTION

Instruction is an essential part of the preventive program if goals for attaining a patient's oral health are to be reached. Personalized patient instruction contributes first to the knowledge, attitudes, and practices of the individual, then through the individual to the family, and the community. The outmoded concept that all teeth eventually must be removed has been replaced by current research evidence that periodontal diseases and dental caries can be prevented or controlled and therefore the teeth can be preserved throughout the lifetime of the individual.

Dental health education is the provision of oral health information to people in such a way that they can apply it in everyday living.[1] To know and believe health facts is not enough; benefits result only when knowledge is put into action. Learning occurs when an individual changes his behavior, and when changes are incorporated as a part of everyday living.

I. Motivation

Instruction is tailored to individual needs and motivations. An individual is motivated to practice behavior that leads to achievement of goals which he values. Dental health instruction can be effective if the patient considers his oral health a valuable asset or goal.

Stimulation of behavior, or motivation, stems from basic physiologic and social needs. Peer group approval and the need to conform to group standards, as well as the fear of disapproval or rejection when appearance of the teeth or odor of the breath is unacceptable, are frequently much higher motivating factors than a health reason such as freedom from infection or the ability to chew food for body cell maintenance. The need for relief from pain can bring a patient to seek immediate dental care, but additional motivation is needed to help the patient realize that through a preventive care program, future pain can be avoided.

Motivation and what the patient will learn and practice are proportional to the sincerity and concern of the dental hygienist. A motivated dental hygienist develops patient-centered systems of instruction that are meaningful to the patient.

I. Patient-Centered Instruction

For most patients major emphasis needs to be placed on control of dental caries or periodontal disease. Attention should also be paid to oral accident prevention particularly related to mouth protectors for contact sports, safety belts for automobiles, and children's accidents which lead to fractured anterior teeth.

Whereas patient instruction of the past connoted teaching the patient how to brush his teeth, usually by means of a model, and in one short session, patient instruction now envelops a wide range of essential areas of learning aimed to develop patients with knowledge, attitudes, and practices for continuing oral health. To be able to interpret and apply current dental research findings requires continuing review through reading and other educational efforts by the dental hygienist.

DENTAL PLAQUE CONTROL

Dental plaque is the most important etiologic factor in the development of dental caries and most periodontal diseases. A direct relationship exists between the degree of oral uncleanliness and the extent of periodontal disease. Epidemiologic investigations have clearly shown that the prevalence and severity of periodontal diseases are significantly less in those persons with clean mouths, that is, with less oral debris, dental plaque, and calculus, regardless of age.[2,3]

Plaque control in the individual is directly related to the measures employed for cleaning the teeth on a regular basis. The most effective means for plaque removal available at present are mechanical, that is, toothbrushing for tooth surfaces which can be reached with the brush, and dental floss or other device for proximal surfaces. Since pellicle begins to form immediately and plaque forms again within a few to 24 hours following its removal (pages 239–240), it is evident that self-care measures for control are necessary on a day-to-day basis.

Personal measures for plaque control need supplementation by professional care measures. The removal of dental calculus and other local irritants is essential to create an environment which can be effectively maintained by the individual. Continuing personal and professional care are mutually interdependent in a successful patient-centered plaque control program. Plaque control in combination with regular periodic scaling for complete calculus removal has been shown to arrest the progress of periodontal disease. In one research study, when a high level of oral hygiene was maintained for three years, the test subjects had less detectable bone loss (determined by radiographs) and less loss of epithelial attachment (measured by probe from the cementoenamel junction to the bottom of the pocket) than the control subjects without the intense oral hygiene program.[4,5]

Oral physical therapy is accomplished by the use of physical agents in the prevention, management, and control of oral diseases. In physical medicine, physical therapy includes the use of various agents particularly light, heat, water, electricity, and exercise. A few of the same agents are used in oral care, and many mechanical devices have been developed for specific application to the teeth and gingiva. The satisfactory use of an oral physical therapy device depends on the patient's understanding of the goals to be attained. Objectives may need reconsideration from time to time depending on new research findings relative to the cause and prevention of oral diseases.

OBJECTIVES

By way of introduction to subsequent chapters, primary objectives for plaque control are listed below. The objectives apply from a preventive or a treatment aspect depending on the status of the patient's health. For the patient undergoing definitive care for periodontal disease, plaque control and oral physical therapy are, first, essential parts of the treatment program, and then equally essential parts of the maintenance phase of care.

For all patients, fulfilling the goals of personal care contributes to prevention of disease. The patient becomes an active participant in obtaining and maintaining his own health, which is in itself the most important objective.

I. Primary Objective: Plaque Control

A. Plaque control involves the following:
  1. Disorganization and reduction of the number of microorganisms through daily removal of plaque.
  2. Prevention of calculus formation by removing the components of calculus prior to calcification.
B. With effective removal of dental plaque from the tooth surfaces, the following benefits can be expected:
  1. Reduction and control of gingivitis and the development of periodontitis.
  2. Reduced incidence of dental caries.

  3. Reduction in sensitivity of exposed root surfaces.
  4. Lessened possibility of halitosis related to oral uncleanliness.
  5. Improved oral comfort, sanitation, and appearance with a refreshed taste, smooth tooth surfaces, and general sense of well-being.

II. Plaque Control and Dental Caries

Control of acidogenic plaque microorganisms is necessary for dental caries prevention as part of a total dental caries control program. Toothbrushing with a dentifrice which contains fluoride combines plaque removal with fluoride application. The application of fluoride by way of a dentifrice is an important objective of toothbrushing.

One research finding pertaining to professionally applied topical fluorides was that the caries-reducing effect of acidulated phosphate fluoride topical applications was greater for children with cleaner mouths (60 percent caries incidence reduction) as compared with children who did not keep their mouths clean (44 percent).[6] Such a study adds a new dimension to the objectives of oral cleanliness.

III. Oral Physical Therapy and Gingival Massage

Gingival massage is the systematic application of a stroking or kneading pressure to the periodontium for the purpose of stimulating the blood circulation to these tissues. It should be realized that as helpful as massage may seem to be in maintaining the health of the gingival tissue, without plaque removal the benefits are not present or at least to a lesser degree.[7] Irritation to the gingiva will persist when plaque bacteria are present, and calculus will accumulate.

Benefits to the gingival tissues which have been considered related to gingival massage include:

1. Improved keratinization to render the gingiva more resistant to trauma.[8,9]
2. Stimulation of circulation.
3. Reshaping of the gingiva: recontouring following disease or surgery.
4. Improved gingival tone.

FACTORS TO TEACH THE PATIENT

I. The relationship between preventive measures and clinical services.
II. Why particular preventive measures were selected for the particular patient.
III. Self-evaluation methods for determining health of gingiva.
IV. Objectives of plaque control.

References

1. Young, W. O. and Striffler, D. F.: *The Dentist, His Practice, and His Community*, 2nd ed. Philadelphia, Saunders, 1969, p. 296.
2. Greene, J. C.: Oral Hygiene and Periodontal Disease, *Am. J. Public Health*, 53, 913, June, 1963.
3. National Center for Health Statistics: Oral Hygiene in Adults, United States—1960–1962. *Vital and Health Statistics.* PHS Publication No. 1000—Series 11—No. 16, Public Health Service, Washington, D. C., United States Government Printing Office, June, 1966.
4. Suomi, J. D., Greene, J. C., Vermillion, J. R., Doyle, J., Chang, J. J., and Leatherwood, E. C.: The Effect of Controlled Oral Hygiene Procedures on the Progression of Periodontal Disease in Adults: Results after Third and Final Year, *J. Periodont.*, 42, 152, March, 1971.
5. Suomi, J. D., West, T. D., Chang, J. J., and McClendon, J.: The Effect of Controlled Oral Hygiene Procedures on the Progression of Periodontal Disease in Adults: Radiographic Findings, *J. Periodont.*, 42, 562, September, 1971.
6. Wellock, W. D., Maitland, A., and Brudevold, F.: Caries Increments, Tooth Discoloration, and State of Oral Hygiene in Children Given Single Annual Applications of Acid Phosphate-fluoride and Stannous Fluoride, *Arch. Oral Biol.*, 10, 453, May-June, 1965.
7. Mackenzie, I. C.: Does Toothbrushing Affect Gingival Keratinization? *Proc. Roy. Soc. Med.*, 65, 1127, December, 1972.
8. Glickman, I., Petralis, R., and Marks, R. M.: The Effect of Powered Toothbrushing and Interdental Stimulation Upon Microscopic Inflammation and Surface Keratinization of the Interdental Gingiva, *J. Periodont.*, 36, 108, March-April, 1965.
9. Toto, P. D.: Electric Toothbrush Effect Upon Keratin Formation, *Periodontics*, 4, 332, November-December, 1966.

Suggested Readings

American Association of Dental Schools, Section on Community and Preventive Dentistry: Preventive Dentistry Curriculum: Minimal Preventive Action, Guidelines for Dental Practice, *J. Dent. Educ.*, 39, 53, January, 1975.

Greene, J. C.: The Case for Preventive Periodontics, *J. Dent. Child.*, 42, 24, January-February, 1975.

Haefner, D. P.: Achieving Public Acceptance of Preventive Dentistry Procedures, *J. Dent. Educ.*, 32, 306, September, 1968.

Heifetz, S. B. and Suomi, J. D.: The Control of Dental Caries and Periodontal Disease: A Fundamental Approach, *J. Public Health Dent.*, 33, 2, Winter, 1973.

Howard, R. L.: Army Motivation Study, *J. Am. Coll. Dent.*, 35, 65, January, 1968.

Katz, S., McDonald, J. L., and Stookey, G. K.: *Preventive Dentistry in Action.* Upper Montclair, N.J., D.C.P. Publishing, 1972, pp. 19–43.

Keyes, P. H.: Present and Future Measures for Dental Caries Control, *J. Am. Dent. Assoc.*, 79, 1395, December, 1969.

Knutson, J. W.: Effective and Practical Preventive Procedures, *Int. Dent. J.*, 24, 66, March, 1974.

Lutz, B. L. and Whisenand, J. D.: A Pilot Program for Dental Disease Control, *J. Am. Coll. Dent.*, 39, 121, April, 1972.

Myers, S. E. and Downs, R. A.: Comparative Findings in School Systems with Differing Approaches to Dental Health Education, *J. School Health*, 38, 604, November, 1968.

Putnam, W. J., O'Shea, R. M., and Cohen, L. K.: Communication and Patient Motivation in Preventive Periodontics, *Pub. Health Reports*, 82, 779, September, 1967.

Robinson, B. A., Mobley, E. L., and Pointer, M. B.: Is Dental Health Education the Answer? *J. Am. Dent. Assoc.*, 74, 124, January, 1967.

Sumnicht, R. W.: Research in Preventive Dentistry, *J. Am. Dent. Assoc.*, 79, 1193, November, 1969.

Suomi, J. D.: Prevention and Control of Periodontal Disease, *J. Am. Dent. Assoc.*, 83, 1271, December, 1971.

World Health Organization: *Dental Health Education.* Technical Report Series, No. 449. Geneva, World Health Organization, 1970, 28 pp.

Chapter 22

Plaque Control: Toothbrushes and Toothbrushing

The toothbrush is the principal instrument in general use for accomplishing plaque removal as a necessary part of plaque control. Many different designs of toothbrushes and supplementary devices have been manufactured and promoted.

Patients who have not previously received professional advice concerning the best brush for their particular oral characteristics very likely have used brushes selected on the basis of cost, availability, advertising claims, family tradition, or habit. Because of the variety in shapes, sizes, textures, and other characteristics, the dental hygienist must become familiar with the many available products in order that patients be advised appropriately.

DEVELOPMENT OF TOOTHBRUSHES[1-4]

Crudely contrived toothpicks, presumably used for relief from food impaction, are believed to be the earliest implements devised for the care of the teeth. Excavations in Mesopotamia uncovered elaborate gold toothpicks used by the Sumerians about 3000 B.C.

The earliest record of the "chewstick," which has been considered the primitive toothbrush, dates back in the Chinese literature to about 1600 B.C. The care of the mouth was associated with religious training and ritual: the Buddhists had a "tooth stick," and the Mohammedans used the "miswak." Chewsticks, made from various types of tasty woods by crushing an end and spreading the fibers in brush-like manner, are still used by many Asiatic and African people.

The Ebers Papyrus, compiled about 1500 B.C. and dating probably at about 4000 B.C., contained reference to conditions similar to periodontal diseases and preparations to use as mouthwashes and dentifrices. The writings of Hippocrates (about 300 B.C.) include descriptions of diseased gums related to calculus, and of complex preparations for the treatment of unhealthy mouths.

It is believed that the first bristled brush was that mentioned in the Chinese literature about 1600. Pierre Fauchard in 1728 in *Le Chirurgien Dentiste* described many aspects of oral health. He condemned the toothbrush made of horse's hair because it was rough and destructive to the teeth and advised the use of sponges or herb roots. Fauchard recommended scaling of teeth, and developed instruments and splints for loose teeth, as well as dentifrices and mouthwashes.

One of the earlier toothbrushes made in England was produced by William Addis around 1780. By the early nineteenth century, craftsmen in various European countries constructed handles of gold, ivory, or ebony, in which replaceable brush heads could be fitted. The first patent for a toothbrush in the United States was issued to H. N. Wadsworth in the middle of the nineteenth century.

Many new varieties of toothbrushes were developed around 1900 when celluloid was available for the manufacture of toothbrush handles. In 1919, the American Academy of Periodontology defined specifications for toothbrush design and brushing methods in an attempt to standardize professional recommendations.[5]

Nylon came into use in toothbrush construction in 1938. World War II complications prevented Chinese export of wild boar bristles and synthetic materials were substituted for natural bristles. Since then, synthetic materials have been improved and manufacturer's specifications standardized. Many current tooth-

brushes are made exclusively of synthet materials. Automatic toothbrushes ha been developed earlier, but it was n until about 1960 that they were active promoted.

MANUAL TOOTHBRUSHES

Although the American Dental Associ tion does not evaluate and classify manu toothbrushes, certain recommendation have been made.[6] Desirable characteri tics of a brush designed primarily promote oral cleanliness are that it

1. Conform to individual requir ments in size, shape, and texture
2. Be easily and efficiently manip lated.
3. Be readily cleaned and aerate impervious to moisture.
4. Be durable and inexpensive.
5. Have prime functional properties flexibility, elasticity, and stiffne in the bristles; and strength, rigid ty, and lightness in the handle.
6. Be designed for utility, efficienc and cleanliness.

I. General Description

A. **Parts** (figure 22–1)
   1. Handle: the part grasped in th hand during toothbrushing.
   2. Head: the working end; that whic holds the bristles or filaments.
      a. Tufts: clusters of bristles or fil ments secured into the head.

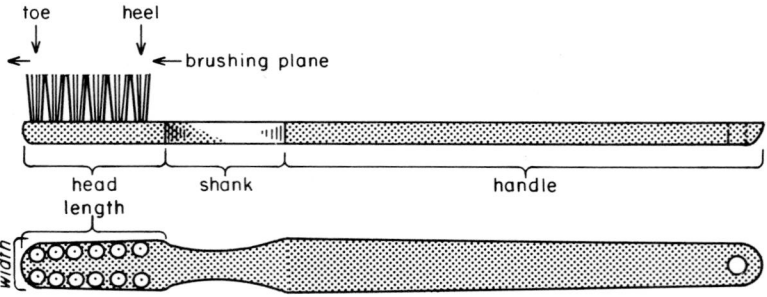

Figure 22–1.   Parts of a toothbrush.

b. Brushing plane: the surface formed by the free ends of the bristles or filaments.

3. Shank: the section which connects the head and the handle.

B. **Dimensions**
1. Total brush length: about six inches; junior and child sizes are smaller.
2. Head: should be only large enough to accommodate the tufts.
   a. Length: 1 to 1¼ inches; width: 5/16 to 3/8 inch.
   b. Bristle or filament height: 7/16 inch.

II. Handle

A. **Composition**
   Nearly all current brush handles are plastics which combine durability, imperviousness to moisture, pleasing appearance, low cost, sufficient rigidity, and smooth surface texture.

B. **Shape**
1. Preferred: straight handle aligned on same plane as the head; with smooth form which is easy to grasp and may be turned as needed but will not slip during manipulation.
2. Variations: a twist, curve, offset, or angle in the shank may frequently be related to new ideas for advertising appeal. Slight deviations may not complicate manipulation or affect control of the brush placement and pressure.
   Bent or thickened handles can be helpful for use by handicapped patients (pages 656–657).

III. Head

A. **Tufts** (figure 22–2)
1. *Tufted Design.* Five or six tufts long and two or three rows wide, spaced for easy cleaning.
2. *Multitufted Design.* Ten or twelve tufts long and three or four rows

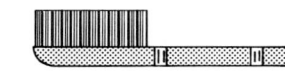

Figure 22–2. Toothbrush design. **A.** Tufted brush, five or six spaced tufts long and two or three rows wide. Tufted brushes are available with bristles or filaments in tapered lengths or all of equal lengths to form a smooth trim as shown. **B.** Multitufted brush, ten or twelve tufts long and three or four rows wide, spaced closely to provide a smooth brushing plane.

wide, spaced closely to provide a smooth brushing plane and to allow the bristles to support each other for longer durability.

B. **Brushing Plane**
1. Preferred: straight, with bristles all of equal length (figure 22–2); permits access to all areas.
2. Uneven planes: brushes are available with variously shaped planes such as with high tufts in the middle position. These arrangements are less efficient and may injure the gingiva or teeth since the longer bristles may be pressed too hard in the attempt to utilize the shorter bristles.

IV. Bristles and Filaments

A. **Natural Bristles**
1. Source: obtained from the hair of hog or wild boar.
2. Uniformity: varies. The bristles are not consistent in texture, size, flexibility, or wearing properties.
3. Stiffness: variations are related to the following:
   a. Diameter of bristle: wider diameters are stiffer. They vary in size from .0035 to .0190 inch depending on the portion of the bristle, the age and life of the animal. Those between .007 and

.010 previously were considered acceptable for use.
    b. Length of trim: shorter bristles are stiffer.
    c. Inherent resiliency: varies with the breed of animal as well as geographic location and season in which the bristles are taken.
4. Properties
    a. Water absorbent: become softened and stay softened longer.
    b. Bristles are hollow tubes which may harbor microorganisms.

B. **Nylon Filaments**
1. Source: manufactured according to federal specifications governing physical properties, composition, and diameter.
2. Uniformity: controlled.
3. Stiffness
    a. Diameter: thinner filaments are softer and more resilient.
    b. Diameter of soft nylon brushes: .006 to .007 inch.
    c. Diameter of regular nylon brushes: .008 inch = soft; .012 inch = medium; .014 inch = hard; .016 inch = extra hard.
4. Properties
    a. Rinse clean and dry rapidly.
    b. Maintain form longer than natural bristles.

V. Toothbrush Selection for the Patient

A. **Influencing Factors** (see also pages 386–387)
    Factors which influence the selection of the proper toothbrush for the individual patient include the following:
1. Ability of the patient to use the brush and remove plaque from all tooth surfaces without damage to the soft tissue or tooth structure.
2. Status of gingival or periodontal health.
3. Anatomic configurations of the gingiva.
4. Method of brushing to be recommended and instructed.
5. Position of teeth: displaced teeth require variations in brush placement.
6. Personal preferences
    a. Professional personnel preferences: dentist and dental hygienist may prefer to instruct certain methods and with certain brushes.
    b. Patient may have preferences and may resist change.
7. Manual dexterity of patient.
8. Motivation, ability, and willingness to follow the prescribed procedures.

B. **Medium or Hard Brush: Tufted**
    Tufted medium or hard brushes were formerly used to a greater extent than currently. They are generally contraindicated because of potential damage to gingiva and teeth while removing plaque from the cervical thirds of the teeth. If they are used, careful supervision by examination for evidences of trauma is needed, and corrections of technique made (pages 324–325).

C. **Soft Nylon Brush: Tufted or Multitufted**
    The following are suggested as advantages for the use of the soft brush with rounded ends:
1. More effective in cleaning the cervical areas, both proximal and marginal.
2. Less traumatic to the gingival tissue, therefore patients can brush at the cervical area without fear of pain or lacerating the tissues.
3. Can be directed into the sulcus for sulcular brushing and into interproximal areas.

4. Applicable around fixed orthodontic appliances, or fixation appliances required in fractured jaw treatment.
5. For overvigorous brushers whose efforts have led to dental abrasion or gingival recession.[7,8]
6. For sensitive gingiva in conditions such as necrotizing ulcerative gingivitis or desquamative gingivitis, or during healing stages following scaling and curettage or periodontal surgery.
7. Small size is ideal for a young child as a first brush on primary teeth.

TOOTHBRUSHING PROCEDURES

Complete toothbrushing instruction for the patient involves teaching many details related to why, what, when, where, and how. In addition to descriptions of specific toothbrushing methods, the succeeding sections will consider the grasp of the brush, the sequence and amount of brushing, the areas of limited access, supplementary brushing for the occlusal surfaces and the tongue, the possible detrimental effects from improper toothbrushing as well as the contraindications, and the care of toothbrushes.

I. Grasp of Brush

A. **Objectives**

Manipulation of the brush for successful plaque removal can be related to the manner in which the brush is held. Most patients need specific instruction in how to hold and place the brush. When they start to brush to remove the dental plaque which has been colored with a disclosing agent, there is realization of the tenaciousness of the plaque and the need for controlled pressure. With a firm, comfortable grasp, the following can be expected:
1. Control of the brush during all movements.

2. Effective positioning at the beginning of each brushing stroke, follow-through during the complete stroke, and repositioning for the next stroke.
3. Sensitivity to the amount of pressure applied.

B. **Procedure**
1. Grasp toothbrush handle in the palm of the hand with thumb against the shank.
   a. Near enough to the head of the brush so that it can be controlled effectively.
   b. Not so close to the head of brush that manipulation of the brush is hindered or that fingers can touch the anterior teeth when reaching the brush head to molar regions.
2. Direct bristles in the direction needed for placement on the teeth: direction is dependent on the brushing method to be used.
3. Adapt grasp for the various positions of the brush head on the teeth throughout the procedure: adjust to permit unrestricted movement of the wrist and arm.

II. Sequence

A. The procedure in brushing, for any method used, should have a definite sequence.
B. To prevent omission of an area, it is recommended that brushing follow from the molar region of one arch around to the opposite side then back around the lingual or facial of the same quadrant.
C. Each brush placement must overlap the previous one for thorough coverage (figure 22–3).
D. Encourage the patient to begin by brushing one of the following which most meets the individual needs:

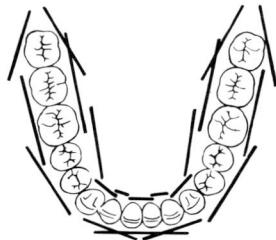

Figure 22–3. Brushing positions. A patient can be instructed to follow a specific order for brushing to prevent omissions. Each brush position, as indicated by a black line, should overlap the previous position. Note placement at canines where the distal of the canine is brushed with the premolars and the mesial is brushed with the incisors. Short lines on lingual anterior indicate brush placed the long narrow way. The maxillary teeth require a similar number of brushing positions.

1. Areas which are most frequently missed.
2. Areas which are most difficult for brush placement and/or manipulation such as the right side for the right-handed brusher or the left side for the left-handed brusher.

E. Suggest that the sequence be changed at least once each day so that the same areas are not always brushed last when the time may be limited and plaque removal may be less complete.

III. Amount of Brushing

A. **The Count System**
For thorough coverage, even distribution of amount of brushing, and to help the patient concentrate on the performance, a system of counting is useful.
1. Count six strokes in each area (or five or ten whichever is most appropriate for the particular patient): for the Rolling Stroke, Modified Stillman, or other method in which a stroke is used.
2. Count slowly to ten for each brush position while brush is vibrated and bristle ends are held in position for the Bass, Charters', or other vibratory method.

B. **The Clock System**
Some patients brush thoroughly while watching a clock or an egg timer for three or four minutes. Timed procedures cannot assure thorough coverage, since single areas which are most accessible may get more time. Patients for whom this system is recommended must be selected carefully.

IV. Frequency of Brushing

Because of individual variations, one set rule for frequency cannot be applied. For the control of plaque, and for oral sanitation and halitosis prevention, more than one brushing and flossing each day is recommended. For patients who have difficulty in changing habits to make oral care a basic necessity, it is probably better for them to have one thorough brushing than several incomplete attempts. When teeth are hastily and partially brushed, it is not unusual for the brusher to omit the same tooth surface each time.

Going to sleep with a clean mouth should be encouraged. For patients who will be using a chewable fluoride tablet, mouthrinse, or custom tray gel application before going to bed, plaque removal before fluoride application is recommended. The fluoride remains on the teeth for a period of time after application.

Suggested recommendations are as follows[9]:

A. Conscientious adult patients who demonstrate their ability to perform complete plaque control measures and who do not have gingival or periodontal disease or evidence of caries susceptibility: one brushing and flossing each day may be sufficient. Such patients usually prefer and are accustomed to more than one brushing, and no change of habits should be recommended.

B. Adult patients with gingival or periodontal involvement under treat ment, or who have been treated for periodontal disease: minimum of two brushings and one flossing with other aids as necessary. A fluoride dentifrice is particularly recommended when there is exposed cementum as an aid in the prevention of root caries.

C. Young patients with gingival disease (or tendency towards gingival involvement): at least two and preferably three brushings, preferably after eating, and one flossing each day.

D. Patients of all ages who show susceptibility to dental caries: thorough brushing after each meal and before going to bed to prevent fermentation of sweet foods left about the teeth. The patient should be reminded that more frequent application of fluoride dentifrice brings greater prevention benefits.

V. Methods

Most toothbrushing methods can be classified into one of seven groups based on the motion applied by the brush.[10] Noted below beside certain categories are names of methods which utilize the designated motion as part or all of their particular procedure. Some of these methods are recorded for descriptive, comparative, or historic purposes only, and are not currently recommended. A few have even been proved detrimental.

A. **Roll:** Rolling Stroke, Modified Stillman's.

B. **Vibratory:** Stillman's, Charters', Bass.*

C. **Circular:** Fones'.

D. **Vertical:** Leonard's.

E. **Horizontal.**

F. **Physiological:** Smith's.

G. **Scrub-brush.**

*The Bass technique is not in the strictest sense a vibratory technique since a tiny back and forth stroke is used (pages 315–316).

THE ROLL or ROLLING STROKE METHOD

I. Purposes and Indications

A. Cleaning gingiva and removal of plaque, materia alba, and food debris from the teeth without emphasis on gingival sulcus.
1. For children and adults with relatively healthy gingiva and normal tissue contour.
2. For general cleaning in conjunction with the use of a vibratory technique (Charters', Stillman's, or Bass).

B. Useful for preparatory instruction (first lesson) for Modified Stillman's technique since the initial brush placement is the same. This can be particularly helpful when there is a question as to how complicated a technique the patient can master and practice.

II. Technique[5,11]

A. **Grasp** brush so that bristles are directed apically (up for maxillary, down for mandibular teeth).

B. **Place** sides of brush on the attached gingiva with bristles directed apically. (When brush handle is level with occlusal or incisal plane, generally the brush will be at the proper height, figure 22–4A).

C. **Press** to flex bristles (gingiva will blanch).

D. **Roll** slowly down over the teeth, turning the wrist slightly, so that bristles remain flexed and will follow the contour of the teeth, therefore permitting the cleaning of the cervical areas. Some bristles will reach interproximally.

E. **Replace** and **repeat** at least five times for each tooth or group. (To remove and replace brush, rotate wrist, move

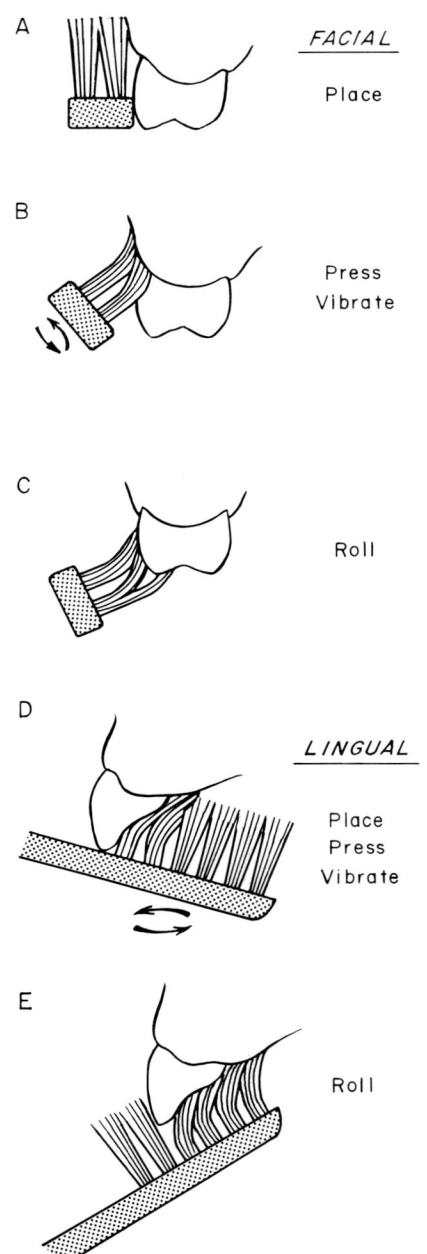

Figure 22–4.   Modified Stillman's method of brushing. **A.** Initial brush placement with sides of bristles or filaments against attached gingiva. **B.** The brush is pressed and angled, then vibrated, with sides of brush ends partly on the gingiva and partly on the tooth. **C.** Vibrating is continued as the brush is rolled over the crown to complete the stroke. **D.** Maxillary anterior lingual placement and activation. The brush is applied the long way. **E.** Vibrating continues as the brush is rolled over the crown and interdental areas. Placement for lingual of mandibular anterior is the same as for maxillary with the brush turned down.

brush away from teeth, stretch cheek buccally with the back of the brush to give space. Take care not to drag the bristle tips over the gingival margin when the brush is returned to the initial position, figure 22–4A).

F. Overlap when moving to the adjacent position.

G. For lingual of maxillary and mandibular anterior components
1. Use the brush the long, narrow way.
2. Hook the heel of the brush on the incisal edge (figure 22–4D).
3. Press down for maxillary (up for mandibular) until the bristles lie flat against the teeth and gingiva.
4. Press and roll (curve up for mandibular, down for maxillary teeth).
5. Replace and repeat five times for each brush width. (Brush placement across the anterior lingual can be compared with the hands of a clock or spokes of a wheel.)

III. Problems

A. Brushing too high during initial placement can lacerate the alveolar mucosa.
B. Tendency for using quick, sweeping strokes results in no brushing for the cervical third of the tooth, since the brush tips pass over rather than into the area; and likewise for the interproximal areas.

THE MODIFIED STILLMAN METHOD

This method as originally described by Stillman[12] was designed for massage and stimulation as well as for cleaning the cervical areas. The brush ends were placed partly on the gingiva and partly on the cervical of the tooth, directed slightly apically, and pressure was applied to effect a blanching. The handle was given a slight rotary motion with the brush end maintained in position on the tooth surface. After several applications, the brush was moved to the adjacent tooth.

In current use, a Modified Stillman incorporates a rolling stroke after the vibratory (rotary) phase. The modifications minimize the possibility of gingival trauma and increase the cleaning effects.[13]

I. Purposes and Indications

A. Dental plaque removal from cervical areas below the height of contour of the enamel and from exposed proximal surfaces.

B. General application for cleaning tooth surfaces and massage of the gingiva.

II. Technique (figure 22–4)

A. **Grasp** brush so that bristles are directed apically (up for maxillary, down for mandibular teeth).

B. **Place** sides of bristles against attached gingiva. (When handle is level with the occlusal or incisal plane, generally the brush will be at the proper height.)

C. **Press** to flex bristles (gingiva will blanch).

D. **Angle** at approximately 45 degrees with long axis of tooth.

E. **Vibrate** gently but firmly: maintain pressure on bristles and keep tips of bristles in position. Count to ten slowly as brush is vibrated by a rotary motion of the handle.

F. **Roll** and **vibrate** brush by turning the wrist, work slowly down over the tooth, making the bristles go between the teeth.

G. **Replace** brush by rotating wrist, remove brush slightly away from the tooth to avoid dragging the bristles over the free margin of the gingiva on the way back to the initial position.

H. **Repeat** at least five times at each position, taking care to overlap placement on the adjacent position.

I. For lingual of maxillary and mandibular anterior components

1. Position brush the long narrow way, as described for the Rolling Stroke technique (figure 22–4D).
2. Another method is to divide the brush over the incisal so that two or three rows of tufts engage the teeth and gingiva on the lingual. Press and vibrate.

III. Problems

A. Without careful brush placement, tissue laceration can result when a hard brush is used. A soft brush used with lighter pressure is preferred.

B. Patient may try to move the brush into the rolling stroke too quickly, and the vibratory aspect may be ineffective in plaque removal at the gingival margin.

THE BASS METHOD: SULCULAR BRUSHING

The Bass technique is widely accepted as the most effective method for dental plaque removal adjacent to and directly beneath the gingival margin. This area around the tooth is the most significant in the control of gingival and periodontal disease. Because of potential damage to the gingival tissue, only a soft nylon brush with rounded filament ends is indicated.

I. Purposes and Indications

A. Dental plaque removal adjacent to and directly beneath the gingival margin.

B. Particularly adaptable for open interproximal areas, cervical areas beneath the height of contour of the enamel, and exposed root surfaces.

C. Useful for the periodontal surgery patient following removal of dressings.

II. Technique[14]

A. **Grasp** brush so that the filaments are directed apically (up for maxillary, down for mandibular). Even though the brush placement calls for directing the filaments at a 45-degree angle, it is usually easier for the patient to adjust

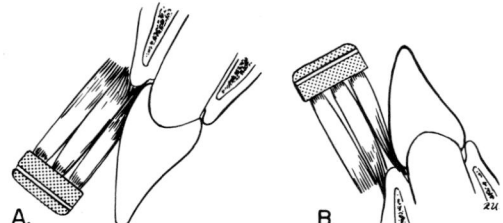

Figure 22–5. Sulcular method of brushing. Filament tips are directed into the gingival sulcus. The filaments are placed at approximately 45 degrees with the long axis of the tooth. **A.** Maxillary facial. **B.** Mandibular facial.

the brush after first placing it parallel to the long axis of the tooth.

B. **Place—Angle:** Place brush with the filament tips directed straight into the gingival sulcus. The filaments will be placed at approximately 45 degrees with the long axis of the tooth (figure 22–5).

C. **Press** lightly so that the filament tips enter the gingival sulci and embrasures and cover the gingival margin. Do not flex the filaments.

D. **Vibrate** the brush back and forth with short strokes without disengaging the tips of the filaments from the sulci. Count ten strokes.

E. **Replace and Repeat:** Apply brush to the next group of two or three teeth; take care to overlap placement with the adjacent position. Follow around each arch until every facial surface and every lingual surface has been brushed.

F. **Lingual Anterior:** Hold brush the long narrow way. Apply toe filaments for sulcular brushing (figure 22–6).

G. **Rinse.**

III. Problems

A. An over-eager brusher may convert the "very short strokes" (note II, D. above) into a scrub-brush technique and cause injury to the gingival margin.

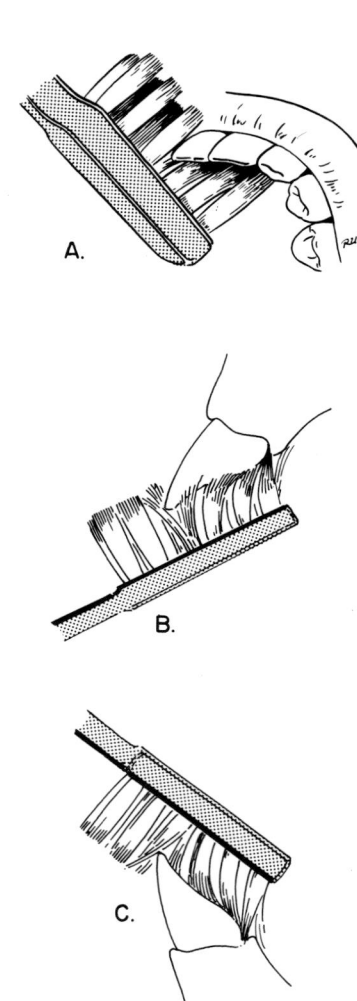

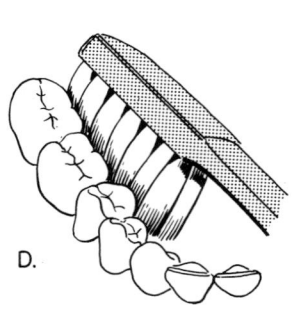

Figure 22–6. Sulcular brushing, lingual surfaces. **A.** Brush positioned for maxillary anterior. **B.** Filament tips are directed into the gingival sulcus. **C.** Lingual of mandibular anterior with filaments in sulcus. **D.** Brush positioned for lingual of posterior.

B. Rolling Stroke procedure may precede the sulcular brushing when a patient believes it helps to clean the teeth. It is recommended that the two techniques are performed separately rather than trying to combine them in what has been referred to as a "modified Bass." The procedure of rolling the brush down over the crown after the vibratory part of the sulcular brush stroke has several disadvantages: (1) too often the brush is hastily and carelessly replaced into the sulcus position, or else the opposite is true and considerable time is consumed in the attempt to replace the brush carefully, (2) gingival margin injury by the constant replacement of the brush is common, and (3) concentration is not on the important objective which is to remove the plaque at the gingival margin. Patients tend to roll the brush down over the crown prematurely and very little sulcular brushing may be accomplished.

THE CHARTERS' METHOD

The original intent, as described by Charters,[15] was to use the toothbrush in a manner which would stimulate the gingival margin "all around each tooth, especially in the inter-dental spaces." The method is generally not used when there are normal interdental papillae since other methods may be easier to teach.

I. Purposes and Indications

A. Loosening of debris and plaque.

B. Massage and stimulation for marginal and interdental gingiva.

C. Indicated for open interdental areas when interproximal tissue is missing as, for example, following periodontal surgery.

D. Adaptable to cervical areas below the height of contour of the crown, and to exposed root surfaces.

E. Useful for cleaning abutment teeth and under the gingival border of a fixed partial denture (bridge), or the under-surface of a sanitary bridge.

F. Aids in cleansing orthodontic appliances (page 360).

II. Technique[16]

A. Instruct in a basic Rolling Stroke technique for general cleaning.

B. Hold brush (outside oral cavity) with bristles toward occlusal or incisal plane (bristle tips are pointed down for application to maxillary and up for application to mandibular arch).

C. **Place** sides of bristles or filaments against the enamel with brush tips toward the occlusal or incisal.

D. **Angle** at approximately 45 degrees with the occlusal plane. Move brush to the position at the junction of the free margin and the cervical third of the teeth (figure 22–7 B).

E. **Press** to flex bristles and force the tips between the teeth. The sides of the bristles press against the gingival margin.

F. **Vibrate** gently but firmly, keeping the tips of the bristles in position. Count to ten slowly as brush is vibrated by a rotary motion of the handle.

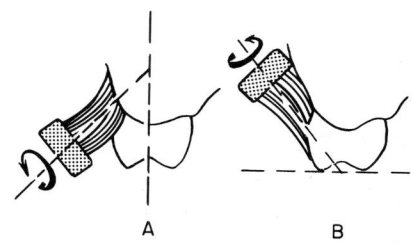

A   B

Figure 22–7. Comparison of brush positions for Stillman's and Charters' methods. **A.** Stillman's. The brush is angled at approximately 45 degrees with the long axis of the tooth. **B.** Charters'. The brush is angled at approximately 45 degrees with the occlusal plane, with brush tips directed toward the occlusal or incisal.

G. **Repeat** several times in each position as defined by the specific needs of the patient.

H. Proceed to adjacent area: make certain that each interproximal embrasure is treated.

I. For fixed partial denture: when placing the brush, check that bristle tips are directed under the gingival border of the pontic.

J. Lingual application: since Charters' brush positioning is difficult to accomplish on the lingual, a Modified Stillman's is frequently advised. When Charters' method is preferred, the position is as follows:
   1. Posterior
      a. With brush tips pointed toward the occlusal, extend the brush handle across the incisal of the canine of the side opposite that to be brushed.
      b. Place the sides of the toe-end bristles against the distal of the most posterior tooth and subsequently at each embrasure.
      c. Press and vibrate.
   2. Anterior
      a. With brush handle parallel with the long axis of the tooth, place the sides of the toe-end bristles over the interproximal embrasure.
      b. Press and vibrate.

K. Rinse thoroughly to remove loosened particles.

III. Problems

A. Brush ends do not engage the gingival sulcus to remove submarginal bacterial accumulations.

B. In some areas, the correct brush placement is limited or impossible; therefore modifications become necessary which add to the complexity of the procedure.

C. Requirements in digital dexterity are high, so few patients continue to use this method indefinitely.

OTHER TOOTHBRUSHING METHODS

The Rolling Stroke, Modified Stillman's, and Bass are probably the methods most used for patient instruction by dentists and dental hygienists. Other methods are and have been used, and few of the well-known ones are included here. As these are reviewed, it will be realized that there is overlap in the technique and intent of some of the methods. Evaluation prior to special instruction generally reveals that a mixture of techniques may be in use by a patient.

I. Circular: The Fones' Method

It is likely that many people, especially school children, received instruction in this method since it was advocated by Fones who founded the first course for dental hygienists. He described the technique in the first dental hygiene text which was used by dental hygiene students throughout the United States for many years.

Although now considered a technique which could be detrimental for adults, particularly when used by a vigorous brusher, it is sometimes recommended as an easy-to-learn first technique for young children. A soft brush with .006 .008" filament diameter is recommended. In abbreviated form, the technique described by Dr. Fones included the following.[17]

A. With the teeth closed, place the brush inside the cheek with the brush tip lightly contacting the gingiva over the last maxillary molar.

B. Use a fast, wide, circular motion which sweeps from the maxillary gingiva to the mandibular gingiva with very little pressure.

C. Bring anterior teeth in end-to-end

contact, and hold lip out when necessary to make the continuous circular strokes.

D. Lingual: use an in-and-out stroke. Brush sweeps across palate on maxillary and back and forth to the molars on the mandibular.

II. Vertical: Leonard's Method

As described by Hirschfeld,[18] the up-and-down stroke is employed when teeth are cleaned with a crude, twig, primitive toothbrush. The true vertical stroke passes from the gingiva over the maxillary to the gingiva over the mandibular, with a vigorous sweeping motion.

Leonard described and advocated a vertical stroke in which maxillary and mandibular teeth are brushed separately. Paraphrased, he described his method as follows.[19]

A. With the teeth edge-to-edge, place the brush with the bristles against the teeth at right angles to the long axes of the teeth.

B. Brush vigorously, without great pressure, with a stroke which is mostly up and down on the tooth surfaces, with just a slight rotation or circular movement after striking the gingival margin with force.

C. Use enough pressure to force the bristles into the embrasure area, but not enough to injure the brush.

D. It is not intended that the upper and lower teeth shall be brushed in the same series of strokes: the teeth are placed in edge-to-edge to keep the brush from slipping over the occlusal or incisal.

III. Horizontal

Horizontal or crosswise brushing is generally accepted as detrimental. An unlimited sweep with a scrubbing motion horizontally will bear pressure on teeth that are most facially inclined or prominent, and with an abrasive dentifrice may produce tooth abrasion. Since the interdental areas are not touched by this method, various gingival and periodontal problems may ensue.

IV. Physiological: Smith's Method

The physiological method was described by Smith[20] and advocated later by Bell.[21] It was based on the principle that the toothbrush should follow the physiological pathway that food does when it traverses over the tissues in a "natural" masticating act.

A soft brush with "small tufts of fine bristles arranged in four parallel rows and trimmed to an even length" was used in a brushing stroke directed down over the lower teeth onto the gingiva and upward over the teeth for the maxillary. Smith also suggested a few gentle horizontal strokes to clean the portion of the sulci directly over the bifurcations of the roots.

V. Scrub-Brush

It can be said that vigorously combined horizontal, vertical, and circular strokes with some vibratory motions for certain areas, comprise a scrub-brush technique. A soft brush with rounded brush ends such as that recommended in particular for the Bass technique, can be used with a very short-stroked scrub-brush technique for plaque removal in the cervical area following periodontal surgery. However, without caution, vigorous scrubbing can encourage gingival recession, and with a dentifrice of sufficient abrasiveness, create areas of tooth abrasion.

AUTOMATIC TOOTHBRUSHES

Automatic brushes are also known as powered, mechanical, and electric brushes. The American Dental Association, Council on Dental Materials and Devices, has the responsibility for the evaluation of automatic brushes.[22] When a device is considered for approval, research evidence must be available that unsupervised use will not be harmful to oral hard or soft tissues or restorations; that it can be used readily by the unsupervised public to provide efficient cleaning when used according to the directions provided by the manufacturer; and that claims in advertising shall be limited to oral cleanliness and not to claims of treatment for existing oral diseases.

The development and promotion of power-driven toothbrushes has stimulated research related to toothbrushing and its effects. Summaries of research[23,24] and a comprehensive consideration of the multiple problems connected with this type of research are available.[25]

Comparisons have been made in research between the automatic and the manual brushes to determine the ability of each type to remove plaque, prevent calculus development, and reduce the incidence of gingivitis. Both types have been shown effective when used correctly. A bibliography of research studies is provided in the *Suggested Readings* at the end of this chapter.

I. Description[26,27]

A. **Head**

The head, connected to the shank, is detachable from the handle and replaceable. In general, automatic brush heads are smaller than manual brushes. They range in size from approximately ¼ to ½ inch wide by ¾ inch long.

B. **Filaments**

Most automatic brushes are multi-tufted with three or four rows of tufts. The diameter of the filaments is from .005 to .007 inch to .010 or .012 inch.

C. **Motion**

The action on different models may be one of the following:

1. Reciprocating: moves back and forth in a line.
2. Arcuate: filament ends follow an arc as they move up and down.
3. Orbital: circular.
4. Vibratory
5. Elliptical: oval.
6. Dual motion: more than one of the above.

D. **Power Source**

1. Direct: cord from electrical outlet connects directly to the toothbrush handle.
2. Replaceable batteries: disadvantage in the nuisance and cost of repeatedly replacing or recharging batteries; also, as the batteries lose their power, the brush is slowed. Corrosion may be a problem if water gets into the case.
3. Rechargeable: the instrument is placed into a stand which contains the recharger and which is connected to the electrical outlet. A few models have a recharger built into the handle.
4. Switches: a few models require that the push button be held down during operation which may present difficulties for some patients such as small children or persons with certain types of handicaps.

E. **Speeds**

Speeds vary with the different models from low to high. Some have the speed coordinated with the filament texture, for example, a soft small brush with a fast vigorous action, or a larger harder brush with a slower, more gentle motion. The number of strokes per minute varies from, for example, as low as 1000 cycles per minute for a replaceable battery type, to about 3600 oscillations per minute for an arcuate model. Between, the rechargeable battery types operate at approximately 2000 complete strokes per minute.

II. Purposes and Indications

A. General Application

For all patients for the removal of dental plaque, materia alba, and food debris. All of the general objectives which apply to plaque control measures and to manual brushes apply to the automatics.

B. Handicapped Patients

Automatic brushes have been shown to be easily handled and manipulated by patients with certain crippling handicaps (page 657).

C. Patients Unable to Brush

The automatic brush is readily handled by a parent, attendant, or other person who cares for the patient.

III. Instruction Compared with Manual

With a manual brush, an individual must learn to use his hand and arm in certain ways in order that each surface of each tooth be reached, slight pressure be applied for a thorough brushing effect, and the stroke be repeated a number of times. With the automatic, the action is built in. The only muscle training required is turning the handle to apply the brush to each surface of each tooth and holding it there for a reasonable length of time in a correct position.

It was observed in one research study[28] that in a group of patients who did not receive specific instruction, the persons with good manual dexterity tended to clean their teeth and remove plaque whether they used the manual or the automatic brush, whereas those with poor dexterity did best with the powered brush. In another experiment[29] where neither the subjects using the manual brush nor those with the automatic were given instruction in how to use the brushes, it was shown that after three months the ones who had used the automatic toothbrush had significantly less gingivitis than those with the manual brush.

Not to underestimate the amount of instruction and practice needed for effective use of an automatic brush, it appears that learning to use a manual brush requires more patience, time, and skill. An automatic brush, on the other hand, seems to be able to overcome some of the problems, at least with some patients.

IV. Methods for Use

The general suggestions presented here are basic and, as with all brushing techniques, need adaptations for an individual mouth. The dental hygienist should become familar with the instructions provided by the manufacturers of various automatic brushes. Other references concerning instruction for use are available in the dental scientific literature for supplementary study.[30,31]

A. Select brush with soft filaments. For sulcular brushing, select extra-soft.

B. Select dentifrice with minimum abrasivity. The extra strokes made by an automatic brush increase the effects of abrasion to the tooth surface.

C. Spread the dentifrice over the teeth and work some between the filaments of the brush to prevent splashing when the power is turned on.

D. Brush position: Nearly all brushing techniques can be applied for use with an automatic brush. For vibratory techniques, wrist motion to change the brush position is not needed.

E. Vary the brush position for each tooth surface: brush each tooth separately.
   1. Apply the brush to the distal, facial, mesial surfaces of each tooth as the brush is moved from the most posterior teeth toward the anterior, quadrant by quadrant.
   2. Hold the brush in one location for a period of time, turn it or move it to reach adjacent areas while keeping the power on.
   3. Angulate for access to surfaces of

rotated, crowded, or otherwise displaced teeth.
4. Retract lip with fingers of other hand, to give access to and visibility of anterior facial surfaces, particularly including prominent canines.
5. Modify brush positions for application to proximal surfaces when there are missing interdental papillae: brush head may be positioned parallel with the long axis and inserted proximally for anterior teeth.

F. Strokes: make strokes slowly, with a slight to moderate steady pressure.

G. Rinse.

H. Precautions: acrylic restorations should be treated without pressure or avoided, as they can wear down under repeated application of the fast-moving filaments with dentifrice.

I. Special application: following periodontal surgery
1. After removal of dressing: use brush without power as a multitufted soft brush for plaque removal during first 12 hours.
2. Use soft brush insert with power and light pressure with regular procedure as soon as possible.

SUPPLEMENTAL BRUSHING

I. Problem Areas

Each surface of each tooth must be brushed. Initial instruction may necessarily be limited to a basic procedure, particularly when it varies from the patient's present procedures. At succeeding lessons, a disclosing agent is used, and the special hard-to-get areas are shown to the patient. Suggestions are made and demonstrated for brush adaptation for areas which were missed. Methods for cleaning the interdental areas and fixed and removable appliances are described in the two chapters following.

Attention in teaching should be given the following:

A. Facially displaced teeth, especially canines and premolars where toothbrush abrasion frequently occurs.

B. Surfaces of teeth next to edentulous areas.

C. Inclined teeth: for example, lingual surfaces of mandibular molars that are inclined lingually.

D. Exposed root surfaces; exposed proximal surfaces.

E. Exposed furcation areas.

F. Right canine and lateral incisor, both maxillary and mandibular, are commonly missed by right-handed brushers; the opposite for left-handed.

G. Distal surfaces of most posterior teeth (figure 22–8).

II. Occlusal Brushing

A. Objectives
1. To loosen plaque organisms packed in pits and fissures.
2. To remove plaque deposits from occlusal surfaces of teeth out of occlusion or not used during mastication.
3. To remove plaque from the margins of restorations.
4. To apply fluoride from fluoride dentifrice.

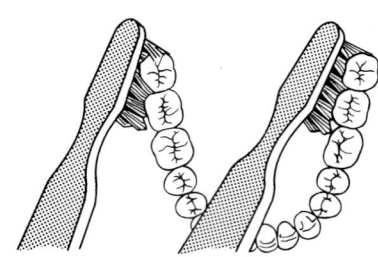

Figure 22–8. Brushing problems. Brush placement to clean the distal surfaces of the most posterior teeth. The distobuccal is approached by stretching the cheek; the distolingual by directing the brush across from the canine of the opposite side.

B. Technique

1. Place brush on occlusal of molar teeth with filament tips pointed into the occlusal pits at a right angle. The handle should be parallel with the occlusal surface. The toe of the brush should be at the distal of the most posterior tooth.

2. Two acceptable strokes are suggested:

   a. Vibrate the brush in a slight circular movement while maintaining the filament tips on the occlusal surface throughout a count of ten. Press moderately so filaments do not bend but go straight into the pits and fissures (figure 22–9).

   b. Force the filaments against the occlusal surface with sharp, quick strokes; lift the brush off each time to dislodge debris; repeat about ten times.

3. Move brush to premolar area, overlapping previous brush position.

4. Rinse thoroughly: the particles were loosened, not brushed away.

C. Precaution

Long scrubbing strokes from anterior to posterior on an occlusal surface contact only the prominent parts of the cusps, which are usually self-cleansing (figure 22–9 B).

III. Tongue Brushing

Total mouth cleanliness includes tongue brushing.

A. Microorganisms of the Tongue

1. Main foci for oral microorganisms.
   a. Dorsum of tongue.
   b. Gingival sulci and pockets.
   c. Dental plaque on all teeth.
2. Microorganisms in saliva are principally from the tongue.
3. Tongue organisms influence the flora of the entire oral cavity.

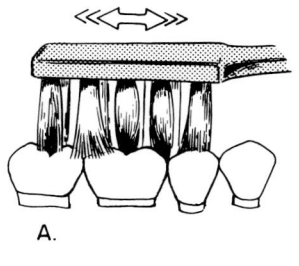

A.

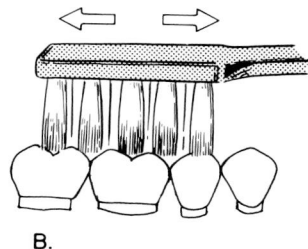

B.

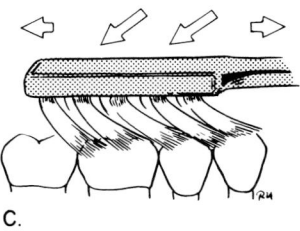

C.

Figure 22–9. Occlusal brushing. **A.** Vibrating brush with light pressure while maintaining the filament tips on the occlusal surface to permit tips to work their way into the pits and fissures. **B.** Long horizontal strokes contact only the cusp tips. **C.** Excess pressure curves filament tips away from pits and fissures and damages the filaments.

B. Effects of Cleaning the Tongue[32,33]

1. Reduction of oral debris.
2. Retardation of plaque formation and total plaque accumulation.
3. Reduction of number of microorganisms. When brushing of the tongue is stopped, the number of organisms increases.
4. Contribution to overall cleanliness.

C. Tongue Anatomy Conducive to Debris Retention

1. Surface papillae: numerous filiform papillae extend as minute projections, while fungiform papillae

are not as high and create elevations and depressions which entrap debris and microorganisms.

2. Fissured tongue: fissures may be several millimeters deep and retain debris.

D. Brushing Procedure

1. Hold the brush handle at a right angle to the midline of the tongue and direct the brush tips toward the throat.
2. With the tongue extruded, the sides of the filaments are placed on the posterior part of the surface.
3. With light pressure draw the brush forward and over the tip of the tongue. Repeat three or four times. Do not scrub the papillae.
4. Rinse.

EFFECTS OF IMPROPER TOOTHBRUSHING

I. Toothbrush Trauma: The Gingiva[34]

A. Acute Alterations

1. *Appearance*
   a. Scuffed epithelial surface with denuded underlying connective tissue.
   b. Punctate lesions which appear as red, pinpoint spots.
   c. Diffuse redness and denuded attached gingiva.
2. *Etiology*
   a. Horizontal or vertical scrubbing toothbrushing method with pressure.
   b. Overvigorous placement and application of the toothbrush.
   c. Penetration of gingiva by filament ends.
   d. Use of toothbrush with frayed, broken bristles or filaments.
   e. Application of filaments beyond attached gingiva.

B. Chronic Alterations

1. *Location*
   a. Usually appear only on the facial gingiva, because of the vigor with which toothbrush is used.
   b. Frequently, inversely related to the right- or left-handedness of the patient.
   c. Areas most often involved are around canines or teeth in labio- or buccoversion.
2. *Recession*[7,8,35]
   a. Appearance: margin of gingiva has receded toward the apex, and the cementum is exposed (page 171).
   b. Predisposing anatomic factors.
      (1) Malposition of teeth: teeth in buccoversion usually have thin alveolar bone covering the buccal surface.
      (2) Narrow band of attached gingiva cannot withstand pressures of brushing.
3. *Changes in gingival contour*
   a. Rolled, bulbous, hard, firm marginal gingiva, in "piled up" or festoon shape (page 171).
   b. Gingival cleft: narrow groove or slit that extends from the crest of the gingiva to the attached gingiva ("Stillman's Cleft," page 171).
4. *Etiology*
   a. Repeated use of a vigorous rotary, vertical, or horizontal toothbrushing method over a long period of time.
   b. Use of a long brisk stroke with excessive pressure, over a long period of time.
   c. Habitual prolonged brushing in one area.
   d. Excessive pressure applied with a worn, nonresilient brush.

C. Suggested Corrective Measures

1. Recommend substitution of a softer toothbrush permanently or at least until the acute phase of alteration subsides and normal tissue tone is restored.

2. Correct the patient's toothbrushing technique or demonstrate a toothbrushing method better suited to his oral condition.

II. Abrasion of the Teeth[36]

Abrasion is the loss of tooth substance produced by mechanical wear other than that by mastication, or, as defined on page 211, it is the pathologic wearing away of tooth substance through some abnormal mechanical process. Factors which are related to abrasion from toothbrushing include the composition of the dentifrice, method of brushing, and the force of brushing.

Several research studies have been made. Tests did not show more abrasion from natural or nylon brushes, but the abrasiveness of the dentifrice made a definite difference.[37] The hardness of the brush is significant. In one study, it was shown that a hard brush caused nearly four times as much wear as a soft brush.[38] In other experiments a manual hard brush was shown to produce more pressure than either a manual soft brush or an automatic soft brush.[39]

A. **Location of Abrasion**
   1. Primarily on facial surfaces especially of canines, premolars, and sometimes first molars, or any tooth in bucco- or labioversion, those most available to the pressure of the toothbrush. The canines are susceptible because of their prominence on the curvature of the dental arches.
   2. Most abraded areas are on the cervical areas of exposed root surfaces, but occasionally may occur on the enamel. When adjacent teeth are involved, the lesions appear in line with each other.

B. **Appearance**
   Saucer-shaped or wedge-shaped indentations with smooth shiny surfaces (figure 13–3, page 212).

C. **Corrective Measures**
   1. Advise a brush with soft-textured bristles or filaments if the patient used a hard one.
   2. Change the angle of brush application.
   3. Recommend a less abrasive dentifrice (page 347).

CONTRAINDICATIONS FOR TOOTHBRUSHING

Even when an unusual oral condition develops, a patient must be encouraged to brush whenever possible to reduce the possibility of infection by decreasing the oral bacterial count. There are no indications for prolonged omission of techniques of plaque removal. Examples of conditions which may indicate a temporary departure from personal care routines are:

A. **Acute Oral Inflammatory or Traumatic Lesions**
   When an acute oral condition precludes normal brushing, the patient should be instructed to brush all areas of the mouth which are not affected, and resume regular plaque control measures on the affected area as soon as possible. When not otherwise contraindicated by instructions from the dentist, rinsing with a warm, mild saline solution can encourage healing and debris removal.

B. **Following Periodontal Surgery**
   Patients will need to receive instructions concerning brushing. Since direct brushing of a periodontal dressing could displace it, brushing of the occlusal surfaces only is advised. Other teeth and gingiva should be brushed as usual. Additional instructions appear in table 35–1, on page 528.

C. **Acute Stage of Acute Necrotizing Ulcerative Gingivitis**
   A major contributing factor in the development of this disease is a lack of

oral cleanliness. During the acute stage, the oral tissues are sensitive to any touch, and toothbrushing will be neglected. Instructions for these patients are on page 601. A very soft brush is indicated along with careful brush placement to avoid trauma.

D. **Following Dental Extraction**

Instructions may be found on page 614 and include brushing all except the surgical wound area. Teeth adjacent to the extraction site need cleaning as soon as possible, to reduce bacterial collections and decrease the possibility of oral infection.

E. **Following Dental Restorations**

Patients will have a tendency to avoid a new crown, newly placed fixed partial denture, or other appliance. Specific instructions should be given at the time of insertion.

CARE OF TOOTHBRUSHES

When discussing the type and features of the brush selected for an individual patient, the number of brushes needed and the frequency of replacement can be included. Perhaps the ideal time to teach cleaning and daily care of brushes would be after a practice session when the brush has to be washed and cleaned for storage at the dental office.

That patients need instruction concerning the care and supply of their brushes is apparent from a survey of family toothbrush practices conducted by the American Dental Association.[40] From the questions asked the 866 participating families (2986 people), about one-half stated they used a toothbrush from four to six months; 20 percent used a brush from 10 to 12 months; and five percent over one year.

The condition of a brush is dependent on many factors including the amount and manner of use, the type of care, as well as the quality of the brush at the start. Toothbrushes in current use were col-

lected from the families in the survey mentioned above and evaluated. Only 44 percent were considered satisfactory for use. The unsatisfactory brushes were worn out, and dangerous for the gingiva because of marked splaying. Many were caked with dentifrice or unsightly deposits, and a few had broken plastic heads.[40]

I. Supply of Brushes

A. Advise at least two brushes for home use and a third portable one for use at work, school, or travel.

B. Brush purchase should be staggered so that all brushes are not new at the same time, but more important that they are not old at the same time so that the gingival condition is maintained at less than optimum.

C. Replace brushes before bristles or filaments become splayed, frayed, or lose resiliency. Worn brushes remove significantly less plaque than new brushes.[41]

II. Cleaning Toothbrushes

A. Clean thoroughly after each use.

B. Hold brush head under strong stream of warm water from faucet to force particles, dentifrice, and bacteria from between the bristles.

C. Tap the handle on edge of sink to remove remaining particles.

D. Use another toothbrush to clean a brush: bristles or filaments can be worked between those of the other brush to remove resistant debris.

E. Rinse completely and tap out excess water.

III. Brush Storage

A. Keep brush in open air with head in an upright position, apart from contact with other brushes, particularly those of another person.

B. Portable brush container should have sufficient holes to give air temporarily until the brush can be completely exposed for drying. A closed container encourages bacterial growth.

References

1. Hirschfeld, I.: *The Toothbrush: Its Use and Abuse.* Brooklyn, N.Y., Dental Items of Interest, 1939, pp. 1–27.
2. Kimery, M. J. and Stallard, R. E.: The Evolutionary Development and Contemporary Utilization of Various Oral Hygiene Procedures, *Periodont. Abstr.,* 16, 90, September, 1968.
3. McCauley, H. B.: Toothbrushes, Toothbrush Materials and Design, *J. Am. Dent. Assoc.,* 33, 283, March 1, 1946.
4. Weinberger, B. W.: *An Introduction to the History of Dentistry.* St. Louis, Mosby, 1948, pp. 43, 140–144.
5. American Academy of Periodontology, Committee Report: The Tooth Brush and Methods of Cleaning the Teeth, *Dent. Items Int.,* 42, 193, March, 1920.
6. American Dental Association, Council on Dental Therapeutics: *Accepted Dental Therapeutics,* 36th ed. Chicago, American Dental Association, 1975, p. 281.
7. Gorman, W. J.: Prevalence and Etiology of Gingival Recession, *J. Periodont.,* 38, 316, July-August, 1967.
8. O'Leary, T. J., Drake, R. B., Jividen, G. J., and Allen, M. F.: The Incidence of Recession in Young Males: Relationship to Gingival and Plaque Scores, *Periodontics,* 6, 109, June, 1968.
9. Katz, S., McDonald, J. L., and Stookey, G. K.: *Preventive Dentistry in Action.* Upper Montclair, N.J., D. C. P. Publishing, 1972, pp. 133–134.
10. Greene, J. C.: Oral Health Care for the Prevention and Control of Periodontal Disease—Review of Literature. Section VII in *World Workshop in Periodontics.* Ann Arbor, American Academy of Periodontology and University of Michigan, 1966, pp. 401–403.
11. Hard, D.: Oral Prophylaxis, in Bunting, R. W.: *Oral Hygiene,* 3rd ed. Philadelphia, Lea & Febiger, 1957, pp. 280–283.
12. Stillman, P. R.: A Philosophy of the Treatment of Periodontal Disease, *Dent. Dig.,* 38, 315, September, 1932.
13. Hirschfeld: op. cit., p. 380.
14. Bass, C. C.: An Effective Method of Personal Oral Hygiene, *J. Louisiana State Med. Soc.,* 106,100, March, 1954.
15. Charters, W. J.: Immunizing Both Hard and Soft Mouth Tissue to Infection by Correct Stimulation with the Toothbrush, *J. Am. Dent. Assoc.,* 15, 87, January, 1928.
16. Charters, W. J.: Home Care of the Mouth. I.

Proper Home Care of the Mouth, *J. Periodont.,* 19, 136, October, 1948.
17. Fones, A. C., ed.: *Mouth Hygiene,* 4th ed. Philadelphia, Lea & Febiger, 1934, pp. 299–306.
18. Hirschfeld: op. cit., pp. 369–371.
19. Leonard, H. J.: Conservative Treatment of Periodontoclasia, *J. Am. Dent. Assoc.,* 26, 1308, August, 1939.
20. Smith, T. S.: Anatomic and Physiologic Conditions Governing the Use of the Toothbrush, *J. Am. Dent. Assoc.,* 27, 874, June, 1940.
21. Bell, D. G.: Home Care of the Mouth. III. Teaching Home Care to the Patient, *J. Periodont.,* 19, 140, October, 1948.
22. American Dental Association, Council on Dental Materials and Devices: *Guide to Dental Materials and Devices,* 7th ed. Chicago, American Dental Association, 1974–1975, pp. 149–151, 272.
23. Greene: op. cit., pp. 408–414, 429–433.
24. Frandsen, A., ed.: *Oral Hygiene.* Copenhagen, Munksgaard, 1972, pp. 37–39.
25. Ash, M. M.: A Review of the Problems and Results of Studies on Manual and Power Toothbrushes, *J. Periodont.,* 35, 202, May-June, 1964.
26. Electric Toothbrushes, *Consumer Reports,* 34, 138, March, 1969.
27. Mumford, J. M.: Electric Toothbrushes, *Brit. Dent. J.,* 118, 127, February 2, 1965.
28. Chaiken, B. S., Goldman, H. M., Schulman, S. M., and Ruben, M. P.: Comparative Cleansing Efficiency of Power-driven and Conventional Toothbrushes, I. Effect in Uninstructed Patients, *Periodontics,* 3, 200, July-August, 1965.
29. Lobene, R. R.: Evaluation of Altered Gingival Health from Permissive Powered Toothbrushing, *J. Am. Dent. Assoc.,* 69, 585, November, 1964.
30. Parfitt, G. J.: Cleansing the Subgingival Space, *J. Periodont.,* 34, 133, March, 1963.
31. Goldman, H. M. and Ruben, M. P.: Methods for Increasing the Efficiency of the Arcuate-motioned, Power-driven Brush in Oral Physiotherapy, *J. Periodont.,* 38, 508, November-December, 1967.
32. Gilmore, E. L. and Bhaskar, S. N.: Effect of Tongue Brushing on Bacteria and Plaque Formed *in Vitro, J. Periodont.,* 43, 418, July, 1972.
33. Jacobson, S. E., Crawford, J. J., and McFall, W. R.: Oral Physiotherapy of the Tongue and Palate: Relationship to Plaque Control, *J. Am. Dent. Assoc.,* 87, 134, July, 1973.
34. Glickman, I.: *Clinical Periodontology,* 4th ed. Philadelphia, Saunders, 1972, pp. 356–357.
35. Grant, D. A., Stern, I. B., and Everett, F. G.: *Orban's Periodontics,* 4th ed. St. Louis, Mosby, 1972, pp. 253–256.
36. Glickman: op. cit., p. 491.
37. Manly, R. S. and Brudevold, F.: Relative Abrasiveness of Natural and Synthetic Toothbrush Bristles on Cementum and Dentin, *J. Am. Dent. Assoc.,* 55, 779, December, 1957.

38. Harte, D. B. and Manly, R. S.: Effect of Five Variables on Dentin Abrasion, *A. A. D. R. Program and Abstracts of Papers*, No. 188, February, 1975, p. 91.
39. Burgett, F. G. and Ash, M. M.: Comparative Study of the Pressure of Brushing with Three Types of Toothbrushes, *J. Periodont.*, 45, 410, June, 1974.
40. American Dental Association, Bureau of Dental Health Education and Bureau of Economic Research and Statistics: Survey of Family Toothbrushing Practices, *J. Am. Dent. Assoc.*, 72, 1489, June, 1966.
41. Kreifeld, J. G., Hill, P. H., and Calisti, L. J. P.: Dependence of Plaque Removal on Brushing Time and Brush Wear, *A. A. D. R. Program and Abstracts of Papers*, No. 191, February, 1975, p. 92.

Suggested Readings

Baer, C. and Baer, P. N.: A Story of the Toothpick, *J. Periodont.*, 37, 158, March-April, 1966.
Berenie, J., Ripa, L. W., and Leske, G.: The Relationship of Frequency of Toothbrushing, Oral Hygiene, Gingival Health, and Caries Experience in School Children, *J. Public Health Dent.*, 33, 160, Summer, 1973.
Gilmore, E. L., Gross, A., and Whitley, R.: Effect of Tongue Brushing on Plaque Bacteria, *Oral Surg.*, 36, 201, August, 1973.
Kelner, R. M., Wohl, B. R., Deasy, M. J., and Formicola, A. J.: Gingival Inflammation as Related to Frequency of Plaque Removal, *J. Periodont.*, 45, 303, May, 1974.
Lang, N. P., Cumming, B. R., and Löe, H.: Toothbrushing Frequency as It Relates to Plaque Development and Gingival Health, *J. Periodont.*, 44, 396, July, 1973.
Sittig, R.: Space Dentistry—A New Science, *Dent. Economics*, 60, 24, July, 1970.

Toothbrushes and Brushing

Anaise, J. Z.: The Toothbrush in Plaque Removal, *J. Dent. Child.*, 42, 186, May-June, 1975.
Bass, C. C.: Optimum Characteristics of Toothbrushes for Personal Oral Hygiene, *Dent. Items of Int.*, 70, 696, July, 1948.
Bay, I., Kardel, K. M., and Skougaard, M. R.: Quantitative Evaluation of the Plaque-removing Ability of Different Types of Toothbrushes, *J. Periodont.*, 38, 526, November-December, 1967.
Berdon, J. K., Hornbrook, R. H., and Hayduk, S. E.: An Evaluation of Six Manual Toothbrushes by Comparing Their Effectiveness in Plaque Removal, *J. Periodont.*, 45, 496, July, 1974.
Cohen, M. M.: A Pilot Study Testing the Plaque-removing Ability of a Newly Invented Toothbrush, *J. Periodont.*, 44, 183, March, 1973.
Curtis, G. H., McCall, C. M., Jr., and Overaa, H. I.: A Clinical Study of the Effectiveness of the Roll and Charters' Methods of Brushing Teeth, *J. Periodont.*, 28, 277, October, 1957.

Fanning, E. A. and Henning, F. R.: Toothbrush Design and Its Relation to Oral Health, *Aust. Dent. J.*, 12, 464, October, 1967.
Frandsen, A. M., Barbano, J. P., Suomi, J. D., Chang, J. J., and Burke, A. D.: The Effectiveness of the Charters', Scrub and Roll Methods of Toothbrushing by Professionals in Removing Plaque, *Scand. J. Dent. Res.*, 78, 459, No. 6, 1970.
Frandsen, A. M., Barbano, J. P., Suomi, J. D., Chang, J. J., and Houston, R.: A Comparison of the Effectiveness of the Charters', Scrub and Roll Methods of Toothbrushing in Removing Plaque, *Scand. J. Dent. Res.*, 80, 267, No. 4, 1972.
Gilson, C. M., Charbeneau, G. T., and Hill, H. C.: A Comparison of Physical Properties of Several Soft Toothbrushes, *J. Mich. Dent. Assoc.*, 51, 347, November, 1969.
Hall, A. W. and Conroy, C. W.: Comparison of Automatic and Hand Toothbrushes: Toothbrushing Effectiveness for Preschool Children, *J. Dent. Child.*, 38, 309, September-October, 1971.
Hansen, F. and Gjermo, P.: The Plaque-removing Effect of Four Toothbrushing Methods, *Scand. J. Dent. Res.*, 79, 502, No. 7, 1971.
Hine, M. K., Wachtl, C., and Fosdick, L. S.: Some Observations on Cleansing Effect of Nylon and Bristle Tooth Brushes, *J. Periodont.*, 25, 183, July, 1954.
Horowitz, A. M. and Suomi, J. D.: A Comparison of Plaque-removal with a Standard or an Unconventional Toothbrush Used by Youngsters, *J. Periodont.*, 45, 760, October, 1974.
Kimmelman, B. B.: Teaching Two Toothbrushing Techniques: Observations and Comparisons, *J. Periodont.*, 39, 96, March, 1968.
McKendrick, A. J. W., McHugh, W. D., and Barbenel, L. M. H.: Toothbrush Age and Wear. An Analysis, *Brit. Dent. J.*, 130, 66, January 19, 1971.
Owen, T. L.: A Clinical Evaluation of Electric and Manual Toothbrushing by Children with Primary Dentitions, *J. Dent. Child.*, 39, 15, January-February, 1972.
Padbury, A. D. and Ash, M. M.: Abrasion Caused by Three Methods of Toothbrushing, *J. Periodont.*, 45, 434, June, 1974.
Puckett, J. B.: Bristles in Hand Manipulated Toothbrushes, *J. Periodont.*, 41, 398, July, 1970.
Robertson, N. A. E. and Wade, A. B.: Effect of Filament Diameter and Density in Toothbrushes, *J. Periodont. Res.*, 7, 346, No. 4, 1972.
Rodda, J. C.: A Comparison of Four Methods of Toothbrushing, *New Zeal. Dent. J.*, 64, 162, July, 1968.
Sangnes, G., Zachrisson, B., and Gjermo, P.: Effectiveness of Vertical and Horizontal Brushing Techniques in Plaque Removal, *J. Dent. Child.*, 39, 94, March-April, 1972.
Swartz, M. L., Phillips, R. W., and Hine, M. K.: Effect of Certain Factors Upon Toothbrush Bristle Stiffness, *J. Periodont.*, 27, 96, April, 1956.
Toto, P. D., Evans, C. L., and Sawinski, V. J.: Reduction of Acidogenic Microorganisms by Toothbrushing, *J. Dent. Child.*, 34, 38, January, 1967.

Automatic Toothbrush

Bechlem, D. N., Saxe, S. R., and Stern, I. B.: A Histologic Study of the Effect Upon the Gingivae of Using an Electric Toothbrush in the Presence of Marginal Periodontitis, *Periodontics*, 3, 90, March-April, 1965.

Chasens, A. I. and Marcus, R. W.: An Evaluation of the Comparative Efficiency of Manual and Automatic Toothbrushes in Maintaining the Periodontal Patient, *J. Periodont.*, 39, 156, May, 1968.

Conroy, C. W.: Comparison of Automatic and Hand Toothbrushes: Cleaning Effectiveness, *J. Am. Dent. Assoc.*, 70, 921, April, 1965.

Conroy, C. W. and Melfi, R. C.: Comparison of Automatic and Hand Toothbrushes: Cleaning Effectiveness for Children, *J. Dent. Child.*, 33, 219, July, 1966.

Glass, R. L.: A Clinical Study of Hand and Electric Toothbrushing, *J. Periodont.*, 36, 322, July-August, 1965.

Harrington, J. H. and Terry, I. A.: Automatic and Hand Toothbrushing Abrasion Studies, *J. Am. Dent. Assoc.*, 68, 343, March, 1964.

Hoover, D. R. and Robinson, H. B. G.: Effect of Automatic and Hand Toothbrushing on Gingivitis, *J. Am. Dent. Assoc.*, 65, 361, September, 1962.

Howell, R. A.: The Automatic Toothbrush as an Aid in Periodontal Treatment, *Dent. Health*, 5, 22, April-June, 1966.

Lefkowitz, W. and Robinson, H. B. G.: Effectiveness of Automatic and Hand Brushes in Removing Dental Plaque and Debris, *J. Am. Dent. Assoc.*, 65, 351, September, 1962.

Lobene, R. R.: Effect of an Automatic Toothbrush on Gingival Health, *J. Periodont.*, 35, 137, March-April, 1964.

Manhold, J. H.: Gingival Tissue Health with Hand and Power Brushing: A Retrospective with Corroborative Studies, *J. Periodont.*, 38, 23, January-February, 1967.

McConnell, D. and Conroy, C. W.: Comparisons of Abrasion Produced by a Simulated Manual Versus a Mechanical Toothbrush, *J. Dent. Res.*, 46, 1022, September-October, 1967.

Muhler, J. C.: Comparative Frequency of Use of the Electric Toothbrush and Hand Toothbrush, *J. Periodont.*, 40, 268, May, 1969.

Powers, G. K., Tussing, G. J., and Bradley, R. E.: A Comparison of Effectiveness in Interproximal Plaque Removal of an Electric Toothbrush and a Conventional Hand Toothbrush, *Periodontics*, 5, 37, January-February, 1967.

Quigley, G. A. and Hein, J. W.: Comparative Cleansing Efficiency of Manual and Power Brushing, *J. Am. Dent. Assoc.*, 65, 26, July, 1962.

Rainey, B. L. and Ash, M. M.: Clinical Study of a Short Stroke Reciprocating Action Electric Toothbrush, *J. Periodont.*, 35, 455, November-December, 1964.

Ritsert, E. F. and Binns, W. H.: Adolescents Brush Better with an Electric Toothbrush, *J. Dent. Child.*, 34, 354, September, 1967.

Sanders, W. E. and Robinson, H. B. G.: Effect of Tooth Brushing on Deposition of Calculus, *J. Periodont.*, 33, 386, October, 1962.

Soparkar, P. M. and Quigley, G. A.: Power versus Hand Brushing: Effect on Gingivitis, *J. Am. Dent. Assoc.*, 68, 182, February, 1964.

Chapter 23

Auxiliary Plaque Control Measures

Auxiliary measures are selected to complement toothbrushing. Since plaque on proximal tooth surfaces is not totally accessible to usual brushing, a means for proximal plaque removal is necessary in complete preventive care. Other objectives and uses are outlined as each auxiliary aid is described in this chapter. Following, in Chapter 24, particular applications are given for care of teeth and tissues related to dental appliances, and in Chapter 25, the mouth with complete rehabilitation.

When the plaque control and oral physical therapy regimen is outlined for an individual patient, the first consideration is given to the specific oral condition and how it can be improved or maintained. Next it is necessary to consider which goals of oral health can be reached by the use of particular implements. For example, certain devices can be expected to remove plaque; whereas others will not remove plaque, but are efficient at removing debris, materia alba, and superficial layers of less tenaciously attached microorganisms over the surface of the plaque.

After matching the available devices with the goals for health of the individual oral condition, teaching, learning, and time must be considered. The simplest possible procedures are selected for the patient's convenience and ease of learning as well as for keeping the daily oral care regimen at a realistic level with respect to the time the patient is able and willing to spend.

INTERDENTAL PLAQUE CONTROL

Normally the interdental gingiva fills the gingival embrasure between two teeth and beneath their contact area. Between posterior teeth there are two papillae, one facial and one lingual, connected by a col which is a depressed concave area (figure 11–5, page 168). Between anterior teeth interdental papillae are generally single, with a pyramidal shape. The epithelium covering the col is thin and less resistant to disease (page 167).

The interdental col area is generally inaccessible for toothbrushing. It is a protected area when the teeth are in normal position. Because of its shape it tends to harbor microorganisms. Most gingival disease starts in the interdental areas and the incidence of gingivitis is highest in the interdental papillae.

When interdental papillae are reduced in height or missing, the proximal tooth surfaces are exposed and the gingiva takes on a different shape, sometimes crater-like. Dental plaque collects on the tooth surfaces and retention of debris in the interproximal area can occur. Irregularities of tooth position such as rotation or alterations related to malocclusion or tooth loss, contribute to differences in the shape of the gingival embrasure, and further complicate the plan for plaque control.

I. Objectives of Interdental Care

The interdental papillae may be missing or reduced in height because of disease such as necrotizing ulcerative gingivitis (Vincent's disease), surgical procedures essential in the treatment of periodontal diseases, or habitual pressure atrophy caused by the use of interdental tips or other devices which are contraindicated when interdental gingiva fill the embrasure. As a result of the exposure of the tooth surfaces, the changes in shape of the interdental tissue, and the general trapping of debris in the unnatural spaces, specific care is needed. The general objectives for plaque control and oral physical therapy apply to this area (page 304). With the judicious use of the various methods and devices available, the following goals may be achieved:

A. Removal of dental plaque to lower the bacterial count and prevent gingivitis, periodontitis and dental caries.

B. Oral physical therapy: reshaping of the interdental gingiva to prevent retention of deposits and allow effective cleaning.

C. Improvement of surface keratinization to increase resistance to trauma and disease.

D. Clean proximal tooth surfaces to permit access for fluoride from self-application preparations (e.g., dentifrice, mouthrinse, gel tray, chewable tablet, pages 439–442).

II. Role of Toothbrushing

Interproximal vibratory and sulcular brushing such as Charters', Stillman's, and the Bass technique, with a soft round-tipped brush, can be successful to some degree in removing dental plaque from the proximal surfaces of the teeth. Research to evaluate the effectiveness of toothbrushing and other methods has shown that all of the proximal plaque is not usually removed by toothbrushing alone.[1,2]

For complete plaque and debris removal from open embrasures, more than the toothbrush is generally needed. Various materials and devices are described in the sections following.

Removal of all calculus and smoothing of the tooth surface increases the effectiveness of devices. The rough tooth surfaces retain plaque and encourage gingival inflammation. Large deposits interfere with the use of devices, for example, dental floss catches and shreds when applied to overhanging margins of restorations or calculus deposits. It is not generally recommended that instruments, which are used to apply pressure for massage or stimulation, be used without first removing submarginal calculus since rubbing the inflamed gingival wall of the pocket over calculus is likely to cause an acute inflammatory reaction.

III. Dental Floss and Tape

When dental floss is applied with firm pressure to a flat or convex proximal tooth surface, plaque can be removed. A concave tooth surface would escape contact with the floss. Figure 23–9 (page 338) illustrates this for the mesial of the maxillary first premolar. In one study in which flossing followed toothbrushing, it was revealed that floss removed nearly all of the plaque left after the brushing, in other words, about 25 percent of the total plaque.[3]

A. **Types of Floss**

1. *Unwaxed.* Frequently recommended because it is thinner and slips through close contacts without pain from pressure, and because it is more absorbent and holds plaque as it is removed.

2. *Waxed.* May be particularly indicated during the initial period of patient care before restorative work

is completed and tooth surfaces are completely scaled and root planed, because the unwaxed floss shreds and tears more easily. The tearing may aggravate the patient and discourage continued use.

B. **Indications**

For most patients dental floss should be used before toothbrushing. Not only does this assure that caries-susceptible proximal surfaces will be de-plaqued, but also that the fluoride from the dentifrice used during brushing will be able to reach the proximal surfaces for caries prevention.

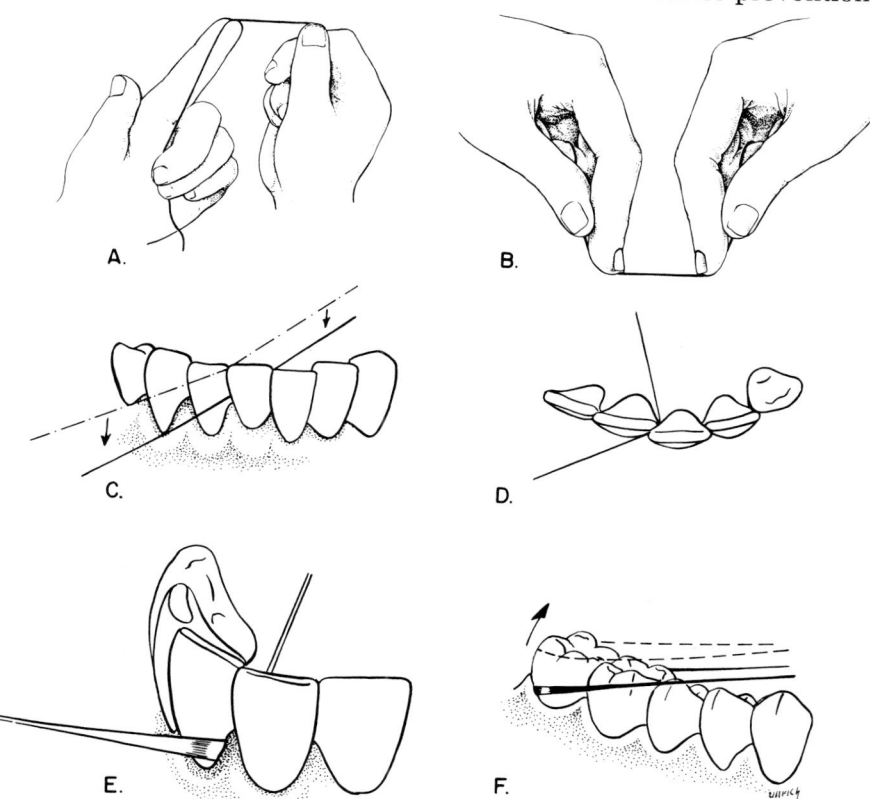

Figure 23–1. Directions for use of floss. **A.** For maxillary insertion hold the floss between thumb and index finger or between thumbs. Grasp the floss firmly. Allow one-half to one inch between fingers. **B.** For mandibular teeth, direct the floss down, guided by the index fingers. **C.** Work the floss slowly between the teeth in a short sawing motion. Avoid snapping through the contact area. **D.** Curve the floss around the tooth in a C-shape. Hold the floss toward the mesial for cleaning the distal surfaces, and toward the distal for cleaning mesial surfaces. **E.** Press the floss firmly against the tooth. Move gently beneath the gingiva until tissue resistance is felt. Slide the floss horizontally and vertically with pressure to remove plaque. **F.** Begin flossing with the distal of the most posterior tooth and work systematically around the arch.

Instruction in the use of floss can be presented after the patient has become adept at toothbrushing. When the patient already has an acceptable brushing procedure, floss instruction is best given first. The use of floss in the care of a fixed partial denture is described on page 357.

During flossing, food debris and materia alba are removed from inter-proximal areas. This contributes to general oral sanitation and the control of halitosis. When there is inadequate contact and the patient indicates that he must use floss or toothpicks to relieve pressure from impacted food, dental attention may be needed and the area should be charted or other-wise brought to the attention of the dentist.

C. Procedure

1. Floss preparation
   a. Hold a 12- to 15-inch length of floss with the thumb and index finger of each hand: grasp firmly with one-half inch of floss be-tween the hands. The ends of the floss may be tucked into the palm and held by the ring and little finger, or the floss may be wrapped around the middle fingers (figure 23–1A and B).
   b. A circle of floss may be made by tying the ends together; the circle may be rotated around as the floss in used[4] (figure 23–2).
2. Application[5]
   a. *Mandibular Teeth.* Direct the floss down by holding the two index fingers on top of the strand. One index finger holds the floss on the lingual and the other on the facial. The side of the finger which is on the lingual is held on the teeth of the opposite side of the mouth to serve as a fulcrum or rest.

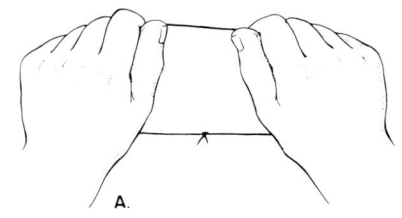

A.

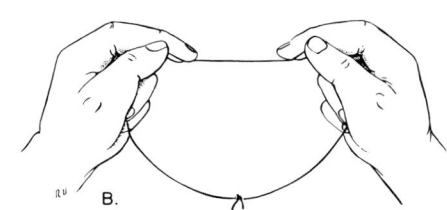

B.

Figure 23–2. Circle of floss. The ends of the floss ar tied together for convenient holding. A child ma be able to manage floss better with this tech nique. **A.** Held for maxillary. **B.** Mandibular.

b. *Maxillary Right.* Pass the strand over the upturned right thumb and the left index finger. Hold the thumb on the facial and the index finger on the lingual as the floss is inserted.
   c. *Maxillary Left.* The left thumb o index finger supports the floss o the facial; right index finger o the lingual.
3. Insertion
   a. Hold floss in a diagonal or ob lique position (figure 23–3).
   b. Ease the floss past each contac area with a gentle sawing mo tion.
   c. Control floss to prevent snappin through the contact area onto th gingival tissue.
4. Cleaning stroke
   a. Clean adjacent teeth separately for the distal aspect hold the flos mesially, and for the mesia aspect hold the floss distall curving around the tooth (figur 23–1,D, E,and F).

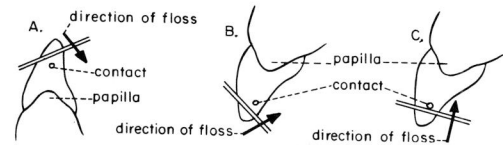

Figure 23–3. Insertion of floss. Hold floss in a diagonal or oblique position. Arrows indicate direction of movement of floss. **A.** Mandibular. **B.** Maxillary. **C.** Incorrect. When floss is held horizontally there is greater possibility for damage to the papilla.

    b. Pass the floss below the gingival margin, press to adapt the floss around the tooth, and slide up the tooth surface. Repeat.

  5. Additional suggestions

    a. When a dentifrice is used, dental tape may retain the dentifrice against the tooth better than floss.

    b. Slide the floss to a new unused portion for succeeding proximal tooth surfaces.

    c. Floss may be used double to provide a wider rubbing surface.

  6. Rinse thoroughly and vigorously to remove food particles and plaque that has been loosened.

D. Precautions

  1. Pressure in col area. The col area is not keratinized and is vulnerable to disease (page 167). Plaque control of the area is of great importance since most gingival and periodontal disease begins in the col area. Too great pressure with floss one or more times daily, particularly very fine floss that tends to cut more easily than thicker floss, can be destructive to the attachment. This may be of particular significance in children while teeth are in the process of eruption.

  2. Prevention of floss cuts.

    a. Location: floss cuts occur primarily on facial or lingual directly beside or in the middle of an interdental papilla. They appear as straight line cuts from the

gingival margin toward the mucogingival junction.

    b. Causes of floss cuts:

      (1) Too long a piece of floss between the fingers when held for insertion.

      (2) Snapping the floss through the contact area.

      (3) Not curving the floss about the teeth; floss held straight across.

      (4) Not using a rest to prevent undue pressure.

E. Use of Floss Holder

  1. Types. Several types of plastic floss holders are available (figure 23–4).

  2. Use. Careful instruction should be provided and supervision given periodically to prevent tissue damage. As threaded into a holder, the floss is in a straight line. To avoid cutting the papilla when applied interproximally, the use of a rest or fulcrum can help prevent snapping through the contact. The floss must be pulled mesially (to clean the distal of a tooth) or pushed distally

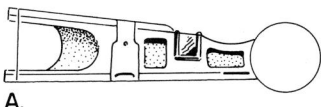

A.

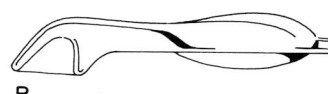

B.

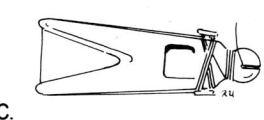

C.

Figure 23–4. Examples of floss holders. **A.** has replaceable floss container. **B.** has replaceable floss cartridge and thin edge for cleaning the tongue. **C.** has threading mechanism which requires a 24-inch length of floss applied at each use.

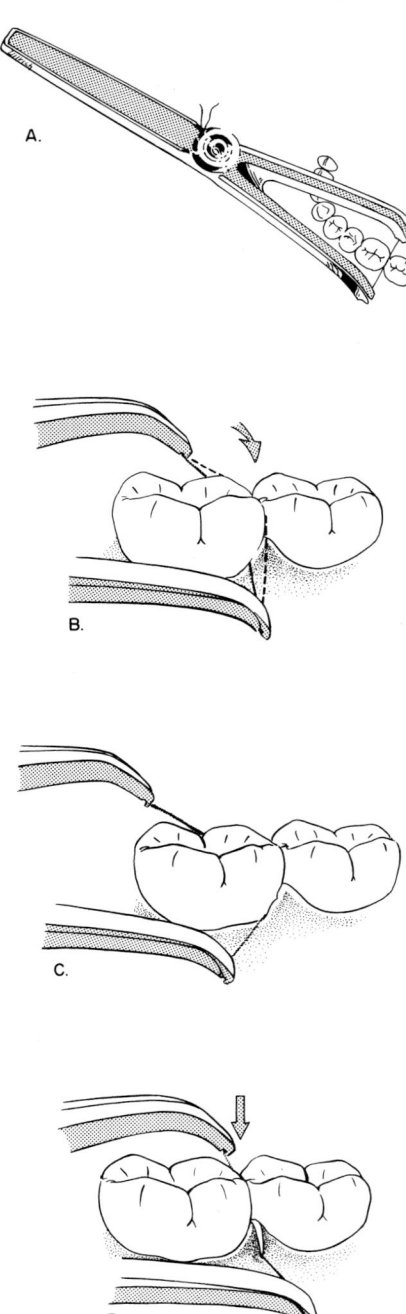

Figure 23–5.   Use of floss holder. **A.** Applied interproximally. **B.** As floss is drawn through the interproximal, the holder should be pulled mesially when the floss is to be applied to a distal surface. **C.** Floss is lowered into sulcus. **D.** Floss cut in papilla resulting from incorrect use.

(to clean mesial surface) to allow floss to be positioned on the side of the papilla (figure 23–5).

IV. Knitting Yarn[6]

A. Indications for Use

For wide proximal surfaces; dental floss is narrow and does not remove plaque fast enough.

1. For mesial and distal abutments of fixed partial dentures (page 357).
2. For isolated teeth or teeth separated by a diastema.

B. Technique

1. Preparation of yarn: fold double about eight inches of three-ply synthetic yarn and loop through about eight inches of dental floss tie floss with one overhand knot.
2. Insert floss through the contact area: draw the yarn into the embrasure (figure 23–6).
3. Clean adjacent teeth separately with a buccolingual back and forth stroke: hold the ends of the yarn distally and then around mesially.
4. For specific areas where a papilla may be high or access is not otherwise sufficient for the wide yarn, the dental floss end of the combination is used.
5. Dentifrice may be used.
6. For closed contacts, use a floss threader (figure 24–3, page 358).

V. Gauze Strip

A. Indications for Use

To clean proximal surfaces of teeth which are widely spaced or adjacent to edentulous areas. Gauze is too thick to pass through contact areas.

B. Technique

1. Prepare strip: cut one-inch gauze bandage into a six-inch length and fold in thirds or down the center.

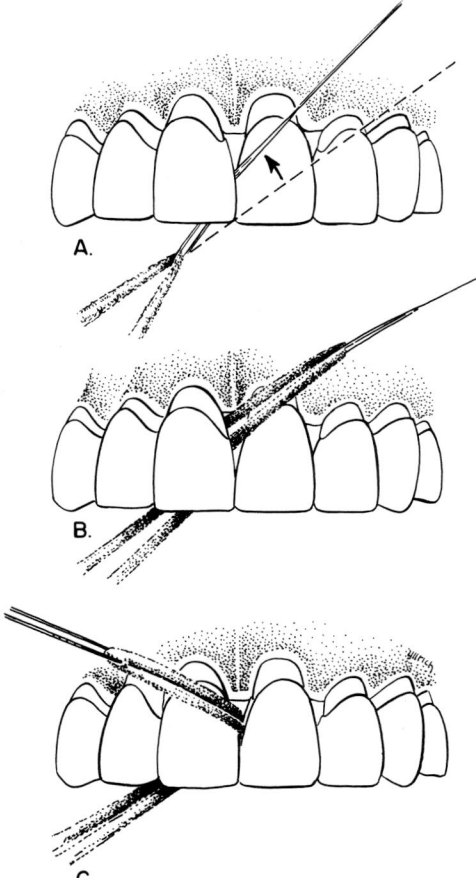

A.

B.

C.

Figure 23–6. Use of knitting yarn in open gingival embrasure. **A.** Yarn is looped through dental floss, and dental floss is drawn through the contact area in usual manner, as shown by arrow. **B.** Yarn is drawn through the embrasure. **C.** Yarn is positioned against the surface of the tooth for plaque removal.

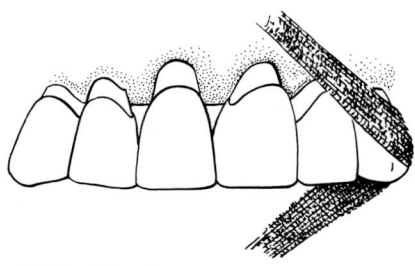

Figure 23–7. Use of gauze strip for surfaces without contact with an adjacent tooth. A six-inch length of one-inch gauze bandage is folded in thirds and placed around the tooth with the folded edge over the cervical third of the tooth. A "shoe-shine" stroke is used to clean the surface.

2. Position the fold of the gauze on the cervical area next to the gingival crest and work back and forth several times; hold ends toward distal to clean a mesial surface, and mesial to clean a distal surface (figure 23–7).

VI. Pipe Cleaner

A. Indications for Use

Proximal surfaces when interdental gingiva is missing; furcation areas.

B. Technique

1. One-third of a regular length pipe cleaner is adequate at a time. Check wire end to prevent damaging the gingiva or scratchng the cemental surface.
2. Carefully work the end of the cleaner through the space with care not to press wire end into the gingiva.
3. Work back and forth pressing toward one surface and then the other.
4. Furcation: slide pipe cleaner through between exposed roots of a furcation. Work back and forth (figure 23–8).

VII. Toothpick Holder (Perio-aid)

A. Indications for Use

1. Periodontal patient: plaque removal at and just under the gingival margin; interdental cleaning particularly for concave proximal tooth surfaces (figure 23–9); exposed furcation area.

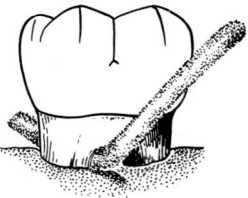

Figure 23–8. Use of pipe cleaner in area between roots where furcation has been exposed.

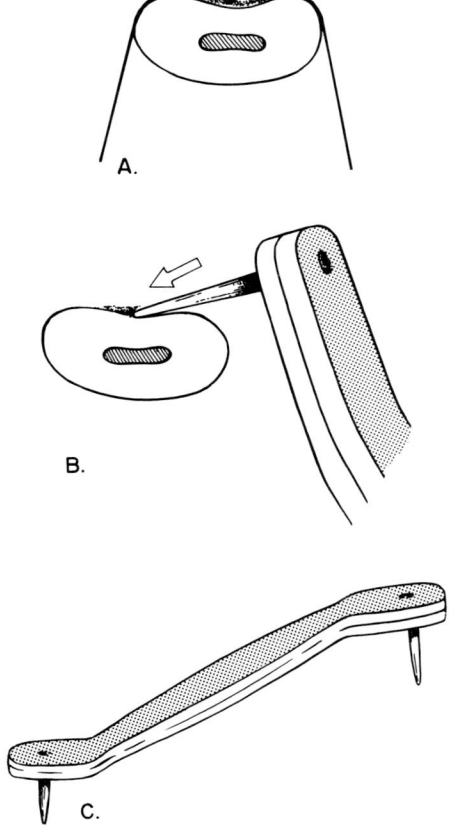

A.

B.

C.

Figure 23–9. Cross section of maxillary first premolar at the cementoenamel junction to show use of Perio-aid on the concave tooth surface. **A.** Note inability of floss to remove plaque from the concavity. **B.** Perio-aid is applied for plaque removal from facial and lingual. **C.** Perio-aid handle angulated for adaptation of one end on facial and the other on lingual.

2. Orthodontic patient: plaque removal at gingival margin above appliance; cleaning around fixed appliances (figure 24–6, page 361).

B. **Technique**
  1. Prepare instrument
    a. Insert round tapered toothpick into the end of the holder. One type of end is angulated for use from the lingual, other type is at a right angle for general application.

b. Twist the toothpick firmly int place. Break off the long en cleanly so that sharp edges car not scratch the inner cheek or th tongue during use.
2. Apply toothpick at the gingiva margin. At a right angle application with moderate pressure, trace th gingival margin around each tooth For removing plaque just below th gingival margin, apply the end a less than 45 degrees, maintain th tip on the tooth surface, and follov around the sulcus or pocket (figur 23–10).
3. After the tip becomes frayed from use, it can be used as a smal cleaning "brush" to rub on tootl surfaces where plaque has col lected. It should be checked fo loose bits of wood which migh become deposited in the sulcus o gingiva. For hypersensitive spots usually at the cervical third of tooth, the patient can use the tip t massage fluoride dentifrice for de sensitization.

VIII. Balsa Wood Wedge

A. **Description**
  Two inches long, wooden "tooth pick" known commercially as th Stim-U-Dent. It is triangular in cros section.

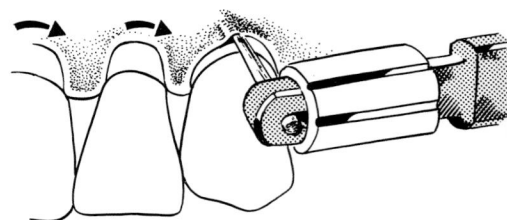

Figure 23–10. Perio-aid applied submarginally. Tip i placed on the tooth surface just below the gingiva margin, and plaque is removed by moving th Perio-aid over the surface around the tooth. Th toothpick tip should be softened in water before use

B. **Indications for Use**
1. For cleaning interdental areas where there are exposed tooth surfaces and missing interdental gingiva. There must be space, otherwise the gingival tissue can be traumatized and the teeth forced apart.
2. As with most interdental devices, it is advised only for the patient who will follow instructions carefully since tissue injury is possible, and the use of the implement after the wood has splayed may force splinters into the gingiva.

C. **Technique[7]**
1. First teach the patient to use his hand as a rest by placing it on his check, chin, or a finger on the gingiva convenient to the place where the tip will be applied. This will help to prevent inserting the wedge with too much pressure.
2. Soften the wood: place the pointed end in the mouth and moisten with saliva.
3. Apply base of the triangular wedge to the gingival border of the interden-

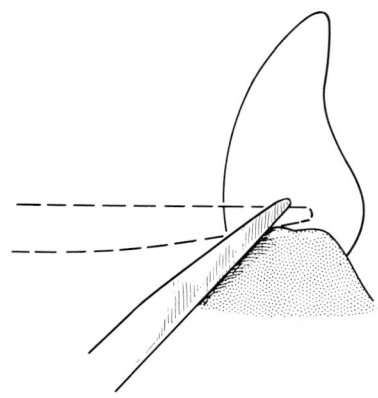

Figure 23–11. Balsa wood wedge. The wedge is used only when there are exposed proximal tooth surfaces and reduced interdental papillae. It is applied at an angle toward the occlusal or incisal to follow the contour of the interdental papilla. The broken line drawing shows horizontal positioning which could flatten the interdental papilla if used regularly.

tal area and insert with the tip pointed slightly toward the occlusal or incisal to follow the contour of the interdental gingiva (figure 23–11). When held horizontally, the interdental tissue can be flattened.
4. Clean the tooth surfaces by moving the wedge in and out while applying a burnishing stroke with moderate pressure first to one side of the embrasure and then the other, about 10 or 12 strokes each.
5. Discard wedge after a few embrasures have been treated or as soon as the first signs of splaying are evident.

IX. **Interproximal Brush[8,9]**

A. **Composition and Design**
1. Soft nylon filaments (.003 to .007 inch diameter) twisted in fine stainless steel wire for insertion into a binangle handle.
2. The small brush is ½ inch long and 3/16 to ¼ inch overall width, with the filaments projecting from all sides to form a round brush.

B. **Indications for Use**
1. Large open interproximal areas and bifurcations or trifurcations.
2. For proximal cleaning and plaque removal.

C. **Technique**
1. Moisten the brush and insert into interdental area or furcation at an angle in keeping with gingival form; brush in and out (figure 23–12).
2. Binangle of handle permits application from the lingual as well as facial.

D. **Care of Brushes**
1. Clean brush during use to remove debris and plaque by holding under actively running water.
2. Clean thoroughly after use and dry in open air.

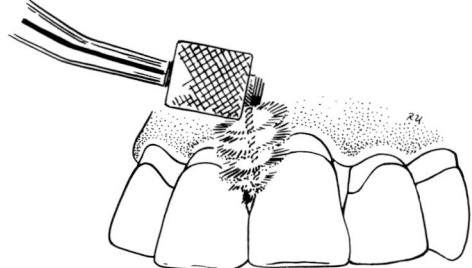

Figure 23–12. Use of interproximal brush. Small soft nylon brush is applied for plaque removal from the facial, and may be applied from the lingual in open embrasures.

X. Interdental Brush

A. **Description:** single tuft approximately six millimeters in diameter, with bristles or filaments mounted in a straight or contra-angled handle.

B. **Indications for Use**
   1. Wide clear interproximal spaces where papillae have been lost.
   2. Dental appliances.
   3. Contraindication: normal papillae which fill the interproximal area.

C. **Technique**
   1. Direct the end of the tuft into the interproximal area.
   2. Combine a rotating motion with intermittent pressure.[10]

XI. Interdental Tip

A. **Composition and Design**
   Conical or pyramidal flexible rubber or plastic tip attached to the end of the handle of a toothbrush, or on a special plastic handle. The soft pliable rubber tip is preferred to the hard, more rigid plastic tip because it can be adapted to the interdental area more easily, and because there is less pain or discomfort for the patient when the instrument is pressed on the tissue.

B. **Indications for Use**
   1. Cleaning debris and materia alba from the interdental area, and, by

rubbing the exposed tooth surface some plaque may be removed.
   2. Reshaping of gingiva followi periodontal surgery or after t damaging effects of acute necrot ing ulcerative gingivitis when c tering has resulted.
   3. Massaging action to stimulate circ lation and improve keratinization increase resistance to trauma.
   4. Adaptation to areas where toot brushing is difficult: for examp exposed furcation areas, mesial mesially inclined teeth, or ab ment teeth.
   5. *Contraindicated.* Clinically he thy gingiva with intact interden papillae. Interdental devices a usually unnecessary and can harmful.

C. **Technique**
   The interdental tip is a diffic instrument to use correctly. Learni to use it may require more patien and time than the average patient w care to give. A mirror should be used show the placement of the tip and t patient should use a mirror for hor practice.
   1. Prepare for application: outside t mouth, hold the handle of t instrument firmly (usually a pa

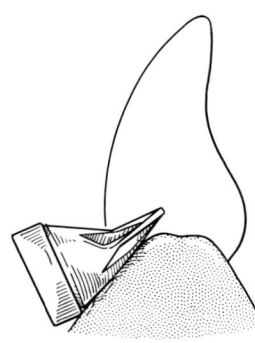

Figure 23–13. Interdental tip. The conical, flexi rubber tip is angled diagonally toward the occlu or incisal to follow the contour of the interder gingiva.

grasp gives best control) with the tip angled up for application to the mandibular and down for the maxillary arch.

2. Insert the tip interdentally, diagonally toward the occlusal or the incisal to follow the contour of the interdental gingiva (figure 23–13).

3. The tip is inserted until it fits the embrasure and touches the sides of the teeth, but it is never pressed forcefully. If forced repeatedly in a horizontal direction, the interdental tissue can be blunted or flattened by pressure, thus increasing the size of the interdental space.

4. Press the side of the tip against the attached gingiva and apply a gentle rotary motion which provides intermittent pressure against the gingival tissue (figure 23–14). The rotary motion is continued to a slow count of ten.

5. When the interdental area is wide, press the tip against one tooth and the attached gingiva for a count of ten, and then slide it over to the side of the adjacent tooth.

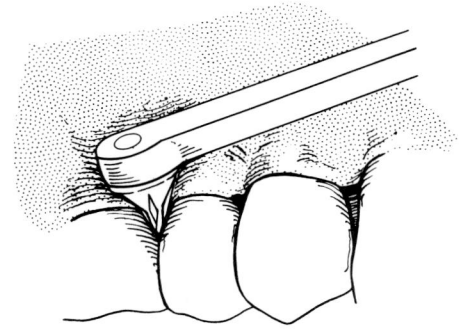

Figure 23–14. Interdental tip. The rubber tip is used when interdental papillae are missing or reduced in height. The tip is inserted until it fits the embrasure and touches the sides of the teeth, but it is not forced interdentally. The side of the tip is then pressed against the attached gingiva and a gentle but firm rotary motion is used to apply intermittent pressure against the gingival tissue.

6. Repeat at next embrasure and on around the arch; apply to lingual when access and visibility permit.

7. For additional cleaning of the proximal surfaces of the teeth, the tip may be rubbed against the teeth as it is moved in and out of the embrasure, and directed toward the part of the tooth surface under the contact area.

8. Rinse the tip as indicated during use to remove debris, and wash thoroughly at the finish.

XII. Automatic Interdental Tip

Several models of automatic brushes carry rubber tip attachments. Because of the tediousness of the use of the manual tip, the automatic tip has been of considerable help to certain patients.

The effectiveness was demonstrated by research in which the use of the automatic tip in conjunction with an automatic brush was shown to reduce the severity of interdental gingival inflammation by an average of 26 percent,[11] which was a markedly greater reduction than was accomplished by the automatic brush alone. In another study[12] the decrease in inflammation was also superior when the tip and brush were both used, and there was an increase in the surface keratinization which was more significant than found by the brush alone.

A. **Description**

A rubber tip is connected to a stalk or shank, which inserts into the automatic toothbrush handle. In general, automatic tips are smaller than manual ones.

B. **Technique**

1. Since the vibration or movement of the automatic tip is rapid, placement and positioning are very important. Patients to whom this device is recommended must be dependable and consistent in their

use of it. Careful patient selection and supervision are needed.

2. Apply the tip close to the gingiva at the interdental area with tip positioned correctly before turning on the power.
3. Hold in place about ten seconds before moving on to the next area.
4. For wide interdental areas, position the tip first against one tooth and then the other.

MOUTH RINSING

Vigorous rinsing to dislodge debris contributes to general oral cleanliness. It has been recommended for after meals and after snacks, particularly "sweet" snacks, when toothbrushing is not possible. The poster distributed by the American Dental Association "IF YOU CAN'T BRUSH AFTER EATING ... SWISH AND SWALLOW"[13] presents an appealing lesson.

A. **Objectives**

The limitations of rinsing should be recognized for although it can aid in removing gross debris, access to submarginal or col areas is not generally possible. The rinse passes over the surface of plaque rather than removing it.

A study in the United States Army Preventive Program[14] compared the use of a toothbrush and dentifrice, a soft balsa wood stick, and vigorous rinsing. The experiment was conducted in a situation simulating self-care practices under field or garrison conditions. Rinsing was the least effective and the least liked by the participants.

Use of a saline solution rinse can be a helpful postoperative procedure following scaling and root planing (page 572). Rinsing is also frequently advised following oral surgery, including tooth removal and periodontal

surgery after dressing remova Mouthwashes for rinsing are consi ered on pages 347–350, and fluoric rinses on page 440.

B. **Procedure for Rinsing**[15]

Many patients, particularly chi dren, should be shown very spe cifically how to rinse, and the metho should be practiced under superv sion. Uninstructed, many patients wi hold water in their mouths and bov the head from side to side, or othe action which cannot force the wate about and between the teeth in manner which will be effective.

1. A small amount of fluid is taken int the mouth; lips are closed.
2. With the teeth kept slightly apar the fluid is forced through th interdental areas with as muc pressure as possible to loosen de bris.
3. A combination of lip, tongue, an cheek action is used as the fluid i forced back and forth between th teeth.
4. The mouth is divided into thre sections and the rinsing should b concentrated on first the anterio then one side followed by the othe
5. Expectorate or swallow.

ORAL IRRIGATION

The use of a forced intermittent c steady stream of water in oral physica therapy is sometimes called hydro therapy. It has proven to be a usefu adjunct to toothbrushing but must not b considered a substitute for brushing o proximal surface plaque removal device since it is not effective in the complete removal of dental plaque.

Oral irrigating devices are examine and studied by the American Denta Association, Council on Dental Material and Devices, and evaluation standard have been outlined. The technical safet f the equipment, the evidence that nsupervised use by the public cannot be armful to the oral hard and soft tissues, hat the implement will produce a high egree of oral cleanliness, and that adver- ising claims be limited to the usefulness s a cleaning device, are factors consid- red for classification as acceptable, provisionally acceptable, or unaccept- ble.[16]

. Objectives

Water irrigation devices have been shown to be valuable aids in maintain- ing the health and cleanliness of the oral cavity. From reported research (see bibliography in *Suggested Read- ings* at the end of this chapter) benefits which may be derived from the use of irrigation include the following:

1. Effective removal of loose unat- tached debris from about the teeth and interdental areas. Attached de- posits (dental plaque or calculus) are not removed.
2. Reduction in numbers of microor- ganisms.
3. Decrease in the incidence of gin- givitis.
4. Promotion of keratinization during healing; does not increase keratini- zation in the col area.
5. Contribution to healing following acute necrotizing ulcerative gin- givitis.

. Types and Description of Irrigators

1. Motor-driven pump unit which generates an intermittent jet of water.
   a. Adjustable dial to regulate water pressure, and a reservoir to main- tain a steady flow.
   b. Hand-held, interchangeable, ad- justable tip which can be turned a complete 360 degrees for ap- plication at various angulations.
2. Single line type which attaches directly to the water faucet.

a. Delivers a continuous stream of water which is adjustable by varying the line pressure.
b. Hand-held interchangeable tip which rotates in a complete 360 degrees for application to all areas.

C. **Technique and Operational Factors**

1. Procedure: the user turns on and adjusts the water jet stream, leans over the washbowl, and directs the tip interproximally in a horizontal direction and along the gingival margins. The stream should not be directed directly into the sulcus or pocket (figure 23–15).
2. Operational factors
   a. Pressure need only be great enough to flush out the interden- tal area.

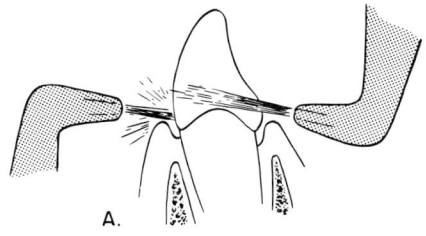

A.

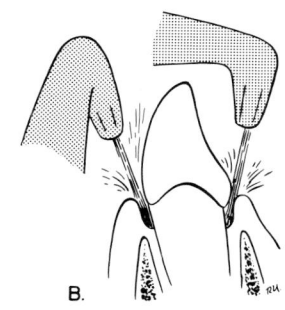

B.

Figure 23–15. Water irrigator. **A.** The water jet stream must be directed horizontally across the gingival margin and through the gingival embrasure. **B.** Incorrect use. Water is directed into the gingival sulcus or pocket and can damage the junctional epithelium and cause periodontal abscess forma- tion. Note correctly positioned horizontally held tip on lingual of **A** compared with vertically downward positioned tip in **B.**

b. Avoid high pressure or prolonged application to a limited or single area. Although adverse effects are uncommon, periodontal abscess formation from water being forced below the junctional epithelium has been reported.

3. Prevention of tissue damage. Tissue damage is in proportion to two factors: the pressure at which the water jet is delivered and the pressure related to the density of the tissues to which the water is applied.[17] For example, a fast forceful water jet on a keratinized firm surface would create no damage, whereas the same forceful jet on thin, less resistant tissue could cause damage.

D. **Indications**

Patients for whom particular benefit can be derived include those with potential food retentive areas:

1. Missing or reduced interdental papillae.
2. Fixed orthodontic appliances.
3. Restorative rehabilitative appliances: fixed partial dentures, splints.

E. **Contraindications**

1. Patients who require antibiotic premedication (see list on page 71). A bacteremia can occur following the use of oral irrigation,[18,19] particularly in patients with untreated gingivitis and periodontitis.
2. Deep periodontal pockets or tissue flaps covering unerupted or partially erupted third molars. Abscesses or periocoronal infections can be induced.
3. Clinically healthy gingiva, with minimum or normal sulcus depths, no bleeding on probing, and a patient who is capable of doing satisfactory plaque removal and cleaning with a toothbrush and

dental floss. In other words, patient who does not need an rigating device for a partic reason should not be encourage purchase and use one. It has been shown by research that stant pressure of the water str over the interdental papilla and area may not act to reduce height of the papilla, which happen when repeated pressur other interdental devices are u such as the interdental tip and b wood wedge.

DENTIFRICES

A dentifrice is a substance used wi toothbrush for the purposes of remov dental plaque, materia alba, and del and for applying specific agents to tooth surfaces for preventive or therap tic purposes. As a result of research, dentist and dental hygienist can ap current knowledge to aid the patien the selection of an appropriate dentif which will benefit or prevent harm to teeth and gingiva.

For a few patients, dentifrice selec can be based on individual preference flavor and cleaning ability, provided dentifrice is not excessively abrasive. most patients, dental caries control i: important factor, and a dentifrice cont ing fluoride is essential.

I. Basic Components[20-22]

Powder dentifrices contain abrasi detergents, flavoring, and sweete Paste dentifrices contain the same binders, humectants, preservative, water. Either may have a coloring age typical formula for a dentifrice would b

Detergent	1–!
Abrasive	20–4
Binder (thickener)	1–!
Humectant	10–:
Flavoring	1–!
Water	20–!

A therapeutic dentifrice has a drug or chemical agent added for a specific preventive or treatment action. In manufacturing products, a major problem is to combine agents that are compatible with each other.

A. **Detergents (Foaming Agents or Surfactants)**
1. Purposes: to lower surface tension, penetrate and loosen surface deposits and stains, emulsify debris for easy removal by the toothbrush, and contribute to the foaming action which many people like.
2. Criteria for use: nontoxic, neutral in reaction, active in acid or alkaline media, stable, compatible with other dentifrice ingredients, no distinctive flavor, and foaming characteristics.
3. Substances used: synthetic detergents

    Sodium lauryl sulfate USP
    Dioctyl sodium sulfosuccinate NF
    Sodium alkyl sulfoacetate
    Sulfocolaurate
    Sodium n-lauryl sarcosinate

B. **Abrasives and/or Polishing Agents**
1. Purposes: an abrasive for cleaning, and a polishing agent to produce a smooth, shiny tooth surface which will resist discoloration and bacterial accumulation and retention. Properties of abrasive agents are described on pages 538–540.
2. Criteria for use: the ideal abrasive is one that cleans well with no damage to the tooth surface and provides a high polish that can prevent or delay the reaccumulation of stains and deposits.
3. Abrasives used:

    Sodium bicarbonate
    Sodium chloride
    Calcium carbonate
    Calcium sulfate
    Calcium pyrophosphate (Crest)
    Calcium orthophosphate
    Dicalcium phosphate dihydrate

Insoluble sodium metaphosphate (IMP) (Cue, Fact, Super Stripe, Colgate with MFP)
Hydrated aluminum oxide
Magnesium carbonates and phosphates
Silicates and dehydrated silica gels

C. **Binders (Thickeners)**
1. Purpose: to prevent separation of the solid and liquid ingredients during storage.
2. Criteria: stable, nontoxic, compatible with other ingredients.
3. Types used: organic hydrophilic colloids

    Alginates
    Synthetic derivatives of cellulose
    Gum Tragacanth USP

    Organic colloids require a preservative to prevent microbial growth.

D. **Humectants**
1. Purposes: to retain moisture and prevent hardening on exposure to air.
2. Criteria: stable, nontoxic.
3. Substances used:

    Glycerol
    Sorbitol
    Propylene glycol

    These agents require a preservative to prevent microbial growth.

E. **Preservatives**
1. Purpose: to prevent bacterial growth.
2. Criteria: compatible with other ingredients.
3. Substances used:

    Alcohols
    Benzoates
    Formaldehyde
    Dichlorinated phenols

F. **Sweetening Agents**
1. Purpose: to impart a pleasant flavor.
2. Criteria: must be nonfermentable sugar.
3. Substances used:

    Artificial non-cariogenic sweetener
    Sorbitol and glycerin, used as humectants, contribute to sweet flavor

G. Flavoring Agents

1. Purpose: to make the dentifrice desirable; to mask other ingredients that may have a less pleasant flavor.
2. Criteria: remain unchanged during manufacturing and storage; compatible with other ingredients.
3. Substances used:

   Essential oils (peppermint, cinnamon, wintergreen, clove)
   Menthol
   Artificial non-cariogenic sweetener

H. Coloring Agents

1. Purpose: attractiveness
2. Criteria: does not stain teeth or discolor other oral tissues.
3. Types: varied; some striped.

II. Prophylactic or Therapeutic Dentifrices

The American Dental Association, Council on Dental Therapeutics evaluates only those dentifrices which claim therapeutic value. To date, a few fluoride dentifrices containing sodium monofluorophosphate or stannous fluoride have been classified as *Accepted*.* There is no evidence to indicate that any particular dentifrice has specific effectiveness in the prevention, treatment, or control of periodontal diseases except in the important role as an aid to plaque removal.

Over the years research on chlorophyll dentifrices, ammoniated dentifrices, dentifrices containing enzyme inhibitors such as sodium-n-lauryl sarcosinate and sodium dehydroacetate, and antibiotics, penicillin and tyrothricin, contributed to the search for a major break into dental caries prevention.[24,25] The fluoride dentifrice research has been shown to contribute the greatest benefits at the present time.

Problems with the fluoride dentifrices primarily have been related to finding

*For a description of American Dental Association classification of products, see *Technical Hints*, page 350.

compatible constituents to be combined with the fluoride in the dentifrice formula. The lack of caries prevention by early sodium fluoride dentifrices has been attributed to the use of abrasives containing calcium which combined with the fluoride and rendered it inactive.[26]

Stannous fluoride suffered similar problems since its instability in paste combination decreased the effectiveness in relatively short time. Additional research was required to find variations in the constituents which could overcome the problem.[27] The benefits derived from fluoride dentifrices are described in the chapter on fluorides, pages 440–441.

III. Dentifrice Selection

The dentifrice that has been used by the patient should be recorded with other information about self-care habits when the dental history is prepared. Later the dentifrice must be evaluated and a change recommended when necessary in accord with the individual oral condition and treatment objectives.

There are specific reasons for recommending particular dentifrices and for discouraging the use of others. The patient looks to the dentist and dental hygienist for professional advice and expects it to be in keeping with current research. The factors described below should be considered in dentifrice selection.

A. Dental Caries Control

The use of a fluoride dentifrice is generally recommended for all age groups and is mandatory for children and caries-prone adults. Fluoride for prevention of cemental caries is necessary after gingival recession and periodontal therapy (page 213). Since some staining is observed when the stannous fluoride dentifrice is used, the sodium monofluorophosphate dentifrice may be advisable for certain patients.

B. Abrasiveness

The patient with exposed cementum or dentin must be advised to use a very mildly abrasive dentifrice. It may be advantageous for the patient with marked recession to use plain water with a soft toothbrush at least a part of the time since that would be the least abrasive of all. Sodium bicarbonate is only slightly abrasive and will usually keep the teeth free from stains. If "salt and soda" are used together, the larger portion should be soda, at least two-thirds soda to one-third salt.

References for the comparative abrasiveness of commercial dentifrices to dentin and enamel are available.[28,29] Although the enamel is resistant to dentifrice abrasion, the repeated use over a long period of time would be undesirable. Dentifrice abrasion is described on page 325.

C. Desensitization

Dentifrices designated specifically for desensitization which are available commercially have not proven their claims sufficiently to gain approval of the Council on Dental Therapeutics. Desensitizing effects of sodium monofluorophosphate dentifrice have been demonstrated (page 564).

D. Cleaning Ability

Selection of a dentifrice on its cleaning ability alone precludes that none of the problems of caries prevention, susceptibility to dentifrice abrasion, or hypersensitivity is present, otherwise the dentifrice must meet dual or triple goals. The cleansing dentifrice is for general oral health and comfort, to improve the appearance, to aid in temporary reduction of mouth odors, to lower the bacterial count, and to control dental plaque. However, the ultimate beneficial effect depends on the frequency and thoroughness of brushing.

MOUTHWASHES

Mouthwashes, for oral rinsing, are classified as cosmetic or therapeutic. Claims for therapeutic value have not been scientifically substantiated, and there may be harm in continued use when a product contains certain chemicals or drugs. Mouthwashes which claim no therapeutic value are not included in the acceptance program of the American Dental Association, Council on Dental Therapeutics.[30] At present, the unsupervised use of medicated mouthwashes by the public cannot be considered to contribute to the oral health, and medicated mouthwashes are classified as *Unacceptable*. Both neutral sodium fluoride and phosphate acidulated fluoride solutions have been accepted as effective agents for use as mouthrinses for reducing the incidence of dental caries.*

When recording information about the oral health practices of a patient as part of the medical and dental history, it is advisable to determine whether a particular mouthwash is used, how frequently, and what the patient believes to be the benefit from its use. If any detrimental effects are suspected after the oral examination, or if adverse effects are known to be possible, the dentist can inform the patient and alternate procedures for rinsing can be recommended.

Rinsing as an aid in plaque control and suggestions for teaching a patient how to rinse were described on page 342.

I. Purposes and Uses

A. Dental Office or Clinic

1. Preoperative rinse to reduce incidence of bacteremia following instrumentation (pages 496–497).[31,32]
2. Preoperative rinse to reduce air contamination during use of handpiece and ultrasonic scaler (page 28).
3. Facilitate impression procedures (page 145).

*J. Am. Dent. Assoc., *91*, 1250, December, 1975.

4. Rinse and refresh the mouth during film placement for radiography and following a dental or dental hygiene procedure.

B. **Patient at Home**
1. Postoperative care
   a. After oral surgery as directed (page 614).
   b. After periodontal surgery: while the dressing is in place, a flavored mouthwash aids in removing debris and freshening the breath.
   c. After submarginal instrumentation: mild hypertonic salt solution may be advised for cleaning the area and encouraging healing.
2. Treatment: during pathologic conditions, for example, acute necrotizing ulcerative gingivitis, to remove debris, encourage healing, and soothe tender gingiva.
3. Cosmetic purposes
   Advertising claims can be misleading and patients need assistance in interpreting what they read and hear. Without advice, people generally select a mouthwash on the basis of flavor and color. Purposes and effects which may be expected from the use of a cosmetic mouthwash are:
   a. Removes loose debris when rinsing is vigorous.
   b. Gives temporary benefit through mechanical reduction in numbers of oral microorganisms.
   c. Imparts a pleasant taste, odor, and stimulating sensation to the oral cavity.
   d. Contributes to a temporary suppression of halitosis when causes are local.
4. Dental caries prevention: the use of sodium fluoride and stannous fluoride mouthwashes for dental caries

control is included in the chapter on fluoride application (page 440)

II. Self-Prepared Mouthwashes

Plain water, saline solutions, or solutions of bicarbonate of soda may be considered the most practical mouthwashes from the point of view of availability, cost, and effectiveness for debris removal and general oral cleanliness. Frequently prescribed or recommended by dentists, they may be helpful in postoperative care following dental and dental hygiene procedures.

When a salt solution is of greater strength than the physiologic salt solution concentration of body cells, by osmotic force fluid is drawn out of the cells to balance the pressure. This can effect reduction of edema and related benefits. The patient history must be checked, as a patient on a low salt or salt-free diet should not use a saline rinse.

A. **Water**

B. **Isotonic Sodium Chloride Solution**
1. Isotonic is normal or physiologic salt solution which is 0.9 percent aqueous solution; same concentration as cellular fluids.
2. Preparation (household measurements): level ½ teaspoonful salt added to one cup (eight ounces) of warm water.

C. **Hypertonic Sodium Chloride Solution**
1. A salt solution the osmotic pressure of which is greater than that of physiologic salt solution is hypertonic.
2. Preparation (household measurements): ½ teaspoonful salt added to ½ cup (four ounces) of warm water.

D. **Sodium Bicarbonate Solution**
Level ½ teaspoonful "soda" added to an eight-ounce glass of water.

E. Sodium Chloride—Sodium Bicarbonate Solution (flavored)

Sodium chloride	2.0 Gm.	½ teaspoonful
Sodium bicarbonate	1.0 Gm.	¼ teaspoonful
Amaranth solution	2.0 ml.	½ teaspoonful
Peppermint water to make	240.0 ml.	8 oz. glass

III. Commercial Mouthwash Ingredients[34,35]

Basic ingredients for both cosmetic and therapeutic types include flavoring, coloring, alcohol, water, and surface active agents.

A. Surface Active Agents
To facilitate cleaning and aid in the solubility of other ingredients.

B. Flavoring
Essential oils and their derivatives (Eucalyptus oil, oil of wintergreen) or aromatic waters (peppermint, spearmint, wintergreen, or others).

C. Alcohol
Ethyl alcohol is used to increase the solubility of the essential oils. The concentration should not exceed 10 percent because of irritation to the tissues. Alcohol acts to lower surface tension, is mildly astringent but is not antibacterial at 10 percent.

D. Water
Makes up the largest percent by volume.

E. Sweetening Agent
Artificial non-cariogenic sweetener

F. Coloring
Which will not discolor oral tissues.

IV. Active Ingredients[34,35]

Commercial mouthwashes generally contain more than one active ingredient and therefore may advertise more than one claim for usefulness. A number of factors influence how effective an agent may be, including the dilution by the saliva, the length of time the agent may be in contact with the tissue or bacteria, and the effect which contact with the organic matter of the mouth may have in changing the action. Agents and products listed below are for information only and should not be considered recommendations.

A. Antibacterial Agents
1. Purposes
   a. To reduce the oral microbacterial count. Although a partial effect is possible, there is inadequate evidence to show that there is any specific benefit from a nonspecific change in the oral flora.[30]
   b. Current research points to the possibility of an antibacterial mouth rinse which will reduce the amount or inhibit the formation of dental plaque and calculus.
2. Limitations of agents to use: many have disagreeable flavors, high cost, or their activity decreases when contact is made with organic matter in the mouth.
3. Active ingredients:

   Hexylresorcinol, thymol, and other phenol derivatives (Chloraseptic, ST 37)
   Quaternary Ammonium Compounds
   Benzethonium chloride (Colgate 100)
   Cetylpyridinium chloride (Scope, Cepacol, Micrin, Reef)
   Boric and Benzoic acid (Listerine, Mi 31)
   Chlorine-liberating compounds (Chlorpactic WCS 60, Kasdenol)
   Hexetidine (Sterisol)

B. Oxygenating Agents
1. Purposes: their effervescence makes them effective in debridement, and they are active against anaerobic microorganisms.

2. Uses: particularly in the treatment of acute necrotizing ulcerative gingivitis.
3. Active ingredients

Hydrogen peroxide (Hydrogen peroxide USP diluted with water)
Perborate (Amosan, Vince)

4. Precaution: continued use of hydrogen peroxide solution as well as most other oxygen-liberating drugs after the treatment of a disease, can lead to sponginess of the gingiva, formation of black hairy tongue, hypersensitiveness of exposed root surfaces and, because an acid is produced when water is added, decalcification of tooth surfaces.

C. **Astringents**
1. Purpose: shrinkage of tissues.
2. Uses: assist during impression making.
3. Active ingredients

Zinc chloride (Lavoris)
Zinc acetate
Alum
Tannic, acetic, and citric acids

4. Precaution: the agents are acid in water solution and can cause tooth decalcification and tissue irritation with repeated use.

D. **Anodynes**
1. Purposes: alleviate pain, soothe sore spots.
2. Uses: temporary pain relief for lesions of mucous membranes; during radiographic film exposure; aid in impression making.
3. Active ingredients

Phenol derivatives (Chloraseptic)
Essential oils

E. **Buffering Agents**
1. Purpose and uses: reduce oral acidity created by the fermentation of food debris; dissolve mucinous films; give relief for soreness of soft tissues.

2. Active ingredients

Sodium Borate Solution NF
Sodium Perborate NF
Sodium Bicarbonate USP

F. **Deodorizing Agents**
1. Purpose: neutralize odors from decomposed oral debris.
2. Uses: lessen possibility of halitosis from local causes.
3. Active ingredients
Chlorophyll and other deodorizing agents (Green Mint)

TECHNICAL HINTS

I. Classification of Products Evaluated by the Council on Dental Therapeutics[36]

American Dental Association

Commercial products are examined either upon the request of the manufacturer or distributor or upon the initiative of the Council. Products are usually accepted for three years. After consideration of a product has been completed, the Council will classify the product as "accepted," "provisionally accepted," or "unacceptable."

Accepted products include those for which there is adequate evidence for safety and effectiveness. They will be listed in *Accepted Dental Therapeutics* and may use the Seal of Acceptance or an authorized statement, unless otherwise provided.

Provisionally accepted will include those products for which there is reasonable evidence of usefulness and safety, but which lack sufficient evidence of dental usefulness to justify being "accepted." These products meet the other qualifications and standards established by the Council on Dental Therapeutics. The Council may authorize the use of a suitable statement to define specifically the area of usefulness of a product classified as "provisionally accepted." It is the policy of the Council to reconsider these products each year on the basis of new evidence which may be produced in their support. Classification in this category is not ordinarily continued for more than three years.

Unaccepted products will include those for which the Council has determined that there is no substantial evidence of usefulness or that a question of safety exists.

II. Inquire and record while preparing the patient's dental history, specific devices, dentifrices, mouthwashes, or other auxiliary aids used, in anticipation of evaluation for professional advice needed.

III. Request that patient bring for demonstration a device used, to assure that no harm is being done which, though not producing symptoms currently, could cause problems after long-term use.

References

1. Powers, G. K., Tussing, G. J., and Bradley, R. E.: A Comparison of Effectiveness in Interproximal Plaque Removal of an Electric Toothbrush and a Conventional Hand Toothbrush, *Periodontics*, 5, 37, January-February, 1967.
2. Keller, S. E. and Manson-Hing, L. R.: Clearance Studies of Proximal Tooth Surfaces. Part II. *In Vivo* Removal of Interproximal Plaque, *Alabama J. Med. Sci.*, 6, 266, July, 1969.
3. Mohammed, C. I. and Monserrate, V.: Dental Plaque Removal by Floss, *J. New Jersey Dent. Soc.*, 36, 419, July-August, 1965.
4. Masters, D. H.: Oral Hygiene Procedure for the Periodontal Patient, *Dent. Clin. North Am.*, 13, 3, January, 1969.
5. O'Leary, T. J. and Nabers, C. L.: Instructions to Supplement Teaching Oral Hygiene, *J. Periodont.*, 40, 27, January, 1969.
6. Smith, J. H., O'Connor, T. W., and Radentz, W.: Oral Hygiene of the Interdental Area, *Periodontics*, 1, 204, September-October, 1963.
7. Manson, J. D.: *Periodontics for the Dental Practitioner*. Chicago, Year Book, 1966, p. 51.
8. Burns, R. L.: A New Approach to Interproximal Hygiene, *Dent. Surv.*, 43, 77, June, 1967.
9. Burns, R. L.: The Most Neglected Aspect of Oral Hygiene, *J. Am. Dent. Hyg. Assoc.*, 42, 34, 1st Quarter, 1968.
10. Bossy, J.: Experiments with a Toothbrush ("Interspace Toothbrush"), *Dent. Health*, 4, 59, October-December, 1965.
11. Glickman, I., Petralis, R., and Marks, R. M.: Effect of Powered Toothbrushing Plus Interdental Stimulation Upon the Severity of Gingivitis, *J. Periodont.*, 35, 519, November-December, 1964.
12. Glickman, I., Petralis, R., and Marks, R. M.: The Effect of Powered Toothbrushing and Interdental Stimulation Upon Microscopic Inflammation and Surface Keratinization of the Interdental Gingiva, *J. Periodont.*, 36, 108, March-April, 1965.
13. American Dental Association: *Swish and Swallow Poster*, American Dental Association Catalog, No. S7.
14. Bernier, J. L., Sumnicht, R. W., Lancaster, J. E., and Monahan, J. L.: A Comparison of Three Oral Hygiene Measures, *J. Periodont.*, 37, 267, July-August, 1966.
15. Everett, F. G. and Bettman, M. M.: Mouth Rinsing, *J. Periodont.*, 23, 213, October, 1952.
16. American Dental Association, Council on Dental Materials and Devices: *Guide to Dental Materials and Devices*, 7th ed. Chicago, American Dental Association, 1974-1975, pp. 151-152, 272.
17. Bhaskar, S. N., Cutright, D. E., and Frisch, J.: Effect of High Pressure Water Jet on Oral Mucosa of Varied Density, *J. Periodont.*, 40, 593, October, 1969.
18. Romans, A. R. and App, G. R.: Bacteremia, a Result from Oral Irrigation in Subjects with Gingivitis, *J. Periodont.*, 42, 757, December, 1971.
19. Felix, J. E., Rosen, S., and App, G. R.: Detection of Bacteremia after the Use of an Oral Irrigation Device in Subjects with Periodontitis, *J. Periodont.*, 42, 785, December, 1971.
20. American Dental Association, Council on Dental Therapeutics: *Accepted Dental Therapeutics*, 36th ed. Chicago, American Dental Association, 1975, pp. 306-309.
21. Kutscher, A. H., Zegarelli, E. V., Hyman, G. A., McLean, P., and Kutscher, H. W.: *Pharmacology for the Dental Hygienist*. Philadelphia, Lea & Febiger, 1967, pp. 233-237.
22. Katz, S., McDonald, J. L., and Stookey, G. K.: *Preventive Dentistry in Action*. Upper Montclair, N.J., D.C.P. Publishing, 1972, pp. 194-204.
23. American Dental Association, Council on Dental Therapeutics: Abrasivity of Current Dentifrices, *J. Am. Dent. Assoc.*, 81, 1177, November, 1970.
24. Mandel, I. D. and Cagan, R. S.: Pharmaceutical Agents for Preventing Caries—A Review, *J. Oral Thera. and Pharm.*, 1, 218, September, 1964.

25. Nolte, W. A., ed.: *Oral Microbiology*, 2nd ed. St. Louis, Mosby, 1973, pp. 330–334.
26. Brudevold, F.: Fluorides in Prevention of Dental Caries, *Dent. Clin. North Am.*, p. 397, July, 1962.
27. Muhler, J. C.: Dentifrices and Oral Hygiene, in Bernier, J. L. and Muhler, J. C., eds.: *Improving Dental Practice Through Preventive Measures*, 2nd ed. St. Louis, Mosby, 1970, pp. 168–169.
28. Ibid., p. 160.
29. Stookey, G. K. and Muhler, J. C.: Laboratory Studies Concerning the Enamel and Dentin Abrasion Properties of Common Dentifrice Polishing Agents, *J. Dent. Res.*, 47, 524, July-August, 1968.
30. American Dental Association, Council on Dental Therapeutics: op. cit., pp. 309–311.
31. Scopp, I. W. and Orvieto, L. D.: Gingival Degerming by Povidone-iodine Irrigation: Bacteremia Reduction in Extraction Procedures, *J. Am. Dent. Assoc.*, 83, 1294, December, 1971.
32. Brennan, H. S. and Randall, E.: Local Degerming with Povidone-iodine. II. Prior to Gingivectomy, *J. Periodont.*, 45, 870, December, 1974.
33. Held, A. J.: Permanent Reaction of Periodontal Tissue by Treatment with Hypertonic Solutions, *J. Periodont.*, 34, 521, November, 1963.
34. Kutscher, et al.: op. cit., pp. 237–239.
35. Rosenthal, M. W.: Mouthwashes, in Balsam, M. S. and Sagarin, E., eds.: *Cosmetics Science and Technology*, 2nd ed., Volume 1. New York, Wiley-Interscience, 1972, pp. 533–563.
36. American Dental Association, Council on Dental Therapeutics: op. cit., p. xvi.

Suggested Readings

Bass, C. C.: The Optimum Characteristics of Dental Floss for Personal Oral Hygiene, *Dent. Items Int.*, 70, 921, September, 1948.
Bergenholtz, A., Bjorne, A., and Vikström, B.: The Plaque-removing Ability of Some Common Interdental Aids. An Intraindividual Study, *J. Clin. Periodont.*, 1, 160, No. 3, 1974.
Cantor, M. T. and Stahl, S. S.: Effects of Various Interdental Stimulators Upon the Keratinization of the Interdental Col, *Periodontics*, 3, 243, September-October, 1965.
Carter, H. G., Barnes, G. P., Bhaskar, S. N., and Woolridge, E. D.: Reduction of Gingival Sulcular Bleeding Using Interproximal Oral Hygiene Aids, *I.A.D.R. Program and Abstracts of Papers*, No. 163, March, 1974, p. 95.
Ceravolo, F. J., Baumhammers, A., and Robin, G.: The Odor Emitted from Dental Floss Used on Flossed Teeth and Non-flossed Teeth for a One Week Time Period, *Periodont. Abstr.*, 21, 155, Winter, 1973.
Frandsen, A., ed.: *Oral Hygiene*. Copenhagen, Munksgaard, 1972, pp. 39–62.

Gjermo, P. and Flötra, L.: The Effect of Different Methods of Interdental Cleaning, *J. Periodont. Res.*, 5, 230, No. 3, 1970.
Hill, H. C., Levi, P. A., and Glickman, I.: The Effects of Waxed and Unwaxed Dental Floss on Interdental Plaque Accumulation and Interdental Gingival Health, *J. Periodont.*, 44, 411, July, 1973.
Radentz, W. H., Barnes, G. P., Carter, H. G., Ailor, J. E., and Johnson, R. M.: An Evaluation of Two Techniques of Teaching Proper Dental Flossing Procedures, *J. Periodont.*, 44, 177, March, 1973.
Saunders, M.: Preventive Periodontics, *Dent. Health*, 10, 7, Spring, 1971.
Simaan, C. and Skarch, M.: Clinical and Histological Evaluation of Gingival Massage in the Treatment of Chronic Gingivitis, *J. Periodont.*, 37, 383, September-October, 1966.
Terhune, J. A.: Predicting the Readiness of Elementary School Children to Learn an Effective Dental Flossing Technique, *J. Am. Dent. Assoc.*, 86, 1332, June, 1973.
Vollmer, D. E.: Preventive Dentistry: Precaution Pays, *J. Am. Soc. Prev. Dent.*, 4, 31, November-December, 1974.

Oral Irrigation

Astwood, L. A. S.: Oral Irrigating Devices; An Appraisal of Current Information, *J. Public Health Dent.*, 35, 2, Winter, 1975.
Brady, J. M., Gray, W. A., and Bhaskar, S. N.: Electron Microscopic Study of the Effect of Water Jet Lavage Devices on Dental Plaque, *J. Dent. Res.*, 52, 1310, November-December, 1973.
Cantor, M. T. and Stahl, S. S.: Interdental Col Tissue Responses to the Use of a Water Pressure Cleansing Device, *J. Periodont.*, 40, 292, May, 1969.
Clynes, J. T. and Wilderman, M. N.: Effectiveness of a Water-pressure Device in Removing Debris from Teeth, *J. Public Health Dent.*, 30, 2, Winter, 1970.
Covin, N. R., Lainson, P. A., Belding, J. H., and Fraleigh, C. M.: The Effects of Stimulating the Gingiva by a Pulsating Water Device, *J. Periodont.*, 44, 286, May, 1973.
Cutright, D. E., Bhaskar, S. N., and Larson, W. J.: Variable Tissue Forces Produced by Water Jet Devices, *J. Periodont.*, 43, 765, December, 1972.
Elliott, J. R., Bowers, G. M., Clemmer, B. A., and Rovelstad, G. H.: II. A Comparison of Selected Oral Hygiene Devices in Dental Plaque Removal, *J. Periodont.*, 43, 217, April, 1972.
Fine, D. H. and Baumhammers, A.: Effect of Water Pressure Irrigation on Stainable Material on the Teeth, *J. Periodont.*, 41, 468, August, 1970.
Gupta, O. P., O'Toole, E. T., and Hammermeister, R. O.: Effects of a Water Pressure Device on Oral Hygiene and Gingival Inflammation, *J. Periodont.*, 44, 294, May, 1973.
Hoover, D. R. and Robinson, H. B. G.: The Comparative Effectiveness of a Pulsating Oral Irrigator as an Adjunct in Maintaining Oral Health, *J. Periodont.*, 42, 37, January, 1971.

Jann, R.: Water Irrigating Devices, *Periodont. Abstr.*, *18*, 6, March, 1970.

Lainson, P. A., Bergquist, J. J., and Fraleigh, C. M.: Clinical Evaluation of Pulsar, a New Pulsating Water Pressure Cleansing Device, *J. Periodont.*, *41*, 401, July, 1970.

Lainson, P. A., Bergquist, J. J., and Fraleigh, C. M.: A Longitudinal Study of Pulsating Water Pressure Cleansing Devices, *J. Periodont.*, *43*, 444, July, 1972.

Lobene, R. R.: The Effect of a Pulsed Water Pressure Cleansing Device on Oral Health, *J. Periodont.*, *40*, 667, November, 1969.

Lobene, R. R.: A Study of the Force of Water Jets in Relation to Pain and Damage to Gingival Tissues, *J. Periodont.*, *42*, 166, March, 1971.

Lobene, R. R., Soparkar, P. M., Hein, J. W., and Quigley, G. A.: A Study of the Effects of Antiseptic Agents and a Pulsating Irrigating Device on Plaque and Gingivitis, *J. Periodont.*, *43*, 564, September, 1972.

O'Leary, T. J., Shafer, W. G., Swenson, H. M., Nesler, D. C., and Van Dorn, P. R.: Possible Penetration of Crevicular Tissue from Oral Hygiene Procedures: I. Use of Oral Irrigating Devices, *J. Periodont.*, *41*, 158, March, 1970.

Wheatcroft, M. G. and Sciantarelli, E.: The Effect of Oral Water Irrigation on the Prevention of Gingival Inflammation, *J. Am. Soc. Prev. Dent.*, *4*, 38, July-August, 1974.

Toto, P. D., Evans, C. L., and Sawinski, V. J.: Effects of Water Jet Rinse and Toothbrushing on Oral Hygiene, *J. Periodont.*, *40*, 296, May, 1969.

Dentifrice

Allen, A. L., Hawley, C. E., Cutright, D. E., and Seibert, J. S.: An Investigation of the Clinical and Histologic Effects of Selected Dentifrices on Human Palatal Mucosa, *J. Periodont.*, *46*, 102, February, 1975.

Berman, E. and McKiel, K.: Is That Toothpaste Safe? *Arch. Environ. Health*, *25*, 64, July, 1972.

Bogle, G. C.: Abrasivity of Dentifrices and Toothbrushes, *Periodont. Abstr.*, *22*, 7, Spring, 1974.

Facq, J. M. and Volpe, A. R.: *In Vivo* Actual Abrasiveness of Three Dentifrices Against Acrylic Surfaces of Veneer Crowns, *J. Am. Dent. Assoc.*, *80*, 317, February, 1970.

Gershon, S. D. and Pader, M.: Dentifrices, in Balsam, M. S. and Sagarin, E., eds.: *Cosmetics Science and Technology*, 2nd ed., Volume 1. New York, Wiley-Interscience, 1972, pp. 423–531.

Heath, J. R. and Wilson, H. J.: The Effect of Dentifrices on Restorative Materials, *J. Oral Rehab.*, *1*, 47, No. 1, 1974.

Heifetz, S. B. and Horowitz, H. S.: An Appraisal of Therapeutic Dentifrices, *J. Public Health Dent.*, *30*, 206, Fall, 1970.

Kowitz, G., Lucatorto, F., and Bennett, W.: Effects of Dentifrices on Soft Tissues of the Oral Cavity, *J. Oral Med.*, *28*, 105, October-December, 1973.

Lobene, R. R.: Effect of Dentifrices on Tooth Stains with Controlled Brushing, *J. Am. Dent. Assoc.*, *77*, 849, October, 1968.

Phillips, R. W.: *Skinner's Science of Dental Materials*, 7th ed. Philadelphia, Saunders, 1973, pp. 635–640.

Robinson, H. B. G.: Individualizing Dentifrices: The Dentist's Responsibility, *J. Am. Dent. Assoc.*, *79*, 633, September, 1969.

Rundegren, J., Fornell, J., and Ericson, T.: *In Vivo* and *In Vitro* Studies on a New Peroxide-containing Toothpaste, *Scand. J. Dent. Res.*, *81*, 543, No. 7, 1973.

Shapiro, I. M., Cohen, G. H., Needleman, H. L., and Tuncay, O. C.: The Presence of Lead in Toothpaste, *J. Am. Dent. Assoc.*, *86*, 394, February, 1973.

Sturzenberger, O. P., Swancar, J. R., and Reiter, G.: Reduction of Dental Calculus in Humans Through the Use of a Dentifrice Containing a Crystal-growth Inhibitor, *J. Periodont.*, *42*, 416, July, 1971.

Suomi, J. D., Horowitz, H. S., Barbano, J. P., Spolsky, V. W., and Heifetz, S. B.: A Clinical Trial of a Calculus-inhibitory Dentifrice, *J. Periodont.*, *45*, 139, March, 1974.

Toto, P. D. and Rapp, G. W.: A Clinical Comparison of a New Low Abrasive Dentifrice with Intermediate and High Abrasive Dentifrices, *J. Periodont.*, *43*, 492, August, 1972.

Volpe, A. R., Mooney, R., Zumbrunnen, C., Stahl, D., and Goldman, H. M.: A Long Term Clinical Study Evaluating the Effect of Two Dentifrices on Oral Tissues, *J. Periodont.*, *46*, 113, February, 1975.

Wictorin, L.: Effect of Toothbrushing on Acrylic Resin Veneering Material. II. Abrasive Effect of Selected Dentifrices and Toothbrushes, *Acta Odont. Scand.*, *30*, 383, September, 1972.

Mouthwash

Ball, D. M. and Ball, E. L.: Comparative Effectiveness of Two Mouthwashes Used after Gingivectomy, *J. Periodont.*, *38*, 395, September-October, 1967.

Carter, H. G. and Barnes, G. P.: Effects of Three Mouthwashes on Existing Dental Plaque Accumulations, *J. Prev. Dent.*, *2*, 6, May-June, 1975.

Duany, L. F., Fitzgerald, R. J., Llorente, M., and Zinner, D. D.: Effects of Povidone-iodine and Isotonic Saline on the Oral Health of Children, *J. Prev. Dent.*, *2*, 22, May-June, 1975.

Gomer, R. M., Holroyd, S. V., Fedi, P. F., and Ferrigno, P. D.: The Effect of Oral Rinses, *J. Am. Soc. Prev. Dent.*, *2*, 6, March-April, 1972.

Griffiths, K. M. E. and Wade, A. B.: The Value of Including Flavouring and Colouring Agents in a Mouth Wash, *Dent. Health*, *4*, 20, April-June, 1965.

Lusk, S. S., Bowers, G. M., Tow, H. D., Watson, W. J., and Moffitt, W. C.: Effects of an Oral Rinse on Experimental Gingivitis, Plaque Formation, and Formed Plaque, *J. Am. Soc. Prev. Dent.*, *4*, 31, July-August, 1974.

Stallard, R. E., Volpe, A. R., Orban, J. E., and King, W. J.: The Effect of an Antimicrobial Mouth Rinse on Dental Plaque, Calculus and Gingivitis, *J. Periodont.*, *40*, 683, December, 1969.

Sturzenberger, O. P. and Leonard, G. J.: The Effect of a Mouthwash as Adjunct in Tooth Cleaning, *J. Periodont.*, *40*, 299, May, 1969.

Chapter 24

Care of Dental Appliances

Total cleanliness of the oral cavity for the health of the teeth and supporting structures involves specific procedures for the care of the natural teeth and all appliances, both fixed and removable. A dental *appliance* is a device used to provide function or for therapeutic purposes. A *prosthesis* is an appliance for the replacement of a missing part of the body by an artificial part.

From the dentist's viewpoint, the success of a dental appliance depends to a large degree on the cooperation of the patient in daily cleaning of the appliance, and plaque control and oral physical therapy for the remaining natural teeth. Likewise, the orthodontist is concerned that appliances be kept clean and periodontal health be maintained.

The patient's cooperation depends on the motivation, information, and sense of appreciation and concern imparted by the dentist and the dental hygienist. For the natural teeth involved, instruction begins early before construction of the partial denture or placement of orthodontic appliances. Instruction is supplemented when an appliance is inserted to demonstrate specific techniques for daily care. Continuing supervision and review of procedures at succeeding appointments and recall appointments are required.

Fixed appliances include fixed partial dentures, space maintainers, periodontal splints, and orthodontic appliances. Examples of removable types are complete and partial dentures, space maintainers, and orthodontic appliances, as well as obturators for closure of palatal defects.

A patient may have more than one prosthesis. For example, there may be a complete maxillary denture, and both fixed and removable partial dentures in the mandibular arch. For this patient, the regimen for personal care involves the natural teeth as well as the fixed and removable dentures. A program of instruction must be worked out for each patient depending on individual needs.

FIXED PARTIAL DENTURES

A partial denture replaces one or more but less than all of the natural teeth.* The fixed partial denture, otherwise called a

---

*All definitions in this chapter which pertain to prosthetic appliances are taken from or adapted from and in accord with the *Glossary of Prosthetic Terms*, 3rd ed., prepared by the Nomenclature Committee of the Academy of Denture Prosthetics, St. Louis, The Journal of Prosthetic Dentistry, Mosby, 1968.

fixed bridge, is one that cannot be re-moved but is permanently attached to natural teeth or roots which furnish support to the appliance.

I. Components of a Fixed Partial Denture (figure 24–1)

A. Abutment
A tooth used for the support or anchorage of a fixed prosthesis is called an abutment tooth.

B. Retainer
An inlay, onlay, or crown which restores an abutment tooth, and is used for fixation and support of the fixed partial denture is called a retainer.

C. Pontic
A pontic is an artificial tooth which replaces a lost natural tooth, restores its function, and usually occupies the space previously occupied by the natural crown.

D. Connector
A connector unites the retainer to the pontic or joins two individual pontics. In a fixed partial denture the connector may be a solder joint or, when the entire bridge is cast as a

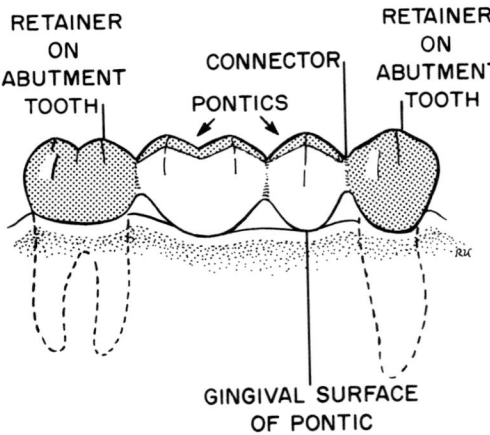

RETAINER ON ABUTMENT TOOTH   CONNECTOR   PONTICS   RETAINER ON ABUTMENT TOOTH

GINGIVAL SURFACE OF PONTIC

Figure 24–1. Parts of a fixed partial denture. Mandibular four unit fixed partial denture to show characteristic parts. Cast gold crowns on abutment teeth serve as the retainers for this bridge.

single unit, the connector may be continuous with the retainer.

E. Surfaces
1. Occlusal: the surface which occludes with opposing teeth.
2. Gingival: the portion or side of the pontic which is adjacent to the edentulous gingiva beneath it.

II. Care Procedures

A. Debris Removal
When suggesting a procedure to follow for cleaning the oral cavity when a fixed partial denture is present, debris removal with an oral irrigator may be recommended as the first step. By removing food and debris, access of the toothbrush and other aids for plaque removal is facilitated. Procedure for use of an oral irrigator is described on pages 342–344.

B. The Abutment Teeth
Nearly all of the methods proposed for plaque control and oral physical therapy in the two previous chapters may be applicable to abutment teeth. The proximal surface and gingiva of an abutment tooth adjacent to a pontic usually require special attention.
1. Toothbrushing: a vibratory technique, or a combination of brushing techniques, is generally indicated. The area of the tooth surface adjacent to and beneath the gingival margin must be kept meticulously free of dental plaque. A nonabrasive dentifrice is indicated to prevent the possibility of abrasion when pontic or crown facings are made of acrylic, when the gold of the partial denture is highly polished and could be scratched, and when there are areas of root exposure on abutment teeth.
2. Additional interdental care: an interdental plaque removal method indicated. This is selected on the

basis of the individual patient or the appliance. The interdental cleaning device is adapted specifically to the distal of the mesial abutment and the mesial of the distal abutment, and from both facial and lingual. The same interdental cleaning procedure can usually be applied to the gingival surface of the fixed partial denture. Interdental cleaning methods and devices are described on pages 331–341.

C. **The Appliance**
1. Areas requiring emphasis: the gingival surfaces of the pontics, and beneath the connectors, are particularly prone to plaque retention.
2. Toothbrushing: a toothbrush in the Charters' position provides one adaptation for cleaning the gingival surface of the pontic from the facial aspect. The filaments can be directed under the pontic to clean the gingival surface.
3. Dental floss
   a. Thread a 12- to 15-inch length between an abutment and pontic, or under the pontic if space permits. The floss may be rigid enough if folded on the end and pressed together, or a plastic or metal floss threader may be more conveniently used. Several types are available (figure 24–2).
   b. Draw the floss through and, using single or double thickness, remove loose debris (figure 24–3).
   c. Apply a new section of the floss with moderate pressure and dentifrice to the undersurface (gingival surface) of the pontics, and then to the proximal surfaces of the abutment teeth, to remove dental plaque. Remove floss and rinse.
   d. Use an additional clean piece of

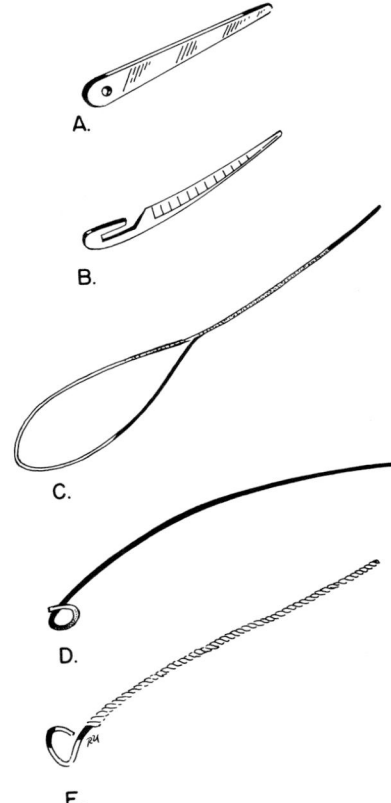

Figure 24–2. Examples of floss threaders. **A.** Clear plastic with closed eye. **B.** Tinted plastic with open eye. **C.** Soft plastic loop. **D.** Flexible wire. **E.** Twisted wire.

floss to remove particles of dentifrice.
4. Knitting yarn: tie yarn to floss in floss threader and pull through under the appliance for a thicker cleaning device than floss alone (page 336).
5. Other interdental devices: the pipe cleaner, interproximal brush, or interdental tip should be recommended and demonstrated as indicated by the needs of the individual appliance.

ORTHODONTIC APPLIANCES

There is a high dental caries rate in teeth with orthodontic appliances, and

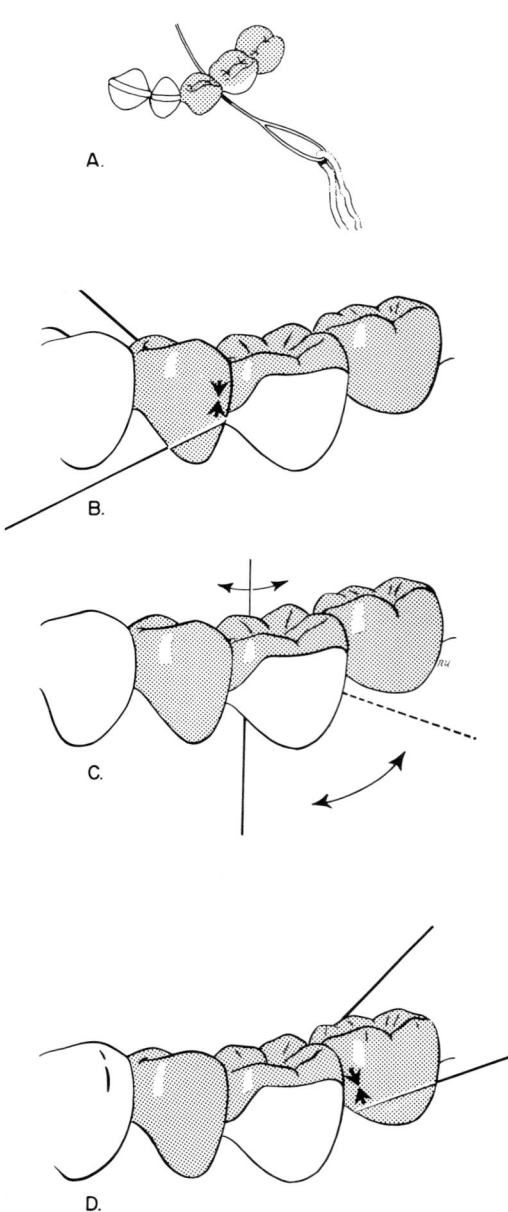

Figure 24–3. Cleaning a fixed partial denture. **A.** Use floss threader to draw floss (or yarn when space permits) between an abutment and a pontic. **B.** Apply floss to the distal surface of the mesial abutment. **C.** Slide floss under pontic. Move back and forth several times as shown by the arrows to remove plaque from the gingival surface of the pontic. **D.** Apply new section of floss to the mesial surface of the distal abutment tooth.

severe gingival and periodontal diseases during and following treatment are not unusual. A rigid preventive program for the patient with fixed orthodontic appliances along with a specific plan of instruction, motivation, and supervision is essential.

The dental hygienist who works with an orthodontist is in a position to perform a highly specialized service. Since the patient will be under care with regular appointments for a long period, frequently over a few years, periodic communication between the patient's referring dentist and dental hygienist is necessary in order that instruction be coordinated along with other necessary dental and dental hygiene care.

I. Complicating Factors

A. **Age**

Most orthodontic patients are pre-teen and teen-age.

1. The incidence of gingivitis is high in this age group; up to 90 percent of patients from ages 9 to 14, with the peak between ages 11 and 13, have gingivitis.[1]

2. At puberty there is a tendency for the gingival tissue to show deviations from normal when hormonal changes may be reflected in the gingiva.

B. **Gingival Enlargement**

Puberty is frequently accompanied by an exaggerated response of the gingiva to local irritation.[2] With orthodontic appliances, the reaction may be compounded, the degree varying from slight to severe enlargement particularly of the papillae. The tissue may greatly enlarge and cover the bands.[3]

C. **Position of Teeth**

Teeth that are irregularly positioned are naturally more susceptible to the retention of deposits and are more difficult to clean. With the severe malocclusions of orthodontic patients, this factor becomes even more significant.

D. **Increased Oral Microbial Flora**

The greater the number of bands on the teeth, the greater increase in microbial counts.[4,5]

E. **Problems with Appliances**[6]
1. Plaque, debris and materia alba are retained.
2. Accidents may cause wires to bend adversely and become imbedded in the gingiva. A loosened band may be forced under the gingiva.
3. Removable appliances or their clasps can press excessively against the gingiva.
4. Rubber bands may slip under the gingiva and detach the junctional epithelium.

F. **Effects on the Periodontium**[7]
1. Increased plaque retention leads to increased gingival and periodontal pocket formation.
2. Excessive forces during too rapid tooth movement may produce necrosis in the periodontal ligament and resorption of alveolar bone.

G. **Self-Care is Difficult**

Even the patient who tries to maintain oral cleanliness has difficulty because the appliances are in the way and interfere with the application of the toothbrush and other devices used for plaque control and oral physical therapy.

II. Toothbrushing

With such a variety of appliances utilized for orthodontic treatment,[8] it is difficult to be too specific in the type of brush and the brushing method which should be selected for an individual patient. As with the selection of procedure for any patient, the severity of the oral condition, the anatomical features of the gingiva, the position of the teeth as well as other factors are the determinants (pages 386–387). Several variations of brush positioning are suggested below.

A. **General Instructions**
1. Perform brushing before a mirror so that brush application is accurate and brushing is thorough.
2. Use a disclosing solution rinse to assist in self-evaluation. Orthodontic patients may find it difficult to chew disclosing wafers without discomfort or pain.[9]
3. Dentifrice: an approved fluoride dentifrice is recommended to aid in dental caries control.
4. Emphasis in brushing should be placed on sulcular brushing and cleaning the area between the orthodontic bands and brackets and the gingiva.

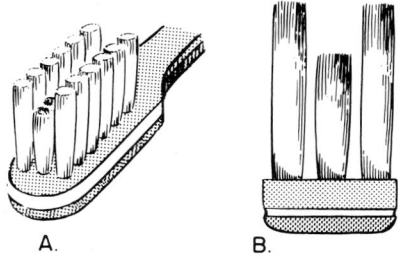

A.   B.

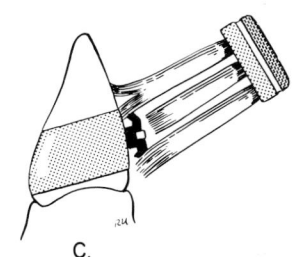

C.

Figure 24–4. Orthodontic toothbrush. **A.** Middle row of filaments trimmed short to fit over fixed appliance. **B.** Cross section. **C.** Illustration of incorrect position of brush. Note that the tipped brush prevents full use of filament tips in cleaning plaque and debris from around bracket and wire.

B. **Manual Brushing**
  1. Brush selection
    a. A soft nylon brush with rounded filaments is generally recommended.
    b. Special orthodontic brush. Designed with two spaced rows of soft nylon filaments with a third middle row which is shorter; it can be applied directly over the fixed appliance and used with a short horizontal stroke (figure 24–4).
  2. Brushing procedure
    a. A vibratory method is needed by most patients for cleaning the appliances and maintaining the gingiva (Modified Stillman, Bass, or Charters', pages 314–318).
    b. Special adaptation for facial surface: place the brush in the Charters' position for over the wire and bracket (or under for mandibular); and Stillman's position for the opposite side (figure 24–5).
    c. To assure cleanliness, it has been suggested that the appliances should be brushed in any way that the filaments can be manipulated: insert the brush from below, over, and above the arch wire, rotate and vibrate to remove plaque and debris.[10]
    d. Lingual: appropriate method which is similar to the basic strokes used on the facial surfaces.

C. **Automatic Toothbrush**
  1. Research: Studies have been reported in which an automatic brush was compared with a manual brush used by orthodontic patients. In one,[11] the brushes were equally effective in preventing or removing dental plaque and calculus, and had an equal effect on gingivitis,

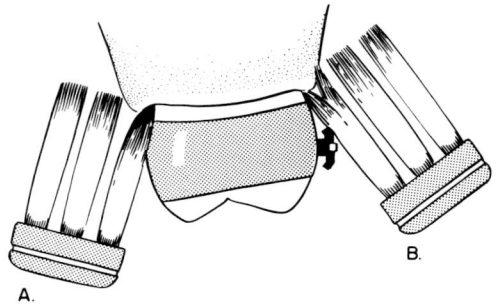

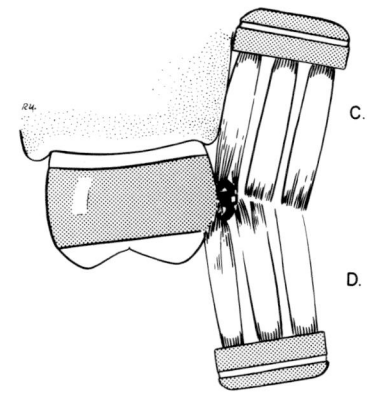

Figure 24–5. Toothbrushing for the patient with fixed orthodontic appliances. Sulcular brushing is advised. **A.** Lingual. **B.** Facial. **C.** Cleaning the appliance: brush in Charters' brushing position for the gingival side, and **D.** in Stillman's position for occlusal side of bracket and wire. An automatic brush can be applied in the same positions.

periodontal disease index, and depth of the gingival sulcus. The other study[12] showed the automatic to be superior in its cleaning efficiency to the manual toothbrush. Both studies indicated that the brushes can be used without an increased incidence of damage or dislodgment of the appliances.
  2. Technique: select softest automatic tip and apply for sulcus brushing and cleaning the appliance (figure 24–5).

III. **Additional Measures**

A. **Interdental Aids**
  The previously described applications of the interdental tip and Perio-

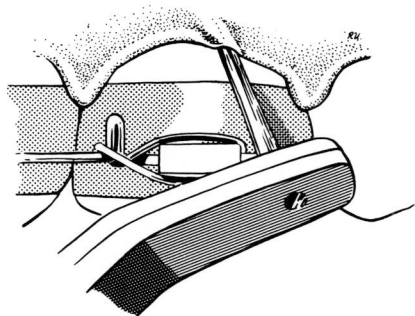

Figure 24–6. Perio-aid for the orthodontic patient. Moistened toothpick end can be applied to clean about appliances and in the submarginal area of gingival sulci and pockets. Directions for use of the Perio-aid are on page 338.

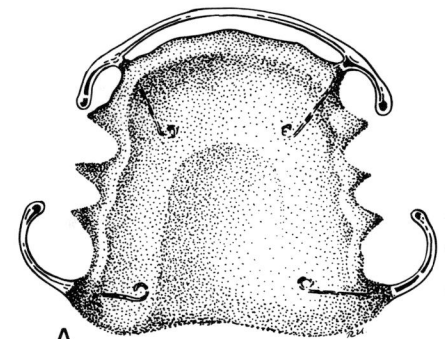

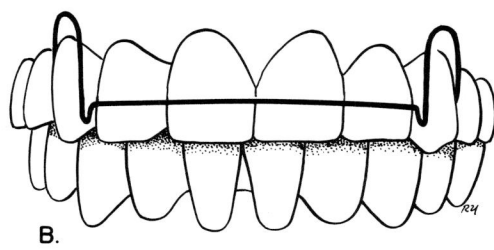

Figure 24–7. Hawley appliance. **A.** Removable acrylic retainer with labial retaining wire and clasps of type worn by orthodontic patient following removal of fixed appliance. **B.** Anterior view of patient showing Hawley appliance in position. Cleaning instructions are the same as for a removable denture (page 369).

aid (pages 337, 340) also apply for care of the orthodontic patient (figure 24–6). A floss threader is needed for plaque removal from proximal tooth surfaces when the appliance prevents passage of floss from the occlusal.

B. **Oral Irrigation**

Most orthodontic patients can benefit from the regular use of an irrigator. From research it was demonstrated that the use of an irrigator will prevent an increase in gingivitis and to some extent decrease gingivitis as well as assist in plaque control.[9,13]

C. **Care of Removable Appliance or Hawley Retainer (figure 24–7)**
1. Clean the appliance after each meal and before retiring. Instructions for cleaning procedures and agents for removable appliances are described with the care of the complete denture (pages 364–365).
2. Teeth and gingival tissue under appliance: brush and rinse each time the appliance is removed. Unless absolutely necessary as directed by the orthodontist, it is best for the health of the underlying tissues if the appliance is not kept in the mouth continuously.

3. Brushing the mucosa under the appliance is frequently advisable. Methods are described on page 366.
4. Keep appliance in a container with water when it is out of the mouth.

COMPLETE DENTURES

Instruction may be for the patient receiving a maxillary and mandibular denture for the first time, for the patient whose dentures have been remade or relined, or for the patient with a single denture which opposes natural teeth. Another patient may be receiving an immediate denture, that is, a denture inserted immediately following removal of natural teeth.

Preliminary instruction must be given the day the appliances are delivered with the exception of the immediate denture which is usually not removed by the patient until after the next appointment. The initial instruction should consist of brief and simple procedures for cleaning the denture and rinsing the mouth. Because on insertion of first dentures the patient may have a number of anxieties relating to appearance, eating, or speaking, the main part of the instruction should be given at succeeding appointments.

It should not be assumed that the patient, who is new to the dental office and is wearing dentures or a denture, knows the proper techniques for caring for the appliances. During questioning for the patient history, information about the method and frequency of denture care is recorded. Later the method of care is reviewed, and alternate cleaning agents, devices, or procedures recommended and demonstrated as indicated.

The need for individual instruction in care of the denture was brought out in a survey of nearly one thousand patients. Of these only 17.5 percent considered their cleaning methods inefficient, but nearly 70 percent exhibited unclean, stained dentures.[14]

I. Components of a Complete Denture (figure 24–8)

To understand the effects of various cleaning agents and devices, information about the structure and material of the parts of a denture is pertinent.

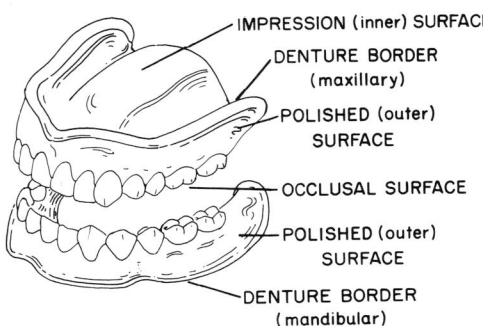

IMPRESSION (inner) SURFACE

DENTURE BORDER (maxillary)

POLISHED (outer) SURFACE

OCCLUSAL SURFACE

POLISHED (outer) SURFACE

DENTURE BORDER (mandibular)

Figure 24–8.   Parts of a complete denture.

A. Denture Base

That part of a denture which rests on the oral mucosa and to which the teeth are attached. Most denture bases are of plastic resin or a metal, for example, chrome-cobalt or gold.

B. Surfaces

1. Impression surface: also called the tissue or inner surface, is the part which lies adjacent to the mucous membrane of the alveolar ridge and immediately associated parts; in the maxillary the tissue surface is adjacent to the hard palate.
2. Polished surface: the external or outer surface, is highly polished and includes everything except the occlusal surface.
3. Occlusal surface: that portion of the surface of a denture which makes contact or near contact with the corresponding surface of the opposing denture or natural teeth.

C. Teeth

The denture teeth may be made of plastic resin or porcelain. Anterior porcelain teeth have metal pins for retention.

II. Purposes for Cleaning

A. Prevent irritants to the oral tissues.
   1. Mechanical irritants: rough deposits of plaque, calculus, thick stains.
   2. Chemical irritants: products of putrefaction of food debris and bacterial metabolic products.

B. Prevent mouth odors.

C. Maintain appearance.

III. Denture Deposits

Accumulation of stains and deposits on dentures varies between individuals in a manner similar to that on natural teeth. The phases of deposit formation may be divided as follows:

A. Mucin and food debris on the denture surface: readily removed by rinsing or superficial cleaning.

B. Dental pellicle and dental plaque: more tenacious, less easy to remove. When left they form the matrix for stain accumulation and calculus formation.

C. Calculus: hard and fixed to the denture surface, generally located on the buccal of the maxillary molars and lingual of mandibular anterior region.

IV. Methods for Cleaning

A. **Rinsing under Running Water**
   Although it would be unusual if a denture could be kept clean by this method only, the use of rinsing after meals when other methods are not possible is necessary.

B. **Brushing**
   With water, soap, or other mild cleansing agent. Coarse abrasives produce scratches.

C. **Immersion**
   The denture is soaked in a solvent or detergent where chemical action removes or loosens stains and deposits which can then be rinsed or brushed away. A sonic device for home use combines immersion in a prepared solution with vibration. From the limited research about this device, it is believed that the cleaning of the denture is more related to the chemical activity of the solution than to the vibratory activity of the device.[15]

V. Classification of Denture Cleaners[14,16]

A. **Solution Cleaners** (Immersion)
   1. *Hypochlorite Solutions*
      a. Active ingredient: dilute sodium hypochlorite.
      b. Example: Clorox.
      c. Disadvantages: odor, corrodes certain metals.

   2. *Alkaline Peroxide Cleaners*
      a. Active ingredient: alkaline peroxide with oxygen-liberating agent.
      b. Examples: Efferdent, Polident, and most other proprietary cleaners.
      c. Disadvantage: will not remove heavy stains or calculus.

   3. *Dilute Acids*
      a. Active ingredient: organic or inorganic acids.
      b. Examples: vinegar, five percent hydrochloric acid; commercially prepared ultrasonic solutions.
      c. Disadvantage: corrosion of chrome alloys (hydrochloric acid).

B. **Abrasive Cleaners**
   1. *Denture Pastes and Powders,* toothpastes and powders.
      a. Active ingredient: an abrasive (see Dentifrices, page 345).
      b. Examples: various commercial products.
      c. Disadvantage: can abrade the plastic resin denture base and acrylic teeth.

   2. *Household Agents*
      a. Active ingredient: detergent and/or abrasive agent.
      b. Examples: salt, bicarbonate of soda, are mildly abrasive; hand soap is cleansing and not particularly abrasive. Scouring powders or other excessively abrasive cleaners should not be used.

VI. General Cleaning Procedures

A. **When to Clean**
   1. Regularly after each meal and before retiring.
   2. Chemical immersion: daily, twice weekly, or weekly, depending on the rate of formation of calculus and stain and the type of solution used.

a. May be at one of the regular cleanings.
b. Suggested: while bathing.
c. May be overnight if denture is removed as instructed by the dentist.

B. **Selection of Method for Cleaning**
    Most people use immersion, brushing, or a combination of the two. When unable to clean, rinsing after eating is advised.

VII. Cleaning by Immersion

A. **Advantages**[17]
1. The solution reaches all areas of the denture for a complete cleaning.
2. Minimizes danger of dropping the appliance: prevents need for handling which is required during brushing.
3. Safe storage when dentures are out of the mouth.
4. Abrasion of the denture material is not possible.
5. Aid to handicapped person with limited ability to manage a brush.
6. When cleaning is distasteful, immersion involves the least handling and observation. This is an advantage particularly for an attendant or nurse who must clean the denture of a helpless patient.

B. **Procedure**
1. Rinse the denture when it is taken from the mouth to remove saliva and loose debris; place in a plastic container with fitted cover which is maintained specifically for this purpose.*
2. Use only warm water for rinsing and for mixing the solution: warm water promotes the action of the cleaner, whereas hot water should never be used because it can distort plastic resin.

*Procedure for removal of a denture for a patient is described on page 549.

3. Cover the denture with solution; cover the container.
4. When the denture is removed, rinse under running water, and brush to remove loosened debris and chemicals before placing in the mouth.

C. **Solutions**
1. *Proprietary.* Purchasable in powder or tablet form.
    a. Preparation: add measured warm water as directed by the manufacturer.
    b. Length of immersion: usually 10 to 15 minutes or as suggested by the manufacturer. Since the action is dependent on the mechanical bubbling effect of released oxygen, the solution has little value after the available oxygen has been released.
    c. Effect: these solutions are only effective against loose debris, and denture cleanliness is dependent on regular daily immersion supplemented by brushing.
2. *Hypochlorite Solution.* Clorox (five percent sodium hypochlorite) and Calgon. Calgon acts as an anticorrosion agent.[18]
    a. Proportions
       1 teaspoonful Clorox
       2 teaspoonfuls Calgon
       ½ glass warm water
    b. Length of immersion: usually 10 to 15 minutes. When stains or calculus form, it may be suggested that the patient soak the denture overnight provided there are no metal parts that can become corroded.
3. *White Household Vinegar*
    a. Indication for use: only when calculus is observed on the denture; not routinely.[17]
    b. Proportion: one or two teaspoonfuls in one cup of warm water.
    c. Length of immersion: the denture may be immersed overnight

when necessary for complete cleaning.

VIII. Cleaning by Brushing

A. **Type of Brush**
   1. *Denture Brush.* A good quality denture brush with rounded filaments is preferable because it is designed for the purpose with two arrangements of filaments: one group in a large round group of tufts permits access to the inner, curved impression surface of the denture. The second group of tufts is arranged to form a rectangular brush for convenient adaptation to the polished and occlusal denture surfaces (figure 24–9).
   2. *Other Brushes.* A few patients prefer not to have a denture brush in their homes for personal reasons. A hand brush can be used, provided the filaments are long enough to

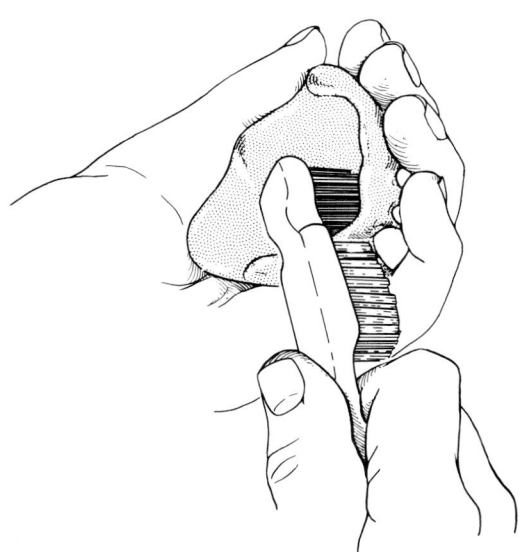

Figure 24–9. Brushing to clean a complete denture. The denture is held securely in the palm of the hand but without a squeezing pressure. A specially designed denture brush is preferred because one group of tufts is arranged to provide access to the inner impression surface of the denture as shown.

reach into the deeper portions of the impression surfaces. Prerequisite is that each area of each surface of the denture must be reached by the brush if dental plaque formation is to be controlled.

If a patient prefers to use an ordinary toothbrush, a multitufted soft nylon brush with rounded ends should be acceptable if access to all of the inner curvatures is possible without undue pressure on certain parts in the attempt to clean others. When the patient wears a single denture, it is advisable to keep separate brushes for the natural teeth and the denture in order that the brush for the natural teeth be in the best condition possible.

B. **Procedure**
   1. Grasp denture in palm of hand securely, but without a squeezing pressure as dentures can be broken (figure 24–9).
   2. Hold the denture low in a sink in which has been placed a towel, wash cloth, or rubber mat spread over the bottom to serve as a cushion should the denture be dropped. The sink should be partially filled with water.
   3. Apply warm water, nonabrasive soap, and brush to all areas of the denture. Particular attention should be paid the impression surfaces where configurations of the surface correspond with those of the oral topography. Rinse thoroughly.

C. **Precautions Related to Brushing**[17]
   1. Overzealous brushing with an abrasive cleaning agent on the impression surface could alter the fit of the denture.
   2. Plastic resin is easily abraded. Scratches make a rough surface; the denture may become more subject to the collection of debris and calculus.

3. Possibility of incomplete coverage during cleaning particularly in the more inaccessible areas.
4. Uneven pressure: brush applied more vigorously to accessible areas.
5. Danger of dropping and breaking the denture is increased when it is soaped, wet, and therefore slippery.
6. Patient who requires eyeglasses should be advised to wear them when brushing: to watch the procedure and to observe the cleanliness of the denture after brushing.

IX. Additional Instructions

A. An appliance made with plastic resin should be immersed in water or cleaning solution when it is not in the mouth.

B. When the denture is kept clean by regular procedures from the time of insertion, accumulation of heavy stains and calculus can be prevented.

C. A denture should never be scraped with a sharp instrument in the attempt to remove calculus deposits. When the cleaning methods recommended in this chapter do not remove deposits, the denture should be taken to the dental hygienist and dentist for professional cleaning. A regular recall plan is advocated.

D. Paste cleaners (dentifrices or denture pastes) may be too abrasive for dentures, but also it is difficult to rinse all traces of the pastes from the denture. Residual chemical agents such as essential oils may cause inflammatory or allergic reactions of the oral mucosa, and phenolic agents can have deleterious effects on plastic resin.[19]

X. The Underlying Mucosa

A. **Rinsing**
Each time the denture is removed, the mouth should be rinsed thoroughly with warm water or a mild salt solution (page 348).

B. **Cleaning**
It is recommended that the edentulous mucosa be brushed at least once daily. A multitufted soft nylon brush is applied in long straight strokes from posterior to anterior.

C. **Massage**
For stimulation of circulation and increasing resistance to trauma, frequent massage is recommended. Studies have shown that massage with a soft automatic toothbrush increased the keratinization of the edentulous alveolar ridge mucosa.[20,21] Methods for massage which may be suggested to the patient are:
1. Digital: place thumb and index finger over the ridge and apply massage with a press and release stroke. The palate may be rubbed with the ball of the thumb.
2. Multitufted soft toothbrush: apply sides of filaments and vibratory motion to each area. Prevent trauma to the tissue by placing the brush carefully and avoiding scrubbing with undue pressure.
3. Automatic brush: apply to each area with smooth, even strokes.

COMPLETE OVERDENTURE

An overdenture is a complete denture supported by both retained natural teeth and the soft tissue of the residual alveolar ridge. It is also known as an overlay denture, coping denture, and tooth-mucosa-supported denture.

I. Purposes[22]

The advantages of an overdenture when compared with a denture in a completely edentulous mouth are that having natural teeth present

A. Helps preserve bone.

B. Allows the remaining teeth to bear occlusal pressures, which reduces the pressures placed on the edentulous areas.

C. Improves stability and retention of the denture.

D. Improves the patient's tactile and proprioceptive senses by having the periodontal ligament present.

E. Increases the patient's psychological acceptance of the denture. The patient does not feel that all natural teeth have been lost.

II. Criteria

The overdenture should be considered for any patient whose treatment plan calls for extraction of all teeth. Teeth to be preserved must meet certain standards of health.

A. **Periodontal Condition**[23]

Since wearing the overdenture brings stress to the periodontium, the tissues must have, or be treatable to obtain, the following:

1. Healthy sulci. There must be no bleeding or other signs of inflammation, minimal sulci depth, and all requirements of health (Table 11–1, page 172).
2. A band of attached gingiva (page 179).

B. **Bone Support.** The bone level following tooth preparation must be adequate to withstand occlusal forces.

C. **Teeth.** Teeth must have minimal mobility. Teeth selected are frequently the mandibular canines and premolars, and maxillary canines.

III. Preparation of the Teeth

A. **Endodontics.** Most preserved teeth need endodontic therapy because the teeth will be reduced.

B. **Periodontics.** Treatment procedures depend on clinical findings, but may include measures to eliminate inflammation and pockets, to increase the zone of attached gingiva, or to reshape the architecture of the bone or gingival tissue.

C. **Restorative**
1. Tooth crowns are reduced to short rounded preparations or in some cases to the level and contour of the gingival margin.
2. There may be only an amalgam restoration to cover the root canals, or the teeth may be protected by a gold coping (figure 24–10). A coping is a cast thin metal covering or cap.
3. The gold coping may be used as a retainer for a retentive attachment.

IV. Dental Hygiene Care and Instruction

The patient must be well-informed concerning the problems of care of the retained teeth and gingiva. A high degree of motivation to want to save the remaining teeth is needed. Supervision by frequent recall appointments for scaling and planing, topical fluoride applications, and motivation and instruction for plaque control will be essential.

A. **Denture Care.** The impression surface of the denture must be kept meticulously free from plaque collection. Denture care is outlined on pages 363–366.

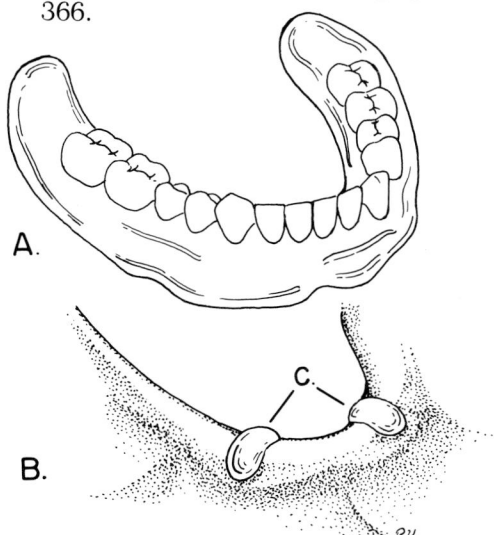

Figure 24–10. Overdenture. **A.** Complete mandibular denture supported by **B.** both mucosa and prepared roots of natural teeth which have been endodontically treated and restored with gold copings (**C**).

B. Gingival Tissue and Natural Teeth

1. Complete plaque control procedures using a soft nylon brush with round ends or an automatic toothbrush (pages 310, 319). Massage of the edentulous gingiva is also recommended.

2. Interdental tip or a Perio-aid should be used daily to trace around each natural tooth to clean submarginally (page 338).

C. Fluoride

A specific fluoride application plan must be included. The requirements depend partly on the past history of dental caries. When the teeth were extracted because of dental caries, caries control measures take on special significance, particularly if dietary habits remain the same. Current dietary habits need to be checked by asking the patient to keep a daily food diary (page 402). Sucrose intake limitations can be recommended accordingly.

1. Fluoride self-application. All patients need to use a fluoride dentifrice. In addition, either a mouthrinse or a gel-tray can be recommended. After cleaning, the patient's denture can be used for a custom tray, and the gel drops can be placed inside at the locations of the natural teeth. Pressure of the denture as it is seated will force the gel about the teeth.

2. Professional topical applications. When daily mouthrinse or gel-tray is not carried out by the patient, topical applications are made. Since frequent recall is needed to check the health of the gingival tissues, an application can be made at each recall. More benefit is derived from the fluoride in direct proportion to the frequency of application.

REMOVABLE PARTIAL DENTURES

The removable partial denture replaces one or more but less than all of the natural teeth and associated structures, and can be removed from the mouth and replaced at will. Depending on the location and number of remaining natural teeth, a partial denture may receive all of its support from the teeth, or it may be partly tooth-borne and partly tissue-borne.

Self-care procedures for the patient with a removable appliance involve much more than cleaning the appliance. The abutment teeth, the gingival tissue, and the mucosa of edentulous areas require regular attention. Gingival health is unfavorably affected by removable partial dentures.[24] When the gingiva is not covered by, or in contact with, the denture there is less problem with tissue response.

Procedures suggested here for care of the removable partial denture apply also to various other removable appliances. Examples of these are removable space maintainers, appliances for orthodontic purposes such as a Hawley biteplate or retainer (figure 24–7), obturators for closure of palatal openings as for cleft palate (page 628) or for replacement of tissue removed in the treatment of oral cancer.

I. Components of a Removable Partial Denture (figure 24–11)

The selection of cleaning agents and procedures for cleaning are complicated by the intricacy of the metallic parts and their relation to the natural teeth as well as by the dental materials used in construction.

A. Denture Base

The part which rests on the oral mucosa and carries the artificial teeth. The base may be made of plastic resin or alloys of gold or chrome.

B. Denture Teeth

Are made of porcelain, plastic resin or metal.

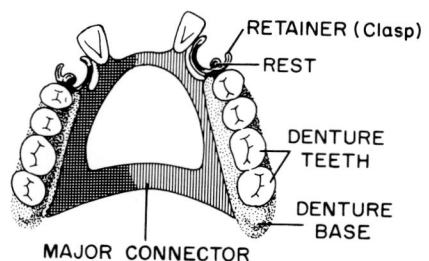

Figure 24–11. Parts of a partial removable denture. A maxillary denture is shown.

C. Major Connectors

Bars of rigid metal which unite the parts of the denture. In the maxillary there can be one or two *palatal bars;* in the mandibular, the *lingual bar.* Minor connectors are between the major connectors and the other units such as clasps and occlusal rests.

D. Retainers

Metal clasps and occlusal rests applied to abutment teeth for the purpose of maintaining the appliance in position.

E. Abutment Teeth

Natural teeth used for the support or anchorage of the appliance.

II. Objectives

A. The Appliance

Because natural teeth are adjacent to the appliance, objectives for cleaning the appliance take on added significance. The same basic objectives applied to the complete denture apply to the removable: remove irritants to the oral tissues, prevent mouth odors, and improve appearance.

B. The Natural Teeth

The objective is to control plaque for the prevention of dental caries and periodontal disease. Other objectives may be found on page 304.

III. Cleaning the Removable Appliance

Rinsing, immersion, and brushing methods, as well as the cleaning agents described for the complete denture on pages 363–365, apply alike to the partial appliance with the few additions noted below.

A. Rinsing

After each meal the denture and the natural teeth should be brushed. When regular cleaning facilities are not available, rinsing is important for both the natural teeth and the removable appliance. While the appliance is out, the tongue can be used to rub the sides of abutment teeth.

B. Immersion

An agent known to discolor metal can be avoided. Procedures for immersion cleaning are described on page 364.

C. Brushing

1. *Recommended Brushes*
   a. *Toothbrush.* One or more should be reserved for the natural teeth. Although not recommended, when a patient does use a regular toothbrush for partial care of a removable appliance, a separate brush is definitely indicated. Brushing the clasps and other metal parts can be destructive to fine toothbrushes.
   b. *Automatic Brush.* An automatic brush is often ideal for the natural teeth of the partial denture patient. However, the automatic brush should not be used in and about the intricate clasps and other parts of a removable appliance because of the danger of catching the brush and damaging the appliance.
   c. *Clasp Brush.* A specially designed narrow, tapered, cylindrical brush about two to three

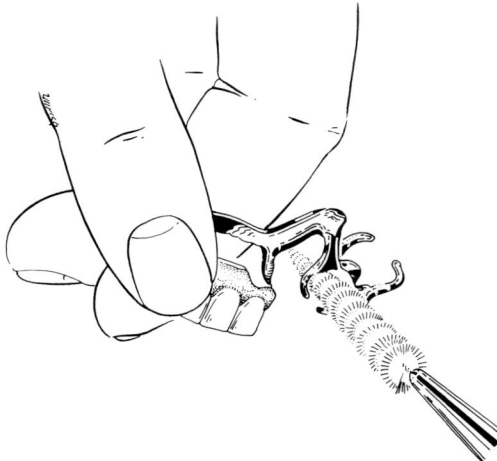

Figure 24-12. Use of a clasp brush for cleaning a partial removable denture.

inches long which can be adapted to the inner surfaces of clasps is recommended (figure 24–12). Clasps and their connectors are closely adapted to the supporting teeth, and the protected internal surfaces are prone to plaque formation. These difficult-to-clean areas require special care.

    d. *Denture Brush.* This was described for the complete denture (figure 24–9) and is an excellent brush for cleaning all of the smooth surfaces and the metal bars of the partial denture.

  2. *Precautions During Brushing.* Too tight a grasp of a partial appliance can result in bending or fracture of clasps or bars. Bristles of a brush can inadvertently catch the appliance and cause it to drop. A liner for the sink is mandatory (page 365).

IV. The Natural Teeth

A. Plaque Control

Toothbrushing and interdental cleaning methods selected for the particular needs of the patient must be

followed meticulously. The longevity of the removable appliance is dependent on the health of the supporting teeth, and in turn the natural teeth are dependent on the cleanliness of the appliance.

B. Dental Caries Control

The topical application of fluoride, the use of a fluoride dentifrice, and other self-applied fluoride measures such as a daily mouth rinse or custom tray, and the control of refined sugars in the diet need to be a definite part of the complete program of oral care for the patient with a removable appliance. The patient must be constantly alert to the control of plaque retention by the appliance and the need for rinsing immediately after eating when brushing is not possible. For the patient who has been caries-susceptible, and whose teeth are missing because of dental caries, a dietary analysis and specific dental caries control program may be indicated (pages 412–415).

TECHNICAL HINTS

  I. Review instruction for each patient with a fixed or removable prosthesis. Do not assume that, because a denture has been in use for a long time, the patient knows how to clean it properly, as well as to care for the soft tissue adjacent to it.

 II. To prevent cross-contamination when receiving a denture from a patient:[26]

    A. Offer a container or disposable napkin in which the patient can place the denture. When the denture is removed by the dental hygienist, rubber gloves should be worn.

    B. Scrub the denture with surgical soap using a disposable or autoclavable scrub brush. Wear rubber gloves.

C. Use disposable or autoclavable denture and/or clasp brush when demonstrating care procedures for patient education.

III. Acrylic restorations, crowns, and pontics are subject to toothbrush attrition and dentifrice abrasion. Select soft brush and nonabrasive cleaning material.

IV. Provide printed instructions for each patient. Personalize the instructions with notations related to particular problem areas of the patient.

V. Sources of educational materials for patients:

American Dental Association, Order Department, 211 East Chicago Avenue, Chicago, Illinois 60611. Request current catalog. Samples of the following booklets related to dentures are available on request: *Immediate Dentures* (G 18) *Dentures: What You Don't Know Can Hurt You* (G 35) *Your New Dentures* (G 4)

American Association of Orthodontists, 747 Delmar Boulevard, St. Louis, Missouri 63130. Request the pamphlet *Orthodontic Tooth Brushing.*

References

1. Parfitt, G. J.: A Five Year Longitudinal Study of the Gingival Condition of a Group of Children in England, *J. Periodont.*, 28, 26, January, 1957.
2. Glickman, I.: *Clinical Periodontology*, 4th ed. Philadelphia, Saunders, 1972, pp. 101–102, 146.
3. Baer, P. N. and Coccaro, P. J.: Gingival Enlargement Coincident with Orthodontic Therapy, *J. Periodont.*, 35, 436, September-October, 1964.
4. Bloom, R. H. and Brown, L. R.: A Study of the Effects of Orthodontic Appliances on the Oral Microbial Flora, *Oral Surg.*, 17, 658, May, 1964.
5. Balenseifen, J. W. and Madonia, J. V.: Study of Dental Plaque in Orthodontic Patients, *J. Dent. Res.*, 49, 320, March-April, 1970.
6. Grant, D. A., Stern, I. B., and Everett, F. G.: *Orban's Periodontics*, 4th ed. St. Louis, Mosby, 1972, pp. 640–644.
7. Glickman: op. cit., pp. 962–965.
8. Stibbs, G. D.: Treatment—Clinical Procedures, in Morrey, L. W. and Nelson, R. J., eds.: *Dental Science Handbook*. Superintendent of Documents, United States Government Printing Office, Washington, D.C., 1970, pp. 190–197.
9. York, T. A. and Dunkin, R. T.: Control of Periodontal Problems in Orthodontics by Use of Water Irrigation, *Am. J. Orthod.*, 53, 639, September, 1967.
10. Graber, T. M.: *Orthodontics, Principles and Practice*, 3rd ed. Philadelphia, Saunders, 1972, pp. 611–617.
11. Kobayashi, L. Y. and Ash, M. M.: A Clinical Evaluation of an Electric Toothbrush Used by Orthodontic Patients, *Angle Orthod.*, 34, 209, July, 1964.
12. Womack, W. R. and Guay, A. H.: Comparative Cleansing Efficiency of an Electric and a Manual Toothbrush in Orthodontic Patients, *Angle Orthod.*, 38, 256, July, 1968.
13. Hurst, J. E. and Madonia, J. V.: The Effect of an Oral Irrigating Device on the Oral Hygiene of Orthodontic Patients, *J. Am. Dent. Assoc.*, 81, 678, September, 1970.
14. MacCallum, M., Stafford, G. D., MacCulloch, W. T., and Combe, E. C.: Which Cleanser? A Report on a Survey of Denture Cleansing Routine and the Development of a New Denture Cleanser, *Dent. Pract. Dent. Rec.*, 19, 83, November, 1968.
15. Nicholson, R. J., Stark, M. M., and Scott, H. E.: Calculus and Stain Removal from Acrylic Resin Dentures, *J. Prosthet. Dent.*, 20, 326, October, 1968.
16. Gallagher, J. B., Jr.: *Handbook for Complete Dentures*. Boston, Tufts University School of Dental Medicine, 1975.
17. Applegate, O. C.: *Essentials of Removable Partial Denture Prosthesis*, 3rd ed. Philadelphia, Saunders, 1965, pp. 315–326.
18. Anthony, D. H. and Gibbons, P.: The Nature and Behavior of Denture Cleansers, *J. Prosthet. Dent.*, 8, 796, September-October, 1958.
19. Smith, D. C.: The Cleansing of Dentures, *Dent. Pract. Dent. Rec.*, 17, 39, October, 1966.
20. Kapur, K. and Shklar, G.: Effects of a Power Device for Oral Physiotherapy on the Mucosa of the Edentulous Ridge, *J. Prosthet. Dent.*, 12, 762, July-August, 1962.
21. Markov, N. J.: Cytologic Study of the Effect of Toothbrush Physiotherapy on the Mucosa of the Edentulous Ridge, *J. Prosthet. Dent.*, 18, 122, August, 1967.
22. Zamikoff, I. I.: Overdentures—Theory and Technique, *J. Am. Dent. Assoc.*, 86, 853, April, 1973.
23. Lord, J. L. and Teel, S.: The Overdenture: Patient Selection, Use of Copings, and Follow-up Evaluation, *J. Prosthet. Dent.*, 32, 41, July, 1974.

24. Bissada, N. F., Ibrahim, S. I., and Barsoum, W.
    M.: Gingival Response to Various Types of
    Removable Partial Dentures, *J. Periodont.*, 45,
    651, September, 1974.
25. Brennon, E. F.: Case Report: Cancer of the
    Antrum, *Dent. Surv.*, 46, 24, January, 1970.
26. Walsh, R. F. and Ames, M. I.: Reinforcing the
    Aseptic Chain in Hospital Dental Practice, *J.
    Hosp. Dent. Pract.*, 6, 57, April, 1972.

Suggested Readings

Dentures

American Dental Association, Council on Dental
    Materials and Devices: *Guide to Dental Mate-
    rials and Devices*, 7th ed. Chicago, American
    Dental Association, 1974–1975, pp. 154–155.
LaVere, A. M.: Denture Education for Edentulous
    Patients, *J. Prosthet. Dent.*, 16, 1013,
    November-December, 1966.
Cooper, T. M. and Ellinger, C. W.: The Overdenture,
    in Ellinger, C. W., Rayson, J. H., Terry, J. M., and
    Rahn, A. O.: *Synopsis of Complete Dentures*.
    Philadelphia, Lea & Febiger, 1975, pp.309–319.
Hall, W. A., Jr.: *Sears' New Teeth for Old*, 5th ed. St.
    Louis, Mosby, 1969, 101 pp.
Hutchins, D. W. and Parker, W. A.: A Clinical
    Evaluation of the Ability of Denture Cleaning
    Solutions to Remove Dental Plaque from
    Prosthetic Devices, *N.Y. State Dent. J.*, 39, 363,
    June-July, 1973.
Muhler, J. C., Stookey, G. K., and Hassell, T. M.: Th
    Development and Evaluation of an Improve
    Denture Cleaning and Polishing Paste, *J. In
    Dent. Assoc.*, 48, 17, January, 1969.
Neill, D. J.: A Study of Materials and Metho
    Employed in Cleaning Dentures, *Br. Dent.
    124*, 107, February 6, 1968.
Wagner, A. G.: Instructions for the Use and Care
    Removable Partial Dentures, *J. Prosthet. Den
    26*, 477, November, 1971.

Orthodontic Appliances

Baer, P. N. and Benjamin, S. D.: *Periodontal Disea
    in Children and Adolescents*. Philadelphia, Li
    pincott, 1974, pp. 109–127.
Dougherty, H. L.: Intraoral Soft Tissue Problems
    Orthodontic Practice, *J. Am. Dent. Assoc.*, 8
    841, April, 1971.
Shannon, I. L. and Miller, J. T.: Caries Risk in Tee
    with Orthodontic Bands: A Review, *J. Acad. Ge
    Dent.*, 20, 24, May, 1972.
Stratemann, M. W. and Shannon, I. L.: Control
    Decalcification in Orthodontic Patients by Dai
    Self-administered Application of a Water-free 0
    per cent Stannous Fluoride Gel, *Am. J. Ortho
    66*, 273, September, 1974.
Zager, N. I. and Barnett, M. L.: Severe Bone Loss i
    Child Initiated by Multiple Orthodontic Rubb
    Bands: Case Report, *J. Periodont.*, 45, 70
    September, 1974.

Chapter **25**

The Patient With Complete Rehabilitation

Complete oral rehabilitation refers to the combined treatment of the teeth and periodontium to restore health, function, and physical form. As generally used, *oral rehabilitation* applies to involved extensive restorative procedures in a mouth which cannot be treated with routine dental care. It is also known as *mouth rehabilitation, occlusal rehabilitation, occluso-rehabilitation, complete reconstruction,* or *periodontal prosthesis.*

The term *periodontal prosthesis* is used to designate restorative and prosthetic treatment which is necessary for the treatment of advanced periodontal disease. The prosthesis used may be a splint, or immobilization or stabilization of a group of teeth or an entire arch, maxillary or mandibular.

Periodontal, restorative, and prosthetic treatments are interdependent. The function and duration of all restorative and prosthetic treatment depend directly on the health of the periodontium which provides the attachment and support necessary for the restored tooth.[1] Likewise, periodontal health is influenced by restorative and prosthetic

treatment. Many predisposing factors which contribute to the initiation, development and progress of periodontal disease are a direct result of untreated dental caries, incomplete or inadequate restorations, unreplaced missing teeth, and inadequate occlusal relationships built into restorations or prostheses.

I. Objectives of Complete Rehabilitation

Objectives for complete rehabilitation involve the same principles as for all oral care and include the need to

A. Restore optimal functional occlusion.

B. Maintain the health of the periodontium.

C. Produce biologically contoured restorations in harmony with normal oral physiology.

D. Replace missing teeth.

E. Provide support to teeth with advanced bone loss and marked mobility.

F. Provide desirable esthetics.

G. Establish acceptable phonetics.

373

II. Components of Treatment

Complete oral reconstruction means total mouth involvement, which brings in many phases of dentistry, often accomplished by individual specialists. The overall treatment plan may include some or all of the following:

A. Extensive periodontal therapy involving various surgical procedures.

B. Occlusal adjustment.

C. Endodontic therapy.

D. Correction of oral habits.

E. Orthodontic tooth movement.

F. Splinting of teeth temporarily or permanently.

G. Restorations involving individual teeth: crowns, inlays, onlays.

H. Replacement of teeth by fixed and/or removable prostheses.

III. Accomplishment of Treatment

Treatment is usually long and involved for the patient who undergoes complete oral rehabilitation. It requires patience, persistence, and dedication of the patient, dental hygienist, and the dentist.

The dental hygiene treatment plan overlaps into every phase of the total treatment beginning with the initial preparation of the patient's mouth. Maintenance and supervision of the patient's self-care program is essential throughout restorative and prosthetic therapy, and continuing into the recall phase.

Specific measures for self-care in terms of plaque removal and dental caries prevention must be selected and supervised. The patient is shown how to self-evaluate, so that minor deviations from normal can be recognized and called to the attention of the dentist.

IV. Characteristics of the Rehabilitated Mouth

To select the appropriate methods for plaque control and caries prevention,

existing conditions must be identifi such as contour and position of gingiva, contour of restorations, and pr lem areas adjacent to fixed prosthe: When these are known, the variety possible techniques and devices plaque removal can be reviewed an plan for care outlined.

A patient who has undergone extens periodontal therapy and restorative prosthetic rehabilitation may have so or all of the characteristics listed he Each condition may require speci; selected or adapted plaque control m

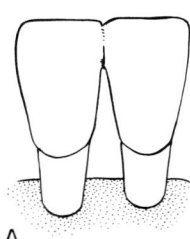

A.

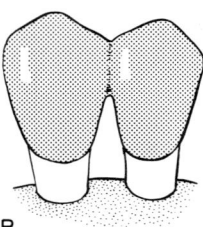

B.

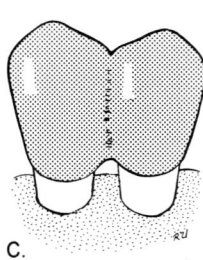

C.

Figure 25–1. Gingival embrasures. A. Wide em sure between two central incisors with mis: interdental papilla and gingival recession wl resulted from periodontal disease. B. Dou abutment with closed contact area to show o embrasure which gives access for plaque rem al. C. Overcontoured crowns of a double al ment showing narrowed embrasure with lim access for cleaning.

sures. Fixed and removable appliances can provide many areas for plaque and debris retention.

A. Periodontal Findings

1. Gingival recession.
2. Exposed root surfaces.
3. Exposed furcation areas.
4. Alterations of gingival contour: the gingival margins may be rolled or rounded.
5. Changes in size and shape of the gingival embrasures.
    a. Missing interdental papillae: wide embrasures with gingival recession and increased root exposure (figure 25–1).
    b. Narrowed embrasures: created by overcontoured restorations or variously shaped pontics (figure 25–2).

B. Fixed Prosthesis

The parts of a fixed prosthesis are described on page 356 and in figure 24–1.

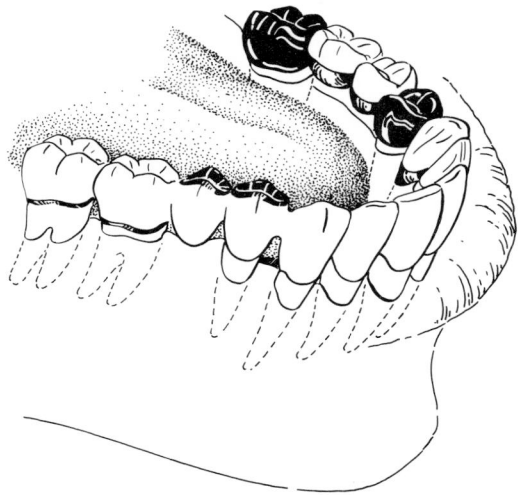

Figure 25–3. Complete arch fixed splint. A continuous therapeutic fixed appliance to stabilize periodontally involved teeth and replace missing components to provide appropriate occlusal relationships. Numerous problem areas for plaque removal exist.

A patient may have:

1. Fixed splinting around long segments of, or an entire, arch (figure 25–3).
2. Abutment teeth with difficult access areas adjacent to a pontic.
3. Closed contacts between teeth involved in a multitooth prosthesis.
4. Gingival surfaces of pontics.
5. Embrasures created by pontics may be wide and triangular, or narrow, unnatural, non-self-cleansing areas created by improperly shaped pontics (figure 25–2B).

C. Removable Prostheses

1. Complete denture may be used in one dental arch opposing natural teeth and partial dentures, fixed or removable.
2. Partial removable denture
    a. Creation of potential areas of plaque and debris retention.
        (1) Alteration of tooth form by clasp, rest, or precision attachment.

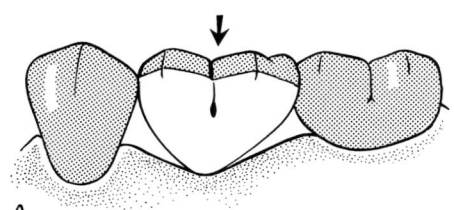

A.

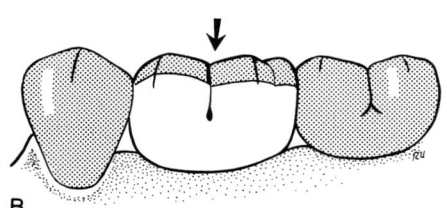

B.

Figure 25–2. Shape of pontics. Mandibular three-unit fixed partial denture to show **A.** "bullet" shape giving wide triangular embrasures for access for cleaning and plaque removal, and **B.** improperly shaped pontic with closed embrasures and wide gingival surface for plaque retention. Arrows indicate pontics.

(2) Improperly contoured edge of partial at the junction of the partial and the abutment tooth.

b. Partial denture may impinge on the gingiva surrounding the abutment tooth.

c. Double abutment (two natural teeth with crowns which are soldered or cast together): closed contact requiring lateral (from facial or lingual) access to the gingival embrasure (figure 25–1 B and C).

d. Mucosa under partial denture may be susceptible to plaque retention.

D. **Single Tooth Restorations**

1. Crowns: gingival margin may appear bluish or bluish/red when the crown margin is below the gingival margin.

2. Various restorative materials.

V. Self-Care of the Rehabilitated Mouth

These special patients require greater than average attention, patience, and teaching skill by the dental hygienist in order to obtain a favorable result which will assure continuing health of the patient's periodontal tissues. Total commitment on the part of the patient is necessary if the selected plan is to meet the requirements for daily care.

Research has shown that when patients with fixed partial dentures had received special instruction and therefore had been influenced to change their tooth cleansing habits, the periodontal condition about the denture was no different from other parts of the same mouth used as a control. On the other hand, patients in the same study who did not receive instruction showed greater periodontal deterioration about the fixed partial dentures than about their control teeth.[2]

A. **Planning the Control Program**[3]

The control program should be planned as a concentrated effort to maintain gingival tissue, the tooth structure which is exposed and, hence, the underlying supporting periodontium as well as the restorations and prostheses. There are two parts to the instructions: first, before the surgical, restorative, and prosthetic treatment and, second, after reconstruction.

1. Part 1: Basic plaque control measures are learned and practiced by the patient during the preparatory phase. The sample treatment plan outlined on page 298 is typical of the procedure which can be used in conjunction with scaling appointments. During these lessons, principles for self-evaluation can be presented.

2. Part 2: After therapy is completed, another set of self-care procedures is required in order to meet the needs of the rehabilitated mouth. Special devices and techniques are selected and tried until the most efficient and thorough procedures are determined.

3. Dietary survey: whether the reasons for need of the rehabilitation were related to extensive dental caries or periodontal disease, dietary counseling is indicated. Every possible means must be taken to prevent carious lesions in the exposed root surfaces about the restorations. Overall diet factors need to be checked to assure support from a nutritional standpoint. Procedures for obtaining the Food Diary and conducting the counseling session are described on pages 402–410.

4. Fluorides

a. Dentifrices: A fluoride dentifrice is needed. One containing

Table 25-1.   Care of the Rehabilitated Mouth

Problem	Device/Method	Special Adaptations
Debris Removal	Water irrigation Toothbrush	Wide embrasures Under fixed partial dentures

Sulcular Brushing	Toothbrush with soft nylon
	  filaments with rounded tips
	
	Supplement: Perio-aid
		Facial and lingual surfaces
		Distals of most-posterior teeth,
		  particularly terminal abutment

Proximal Surfaces Plaque Removal	Floss Floss with threader Yarn with floss and/or threader Perio-aid Pipe cleaner Interproximal brush	Abutment teeth Proximal root surfaces Pontic surfaces Narrowed embrasures

Proximal Surfaces
  without contact
  with adjacent tooth
	Gauze strip
	Yarn
		Terminal abutment of removable
		  partial denture
		Distals of most-posterior teeth
		  in the dental arch

Exposed Furcation of Molars	Pipe cleaner Floss/yarn in threader Interproximal brush Interdental rubber tip	Rotated tooth

Exposed Furcation of
  Maxillary First
  Premolar
	Perio-aid
	Interdental rubber tip
		Fused root with groove

Exposed Root Surfaces	Perio-aid with dentifrice con- taining monofluorophosphate	Desensitization

Fixed Partial Denture	Toothbrush (soft nylon)
	Floss threader with floss/yarn
	Any other proximal surface
	  procedures as applicable
		Gingival surfaces of pontics
		Proximal surfaces of pontics
		  and retainers

Edentulous Gingiva
  under Removable
  Denture
	Toothbrush (soft nylon)
	  (manual or automatic,
	  page 366)
		Stimulation and plaque
		  removal

Tongue Brushing	Toothbrush (soft nylon), page 323	Fissures
Removable Denture	Denture brush Clasp brush Chemical cleaner for immersion	Clasps

monofluorophosphate would generally be selected because of the desensitizing properties (page 564), and because exposed cementum and tooth color restorations could be discolored by a stannous fluoride dentifrice.

b. Self-application: A daily mouth-rinse or custom-tray gel application would be advised to prevent the development of root caries.

c. Topical applications in the dental office: When self-treatment methods are not used on a regular basis, professional topical applications are made at each recall appointment.

B. **Plaque Control: Selection of Methods**

Any of the methods and techniques described in Chapters 22, 23, and 24 may be needed in the care of the oral soft tissues, tooth surfaces, restorations, and fixed and removable prostheses. Methods selected must accomplish complete daily plaque removal from each area around every tooth or replacement. A summary of devices and methods is provided in table 25–1.

Most patients need a method for each of the following:

1. Debris removal, particularly from interproximal areas and around fixed prostheses.
2. Sulcular brushing.
3. Interdental plaque removal.
   a. Proximal surfaces of natural and restored teeth including exposed roots where there is access from the incisal or occlusal.
   b. Proximal surfaces of abutment teeth under closed contact areas (figure 25–4).
   c. Mesial and/or distal surfaces of teeth without proximal contact.
4. Fixed partial denture: cleaning and plaque removal.

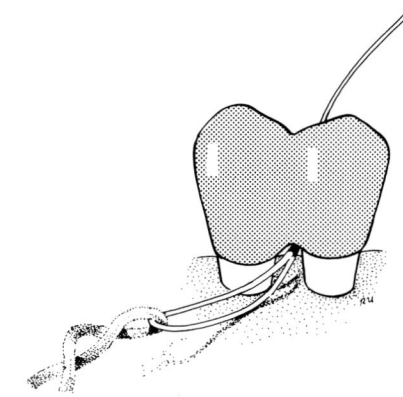

Figure 25–4. Use of floss threader to pull nylo yarn through embrasure created by doubl abutment. Narrowed embrasure from overco abutment. Narrowed embrasure from overco toured crowns increases plaque and debr retention and makes cleaning difficult. Proc dures for use of nylon yarn are on page 336.

a. Gingival surfaces of pontics.
b. Proximal surfaces of pontics.
5. Removable prosthesis: cleaning.

C. **Procedure**

No fixed procedure can be state which will apply to every patient. personalized sequence must l worked out, often by trial and error

1. Outline a possible sequence.
   a. Select methods and devic which can meet the requir ments of the individual o characteristics (IV, above).
   b. Demonstrate the use of tl methods and have patient pra tice under supervision. Avo presenting too many procedur in one lesson which can confu and discourage the patient.
   c. Provide step-by-step written rections for home reference.
2. Recheck successes within a f days and at least by one week.
   a. Evaluate gingival tissue (ta 11–1, page 172), plaque, a technique performance.
   b. Observe patient's dexterity managing the techniques.

c. Make necessary adjustments to simplify, clarify, and assure that all areas are completely de-plaqued daily.

3. Reevaluate weekly or as frequently as needed to maintain the patient's motivation, follow the health of the gingival tissues, and to recognize a need for changes in the procedure used.

D. **Sample Procedure**

The patient described below has a complete maxillary fixed partial denture (splint), which has several natural teeth as abutments and four areas of double pontics; a mandibular removable partial denture with double abutments connecting mandibular canines and first premolars on each side; and wide embrasures between mandibular incisors caused by previous periodontal disease which has since been treated with periodontal surgery.

The patient might use the following procedure:

1. Morning after eating
   a. Complete brushing with automatic brush (containing softest filaments available), applying the brush to proximal surfaces.
   b. Brush partial removable denture and rinse thoroughly.
2. Noon after eating (away from home)
   a. Rinse partial under running water.
   b. Use manual toothbrush, covering all surfaces as thoroughly as possible.
   c. Rinse carefully, forcing the water under fixed partial denture areas.
3. Evening, after all eating.
   a. Remove partial denture, rinse under running water, and place in cleansing solution. (Complete procedure for partial removable denture is described on page 369.)
   b. Use water irrigator to remove debris from all parts of fixed splint and from all proximal surfaces of mandibular teeth.
   c. Use toothbrush for facial and lingual sulcular brushing, applying the brush interdentally as much as possible. Use fluoride dentifrice.
   d. Brush tongue and edentulous gingiva under removable dentures.
   e. Use dental floss and/or nylon yarn for proximal surfaces accessible from incisal.
   f. Use floss and nylon yarn with floss threader for all proximal surfaces not accessible from incisal or occlusal. Clean all gingival surfaces of fixed partial denture. Interproximal brush may be needed for certain wide embrasures.
   g. Use nylon yarn or gauze strip for distals of the abutment teeth for the mandibular removable denture (mandibular premolars).
   h. Use Perio-aid with fluoride dentifrice containing monofluorophosphate to massage hypersensitive areas of exposed roots.
   i. Rinse with fluoride mouthrinse.
   j. Clean partial denture using denture brush and clasp brush, and rinse the denture thoroughly.

VI. Recall

Continuing supervision of the patient with oral rehabilitation is an absolute essential. The well-informed and conscientious patient who devotes up to an hour each day on personal care procedures expects a recall review appointment which thoroughly evaluates the gingival tissue, the rehabilitation appliances, and the completeness of plaque control efforts.

Everything listed on page 574 for inclusion within the recall examination applies with special meaning and emphasis to the rehabilitated patient. What could seem like a minute area of gingival bleeding on probing, whether the pocket is shallow or has started to deepen, should be a warning signal that an area may not be covered by present self-care procedures and needs some form of treatment. Each millimeter of sulcus-pocket must be probed carefully to detect incipient changes.

FACTORS TO TEACH THE PATIENT

I. The health of the periodontal tissues and the duration of the restorations and prostheses depend on the daily self-care by the patient.

II. More thought and concentration are required to maintain the mouth with advanced restorative dentistry or periodontal prosthesis than are needed for an average mouth.

III. It takes longer to clean a mouth with complex restorations. Time must be allotted in the daily schedule for complete cleaning and plaque removal once each day, supplemented by cleaning at least three times each day, or after each meal.

IV. Do not *go easy* with the brush and other devices in the attempt to protect the restorations from breakage. *Protection* is for the gingival tissues and the preservation of the periodontium, and is accomplished only by thorough plaque removal about every tooth.

V. The need for frequent, regular recall appointments.

References

1. Glickman, I.: *Clinical Periodontology*, 4th ed. Philadelphia, Saunders, 1972, pp. 890–927.
2. Silness, J. and Ohm, E.: Periodontal Conditions in Patients Treated with Dental Bridges, V. Effects of Splinting Adjacent Abutment Teeth, *J. Periodont. Res.*, 9, 121, No. 2, 1974.
3. Bradbury, E.: Harvard University School of Dental Medicine, Boston, Massachusetts, personal communication.

Suggested Readings

Calagna, L. J.: A Comprehensive Treatment Rationale Combining Prosthodontics and Periodontics, *J. Prosthet. Dent.*, 30, 781, November, 1973.
Grant, D. A., Stern, I. B., and Everett, F. G.: *Orban's Periodontics*, 4th ed. St. Louis, Mosby, 1972, pp. 673–679.
Goldman, H. M. and Cohen, D. W.: *Periodontal Therapy*, 5th ed. St. Louis, Mosby, 1973, pp. 969–976, 977–1013.
Lytle, J. D.: Periodontal Prosthesis, in Goldman, H. M., Gilmore, H. W., Irby, W. B., and Olsen, N. H.: *Current Therapy in Dentistry*, Vol. 5. St. Louis, Mosby, 1974, pp. 261–265.
Ramfjord, S. P.: Periodontal Aspects of Restorative Dentistry, *J. Oral Rehab.*, 1, 107, No. 2, 1974.
Silness, J.: Periodontal Conditions in Patients Treated with Dental Bridges. IV. The Relationship between the Pontic and the Periodontal Condition of the Abutment Teeth, *J. Periodont. Res.*, 9, 50, No. 1, 1974.
Silness, J.: Periodontal Conditions in Patients Treated with Dental Bridges. II. The Influence of Full and Partial Crowns on Plaque Accumulation, Development of Gingivitis and Pocket Formation, *J. Periodont. Res.*, 5, 219, No. 3, 1970.
Silness, J.: Periodontal Conditions in Patients Treated with Dental Bridges, *J. Periodont. Res.*, 5, 60, No. 1, 1970.

Chapter 26

Disclosing Agents

A disclosing agent is a preparation in liquid, tablet, or lozenge form which contains a dye or other coloring agent. In dentistry a disclosing agent is used for the identification of soft deposits for instruction, evaluation, and research.

When applied to the teeth, the agent imparts its color to soft deposits but can be rinsed readily from clean tooth surfaces. After staining, the deposits can be distinctly seen, which provides a valuable visual aid in patient instruction. This procedure can demonstrate dramatically to the patient the presence of deposits and the areas which need special attention during personal oral care.

I. Purposes

A disclosing agent clearly demarcates soft deposits which might otherwise be invisible, and therefore facilitates

A. Personalized patient instruction in the location of soft deposits and the techniques for removal.

B. Self-evaluation by the patient on a daily basis during initial instruction and periodic checks thereafter.

C. Continuing evaluation by the dental hygienist of the effectiveness of the instruction for the patient
   1. To determine the need for revisions of the plaque control procedures.
   2. To study the long-term effects over successive recall appointments.

D. Preparation of plaque indices (pages 276, 279).

E. Performance of clinical services by the dental hygienist
   1. To identify location of deposits before scaling and polishing.
   2. To evaluate completion of scaling and polishing.

F. Research studies to gain new information about the incidence and formation of deposits on the teeth, the effectiveness of specific devices for plaque control, antiplaque agents, and to evaluate clinical and instructional group health programs.

II. Properties

A. **Intensity of Color**

   A distinct staining of deposits should be evident. The color should contrast with normal colors of the oral cavity.

B. **Duration of Intensity**

The color should not rinse off with ordinary rinsing methods, or be removable by the saliva for the period of time required to complete the instruction or clinical service. It is desirable for the color to be removed from the gingival tissue and lips by the completion of the appointment, as the patient may have a personal reaction to color retained for a long period of time.

C. **Taste**

The patient should not be made uncomfortable by an unpleasant or highly flavored substance, since his cooperation may be decreased.

D. **Irritation to the Mucous Membrane**

The patient should be questioned concerning the possibility of an idiosyncrasy to an ingredient. When this information is obtained it should be entered on the patient's permanent history record. Because of the possibility of allergy, more than one type of disclosing agent should be available for use.

E. **Diffusibility**

A solution should be thin enough so it can be applied readily to the exposed surfaces of the teeth, yet thick enough to prevent its prompt diffusion over the gingival tissues to the mucobuccal folds and tongue.

F. **Astringent and Antiseptic Properties**

These properties may be highly desirable in that the disclosing agent may contribute other factors to the techniques. It is frequently recommended that an antiseptic be applied prior to scaling, and if an antiseptic disclosing agent is used, one solution serves a dual purpose.

One example is erythrosin which has been shown to inhibit the growth of a variety of organisms.[1,2] In quantitative plaque research studies, therefore, it would be necessary to use other disclosing agents.

III. Formulae

A wide variety of disclosing agents has been used. Skinner's Iodine Solution has been perhaps the most classic and widely used. In general, iodine solutions are less desirable because of their unpleasant flavor.

Aniline dyes have been shown to have carcinogenic potential. Therefore, the use of basic fuchsin and beta rose (flavored basic fuchsin) has been discouraged.

The formulae of a few of the more commonly used disclosing agents are included in this chapter. Other well-known ones are Buckley's, Berwick's, Talbot's Iodo-glycerol, and Metaphen solutions.

A. **Iodine Preparations**
   1. Skinner's Solution

Iodine crystals . . .	3.3	Gm.
Potassium Iodide .	1.0	Gm.
Zinc Iodide	1.0	Gm.
Water (distilled) . .	16.0	ml.
Glycerin	16.0	ml.

   2. Iodine Disclosing Solution

Potassium Iodide .	1.6	Gm.
Iodine crystals . .	1.6	Gm.
Water (distilled), . .	13.4	ml.
Glycerin . . to make	30.0	ml.

   3. Diluted Tincture of Iodine

Tincture of Iodine .	21.0	ml.
Water (distilled) . .	15.0	ml.

B. **Mercurochrome Preparations**
   1. Mercurochrome Solution (5%)

Mercurochrome . .	1.5	Gm.
Water (distilled) to make	30.0	ml.

2. Flavored Mercuro-
    chrome Disclosing
    Solution

Mercurochrome . .	13.5	Gm.
Water (distilled) . .	3.0	l.
Oil of Peppermint .	3	drops
Artificial non-cario-		
genic sweetener		

C. **Bismarck Brown (Easlick's Disclosing Solution)**

Bismarck Brown . .	3.0	Gm.
Ethyl Alcohol . . .	10.0	ml.
Glycerin	120.0	ml.
Anise (flavoring) . .	1	drop

D. **Merbromin**

Merbromin, N.F.. .	450.0	mg.
Peppermint oil . .	1	drop
Distilled water		
to make	100.0	ml.

E. **Erythrosin**
   1. Concentrate for application by rinsing

F.D.C. Red No. 3 . .	6.0	Gm.
Water . . . to make	100.0	ml.

   2. For direct topical application

Erythrosin	0.8	Gm.
Water (distilled) . .	100.0	ml.
Alcohol (95%) . . .	10.0	ml.
Oil of Peppermint .	2	drops

   3. Tablet[3]

F.D.C. Red No. 3 . .	15.0 mg.
Sodium chloride . .	.747%
Sodium sucaryl . .	.747%
Calcium stearate . .	.995%
Soluble saccharin .	.186%
White oil	.124%
Flavoring	2.239%
Sorbitol to make a 7 grain tablet	

F. **Fast Green**
   F.D.C. Green No. 3 . 5% or 2.5%

G. **Fluorescein[4]**
   F.D.C. Yellow No. 8 (used with a special light source to make the agent visible)

H. **Two-tone[5]**
   F.D.C. Green No. 3
   F.D.C. Red No. 3

IV. Technique for Application

A. **Solution for Direct Application**
   During or following dental hygiene instrumentation an application may be made to each quadrant of the teeth as a guide to, or for evaluation of, techniques.
   1. Dry the teeth with compressed air, retracting cheek or tongue.
   2. Use very small cotton pellet with cotton pliers to carry the solution to the teeth.
   3. Apply solution to the crowns of the teeth only.
   4. Remove excess solution.
      a. Request the patient to rinse.
      b. When the flavor of the disclosing solution is unpleasant to the patient, it may be desirable to remove the excess solution by blotting with a cotton roll.
   5. Apply compressed air and inspect.
   6. Polish disclosed areas as required to remove visible deposits.

B. **Rinsing**
   A few drops of a concentrated preparation are placed in a paper cup and water is added for the appropriate dilution. Instruct the patient to rinse the solution over all tooth surfaces.

C. **Tablet or Wafer**
   The patient chews the wafer (one-half may be sufficient for some patients), swishes it around for 30 to 60 seconds, and rinses.

D. **Effect**
   Clean tooth surfaces do not absorb the coloring agent; when pellicle and dental plaque are present they absorb the agent and are disclosed. Pellicle stains as a thin, relatively clear covering, whereas dental plaque appears darker, thicker, and more opaque.
   The oral mucous membrane and lips may retain the color from certain disclosing agents. Application of petrolatum or other coating substance may prevent absorption of the color by the lips.

TECHNICAL HINTS

I. Avoid using disclosing or antiseptic solutions on teeth which have silicate cement or resin restorations as these materials may be stained by coloring agents.

II. Purchase solutions in small quantities. Do not keep solutions containing alcohol longer than two or three months since the alcohol will evaporate and render the solution too highly concentrated.

III. Use small bottles with dropper caps for solutions. Transfer solution to a dappen dish for use. Do not contaminate the solution by dipping cotton pliers with pellet directly into the container bottle.

IV. Use only small, unsaturated, cotton pellets with adequate retraction of cheeks and tongue to prevent staining of tongue and alveolar mucosa.

V. Maintain a list of methods for spot removal in case the dye-containing solutions are inadvertently spilled.

VI. Request local druggists to stock disclosing tablets for patients to purchase. Advise patients of the stores where the agents may be purchased.

FACTORS TO TEACH THE PATIENT

I. Purposes for use of disclosing agents: the appearance of stained dental plaque and the methods of daily care necessary to keep plaque controlled.

II. Self-evaluation of plaque control methods by using a disclosing agent.

III. For the parent: method of application of a disclosing agent to a small child's teeth to evaluate for the presence of plaque.

References

1. Beque, W. J., Bard, R. C., and Koehne, G. W Microbial Inhibition by Erythrosin, *J. Den Res.*, 45, 1464, September-October, 1966.
2. Caldwell, R. C. and Hunt, D. E.: A Comparise of the Antimicrobial Activity of Disclosir Agents, *J. Dent. Res.*, 48, 913, Septembe October, 1969.
3. Arnim, S. S.: Use of Disclosing Agents f Measuring Tooth Cleanliness, *J. Periodon* 34, 227, May, 1963.
4. Lang, N. P., Østergaard, E., and Löe, H.: Fluorescent Plaque Disclosing Agent, *Periodont. Res.*, 7, 59, No. 1, 1972.
5. Block, P. L., Lobene, R. R., and Derdivanis, J. P A Two-tone Dye Test for Dental Plaque, *Periodont.*, 43, 423, July, 1972.

Suggested Readings

American Dental Association, Council on Dent Therapeutics: *Accepted Dental Therapeutic* 36th ed. Chicago, American Dental Associatio 1975, p. 283.
Bellini, H. T., Ånerud, Å., and Moustafa, M H Disclosing Wafers in an Oral Hygiene Instructic Program, *Odontol. Revy*, 25, 247, No. 3, 1974.
Bennett, C. G.: Disclosing Solutions for Pedodo tics, *J. Dent. Child.*, 31, 131, 2nd Quarter, 196
Cohen, D. W., Stoller, N. H., Chace, R., and Laste L.: A Comparison of Bacterial Plaque Disclosan in Periodontal Disease, *J. Periodont.*, 43, 33 June, 1972.
DeMarco, T. J. and Sokolof, M. L.: The Effect Sodium Fluorescein on the Mucosa of tl Hamster, *J. Periodont.*, 44, 640, October, 1973
Downton, J. M. and Castaldi, C. R.: A Study of Fo Disclosing Solutions, *Can. Dent. Hyg.*, pp. 6–1 Fall, 1967.
Edwards, R. C. and Sullivan, W. W.: An Evaluation Plaque Disclosants: Clinical Significance, *U. Navy Med.*, 62, 28, July, 1973.
Goldman, H. M. and Cohen, D. W.: *Periodont Therapy*, 5th ed. St. Louis, Mosby, 1973, p 427–429, 966, 1026.
Goldman, R. S., Abelson, D. C., Mandel, I. D., an Chilton, N. W.: The Effect of Various Disclosan on Plaque Accumulation in Human Subjects, *Periodont. Res.*, 9, 381, No. 6, 1974.
Hefferren, J. J., Cooley, R. O., Hall, J. B., Olsen, N. H and Lyon, H. W.: Use of Ultraviolet Illuminatio in Oral Diagnosis, *J. Am. Dent. Assoc.*, 82, 135 June, 1971.
Squillaro, R. C., Cohen, D. W., and Laster, L.: Comparison of Microbial Plaque Disclosan After Personal Oral Hygiene Instruction an Prophylaxis, *J. Prev. Dent.*, 2, 3, March-Apr 1975.

Chapter 27

Plaque Control: Instruction Procedures

People will learn and adhere to the principles and details of methods for the prevention and control of dental caries and periodontal diseases in proportion to the dental hygienist's concern and professional enthusiasm shown for their future oral health. Specialized knowledge of dental and periodontal diseases and skill in teaching foster confidence, but of greatest importance is *conviction* that careful treatment and teaching for the particular patient is worthwhile.

An effective teaching program provides both detailed information and principles to guide and motivate the patient to cooperate in his own optimal management. The overall teaching objective is to assist the patient to acquire knowledge, attitudes, and practices which will aid him in attaining and maintaining oral health.

I. Planned Instruction

Instruction needs to be planned if it is to stay directed toward goals, utilize available time efficiently, and help the patient to learn sequentially, from the simpler to the more complex. The design of instruction may be divided into certain basic steps:

A. **Objectives**

What knowledge and skills will be expected of the learner-patient after instruction?

B. **Presentation**

What knowledge-content must be included? How will the patient be oriented to the overall requirements for reaching the goals? Which instructional methods can be most helpful? What teaching aids will be most efficient?

C. **Demonstration**

What mode of demonstration will be most meaningful to this patient? What is the sequence of steps in the procedures to be learned? How can the steps be shown for sequential learning?

D. **Practice**

How will the procedures be practiced? How much practice will be needed? How can knowledge and skill-practice be integrated?

E. **Evaluation**

Can the patient demonstrate the procedures for self-care? Do the teeth and gingiva show the benefits of his

385

learning? Does the patient show basic understanding and motivation for continuing care?

The suggested procedure for patient instruction outlined in this chapter will follow these five steps. There are numerous modes of presentation, demonstration, and practice which can be used, but it is not possible to describe and evaluate all of them in this chapter.

Each dental hygienist will develop patient-centered systems of instruction which prove effective, and which are in accord with the policies and beliefs of the dentist. The important considerations for the methods used are that they are based on current, sound, scientific knowledge, and that they are applied efficiently so that the patient acquires the skill and know-how for adequate self-care.

II. Principles of Learning[1]

A. Learning is more effective when an individual is physiologically and psychologically ready to learn.

B. Individual differences must be considered if effective learning is to take place.

C. Motivation is essential for learning.

D. What an individual learns in a given situation depends upon what he recognizes and understands.

E. Transfer of learning is facilitated by recognition of similarities and dissimilarities between past experiences and the present situation.

F. An individual learns what he actually uses.

G. Learning takes place more effectively in situations where the individual derives feelings of satisfaction.

H. Evaluation of the results of instruction is essential to determine whether or not learning is taking place.

INDIVIDUAL PATIENT PROGRAM

Each patient has his own requirement for self-care, and objectives to fulfill these requirements must be related realistically to his individual needs, interests, and ability level. If the patient is to participate effectively in the learning process, he must be actively involved in setting his own goals.

The general objectives for plaque control and oral physical therapy described on page 304 provide the basis for the goals of an individual patient. The primary goal is plaque control, and the objectives for action are selected to accomplish this.

I. Selection of Objectives

From the patient history, oral inspection, radiographs, study casts, and all other data collected during the initial evaluation, and the diagnosis, details of the self-care program are evolved. The factors considered for toothbrush selection (page 310) are included for the total program. The items listed below summarize factors which must be considered. Plaque retention factors are of primary significance (pages 268–271).

A. **The Gingiva**
1. Current status of gingival health as evidenced by the color, size, contour, consistency, surface texture and tendency to bleed.
2. Treatment plan: whether to be treated by scaling, curettage, or will require more complicated periodontal therapy.
3. Specific anatomical features
    a. Open interdental areas or intact interdental gingiva.
    b. Recession with root exposure.
    c. Evidence of previous detrimental practices.

B. **The Teeth**
1. Position
    a. Malrelations such as crowding

overbite, crossbite, or malpositions of individual teeth; normal alignment.
b. Teeth adjacent to edentulous areas.

2. Abutment teeth.
3. Dental appliances: fixed, removable, orthodontic.

C. **General Health**
1. Chronic disease or other systemic condition which may limit the ability to perform certain tasks, or which may cause an exaggerated response of the gingiva to local irritants and require more intensive care.
2. Ability of patient to care for himself: physical and mental handicaps which require that another person perform his plaque control procedures for him.

D. **Age**
1. Preschool child requires parental assistance.
2. Motivation varies with age.

E. **Dexterity**
1. Occupation which requires manual or digital dexterity may contribute to increased facility in the manipulation of oral care devices.
2. For most patients, dexterity cannot be detected until after instruction has begun.

F. **Motivational Factors**
1. Immediate evaluation: previous oral health habits can reveal present attitudes and motivation, but frequently a lack of oral cleanliness can be attributed to a lack of knowledge. Many people have had very little or no instruction in how to care for their mouths.
2. Long-range motivation: prejudging a patient's motivation and willingness to carry out prescribed procedures is rarely possible. Some people show tremendous enthusiasm which may be short-lived; others reveal little interest at first, but prove to be highly conscientious.
3. Motivation is directly related to the dental hygienist's concern and enthusiasm.

II. Program Outline

A. **Program Planning**
All of the above factors which apply to an individual patient are matched with the available plaque control and oral physical therapy procedures. These include the selection of a toothbrush, toothbrushing method, interdental care devices and methods, dentifrice, and applied techniques for fixed and removable dental appliances.

With a clear definition of the needs of the patient, a recommended regimen or program can be outlined. The patient is shown his oral condition, changes and benefits which can be expected are explained, and cooperation is solicited. In this framework, the patient helps to formulate his own objectives.

B. **Immediate and Long-Range Programs**
Immediate and long-range programs are usually indicated. The immediate program is related to the treatment phase, whereas the long-range program is related to the maintenance phase of care. The immediate program may need to be more complicated and intensified than the long-range program. It may seem more complicated to the patient because of the anxieties generally associated with learning new procedures and changing former habits.

The new habits and attitudes acquired during the immediate program phase may aid the transition to the long-range program. With continuing reinforcement of instruction and encouragement, plaque control measures become a part of the daily routine and the health of the oral cavity can be maintained.

C. **When to Teach**

Unless a patient has an unusual amount of calculus, the initial instruction is best given *first*, before any clinical treatment. Reasons related to the educational aspects are:

1. *Emphasis on Importance of Self-Care.* Clinical professional services have only short-term effectiveness if the patient does not maintain the plaque control program. If considered first, and first in succeeding appointments, the degree of importance placed on self-care procedures by the dentist and dental hygienist will become apparent to the patient.

2. *Teaching Is More Effective.* If instruction is delayed until after the clinical procedures in an appointment:
   a. Time may be limited.
   b. The gingival margin may be sensitive from instrumentation.
   c. Blood clots forming in sulci after scaling and curettage should not be disturbed.
   d. Patient may be tired, anxious to leave, and less receptive to instruction.

3. *Plaque on Patient's Teeth.* With removal of tooth deposits during scaling, the opportunity to utilize the patient's plaque as a demonstrative educational aid is missed. Instruction is more effective when it is specifically concerned with the patient's own oral condition. Several principles of learning can be applied to the use of this system of teaching (see Principles of Learning, page 386).

PRESENTATION, DEMONSTRATION, PRACTICE

With the use of a disclosing agent, a method of instruction is available which can clearly and dramatically show the patient what he is trying to accomplish. Dental plaque is not visible on most teeth without staining. Words fail to impress upon patients that there are bacterial colonies on their teeth, and these multitudes of microorganisms, also called microcosms,[2] are the responsible agents for dental and periodontal diseases.

Because of the need for the light and rinsing facilities during the demonstration, instruction may best be given at the dental chair. Without an extensive display of instruments and other equipment to distract the patient, and with the dental hygienist seated beside the dental chair at the patient's eye level, an atmosphere conducive to learning can be created.

A specific area may be set aside and furnished for plaque control instruction in a dental office or clinic. Such an area should be planned with mirrors for the patient to use to observe the stained plaque on posterior teeth and distal surfaces. The patient should also be able to see placement of the toothbrush and floss in all areas of his mouth.

A suggested outline for conducting the plaque control program follows. Various adaptations can be made to adjust the plan to individual patients. A Gingival Index (GI), Plaque Index (Pl I), or other plaque control record can be educational and motivating for patients.[3-5] Indices are described in Chapter 19.

I. **First Lesson**

A. **Objective**

Orientation to dental plaque removal.

B. **Describe**

The formation and composition of dental plaque, its relationship to oral disease, and specifically its relationship to the patient's present condition. Present an overview of the plaque control program, what it can accomplish, and its purposes in relation to professional treatment.

C. **Illustrate**

Sketch on a pad of paper or use prepared materials. Show a tooth with gingiva and point out where the bacterial masses collect to form plaque. Explain how inflammation develops in the gingiva. The complete description should be divided over more than one instruction period. Too long a "lecture" with too many facts and details at one time may mean the patient cannot absorb any of them.

1. Patient with gingivitis: show and explain the formation of dental calculus and how periodontal disease can develop if gingivitis is left untreated.

2. Patient with periodontitis: introduce pocket formation and the reasons for pocket elimination.

3. Patient whose most severe problem is dental caries: when a dietary survey will be made, orientation to the preparation of the survey precludes discussion of plaque, sucrose, and dental caries, until the dietary record is obtained (pages 402–403).

D. **Demonstrate**

1. While the patient observes in a hand mirror, a healthy area of gingiva and an inflamed area can be compared.

2. A periodontal probe can be used to show the gingival sulcus and increased pocket depth related to periodontal involvement.

3. Remove a sample of plaque with a curet to demonstrate the thickness and consistency of plaque, to use in a test for acid formation (Methyl

Red Spot Plate Test, or Snyder Test, pages 416–417) and to use for a phase microscope demonstration.[6–8]

E. **The Disclosing Agent**

1. Explain its purpose: discoloration of plaque to show where the masses of bacteria accumulate.

2. Apply disclosing agent by topical application, provide diluted concentrate for a rinse, or request the patient to chew a tablet, swish for approximately one minute, and rinse.*

3. Examine the teeth with the patient, point out the stained plaque, and explain how these areas (generally the proximal surfaces and cervical third of the teeth) are adjacent to the gingiva, and therefore the bacteria must be removed to control inflammation.

4. Evaluation of the location of disclosed plaque will guide the instruction for plaque removal. Most patients will benefit from learning to floss before brushing.

F. **Plaque Removal Instruction**

1. Keep instruction simple. It is usually better not to teach both flossing and brushing during the first control lesson.

2. Floss first.
   a. Review objective.
   b. Show manner of holding the floss, inserting proximally, pressing around the tooth, and activating for plaque removal (figure 23–1, page 333).
   c. Examine in mirror to observe proximal areas where plaque has been removed.

3. Brush. Give the patient a soft brush and ask him to remove the stained plaque. No specific brushing in-

*Disclosing agents are described on pages 382–383.

structions may be given at this time so that the patient can concentrate on the single objective related to plaque removal.

4. After brushing, examine the teeth with the patient: the patient will see that he was able to remove accessible plaque.

5. Explain that the use of a toothbrush is the most effective means for plaque control for facial and lingual surfaces, and floss for proximal surfaces.

G. **Summary of Lesson I**

1. Review the basic objectives: to learn about plaque composition, occurrence, and relationship to oral disease; to learn about the use of a disclosing agent to aid in plaque detection and removal.

2. At the first lesson a specific tooth-brushing method is not generally presented so that the basic objectives are not obscured by inclusion of excess information or diversion of the patient's thinking by requiring his concentration on details of brush position. There are exceptions, for example:

a. The patient who demonstrates an acceptable brushing technique, whose mouth has been kept reasonably clean and shows no signs of detrimental brushing, may only need to be shown a few special adaptations for the difficult-to-reach areas or other improvements.

b. The patient who demonstrates a brushing method which is detrimental such as a vigorous horizontal stroke or a haphazard scrub-brush method, and whose teeth and/or gingiva show the effects of harmful brushing, may need an introduction to the method recommended for his personal care.

H. **Continuation of Appointment**

Usually instruction and practice in plaque removal should occupy the first appointment, and clinical services should not be started until the gingival inflammatory clinical signs have been lessened and the patient shows good progress in learning self-care. When calculus removal is initiated, the relation of clinical procedures to plaque control should be made clear to the patient. The satisfactory long-range outcome of scaling, curettage, and other professional treatment is dependent on complete daily plaque removal.

I. **End of Appointment Instruction**

1. Use of disclosing agent at home: provide patient with tablets or instructions for purchasing. Suggest using a tablet for daily plaque checks.

2. Emphasize the need for cleaning regularly for complete daily plaque removal. Discuss carrying a toothbrush for use when not at home.

3. When extra brushes cannot be supplied, explain that the toothbrush that has been used that day will be kept in the office for use during future appointments. Write down the name (number) of the brush for the patient to purchase for home use.

J. **Patient Records**

Methods, procedures, and patient progress and problems should be recorded following each appointment. The documented record can be reviewed prior to each appointment as a guide to continuing instruction.

II. **Second Lesson**

A. **Objectives**

To evaluate patient's success to date and to review and expand the knowledge-content of the previous lesson.

B. **Evaluation**
   1. Examine the gingival tissue with the patient. Evaluate and compare with notes recorded from previous examination (table 11–1, page 172).
   2. Apply the disclosing agent, and evaluate the plaque with the patient as he self-evaluates, using the hand mirror, his improvement in care as tested by the stained plaque. Chart plaque index or other record.

C. **Review and Expand Knowledge**
   1. Invite patient questions concerning plaque formation and gingival and periodontal diseases to determine how clearly information from the previous lesson was understood and retained.
   2. Discuss dentifrice recommendation when information from the dental history and the oral examination indicates the need for a change.
   3. Explain why the patient needs a more scientific brushing method (or how a few alterations in the previous method can improve his oral condition).
   4. Relate brushing to the treatment phase of oral care.

D. **Demonstrate**
   When not previously done, demonstrate the brushing technique of choice for this particular patient.
   1. Show the basic stroke on the anterior teeth where the patient can observe brush position and activation. Explain each step.
   2. For certain patients, only the facial aspects are demonstrated and practiced and the lingual is presented in a separate lesson. Instruction is divided appropriately to permit the patient to learn at a comfortable pace. When a patient has an automatic brush, it is recommended that initial instruction be given with the manual brush so that profi-

ciency can be attained with both. The patient should be asked to bring the automatic brush to the next appointment for demonstration and instruction.

E. **Practice**
   1. Each position around each arch must be practiced because of the variations in grasp of brush and hand positions, the difficulty of access, and the individual tooth positions, particularly malpositions.
   2. A recommended sequence for brushing which will include all areas and the tongue is discussed with the patient.

F. **Instructions for Home Procedures**
   Use disclosing agent after flossing and brushing to test completeness of plaque removal. A mouth mirror for the patient to use at home can be helpful. Inexpensive plastic mirrors are available for this purpose.

III. Third Lesson

A. **Objectives**
   1. Patients with reasonable mastery of the flossing and brushing methods and who need auxiliary plaque control and oral physical therapy measures (interdental, dental appliances, or other) will begin the third phase of their instruction.
   2. When a patient is not ready and cannot show reasonable skill with the floss and brush, introduction of new material is postponed, and previous instruction is reviewed and practiced.
   3. Many dentists will postpone therapy until the patient shows that an effective plaque control program can be carried out and an acceptable level of oral cleanliness can be maintained.

B. **Evaluation and Review**
  1. *Evaluate Gingiva.* Inspect with the patient for color, size, and other characteristics (table 11–1, page 172). Probe to detect bleeding. Review the features of normal gingiva and commend improvements.

     Question the patient relative to changes observed during the past week or since the previous appointment, such as less bleeding when brushing and an overall feeling of cleanliness. Emphasize the role of self-care in accomplishing the improvements rather than the effects of professional treatment.
  2. *Evaluate Plaque.* Apply disclosing agent and inspect for areas that need additional instruction. Relate areas of persistent gingival redness to areas inadequately flossed and brushed.
  3. *Evaluate Brushing.* Patient demonstrates. Ask him to show how he brushes the areas missed as revealed by gingival and disclosing agent inspections. Help him to evaluate and make his own corrections. Supplement as needed with demonstration.

C. **Introduce New Material**
   Demonstrate auxiliary interdental or other methods; explain the purposes and procedures for each method selected for this patient (pages 331–344).

D. **Practice**
   Continued instruction is usually needed for most interdental methods. A specific appointment to check the method of use is particularly important at least by the end of the first week, since incorrect habits may become permanent if allowed to persist.

IV. Continuous Instruction

A. **Number of Lessons**
   It is not possible to predict in advance the number of specific teaching sessions a patient will need to demonstrate mastery of the recommended procedures, and to show by the appearance of the teeth and gingiva that the practices have been carried out daily. When additional supervision is indicated after dental hygiene professional treatment has been completed, short appointments may be scheduled in conjunction with dental appointments.

   One teaching-learning experience is rarely adequate. When a patient has been able to maintain relatively clean teeth and clinically healthy gingiva and can demonstrate an acceptable toothbrushing method, a review of difficult-to-reach areas can be made and reevaluated at a follow-up appointment.

B. **Relationship to Gingival Health**
   When areas of gingival marginal redness and sponginess persist, tooth surfaces are checked carefully for residual calculus, and scaling and planing are completed as indicated. When the patient consistently fails to remove dental plaque in certain areas, a reevaluation of the program is made. Perhaps the selected procedures are too difficult for the patient to accomplish, or perhaps supplementary measures are needed.

C. **Recall**
   The first recall after the initial instruction series is best scheduled after a shorter interval than may be used for succeeding recall appointments. It is necessary to evaluate the patient's ability to continue adequate self-care, and to determine whether true learning has resulted and new habits have been adopted. Learning means that a change in behavior has occurred.

   At the recall appointment, patient and dental hygienist evaluate together: the gingival characteristics, the occurrence of dental plaque (disclosed), and the performance of brushing and other measures. The complete procedures for the recall appointment are described on pages 573–575.

V. Instruction Adaptability

The methods for presentation, demonstration, practice, and evaluation described in the previous pages can be adapted readily to various age levels. Awareness of the changing motivation and interests from the young to the elderly, and adaptations of terminology with respect for the patient's level of understanding, ease the transition from patient to patient.

Others for whom instruction is provided are the nurses or family members who attend patients who are unable to care for themselves. In Section VI, the various chapters which pertain to the helpless, handicapped, or otherwise afflicted include suggestions for patient care. For many of these patients an automatic brush has been especially useful.

THE PRESCHOOL CHILD

The establishment of positive health habits and attitudes in the adult has its beginnings in childhood. Even before birth and during the first year after birth, the parent's education for prevention of dental caries and gingival disease should begin.

After birth regular daily systemic fluoride in the absence of fluoridation, as well as attention to the control of dietary sucrose can mean a great deal to the future health of the child. Nursing bottle caries was described on page 215. Information about plaque control for gingival health has application while the child's primary teeth are erupting.

I. Early Plaque Control

Conditioning a child to associate cleaning of the oral cavity with total body cleanliness can begin when the first teeth erupt. A small, soft toothbrush may be used or, at first, the parent can rub the teeth and gingiva with a cloth wrapped over a finger.

As time goes on and the child grows, he will want to use the brush himself, particularly if he is given the opportunity to watch his parents brush their teeth. At first a tiny child may only chew on the brush, but eventually he may try to imitate the parents. Gradually an actual brushing procedure can be encouraged which frequently may resemble a scrub-brush technique (page 319).

For several years the parents will have the responsibility for brushing after meals and before the child retires. The age varies with the individual child relative to when the child can take on the responsibility himself. It has been suggested that when a child attends to bathing himself, he is probably ready to do all of his own toothbrushing. Parental supervision and encouragement must continue for a few more years for most children.

II. Professional Instruction

A. The First Dental Appointment

Early visits to the dental office for orientation and getting acquainted are to be encouraged. If the child has not had a dental emergency which brought him to the dental office earlier, oral inspection and necessary treatment are indicated between two and three years of age. It is recommended that the first appointment with the dental hygienist be reserved for instruction in plaque control.

B. Effect of Age

There is a great deal of difference with each year of age of preschoolers. The child at two years may be cooperative and well-behaved, but at about two and one-half he can be contrary and difficult; by three, amiable and in good control, yet at four be difficult and dogmatic.[9] The general suggestions made below need application to the individual child, and are presented only as a basis from which instruction can be planned.

C. **Instruction for the Child**
1. Toothbrush selection: a child-sized, soft nylon brush is recommended. When possible, let the child select his own from assorted colors.
2. Method: Control of dental plaque at the gingival margin and on proximal tooth surfaces requires the same emphasis in the very young as at other ages. Although the very young child will have a short interest span for specific instruction, the mother can be coached to assist with supplementary home instruction. Many dentists favor instruction in a scrub-brush method for preschool children.

III. Instruction for the Parent

The parent who is a patient in the same dental practice may be already familiar with the teaching methods used and well-oriented to the importance of plaque control. Transfer of knowledge and skills to care of the child can be relatively easy. When the child is a patient in a pedodontic specialty practice or the parent is a patient elsewhere, orientation will be needed in accord with the parent's present knowledge.

A. **Disclosing Agent**
1. When the child will chew a tablet, it is preferable so that he will learn to use the tablets at home for the parent to evaluate. One-half tablet is sufficient. When a young child cannot understand about chewing the tablet, disclosing solution can be applied.
2. Inspection: the child is given a mirror to "watch" his teeth. The plaque deposits are pointed out and discussed with the parent, and a little plaque removed with a probe to illustrate.

B. **Demonstration**

The selected brushing method of choice is shown to the parent while the child is in the dental chair under the light.

C. **Procedure and Practice**
1. Demonstration is given with the child and parent standing to simulate the home setting.
2. Show the parent how, if he brushes the child's teeth from the front, the child's head falls back, unsupported, and it is difficult to see into the mouth.
3. Recommended position: child stands in front of parent and leans back against him.[10] The dental hygienist demonstrates, and then the parent practices.
4. Parent cradles the child's head with his left arm and brings his left hand around to hold the chin in the palm of his hand and to retract the lips and cheek with his fingers.
5. Brush mandibular teeth: retract lip for anterior and cheek for posterior. The back of the brush head will retract the tongue.
6. Maxillary teeth: child is asked to tip his head back so that the parent can look in the mouth while fingers retract the upper lip for anterior and the cheek for posterior.
7. Dental floss: with the child's head supported as described above for brushing, the parent can be shown how finger and hand rests (fulcrums) can be maintained while floss is applied. When primary teeth are widely spaced, brushing may be adapted to remove plaque from all surfaces without a need for flossing. If necessary the parent can use nylon yarn for proximal surfaces (page 336). Flossing may not be recommended for all children (page 335).
8. Dentifrice recommendation: a

fluoride dentifrice is preferred, even when there is fluoride in the drinking water.

D. **Summary**

Instructions include brushing after each meal and using the disclosing test before one of the brushings.

E. **Second Appointment**

Procedure follows that of an adult. The gingiva are examined and evaluated, plaque is disclosed and areas with stain are discovered, the child demonstrates brushing, and then the parent. Suggestions for improvement are offered.

As needed, calculus and stain are removed professionally. Brushing demonstration precedes each succeeding restorative appointment until proficiency is demonstrated.

IV. Recall

Instruction continues with each four to six months' recall appointment.

THE TEACHING SYSTEM

A simple direct approach such as has been described, with specific content and unembellished with excess distracting material, focuses the attention of the patient-learner on the central theme: plaque control. The more practical, realistic, and goal-centered the components of instruction can be, the more effective the outcomes will be in terms of treatment and prevention of recurrence of disease. An *informed*, knowledgeable patient will have reasons for *practicing* appropriate, scientifically based, self-care measures.

A teaching system must be reevaluated from time to time particularly as new research reveals new aspects of prevention and treatment. New devices for plaque removal and gingival care may become available and these need study before recommendations to patients can be made.

The teaching system presented in this chapter has a built-in evaluation of patient learning. The outcomes of learning are shown by examination and demonstration: examination for the gingival characteristics consistent with health, demonstration of disclosable plaque, and the demonstration of the patient's ability to use floss and brush for plaque removal without harm to the oral tissues.

Since the ultimate objective of plaque control is to prevent dental caries and periodontal diseases, the oral health history of the patient over several years will document a true evaluation. The teaching system must involve development of the patient's attitudes relative to continuing professional supervision and regular appointments for examination and treatment.

EVALUATION OF TEACHING AIDS

I. General Characteristics

Evaluation of teaching aids involves consideration of their

A. **Simplicity**

Ease of management, ready obtainability, easy understanding by the patient.

B. **Content**

Practical, scientifically sound, meaningful.

C. **Level of Orientation**

Appropriate to the individual patient.

D. **Durability**

If reusable, they must maintain their cleanliness and freshness.

E. **Cost**

Reasonable. Cost relates to their essential value in reaching goals.

F. **Objectives**

1. Objective of a teaching aid must be clear and readily understood by the patient.
2. In teaching, activities should be reality-centered not fantasy-

centered.[11] A well-intentioned visual aid may provide entertainment rather than education, and have no transfer value, in terms of the actual oral health lesson, to the behavioral pattern of the patient.

II. Reading Material for the Patient

Effectively presented, informational books and leaflets can supplement and reinforce individually presented instruction. Selected with a purpose, a booklet or other printed material may be presented to the patient to read while at the dental office or it may be given for "homework." The booklet's contents must be reviewed with the patient and particular sections may be marked to personalize the instruction and encourage reading. Indiscriminate distribution of printed materials is pointless.

Obtaining copies and reviewing newly available materials are essential parts of the dental hygienist's work, even as a teacher reviews new textbooks and materials for possible use in a classroom. The professionally prepared materials from the American Dental Association are recommended. The address is included under *Technical Hints.*

Instruction sheets and leaflets can be custom-made by the dental hygienist with the cooperation and recommendations of the dentist. It is especially helpful to have postoperative instructions, plaque control, and oral physical therapy procedures outlined so that the patient will have a reference for home use. Materials can be personalized by writing the patient's name and special procedures or reminders.

III. Use of Models

A. Patient's Study Cast

The cast can be useful to explain oral conditions or restorations such as the need to replace missing teeth. With certain patients, aspects of plaque control and oral physical therapy can be demonstrated provided the patient is properly oriented to associate the cast with his own teeth.

B. Commercially Available Models

Although plastic models (dentoforms) have been used extensively for teaching toothbrushing methods, their meaningfulness to the patient has not been demonstrated. When a toothbrush is to be available for the patient to practice brushing in his mouth, the usefulness of the time spent to demonstrate on a model first may be questioned. When teaching is by means of the model and brush only, and particularly when the oversized model will be used, the patient's learning should be carefully evaluated. It is suggested that all three of the patient evaluation methods described in this chapter (gingival status, disclosed plaque, and ability of patient to brush) be utilized.

It is probable that the model and the toothbrush do not represent a problem to the patient and that most patients can imitate the movements of the toothbrush on the model quite accurately when asked.[12] The difficulty comes in transferring the motions to the mouth, and the more complex the technique, the greater the difficulty of transfer.

TECHNICAL HINTS

Sources of Educational Materials
1. American Dental Association, Order Department, 211 East Chicago Avenue, Chicago, Illinois 60611. (Request current year's catalog)
2. American Academy of Periodontology, Public and Professional Relations Committee, 211 East Chicago Avenue, Chicago, Illinois 60611. (Request *Periodontal Health Catalog*)
3. Information Office, National Institute

of Dental Research, National Institutes of Health, Bethesda, Maryland 20014. (Request sample copies of Plaque and Periodontal Disease leaflets)

References

1. Sand, O.: *Curriculum Study in Basic Nursing Education.* New York, Putnam's, 1955, pp. 53–60.
2. Arnim, S. S. and Williams, Q. E.: How to Educate Patients in Oral Hygiene, *Dent. Radiogr. Photogr.,* 32, 61, No. 4, 1959.
3. O'Leary, T. J., Drake, R. B., and Naylor, J. E.: The Plaque Control Record, *J. Periodont.,* 43, 38, January, 1972.
4. Barrickman, R. W. and Penhall, O. J.: Graphing Indexes Reduces Plaque, *J. Am. Dent. Assoc.,* 87, 1404, December, 1973.
5. Garnick, J. J.: Use of Indexes for Plaque Control, *J. Am. Dent. Assoc.,* 86, 1325, June, 1973.
6. Katz, S., McDonald, J. L., and Stookey, G. K.: *Preventive Dentistry in Action.* Upper Montclair, N.J., D. C. P. Publishing, 1972, pp. 148–149.
7. Wren, L. A. and Corrington, J. D.: *Understanding and Using the Phase Microscope.* Unitron Instrument Company, 66 Needham Street, Newton Highlands, Massachusetts, 59 pp.
8. Wheatcroft, M. G.: Instructions for the Use of the Phase Microscope, in DiOrio, L. P. and Madsen, K. O.: *A Personalized Program. Educating the Patient in the Prevention of Dental Disease.* Chicago, March Pub., 1972, pp. 58–60.
9. Finn, S. B.: *Clinical Pedodontics,* 4th ed. Philadelphia, Saunders, 1972, p. 32.
10. Starkey, P. E.: Instructions to Parents for Brushing the Child's Teeth, *J. Dent. Child.,* 28, 42, 1st Quarter, 1961.
11. Young, M. A. C.: Dental Health Education—Whither? *J. Am. Dent. Assoc.,* 66, 821, June, 1963.
12. Henning, F. R. and Fanning, E. A.: Instruction in Oral Hygiene, *Aust. Dent. J.,* 13, 40, February, 1968.

Suggested Readings

Akst, H., DeMarco, T. J., Duchon, S., Meclovsky, E., and Resnick, J.: A Profile of Clinical Preventive Practice, *J. Am. Dent. Assoc.,* 87, 857, October, 1973.

Arnim, S. S.: The Effect of Thorough Mouth Cleansing on Oral Health—Case Report, *Periodontics,* 6, 41, February, 1968.

Ayer, W. A.: Efforts to Improve Oral Hygiene Practices: A Review and Critical Evaluation, *J. Am. Dent. Hyg. Assoc.,* 46, 437, November-December, 1972.

Barnes, G. P. and Perkins, B. E.: Plaque Control and Oral Hygiene Status of Dental Auxiliary Personnel, *Dent. Hyg.,* 49, 63, February, 1975.

Durlak, J. A. and Levine, J.: Seeing Oral Health Patients in Groups, *J. Am. Dent. Assoc.,* 90, 426, February, 1975.

Gift, H., Muller, T., and Newman, J.: Characteristics of Dental Oral Hygiene Education in Private Practice, *J. Prev. Dent.,* 2, 37, January-February, 1975.

Goldman, H. M. and Ruben, M. P.: Methods for Increasing the Efficiency of the Arcuate-motioned, Power-driven Brush in Oral Physiotherapy, *J. Periodont.,* 38, 508, November-December, 1967.

Minnich, W. and Latimer, L.: Dental Health Education Methods—A Comparison of Their Effectiveness, *J. Am. Dent. Hyg. Assoc.,* 44, 40, 1st Quarter, 1970.

O'Leary, T. J. and Nabers, C. L.: Oral Physiotherapy, in Goldman, H. M. and Cohen, D. W.: *Periodontal Therapy,* 5th ed. St. Louis, Mosby, 1972, pp. 427–445.

Sangnes, G.: Effectiveness of Vertical and Horizontal Toothbrushing Techniques in the Removal of Plaque, II. Comparison of Brushing by Six-year-old Children and Their Parents, *J. Dent. Child.,* 41, 119, March-April, 1974.

Telford, A. B. and Murray, J. J.: The Effect of Systematic Chairside Oral Hygiene Instruction on Gingivitis and Oral Cleanliness in Children, *Community Dent. Oral Epidemiol.,* 2, 50, No. 2, 1974.

Toto, P. D.: Effective Toothbrushing Requires Instruction, *J. Dent. Child.,* 34, 296, July, 1967.

Vande Voorde, H. E.: A Movie vs. Chairside Instruction to Present Preliminary Oral Hygiene Information, *J. Periodont.,* 43, 277, May, 1972.

Dental Health Programs

Berk, G.: The Effectiveness of a Dental Hygiene Education Program on Oral Hygiene, *Dent. Hyg.,* 49, 161, April, 1975.

Dunning, J. M. and Sanzi, S.: Changes in Dental Care Following Dental Health Program in Boston Schools, *J. Dent. Educ.,* 37, 26, February, 1973.

Heifetz, S. B., Bagramian, R. A., and Suomi, J. D.: Programs for the Mass Control of Plaque: An Appraisal, *J. Public Health Dent.,* 33, 91, Spring, 1973.

Hudson, L. C.: A School Plaque Control Program for First Grade, *Dent. Hyg.,* 48, 299, September-October, 1974.

Ingalls, J. A.: The Dental Hygienist as Home Consultant, *J. Am. Dent. Hyg. Assoc.,* 47, 38, January-February, 1973.

Podshadley, A. G. and Schweikle, E. S.: The Effectiveness of Two Educational Programs in Changing the Performance of Oral Hygiene by Elementary School Children, *J. Public Health Dent.,* 30, 17, Winter, 1970.

Podshadley, A. G. and Shannon, J. H.: Oral Hygiene Performance of Elementary School Children Following Dental Health Education, *J. Dent. Child.,* 37, 298, July-August, 1970.

Raynor, J. F. and Cohen, L. K.: A Position on School Dental Health Education, *J. Prev. Dent.*, 1, 11, July-August, 1974.

Silverstein, S., Gold, S., Heilbron, D., Nelms, D., and Wycoff, S.: Effect of Supervised Deplaquing on Gingivitis and Plaque, *A. A. D. R. Program and Abstracts of Papers*, No. 607, February, 1975, p. 197.

Stolpe, J. R., Mecklenburg, R. E., and Lathrop, R. L.: The Effectiveness of an Educational Program on Oral Health in Schools for Improving the Application of Knowledge, *J. Public Health Dent.*, 31, 48, Winter, 1971.

Terhune, J. A.: Predicting the Readiness of Elementary School Children to Learn an Effective Dental Flossing Technique, *J. Am. Dent. Assoc.*, 86, 1332, June, 1973.

Young, M. A. C.: Dental Health Education. An Overview of Selected Concepts and Principles Relevant to Programme Planning, *Int. J. Health Educ.*, 13, 2, January-March, 1970.

Motivation

Baseheart, J. R.: Nonverbal Communication in the Dentist-patient Relationship, *J. Prosthet. Dent.*, 34, 4, July, 1975.

Counsel, L. A.: The Implications of the Behavioral Sciences for Dental Health Education, *J. Public Health Dent.*, 30, 38, Winter, 1970.

Derbyshire, J. C.: Motivation of Patients, in Goldman, H. M. and Cohen, D. W.: *Periodontal Therapy*, 5th ed. St. Louis, Mosby, 1972, pp. 446–462.

Dummett, C. O.: Understanding the Underprivileged Patient, *J. Am. Dent. Assoc.*, 79, 1363, December, 1969.

Evans, R. I.: The Social Psychology of Persuasion: The Use of Fear and Other Problems, *J. Am. Soc. Prev. Dent.*, 2, 18, July-August, 1972.

Ferris, R. T. and Winslow, E. K.: Reinforcing Desired Behavior with Periodontal Patients, *Dent. Clin. North Am.*, 14, 279, April, 1970.

Gold, S. L.: Establishing Motivating Relations in Preventive Dentistry, *J. Am. Soc. Prev. Dent.*, 4, 17, November-December, 1974.

Jackson, E.: Effective Persuasion in Dental Practice, *J. Am. Soc. Prev. Dent.*, 5, 15, May-June, 1975.

Legler, D. W., Mayhall, C. W., and Bradley, E. L.: Behavioral Characteristics of Disadvantaged Adult Patients, *J. Public Health Dent.*, 32, 15, Winter, 1972.

Parker, M. W.: Patient Motivation—A Systematic Approach, *J. Am. Soc. Prev. Dent.*, 2, 36, November-December, 1972.

Podshadley, A. G.: The Essential Elements in Educating Patients, *J. Public Health Dent.*, 28, 249, Fall, 1968.

Ramirez, A., Lasater, T. M., Anderson, R. L., Cameron, B. G., Connor, R. B., Davis, J. C., and Meon, M. J.: Use of Fear Appeals in Dental Health Education, *J. Am. Dent. Assoc.*, 83, 1086, November, 1971.

Shulman, J.: Current Concepts of Patient Motivation Toward Long Term Oral Hygiene: A Literature Review, *J. Am. Soc. Prev. Dent.*, 4, 7, November-December, 1974.

Stacey, D. C., Abbott, D. M., and Jordan, R. D.: Improvement in Oral Hygiene as a Function of Applied Principles of Behavioral Modification, *J. Public Health Dent.*, 32, 234, Fall, 1972.

Stewart, R. T., Parr, R. W., Block, P. L., Johnson, W., Niver, F., and Antelyes, A.: What Is the Most Effective Means of Changing Patients' Plaque Control Behavior? *Periodont. Abstr.*, 21, 63, Summer, 1973.

Sword, R. O.: Oral Neglect—Why? *J. Am. Dent. Assoc.*, 80, 1327, June, 1970.

Weisenberg, M.: Behavioral Motivation, *J. Periodont.*, 44, 489, August, 1973.

Wentz, F. M.: Patient Motivation: A New Challenge to the Dental Profession for Effective Control of Plaque, *J. Am. Dent. Assoc.*, 85, 887, October, 1972.

Winslow, E. K. and Ferris, R. T.: Developing Desired Patient Behavior, *Dent. Clin. North Am.*, 14, 269, April, 1970.

Chapter 28

Nutrition, Diet, and Dietary Analysis

Planning for a total preventive program for an individual patient involves consideration of dietary and nutritional factors. The status of oral health can be affected by nutrition, diet, and food habits. Since proper nutrition improves general health, it follows that improved general health can produce a higher degree of oral health.

Instruction relating to diet is coordinated with other phases of teaching. To give information about a diet conducive to oral health is a responsibility, and to help motivate a patient to adopt new eating patterns, a challenge.

Food selection by an individual is influenced by age, sex, geographical location, economic status, available foods, family traditions, religion, cultural habits, prejudices, fallacies, and advertising, as well as emotional and social factors. Instruction must be made practical and possible to apply if it is to have impact on these forceful influences.

I. Definitions

A. Nutrition
The combination of processes by which the living organism receives and utilizes the materials (food) necessary for the maintenance of its functions and for the growth and renewal of its components.

B. Diet
The total food and drink regularly consumed.

C. Nutrients
Those chemical substances in food that are needed by the body. They are divided into six classes: proteins and amino acids, fats and fatty acids, carbohydrates, mineral elements, vitamins, and water.

D. Nutritional Deficiency
An inadequacy of nutrients in the tissues. A deficiency may be the result of inadequate dietary intake, or impairment in digestion, absorption, transport metabolism, or excretion.

II. Periodontal Tissues[1,2]

A. Nutritional Deficiencies
1. Protein, vitamins, and other nutrients are essential to the health of the periodontal tissues, just as they are for the tissues throughout the body.

2. A nutritional deficiency has never been shown to be the specific cause of periodontal pocket formation, gingivitis, or periodontal disease. For these conditions to develop, local irritants must be present, particularly plaque.
3. Certain nutritional deficiencies (protein, ascorbic acid (vitamin C), and B Complex particularly) modify the gingival tissue resistance so that an inflammatory condition (initiated by local irritants) may be accelerated or increased in intensity.
4. The effects of periodontal disease can alter the capacity of the tissues to utilize available nutrients and therefore the potential for repair is modified.

B. **Consistency of Food**
1. Soft sticky foods cling to the teeth and gingiva and encourage food and debris accumulation, increased dental plaque, and calculus formation.
2. Firm fibrous foods stimulate the tissues and improve circulation.
   a. Fibrous foods (particularly uncooked fruits and vegetables) tend to clear away loose debris and impart a generally clean sensation. They do not remove plaque from the cervical area.[3,4]
   b. Chewing is important to health: normal use of tissues promotes keratinization and improves circulation.

C. **Dietary Analysis**
Patients with acute gingival disease, necrotizing ulcerative gingivitis, and most patients undergoing periodontal therapy, need specific instruction in diet selection. A dietary survey with analysis is important if a true idea of the patient's diet is to be available for study. Procedures for the survey and analysis are described later in this chapter.

III. Mucous Membranes

A. **Nutritional Deficiencies**
Severe nutritional deficiencies are rare except in underdeveloped areas of the world. Deficiencies tend to produce symptoms of mixed clinical entities but infrequently of a severe acute disease. When certain oral symptoms suggest nutritional deficiencies, the patient would most likely be suffering from multiple deficiencies.

Ordinarily the effects of a deficiency would be chronic in nature and run a slow, gradual course. The clinical manifestations are influenced by trauma, local irritation, or systemic factors such as a chronic disease, which act on tissue resistance.

B. **Oral Lesions**
Types of oral lesions which suggest the possibility of an underlying nutritional deficiency are stomatitis, glossitis, cheilitis, and localized ulcerations and areas of atrophic change.[5] Definitive diagnosis by the dentist is difficult or impossible even with the patient history, a dietary analysis, and laboratory tests. Nutrients which are considered particularly associated with the health of the oral mucosa are iron, ascorbic acid, and various B vitamins.

C. **Instruction**
Assistance to patients through recommendations for an adequate diet for general health will contribute to preserving the integrity of the oral mucosa.

IV. Dental Caries

A. **Prevention**
The nutrient fluoride is the essential tooth component for dental caries

prevention. Calcium, phosphorus, and vitamin D which is necessary for the utilization of calcium and phosphorus, are implicated in tooth formation, but there is no conclusive evidence that dental caries is influenced specifically by the nutrients involved in tooth development other than fluoride.

B. Role of Sucrose

Dental caries is the result of action on the external surface of the tooth. Instead of being a deficiency disease, it can be considered the result of an excess food component, carbohydrate, and specifically sucrose. Dietary sucrose produces acids when acted upon by specific streptococci, and also contributes to the storage of dextrans and levans in dental plaque. Dextrans and levans act as reservoirs for the continuing production of acid. These factors were discussed in connection with dental plaque, pages 239–244.

C. Dietary Analysis

The use of a dietary analysis in the instruction of patients and their parents relative to dental caries control has proven very helpful to many people. The dental caries control study is described later in this chapter.

DAILY FOOD REQUIREMENTS

Patient instruction by the dental hygienist centers around helping patients learn the foods which make an adequate diet, and improve their food selection. Poor food habits, such as missed meals, omission of essential foods, regular use of non-nutritious snacks, or illogical unsupervised dieting, frequently are important to recommendations related to nutritional practices for oral health. Generalities may be useful to a degree, but for daily application specific suggestions for meal planning and food selection are needed.

The information in this chapter and the suggestions for application assume that each dental hygienist has had the opportunity before entering practice to study the science of nutrition somewhat comprehensively. It is also expected that reference books and other materials are available. Knowledge of sources of informational leaflets which can be made available to provide patients with useful, practical facts about diet and meal planning is necessary. Continued review of new materials constitutes an important phase of teaching.

I. Recommended Dietary Allowances[6]

A standard of dietary adequacy was prepared by the United States National Research Council for certain nutrients. For example, for an average adult, daily recommended dietary allowances to maintain health include protein, 56 grams for males, 46 grams for females; vitamin A, 5000 I.U. for males, 4000 I.U. for females; ascorbic acid, 45 milligrams; calcium, 800 milligrams; and iron, 10 milligrams for males, 18 milligrams for females. During school years, adolescence, and pregnancy, 400 I.U. of vitamin D are needed.

Recommended daily dietary allowances are not the same for all, are not recommended as an ideal diet, and do not include special needs such as during illness. The figures are intended as a guide. From the examples given above, it can be seen that such designations of the amounts of nutrients are impractical for patient instruction. To be meaningful, nutrients must be expressed in terms of the foods which contain them and how much of these foods must be used daily to meet the requirements.

II. The Food Groups

To fulfill minimum requirements of nutrients for the maintenance of health and resistance to disease is not a problem when a wide variety of foods is included in the diet each day. The foods which contain the essential nutrients, called foundation or protective foods, have been divided into four food groups: the milk group, the meat group, the vegetable-fruit group, and the bread-cereal group.

The leaflet *Food for Fitness . . . A Daily Food Guide*, prepared by the United States Department of Agriculture,[7] is arranged for conveniently teaching about the four food groups. Table 28–1 provides a summary of the groups, examples of foods included in each, the recommended daily servings, and the major nutrients which each group contributes to the diet.

III. Applications

The size of the servings of the protective foods (table 28–1, middle column) varies with age and physiological states. Servings for children will be smaller, for teen-agers extra large or increased in number. Nutritional requirements for teen-age boys are higher than at any other time in their lives, and for girls the only time they will be higher will be during pregnancy or lactation. Dietary requirements for pregnancy are summarized in the chapter on prenatal care, page 718.

With old age, total requirements decrease, but the components of the daily requirements remain the same. Tissue building and repair continue throughout life, and nutrients must be supplied accordingly. Problems of the diet of aging persons are summarized on pages 592–594.

THE DIETARY ANALYSIS

A dietary analysis is used as a guide for patient instruction.* Whether the analysis is made to help a patient whose major oral health problem is dental caries or periodontal disease, the same general procedures can be followed.

*The word "patient" is used to mean the patient and the parent when the patient is a child.

The type of dietary analysis made i sometimes referred to as *qualitative*. I takes into consideration the general foo groups essential or detrimental to goo oral health and does not pretend to sho precise mathematical calculations of th chemical constituents, as does the *quan titative* type of dietary analysis. Th nutritionist is skilled in making detaile quantitative diet analyses and work under the direction of the physician t provide specific therapeutic diets fo physiologic and pathologic conditions.

I. Objectives of a Dietary Analysis

A. To give a patient an opportunity t study, objectively, personal dietar habits.

B. To obtain an overall picture of th types of food in the patient's diet, foo preferences, and the quantity of foo eaten.

C. To study the food habits with particular reference to frequency and regularity of eating and the order in which food is taken.

D. To compare the frequency of eating carbohydrates with the caries activit test results and clinical and radiographic findings.

E. To determine which fibrous foods are regularly included in the diet and the relationship of their position in the diet to the position of fermentable carbohydrates.

F. To provide a basis for making individual recommendations for changes in the diet important to the health of the oral mucosa and the periodontium and to the prevention of dental caries.

II. The Food Diary

A. **Types**
  1. *Short.* A record of the food eaten by the patient over the previous 24

Table 28–1. Food for an Adequate Diet

Food Group	Recommended Daily Amount		Contribution to Diet
Milk Group		*Servings**	
Milk: whole, evaporated, skim, dry, buttermilk **Cheese** and other milk products	Children under 9 Children 9 to 12 Teen-age Adults Pregnant women Nursing mothers	2 to 3 3 or more 4 or more 2 or more 3 or more 4 or more	Calcium Protein Riboflavin Vitamin A (whole milk) Vitamin D (when fortified) Thiamine
Meat Group **Meats,** fish, poultry **Eggs** **Alternates:** vegetable protein (dry beans, dry peas, lentils, nuts)	2 or more servings to include 3 to 5 eggs weekly		Protein Iron Thiamine Riboflavin Niacin Vitamin A (egg yolk, liver)
Vegetables—Fruit Group **All vegetables and fruits** Divided between Dark green or yellow vegetables and Citrus fruits Includes potato	4 or more servings		Vitamin A (deep yellow and green vegetables) Ascorbic acid (citrus fruits) Other minerals and vitamins
Bread—Cereal Group **All breads and cereals** that are whole grain, enriched or restored	4 or more servings		Protein Iron B vitamins Food energy
Other Foods **Butter,** margarine **Other** fats	To round out meals and meet energy needs		

*Servings: *Milk group:* one serving is one 8-ounce glass of fluid milk or its calcium equivalent in cheese and other milk products.

  Meat group: one serving is two to three ounces of lean meat, fish, poultry, two eggs, or one cup cooked dried beans or peas.

  Vegetables—Fruits group: one serving is one-half cup or portion normally used such as one apple, orange, potato.

  Bread—Cereal group: one serving is one slice of bread, one-half cup cooked cereal, rice, pasta, etc.

hours can be obtained by interview. Although of assistance for discussion during instruction, a truer picture of the patient's usual diet can be obtained from a food diary kept for a week or at least five days.

2. *Week-long.* The week or series of consecutive days selected should be typical of ordinary daily living uncomplicated by illness, holidays, fasting, or other unusual events.

B. **Characteristics of Forms to Use**
1. Simple, with ample spacing.
2. Space indicated for patient's name, the day, and the date on each page.
3. Blocked off areas for each meal and between-meal.
4. Space to indicate time of eating.
5. Column to record food item and amount (figure 28–1).
6. Cover page with sample procedure for entering items (figure 28–2).

III. Presentation to Patient

Result obtained can be expected to be directly proportional to the care taken in presentation.

A. **Explain the Purpose**
Avoid mention of specific foods and their relationships to oral health: the patient may not provide a true diary if he knows what will be checked.

B. **Explain the Form**
Discuss the cover page suggestions for listing various foods, and the use of household measurements for indicating quantity.

C. **Complete the Current Day's Diary with the Patient**
To illustrate how to itemize and how to list the foods in the order in which they were eaten.

D. **General Directions**
1. Emphasize importance of completing each meal's record as soon after eating as possible to avoid forgetting.

2. Explain need for recording what was actually eaten in contrast to recording everything served.
3. Review details of recording the component parts of a combination dish such as a salad, sandwich, casserole.
4. Indicate need for recording vitamin concentrates, prescribed medicines, water.
5. Request that meals eaten other than at home be identified by writing "restaurant," "guest at friend's home," or "party."

IV. Receiving the Completed Food Diary

The appointment for receiving the food diary should follow soon after its completion.

A. Question the patient and record additional information
1. Whether the diary represents that of a typical week.
2. Appetite.
3. Food likes and dislikes; preferences.
4. Allergies.
5. Specially prescribed diets for the patient or other members of the family.

B. Review with the patient each day's recorded food list and supplement details which have been omitted.
1. Identify additions by using ink if the diary has been kept in pencil or *vice versa.*
2. Common omissions
   a. Garnishes: frosting, whipped cream, butter or oleomargarine on vegetables, salad dressings?
   b. Size of drinking glass: four ounce, eight-ounce?
   c. Bread or toast: white, enriched wheat?
   d. Chewing gum: sugarless, amount?
   e. Canned fruit: packed in water or heavy or light syrup?

f. Fruit salad: canned, fresh?
g. Cereal: kind, milk, cream, sugar, quantity?
h. Potato: baked, buttered, fried?
i. Doughnut: sugared, glazed, plain?

. Summary and Analysis

The three principal parts to analyze are foods from the four food groups, texture and consistency of foods, and the foods containing sugar (sucrose). For convenience, check sheets should be devised for recording the frequency of use of each of the three.

. Protective Foods
1. Analysis of overall content of the diet.
   a. Comparison with four food groups (table 28–1).
   b. Approximate proportion of foods containing primarily fermentable carbohydrate compared with proportion of protective foods.
2. Suggested procedure: use check sheet to mark daily portions of each food group (figure 28–3).
   a. Total for the week may be summarized for each category.
   b. Gross excesses and deficiencies can be identified readily.

. Fermentable Carbohydrate
1. Types of sugar-containing foods included.
2. Frequency of use
   a. Daily or occasionally.
   b. Number of between-meal snacks and how many of these include sweets.
3. Time of use.
4. Consistency of sugar-containing foods: related to probable length of time food might remain on the tooth surfaces.
5. Quantity: related to frequency more than size of individual serving (page 410).

6. Water taken at times when it could aid in rinsing sucrose from the tooth surfaces.
7. Underline in red on the food diary the foods which contain sugar, or during the counseling appointment ask the patient to underline them to help him learn more about the extent of his problem. The experience can be impressive to the patient, since people usually do not realize how many of the foods they are eating contain sucrose.

C. **Consistency of Diet: Detergent Foods**
1. Types of fibrous foods used: primarily uncooked, crisp, juicy fruits and vegetables.
2. Frequency of use: daily or occasionally.
3. Time of use
   a. During meal, end of meal, or between-meals.
   b. Relationship to providing cleansing mechanism for sugar contained in other foods.

D. **Analysis**
1. The patient can identify desirable and undesirable practices.
2. Compare findings with clinical findings and the patient's oral health problems.

PATIENT COUNSELING

I. **Preparation**

A. **Define Objectives**
1. To help the patient study his individual oral problems and understand the need for changing habits.
2. To explain specific changes in the diet necessary for improved general and oral health.
3. For dental caries control, to promote the elimination of sugar-containing foods, particularly those between meals, and the substitution of protective foods.

THE DAY'S FOOD DIARY

NAME__________

DAY______ DATE______

	AMOUNT		AMOUNT
BREAKFAST______ A.M. Finished______ A.M.		BETWEEN LUNCH AND DINNER______ P.M.	
BETWEEN BREAKFAST AND LUNCH______ A.M.		DINNER______ P.M. Finished______ P.M.	
LUNCH______ A.M. Finished______ P.M.		BETWEEN DINNER AND RETIRING______ P.M.	

Figure 28–1. Food diary: form used by patient to record daily diet. A booklet for a week's record is made by fastening seven of these forms together. The cover for the booklet is shown in Figure 28–2.

AGE_____ WEEK OF_____

SUMMARY

EXAMPLE OF HOW FOODS SHOULD BE LISTED

BREAKFAST 7:30 A.M.

Oatmeal	1 cup
with milk	½ cup
with brown sugar	2 teasp.
Milk	1-8 oz. glass
Toast - whole wheat bread	2 slices
with butter	generous
Egg - boiled	1
with butter	½ teasp.
Prunes - stewed -- with syrup	6 large

Finished 7:45 A.M.

BETWEEN BREAKFAST AND LUNCH 10:00 A.M.

Coffee	1 cup
with cream	1 teasp.
with sugar	2 teasp.
Water (around 11:00)	1 paper cup

Food eaten at lunch and dinner should be listed just as carefully as the breakfast shown above. If sandwiches are eaten, list the contents of the filling, such as egg, beef, lettuce, dressing.

Please show the approximate amounts of every kind of food that you ate. Do not mention any food that is served unless you ate it.

Please record all candy, cough drops, milk shakes, soft drinks, ice cream cones, popcorn, fruit (kinds), or cookies that you ate between meals. Also record vitamin concentrates or medicaments related to diet.

Figure 28-2. Food diary: cover page for patient's dietary record. Examples of how to list foods and indicate household measurements are provided on the left. The blank space on the right is for summary. The cover is fastened with seven copies of the form for recording a day's food diary as shown in Figure 28-1.

DIETARY ANALYSIS

Name____________________

Age_____ Date______________

FOOD GROUPS		Day 1	2	3	4	5	6	7	Daily Average	Recommended Daily Amounts	Ade-quate	Inade-quate
MILK GROUP	Milk									Child 2-4; Adol. 4+more; Adult 2+more		
	Milk Products											
MEAT GROUP	Meat, Fish Poultry									2 or more servings		
	Eggs									(Eggs: 3-5 per week)		
VEGETABLE	Yellow & Dark Green									4 or more servings		
	Other									including		
	Potato									1 yellow or dark green vegetable		
& FRUIT	Raw- Citrus									1 citrus fruit		
	Other											
	Cooked											
BREAD & CEREALS GROUP										4 or more servings		
SWEETS									Total	NOTES AND RECOMMENDATIONS		
Liquid	With Meal											
	End of Meal											
	Between Meal											
Soft (Sticky Retentive)	With Meal											
	End of Meal											
	Between Meal											
Hard (Sucked-Long-Lasting)	End of Meal											
	Between Meal											

Figure 28–3. Dietary analysis: form used with patient to summarize his diet. From the food diary kept by the patient (Figures 28–1 and 28–2)

B. Factors for Planning

1. Consider patient's willingness and ability to cooperate in relation to other demonstrations, such as conscientiousness in keeping appointments and following personal oral care procedures.
2. Identify problems which arise in presenting changes in the diet as they apply to this particular patient.
   a. Difficulty in change of any habit.
   b. Patient may feel dissatisfied without the foods to which he has been accustomed.
   c. Lack of appreciation of need for change because of limited knowledge concerning diet, nutrition, and their relationship to oral health.
   d. Common misconception that concentrated sugar is an indispensable source of energy.
   e. Degree of emphasis: dental disease does not kill anyone and nothing drastic is going to happen if minor deviations from the recommended diet occur.
   f. Social prejudices against coarse, raw, or unrefined foods.
   g. Cultural patterns.
   h. Financial considerations.
   i. Emotional disturbances which have led to or contributed to a craving for sweets.
   j. Parental attitude that removal of sweets from a child's diet would be depriving him of normal childhood pleasures.

C. Select Appropriate Teaching Aids

1. Patient's radiographs, charting, and food diary.
2. Diagrams, models, or charts applicable to material to be presented.
3. Instructive leaflets to illustrate patient's special dietary or oral health needs. (*Food for Fitness . . . A Daily Food Guide*[7] useful for discussion of basic food groups.)
4. Printed outline of diet plan with specific suggestions for food substitutes.
5. Printed list of snack suggestions.

D. Review

Review data and recommendations with dentist for additions and suggestions.

II. Conference Procedures

The conference should be held in a setting free from interruptions and distracting background sounds. Participants seated comfortably in a group will contribute to an atmosphere conducive to learning.

For the child patient, both parents should be encouraged to be present since both may supervise the child's eating and plaque control activities. For any age, it is particularly important for the person who plans and prepares the family meals to be present. To emphasize the importance of the conference and the concern of the entire dental group for the patient's problem, the dentist should participate by opening the conference and reviewing factors related to the treatment plan.

Some pointers for the success of the conference are the following:

A. Be prepared—on time.
B. Plan for only a few simple visual aids.
C. Encourage parents to exclude small children (other than patient) from the conference, as they create distraction.
D. Develop a permissive atmosphere.
E. Take care not to follow a written outline of recommendations so rigidly that the conference lacks informality.
F. Include all people present in the discussion.
G. Use a conversational tone of voice.
H. Make certain that all questions from patient or parent are discussed adequately.

I. Avoid note taking during the conference as much as possible.

III. Presentation

A. Review of Purposes

Extent of detail included depends on whether parents attending conference have already participated in previous appointments. A teen-age patient may have been coming for appointments unattended, hence the need for clear review for understanding of all details by the parents.

B. Examine the Patient's Food Diary and Summary

Discuss deficiencies and excesses, defining the role of the various food groups, fibrous foods, and carbohydrates in dental caries initiation or prevention.

To make major changes in food habits is difficult, if not traumatic, for any individual. Application of the knowledge of the principles of learning (page 386) and the skills of a counselor are essential. The attempt must be made to retain as many as possible of the patient's present food habits, and to make recommendations which can be adapted into the patient's pattern of living.

1. Discuss foods from each food group that are liked by the patient and can be added to the diet or substituted for less desirable foods used.
2. Guide the patient to select those items from his present diet which need changing, and to make suggestions for appropriate substitutes.

C. Follow-up

All teaching needs review and reinforcement. A single learning experience is rarely effective in producing lasting change. With each appointment and recall, continued efforts to help the patient can be made.

DIET CONTROL PROGRAM

For the caries-susceptible patient, control of the sucrose in the diet is essential. The plan for the patient is to make immediate changes which will remove all excess sucrose-containing foods, particularly those ordinarily consumed between meals, and to substitute foods from the four food groups. It is expected that the appetite will be satisfied, and cravings for sweet foods will diminish gradually over the first three weeks of the program so that the new eating pattern will continue indefinitely.

A suggested plan for presenting the problem and initiating discussion with the patient or parents to motivate interest in changing the diet is outlined below.

I. Dental Caries and Sucrose

It should be obvious that the patient cannot be told simply to "cut out the sweets in the diet." The meaning of "sweets" must be made clear, and specific suggestions provided for "cutting them out."

A. Define what is meant by a fermentable carbohydrate and use specific examples from the patient's dietary survey.

B. Discuss principles for understanding the role of sucrose in dental caries initiation.
1. Sugar on the tooth surface is changed to acid within five minutes.
2. Acid left undisturbed is not cleared from the mouth for one and one-half to two hours.
3. *Amount* of sugar consumed is not as important as *when* it is consumed; large amounts of sweet foods with a meal are not as detrimental as small amounts at intervals between meals.
4. Natural sugars are just as detrimen-

tal as refined ones (examples: maple syrup, honey).

5. *Significance of Length of Time Food Is Retained in the Mouth*
   a. Sugar in liquid form is retained in the mouth for less time than solid.
   b. Texture of the food which contains the sugar influences the length of time it will stay in the mouth (whether sticky or combined with a sticky substance).
   c. Vigorous rinsing after eating a concentrated sweet helps to remove it from the mouth.
   d. Sweet food taken before going to bed is not cleared readily from the mouth since salivary flow decreases during sleep.

II. Presentation of Specific Dietary Recommendations

The suggestions listed below represent basic principles to be applied. More specific recommendations should be added as they relate to the individual family. Directions must be simple and specific as the interpretation of many new ideas is difficult for the patient.

A. Incorporate foods from the basic groups to complete the patient's dietary. A diet high in protective foods frequently may imply a diet low in fermentable carbohydrate.

B. Limit the use of fermentable carbohydrates to mealtimes, paying particular attention to the final food used in the meal which may remain on the teeth if immediate toothbrushing is not possible.

C. Omit sweet foods even at mealtime when a very high dental caries rate is evident, and limit the diet to foods from the meat, milk, and vegetable-fruit groups (table 28-1). Selections from the bread and cereals groups

should be limited to dark bread and whole grain and enriched cereals.

D. Select between-meal snacks from protective noncariogenic foods such as unsweetened milk, fresh fruits, and raw vegetables.

E. Use as little concentrated sweet in the preparation of foods as possible, and observe care in the purchase of prepared foods. Examples: unsweetened fruit juice, dietetically prepared canned fruits, and sugar-free ice cream.

F. Eat well at mealtime to lessen desire for between-meal snacks. Protein and fat-containing foods digest more slowly and need to be included at each meal to prevent between-meal hunger.

G. Emphasize need for rigid adherence to the diet features: even occasional deviations can affect the results.

III. Summary

At the end of the teaching conference the entire study needs to be reviewed and the parts correlated into a meaningful program for the patient. Exactly how a particular patient (and/or parent) will learn to apply the principles of diet control of sugar which can influence the incidence of dental caries, cannot be predicted. Frequently a variety of teaching methods needs to be tried over a period of time.

Patient participation is very important. Using the patient's own food diary as a pattern, the patient provides suggested substitutes for foods containing sugar, particularly the retentive foods—those that will cling to the teeth. Substitutes selected from the basic food groups are needed, and as the patient makes the suggestions, they can be written down for the patient to take home for reference. When time permits it may be possible to compose a full week's diary of the foods known to be liked by the patient. Additional meal plan suggestions in printed form can be provided by the dental hygienist.

A snack list can also be discussed and prepared. When a snack list has been prepared and printed in advance, it must be discussed, and additions made at the patient's suggestion. If a patient responds with foods which are cariogenic, it may be evident that the principle has not been understood and further interpretation of which foods are to be avoided must be made.

DENTAL CARIES CONTROL STUDY

Patients who are subject to marked dental caries activity are a particular responsibility of the members of the dental profession. These patients, and their parents when the patient is a child, need special help in coping with the problem which, if left unattended, may well lead to an extensive and premature loss of teeth. To instigate a program of dental caries control requires thought, effort, and patience on the part of the dentist and dental hygienist in determining the method of approach.

A dental caries control study may be described as a planned effort to help the patient analyze the problem and initiate an effective preventive program. This educational effort includes in part much of the same information provided for all patients. In a caries control study, the instruction becomes more intensified as the patient is counseled to put into effect a specific program for diet and personal care.

To the pertinent information obtained through patient history, oral inspection, radiographic survey, charting, and other initial evaluation procedures, is added a study of the diet made through use of a week-long diary kept by the patient. A dental caries activity test may be used as

an instructional device to monitor the progress made.

A critical review of all information obtained leads to the preparation of a plan for the elimination of foods with high sucrose content, and for the limitation of all carbohydrates, in the attempt to curb the process of dental caries. Meticulous procedures for the patient's personal oral care are emphasized. Through dental health instruction the patient comes to learn the purposes of each step in the study and to accept responsibility in carrying out his part of the program of action.

The success of dental caries control measures is dependent on the patient's clear understanding and appreciation of the procedures, as well as his ability and willingness to cooperate. In turn, the dental hygienist applies knowledge of the physical and emotional problems at various age levels to try to understand and motivate the patient.

I. Patient Selection

The study can be proposed as a result of the initial diagnosis and treatment planning by the dentist, or preferably at a recall appointment when the patient has shown real concern for the problem and has demonstrated a cooperative attitude in having necessary restorations completed. Interest in participation in a study can and should be developed in patients who need help.

A patient of any age who has dental caries activity can benefit from the study. A number of factors are involved to determine the probability of success.

A. Acceptance of Responsibility
1. Dentist and dental hygienist: must sincerely demonstrate their desire for better oral health for the patient.
2. Patient
   a. Young children: parents bear weight of responsibility.
   b. Intermediate children: child

will have certain responsibilities along with the parents.

  c. Teen-agers: patient will have responsibility, but parent cooperation is essential, particularly in relation to food preparation.

  d. Adult: has own responsibility, but family cooperation will contribute.

B. Patient Evaluation

    It is difficult to determine whether interest and enthusiasm evidenced at the beginning will carry on throughout a study. Continued acceptance and enthusiasm of dental personnel contribute much to patient motivation.

II. Preparation for the Study

A. Review physical and emotional characteristics of the patient's age group.

B. Plan the approach to the patient in accord with the appraisal of his individual characteristics.

C. Outline objectives for the patient in terms of his basic oral health needs.

APPOINTMENT PLANNING

    There is no standard or uniform procedure which can be applied for all patients. A number of factors will enter into the determination of the number and length of appointments, particularly the patient's capacity for learning. Overcrowded, hurried appointments with too much material presented at one time will make it difficult for the patient to absorb the material and follow instructions.

    A series of appointments permits time to review and to encourage the patient to ask questions. A suggested procedure is presented here.

I. First Appointment

A. Explanation of Procedures

    The final outcome frequently depends on the preliminary understanding by the patient of the objectives and expected effects. A well-informed patient is more cooperative and appreciative. At the outset at least the four factors listed below should be described, discussed, and clarified by encouraging patient (and parent) questions.

  1. Purposes and general objectives in terms of better oral health and the social and economic advantages.

  2. An outline of the procedures involved.

  3. Description of the time involved and suggestions concerning appointment planning.

  4. Need for mutual cooperation.

B. Obtain Saliva Sample for Dental Caries Activity Test (Tests are described on pages 416–417).

C. Explain and Record Indices To Be Used: Gingival Index (GI) and Plaque Index (Pl I) are described on pages 275–280.

D. Take Plaque Sample when a plaque pH test[8] or Methyl-Red-Plaque-Sugar test (page 417) is used.

E. Introduce Plaque Control Procedures.

  1. Follow *First Lesson* as described on page 388.

  2. Omit reference to diet control for dental caries so the patient will be unprejudiced while preparing the food diary.

F. Introduce the Food Diary (page 402).

G. Make Impressions for Study Casts if the use of custom-trays for daily application of fluoride is to be recommended.

H. Following Dismissal of Patient

    Enter material for case history record in the patient's permanent record (page 414). Following each appointment, additions are made.

II. Second Appointment

A. **Receive and Review the Food Diary**
   Discuss the entries and record additional information where needed (page 404).

B. **Patient Counseling**
   1. Follow Summary and Analysis Procedures, page 405.
   2. Guide patient to complete the analysis form, figure 28–3.
   3. Explain dental caries and the diet control program (page 410). Tie in the results of the caries tests made at the previous appointment.
   4. Assist patient in preparing suggestions for the new diet that must be followed.

C. **Continue Plaque Control Instruction**
   1. Follow *Second Lesson* as described on page 390.
   2. Relate plaque control with diet procedures previously described.

D. **Describe and Give Instructions for Self-Applied Fluoride:** dentifrice and mouthrinse or custom-tray.

E. **Following Dismissal of Patient**
   1. Make entries in the case history.
   2. Discuss case with the dentist.
   3. Telephone patient in three or four days to give encouragement and to clarify questions about the expected procedures.

III. Third Appointment

A. **Make Inquiries**
   Inquire concerning all procedures, particularly the sugar-control diet. Commend and encourage. Provide informal question–references to the instruction given to determine any misconceptions.

B. **Continue Plaque Control Instruction**
   1. Follow *Third Lesson*, page 391.
   2. Explain the relation of professional treatment to plaque control and diet control.

C. **Scaling.** The extent of the calculus and the depth of the pockets will determine the time needed. When there is extensive scaling to be done by quadrants and under anesthesia, four appointments are planned, each to be preceded by an evaluation of gingiva, plaque, bleeding, and, as needed, demonstration of toothbrushing, flossing, or other aids. As the condition of the gingival tissue continues to improve, other parts of the treatment plan are undertaken.

IV. Fourth Appointment (three to four weeks after start of special diet)

A. **Obtain saliva sample for caries activity test.** In a mouth with many large carious lesions, this is not done until restorative dentistry has been initiated and, in some instances, completed. Since there are many acid-forming organisms held within a carious lesion, a positive response can always be expected when the lesions are present.

B. **Evaluation of Personal Care Procedures**
   Gingival tissue, plaque, and toothbrushing (page 392).

C. **Give Encouragement**
   Encourage continuation of sugar-control diet and personal oral care measures.

D. **Plan the Recall in Three to Four Months**

E. **Following the Appointment**
   Telephone to tell patient results of the dental caries activity test.

CASE HISTORY RECORD

The written history of the dental caries control study relates and integrates the events which have occurred with observations made during the study. Interpretation of the facts should be done as objectively as possible.

The case history becomes a part of the patient's permanent record. Careful and complete recording is important in order that the text of the report will be meaningful and clear for follow-up reference.

I. General Instructions

A. Date Each Recorded Entry

B. Record Events As Soon As Possible After They Occur

1. Make brief notes during the appointments as an aid to writing the case history. Note taking should be done inconspicuously so it does not distract the patient.
2. Record in the history all contacts with the patient during the study, including telephone conversations.
3. Include specific quotes from conversations if they reflect attitudes, habits, or acquired knowledge.

II. Observations of Patient's Personality and Development

The study provides an excellent opportunity to gain insight into the personality and development of the patient. Knowledge acquired can greatly augment understanding of the young patient and the parental influences. Suggested questions for consideration while making observations are listed below.

A. Observing Intellectual Development

1. Is patient's vocabulary average, below average, or above average for his age? Quote sample sentences in the patient's record.
2. Does he understand what is told him when words that he should understand are used? How does he show this?
3. Does he show intellectual curiosity about the techniques and services which are performed for him? What questions does he ask?
4. What does he tell about his success in school?

B. Observing Physical Development

1. Does anything in the patient's medical history indicate abnormal physical development?
2. Is he apparently of normal height and weight for his age, structure, and heredity?
3. Is his coordination good? Does he learn to brush his teeth readily as might be expected for his age group?
4. Does he have enough hours of sleep and rest?

C. Observing Emotional Development

1. What is the patient's reaction to his parents' authority? To the authority of the dentist or dental hygienist when no parent is present? Is he at ease, apprehensive, obedient, or submissive? How does he show this?
2. What does he say about his family?
3. Does he express affection toward his parents? How?
4. What fears, if any, does he exhibit?
5. Does he show indications of self-discipline? Does his parent indicate that he brushes his teeth without being told? Did he help to complete the dietary survey? Does he accept the services done for him with a pleasant and cooperative attitude?

DENTAL CARIES ACTIVITY TESTS

A dental caries activity test may be used as an instructional and motivational aid to guide the patient toward practicing habits conducive to the prevention of dental caries. The use of test results for a visual aid can be helpful since changes in results of a series of tests can show dramatically the effects of the patient's personal efforts in carrying out dietary and oral care preventive procedures.

A caries activity test is used to monitor the progress of diet therapy; therefore, it is important that plaque control and various treatment procedures be done. The acid-forming organisms will be present in carious lesions, and only a very drastic, rigid, sucrose-free diet will make a difference in a successive caries activity test. Control of dental caries by diet should follow and supplement plaque control procedures and the restoration of carious lesions.[9]

Caries activity tests provide information about the current oral environment. The tests are not "susceptibility" tests to predict what may occur at some future time. Various types of tests have been devised to detect dental caries activity. Evaluation is made by counting the numbers of acid-forming bacteria or determining the acid produced or other specialized activity of the microorganisms.

Studies of the oral bacteria show that they are not distributed evenly. Microorganisms in the dental plaque on tooth surfaces contribute very little to the pool of bacteria obtained when a saliva sample is collected. A large part of the organisms in the saliva are from the tongue. Such findings provide at least a partial explanation for the inconsistencies of dental caries activity tests.

I. Snyder Colorimetric Test[10]

The Snyder Test Agar contains the indicator brom-cresol-green and is adjusted to a pH of 5.0. Acid formation by bacteria from the saliva sample added to the medium lowers the pH. At the lowered pH, the brom-cresol-green changes from green to yellow. It is the rapidity of color change that indicates the caries activity at that time.

A. Obtain Saliva Sample

The patient chews a piece of paraffin for three minutes and expectorates into a sterile bottle.

B. Laboratory Procedures

1. Place tube of Snyder Test Agar in boiling water until agar melts; cool until it can be held comfortably against the cheek.
2. Shake the saliva sample well to distribute bacteria, and pipette 0.2 ml. into the agar. Mix by gentle rotation.
3. Allow to solidify and incubate at 37° C.
4. Examine daily for three days and record changes in color compared with uninoculated control. Hold tubes against a white background when making observations.

C. Interpretation of Results

The rate of color change from green to yellow is related to the degree of caries activity. In the process of changing color the agar will appear light green, then greenish-yellow, and finally appear a definite yellow.

No change in color indicates little or no caries activity whereas a prompt change to yellow within 24 hours indicates marked acid formation or caries activity. The significance of the color changes is summarized in table 28–2.

II. Modified Snyder Test[11]

A miniature version of the standard Snyder test has been used which is simpler, less expensive, and occupies less space, particularly during incubation.

Table 28–2.   Color Changes in the Snyder Test

Color of Snyder Test Agar after Incubation			Suggested Degree of Caries Susceptibility
24 hours	48 hours	72 hours	
Green	Green	Green	Little or none
Green	Light green	Yellow	Slight
Green	Yellow		Moderate
Yellow			Marked or rampant

A. **Obtain Saliva Sample** (I.A above)

B. **Laboratory Procedures**
1. Shake specimen of saliva and use wire loop (flamed for sterility) to withdraw saliva (loop holds about .0113 ml.). Stab loop into the agar for inoculation.
2. Culture medium: Snyder test agar with the concentration of bromcresol-green increased to facilitate the observation of the color change in the small amount of agar (0.2 ml.).
3. Incubate at 37° C. for 24, 48, and 72 hours.
4. Examine daily.

C. **Interpretation of Results**
See table 28–2. The results are easier to read than the standard Snyder because the whole of the small amount of agar changes color.

III. Swab Test[12]

The Swab test is also a modified Snyder test. Time is saved in that a saliva sample is not obtained, and the test results are evaluated after 48 hours.

A. **Obtain Sample**
Stroke the buccal gingival areas of the teeth in each of the four quadrants with a sterile cotton applicator.

B. **Laboratory Procedures**
1. Remove cap from a vial of the special medium, insert the applicator to the bottom, and rotate it about five times. Raise the applicator and break off the stick against the lip of the vial, let it drop down, and replace the cap firmly.
2. Incubate at 37° C. for 48 hours.
3. Make pH reading by a color comparator or electric pH meter.

C. **Interpretation of Results**
1. Color comparator: the bromcresol-green changes from green to yellow as the pH declines.
2. Measurement and significance of pH (meter method)

Rampant:	pH below 4.1
Active:	pH 4.2 to 4.4
Slightly active:	pH 4.5 to 4.6
Inactive:	pH over 4.6

IV. Salivary Reductase Test[13]

This test measures the activity of the reductase enzyme present in salivary bacteria.

A. **Obtain Saliva Sample** (I.A. above)

B. **Laboratory Procedures**
1. Saliva sample is mixed with the dye diazoresorcinol (Resazurin Reagent) and allowed to stand 15 minutes.
2. The color changes as the dye is reduced, and the caries conduciveness is interpreted after fifteen minutes at room temperature.

C. **Interpretation of Results**
See table 28–3.

V. Methyl Red-Plaque-Sugar Test[14]

This test is also known as the Spot Plate Colorimetric Test. A dramatic change in the color of the methyl red from yellow to red occurs as the pH changes from about 6.3 to 4.2. Lowering of the pH is accomplished by the acid-producing bacteria in the plaque acting on sucrose.

A. **Obtain Plaque Sample**
With a curet, scrape plaque from the distobuccal of maxillary molars, lingual of mandibular molars, or other surfaces with thick plaque. Collect

Table 28-3. Color Changes in the Salivary Reductase Test

Color	Caries Conduciveness
Blue in 15 minutes	Nonconducive
Orchid in 15 minutes	Slightly conducive
Red in 15 minutes	Moderately conducive
Red immediately on mixing	Highly conducive
Colorless in 15 minutes	Extremely conducive

enough plaque to cover the working end of the curet.

B. **Test Procedure**
1. Arrange the plaque sample in a small circle (about one-fourth inch diameter) on a white porcelain tile.
2. Cover with two to three drops of methyl red indicator. Sprinkle a few crystals of sugar (sucrose) into the center of the circle. A second method for accomplishing the same result is to use a two percent sucrose sodium salt methyl red solution. Explain to the patient that it contains sucrose.
3. Wait 10 to 30 minutes for the color change.

C. **Interpretation**
1. The following criteria for scoring the color change may be used. The amount of red present determines the degree of acid production.
   0 = Yellow
   +1 = Yellow with a small red circle
   +2 = Yellow with a red circle one-half of the area
   +3 = Yellow with a red circle covering all but the edges
   +2 and +3 indicate the presence of a significant number of plaque bacteria that are acid producing
2. Record results in patient's record.

EVALUATION OF PROGRESS

The success of the dental caries control study is dependent upon learning by the patient. Learning implies a change of behavior and progress toward goals which are clearly understood by the learner.

I. Immediate Evaluation

A. A lowered caries activity test result at the end of the three to four-week test period of restricted diet may indicate success to that date.

B. The patient's expressed interest and demonstration of cooperation in the caries control program indicate that at least temporarily the patient is motivated.

II. Overall Evaluation

A. Consistent reduction in dental caries rate in the years following the study shows sustained change in habits.

B. Patient's and parents' attitudes toward maintaining adequate oral health habits of personal care, diet containing minimum fermentable carbohydrate, and routine professional dental care indicate application of learning.

RECALL

I. Three Months' Follow-up

A. Obtain saliva sample for caries activity test.

B. Request patient to keep a five- to seven-day food diary for analysis and evaluation.

C. Review plaque control procedures and provide suggestions as needed.

D. Recommend return to restricted carbohydrate diet when indicated.

II. Six Months' Recall

A. Obtain saliva sample for caries activity test.

B. Inspection and clinical procedures
1. Scaling when needed.
2. Topical application of fluoride depending on self-applied fluoride program.
3. Charting.

C. Compare dental caries incidence with previous chartings and completed restorative dentistry.

D. Make dietary recommendations in accord with results from the test.

References

1. Glickman, I.: *Clinical Periodontology*, 4th ed. Philadelphia, Saunders, 1972, pp. 103, 365–382.

2. American Dental Association, Council on Dental Therapeutics: *Accepted Dental Therapeutics*, 36th ed. Chicago, American Dental Association, 1975, pp. 88–92.
3. Arnim, S. S.: The Use of Disclosing Agents for Measuring Tooth Cleanliness, *J. Periodont.*, 34, 227, May, 1963.
4. Lindhe, J. and Wicén, P-O.: The Effects on the Gingivae of Chewing Fibrous Foods, *J. Periodont. Res.*, 4, 193, No. 3, 1969.
5. McCarthy, P. L. and Shklar, G.: *Diseases of the Oral Mucosa.* New York, Blakiston Division, McGraw-Hill, 1964, pp. 236–245.
6. National Research Council, Food and Nutrition Board: *Recommended Dietary Allowances*, 8th ed. Washington, D.C., National Academy of Science, 1974, p. 129.
7. United States Department of Agriculture, Agricultural Research Service: *Food for Fitness . . . A Daily Food Guide.* Leaflet No. 424, Revised 1971. Superintendent of Documents, U.S. Government Printing Office, Washington, D.C. 20402.
8. Katz, S., McDonald, J. L., and Stookey, G. K.: *Preventive Dentistry in Action.* Upper Montclair, N.J., D. C. P. Publishing, 1972, pp. 65–69.
9. Sims, W.: The Interpretation and Use of Snyder Tests and Lactobacillus Counts, *J. Am. Dent. Assoc.*, 80, 1315, June, 1970.
10. Snyder, M. L.: A Simple Colorimetric Method for the Estimation of Relative Numbers of Lactobacilli in the Saliva, *J. Dent. Res.*, 19, 349, August, 1940.
11. Sims, W.: A Modified Snyder Test for Caries-activity in Humans, *Arch. Oral Biol.*, 13, 853, August, 1968.
12. Grainger, R. M., Jarrett, M., and Honey, S. L.: Swab Test for Dental Caries Activity: An Epidemiological Study, *J. Can. Dent. Assoc.*, 31, 515, August, 1965.
13. Rapp, G. W.: Fifteen Minute Caries Test, *Ill. Dent. J.*, 31, 290, May, 1962.
14. Arnim, S. S. and Sweet, A. P.: Acid Production by Mouth Organisms. Use of Aqueous Methyl Red for Patient Education, *Dent. Radiogr. Photogr.*, 29, 1, No. 1, 1956.

Suggested Readings

Bibby, B. G.: The Cariogenicity of Snack Foods and Confections, *J. Am. Dent. Assoc.*, 90, 121, January, 1975.
Brook, M.: Sugar Substitutes and Their Significance for Dental Health, *Dent. Health*, 9, 46, July-September, 1970.
Enwonwu, C. O.: Role of Biochemistry and Nutrition in Preventive Dentistry, *J. Am. Soc. Prev. Dent.*, 4, 6, September-October, 1974.
McBean, L. D. and Speckmann, E. W.: A Review: The Importance of Nutrition in Oral Health, *J. Am. Dent. Assoc.*, 89, 109, July, 1974.
McDonald, J. L.: Surprising but True: Nutrition and the Dental Hygienist, *J. Am. Dent. Hyg. Assoc.*, 45, 176, May-June, 1971.
Newbrun, E.: The Role of Food Manufacturers in the Dietary Control of Caries, *J. Am. Soc. Prev. Dent.*, 4, 33, September-October, 1974.
Nikiforuk, G.: Posteruptive Effects of Nutrition on Teeth, *J. Dent. Res.*, 49, 1252, November-December, 1970.
Palmer, C. A.: The Human Touch in the Dental Office, *Dent. Assist.*, 44, 28, March, 1975.
Parfitt, G. J. and Speirs, D. M.: Role of Nutrition in the Prevention and Treatment of Periodontal Disease, *J. Can. Dent. Assoc.*, 36, 224, June, 1970.
Randolph, P.: The Continuing Vitamin C Controversy, *J. Prev. Dent.*, 2, 18, May-June, 1975.
Shannon, I. L. and Edmonds, E. J.: Dietary Sucrose: Dental Dilemma, *Dent. Hyg.*, 49, 257, June, 1975.
Shaw, J. H.: Preeruptive Effects of Nutrition on Teeth, *J. Dent. Res.*, 49, 1238, November-December, 1970.
Volker, J. F. and Caldwell, R. C.: Food and Dental Caries, in Finn, S. B.: *Clinical Pedodontics*, 4th ed. Philadelphia, Saunders, 1972, pp. 518–536.
Weiss, R. L. and Trithart, A. H.: Between-meal Eating Habits and Dental Caries Experience in Preschool Children, *Am. J. Public Health*, 50, 1097, August, 1960.

Diet Counseling

Alban, A. L.: Dental Office Nutrition Counseling, *J. Am. Soc. Prev. Dent.*, 5, 27, May-June, 1975.
DiOrio, L. P. and Madsen, K. O.: *Educating the Patient in Prevention of Dental Diseases.* Chicago, March Publishing, 1972, pp. 13–57.
Holloway, P. J., Booth, E. M., and Wragg, K. A.: Dietary Counseling in the Control of Dental Caries, *Br. Dent. J.*, 126, 161, February 18, 1969.
Katz, S., McDonald, J. L., and Stookey, G. K.: *Preventive Dentistry in Action.* Upper Montclair, N. J., D. C. P. Publishing, 1972, pp. 241–267.
Nizel, A. E.: *Nutrition in Preventive Dentistry: Science and Practice.* Philadelphia, Saunders, 1972, pp. 356–426.
Nizel, A. E.: Where Are We? Where Are We Going? The Practice of Nutrition in Dental Caries Prevention, *J. Am. Soc. Prev. Dent.*, 5, 32, January-February, 1975.
Owens, B. A.: Nutritional Counseling in the Dental Office, *Dent. Hyg.*, 48, 288, September-October, 1974.
Palmer, C.: The Art of Communication and Counseling, in Nizel, A. E.: *Nutrition in Preventive Dentistry: Science and Practice.* Philadelphia, Saunders, 1972, pp. 343–355.
Strieff, M., Seglins, B., Marshall, G., Finstad, S., and Borgendale, G.: The Caries Control Study, *J. Am. Dent. Hyg. Assoc.*, 29, 143, October, 1955.

Detergent Foods

Birkeland, J. M. and Jorkjend, L.: The Effect of Chewing Apples on Dental Plaque and Food Debris, *Community Dent. Oral Epidemiol.*, 2, 161, No. 4, 1974.
Longhurst, P.: Apples and Gingival Health, *Br. Dent. J.*, 134, 475, June 5, 1973.
Reece, J. A. and Swallow, J. N.: Carrots and Dental Health, *Br. Dent. J.*, 128, 535, June 2, 1970.

Wade, A. B.: Effect on Dental Plaque of Chewing Apples, *Dent. Pract. Dent. Rec., 21,* 194, February, 1971.

Caries Activity Tests

Alban, A.: An Improved Snyder Test, *J. Dent. Res., 49,* 641, May-June, 1970.

Bowen, W. H.: Caries Activity Tests, *Int. Dent. J., 19,* 267, June, 1969.

Shory, N. L.: Comprehensive Field Evaluation of the Treatex Test, *J. Am. Dent. Assoc., 72,* 899, April, 1966.

Stolpe, J. R.: Chemical and Bacteriological Tests for Determining Susceptibility to, and Activity of Dental Caries: A Review, *J. Public Health Dent., 30,* 141, Summer, 1970.

Adolescents

Baer, P. N. and Benjamin, S. D.: *Periodontal Disease in Children and Adolescents.* Philadelphia, Lippincott, 1974, pp. 271–286.

Huenemann, R. L., Shapiro, L. R., Hampton, M. C. and Mitchell, B. W.: Food and Eating Practices of Teen-agers, *J. Am. Diet. Assoc., 53,* 17, July, 1968.

Mickelsen, O.: Adolescent Nutrition, *J. Periodont., 42,* 460, August, 1971.

Nizel, A. E. and Shulman, J. S.: The Science and Art of Inhibiting Caries in Adolescents Via Personalized Nutritional Counseling, *Dent. Clin North Am., 13,* 387, April, 1969.

Edentulous Patients

Hartsook, E. I.: Food Selection, Dietary Adequacy and Related Dental Problems of Patients with Dental Prostheses, *J. Prosthet. Dent., 32,* 32, July, 1974.

Nizel, A. E.: *Nutrition in Preventive Dentistry: Science and Practice.* Philadelphia, Saunders, 1972, pp. 456–459 (Denture patient).

Ramsey, W. O.: The Role of Nutrition in Conditioning Edentulous Patients, *J. Prosthet. Dent., 23,* 130, February, 1970.

Chapter 29

Fluorides

The use of fluorides in preventive dental care is based on the knowledge that when the fluoride content of the teeth, particularly of the surface enamel, is increased to an optimum level, there is marked resistance to dental caries. Fluoride is a mineral nutrient essential to the formation of sound teeth and bones, just as are calcium, phosphorus, and other minerals obtained from food and water.

Fluoride is made available to the tooth structure by two general means: *systemically* by way of the circulation to developing teeth, and *topically*, directly to the exposed surfaces of erupted teeth. Fluoride as a systemic nutrient is available from the community drinking water, either naturally or by fluoridation, or from prescribed dietary supplements.

Fluoride can be made available for uptake at the surface of the erupted tooth by professional applications of fluoride solutions or gels, as well as by self-application including mouthrinses, chewable tablets, and dentifrices. Fluoride is also taken up at the tooth surface from the drinking water as it passes over the teeth.

Fluorides have had a significant impact on clinical practice of dentistry and dental hygiene. With less dental caries, fewer extractions, and more complete dental service possible for more patients, increased emphasis can be placed on preventive care.

FLUORIDE ACTION

There are two basic factors believed responsible for the remarkable action of fluoride against dental caries. These are related to the amount of fluoride contained in the surface of the tooth and the antibacterial or enzyme-inhibiting effects of the fluoride within dental plaque.

I. Fluoride and Tooth Development[1]

Resistance to dental caries is proportional to the amount of fluoride in the tooth surface present as fluorapatite. The teeth can acquire fluoride during three periods: during the *calcification stage* of tooth development, *after calcification* and before eruption, and *after eruption*. At this point of study, a review of the histology of tooth development and calcification can be helpful to supplement the information included here.[2,3]

421

A. **Pre-eruptive: Calcification Stage**
1. Fluoride is deposited during the formation of the enamel crystals, starting at the dentinoenamel junction after the enamel matrix is laid down by the ameloblasts (figure 29–1 A).
2. Fluoride is incorporated as fluorapatite during calcification.
3. Fluoride is available to the developing teeth by way of the blood stream to the tissues surrounding the tooth buds.
4. Source of fluoride: drinking water and other ingested fluoride such as from tablets or drops.
5. During calcification, when there is excess fluoride, the normal activity of the ameloblasts may be inhibited and a defective enamel matrix can form. This is the fundamental mechanism of dental fluorosis.

B. **Pre-eruptive: Maturation Stage**
1. After calcification is complete and before eruption, fluoride deposition continues in the surface of the enamel (figure 29–1 B).
2. Fluoride is taken up from the nutrient tissue fluids surrounding the tooth crown. Much more fluoride is acquired by the outer surface during this period than in the underlying layers of enamel during calcification. Children who are exposed to fluoride for the first time within the two years prior to eruption benefit from fluoride acquired during this pre-eruptive stage.

C. **Posteruptive**
1. After eruption and throughout the life span of the teeth, fluoride is taken up from the drinking water, food, and saliva (figure 29–2).
2. Uptake is rapid on the enamel surface during the first years after eruption and is greater at high than

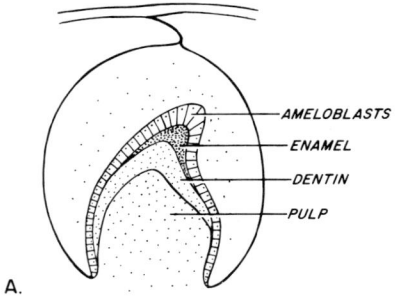

A.

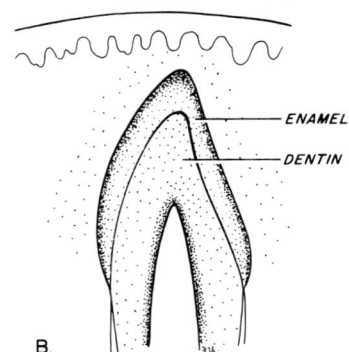

B.

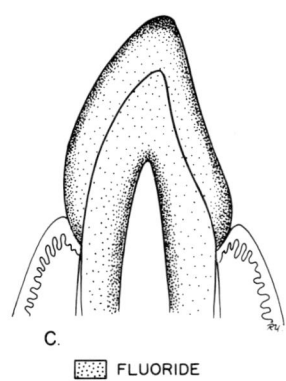

C.

▓ FLUORIDE

Figure 29–1. Systemic fluoride. Dots represent fluoride ions in the tissues and distribution throughout the tooth. **A.** Developing tooth during calcification to show fluoride from drinking water and other systemic sources deposited throughout the enamel and dentin. **B.** Maturation stage prior to eruption when fluoride is taken up from the tissue fluids surrounding the crown. **C.** Erupted tooth continues to take up fluoride on the surface from external sources. Note that the fluoride deposition is concentrated on the surface of the enamel and on the pulpal surface of the dentin.

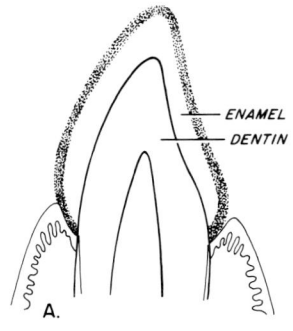

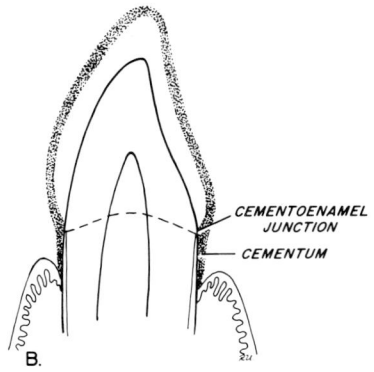

Figure 29–2. Fluoride acquisition after eruption without the benefit of systemic fluoride during tooth development. **A.** Fluoride on surface taken up from topical application, chewable tablets, mouthwash, and other external sources. **B.** When there is recession, exposed cementum benefits by acquiring surface fluoride to aid in the prevention of root caries and sensitivity.

at low levels of fluoride in the drinking water.

3. Fluoride concentration decreases from the enamel surface to the dentinoenamel junction. The fluoride concentration then increases from the dentinoenamel junction to the pulpal surface where fluoride can still be added from the systemic source.

II. Tooth Surface Fluoride

A. Fluoride associated with caries prevention is deposited in the enamel, dentin, cementum, and bone as fluorapatite.

B. The unit crystal is hydroxyapatite. The fluoride ions substitute for the hydroxy radical and fluorapatite is formed. Fluoride is confined to the surface of the crystals.

C. Uptake of fluoride depends on the amount of fluoride ingested and the length of time of exposure.

D. Amount of fluoride in the enamel surface: extracted teeth have been analyzed from people who had used water with fluoride all their lives. The parts per million (ppm) fluoride in the enamel are shown by the following:[4]

Fluoride in Water	Fluoride in Enamel	
	Under Age 20	Over Age 50
0.1 ppm	500 ppm	1200 ppm
1.0 ppm	900 ppm	1500 ppm
3.0 ppm	1900 ppm	2300 ppm

Fluoride is a natural constituent of enamel; even at minimal fluoride exposure (0.1 ppm) there is 500 to 1200 ppm fluoride in the enamel.

E. Decalcified white areas. When fluoride is applied to the surface, it diffuses deeper into decalcified areas than on intact enamel. The caries process is slowed because the fluoride encourages remineralization.

III. Topical Agents

A. Effectiveness of topical agents depends on their ability to deposit fluoride as fluorapatite in the tooth surface.[5]

B. Reaction to application: calcium fluoride and fluorapatite are formed on the tooth surface immediately after application. Calcium fluoride and any unused fluoride which did not react during the application are gradually leached away, but fluorapatite remains. The loss of fluoride may occur over several days.[5] These factors explain why the patient should be instructed not to rinse, eat or brush for as long as possible after an application and why chewable tablets should be used just before going to bed, after brushing.

C. The most fluoride is taken up from topical preparations applied soon after eruption.

IV. Plaque Fluoride

A. Dental plaque contains variable concentrations of fluoride which are related to the amount of fluoride in the drinking water and the use of fluoride dentifrice and mouthrinse (page 240).[6]

B. Less than five percent of the fluoride in plaque is in a free form (ions) and it is believed that most of the plaque fluoride is bound within the cells of plaque bacteria.[7]

C. Antibacterial effects of fluoride probably relate to inhibition of enzymes involved in the acid production which is part of the process of dental caries initiation (pages 243–244).

FLUORIDATION

Fluoridation is the adjustment of the fluoride ion content of a domestic water supply to the optimum physiologic concentration which will provide maximum protection against dental caries and enhance the appearance of the teeth with a minimum possibility of producing objectionable enamel fluorosis.[8] Fluoridation has been established as the most efficient, effective, reliable, and inexpensive means for improving oral health.

I. Historical Aspects[9,10]

A. **Mottled Enamel and Dental Caries**
    Early in this century Dr. Frederick S. McKay began his extensive studies to find the cause of "brown stain" which later was called mottled enamel, and now is known as dental fluorosis. He observed that people with mottled enamel had much less

dental caries.[11] He associated the condition with the drinking water, but tests were inconclusive until 1931 when Churchill pinpointed fluorine as the specific element related to the tooth changes.[12]

B. **Background for Fluoridation**
    Epidemiological studies of the 1930s sponsored by the United States Public Health Service and directed by Dr. H. Trendley Dean led to the conclusion that the level of fluoride in the water optimum for dental caries prevention is one ppm. Clinically objectionable dental fluorosis is associated with levels well over two ppm.[13]
    From this knowledge and the fact that many healthy people had lived long lives in communities where the fluoride content of the water was much greater than one ppm, the concept of adding fluoride to the water developed. It was still necessary, however, to show that the benefits from controlled fluoridation could parallel those of natural fluoride.

C. **Fluoridation—1945**
    The first communities were fluoridated in 1945. Research in the communities began before fluoridation was started to obtain base-line information, and continued over the years with detailed examinations and reports in the following communities and their scientific controls:

Fluoridation	Control City
Grand Rapids, Michigan (January, 1945)	Muskegon, Michigan
Newburgh, New York (May, 1945)	Kingston, New York
Brantford, Ontario (June, 1945)	Sarnia, Ontario
Evanston, Illinois (February, 1947)	Oak Park, Illinois

Aurora, Illinois, where the natural fluoride level is optimum (1.2 ppm), was used to compare the benefits of natural fluoride in the water supply with those of fluoridation, as well as with a fluoride-free city, Rockford, Illinois.

The research conducted in the above cities, as well as other research throughout the world, has documented the influence of fluoride on oral health. The effects and benefits itemized below summarize important features of fluoridation; examples of research findings are given for illustration.

II. Fluoride Level

One part per million is considered the optimum fluoride level for water in temperate climates. For warmer and colder climates the amount can be adjusted from approximately 0.6 ppm to 1.2 ppm, adapted in accord with the amount of water consumed.[8]

In the United States, close to 9,000,000 people live in communities where natural fluoride occurs in the drinking water at 0.7 ppm or more,[14] a level which is sufficient to prevent dental caries. In approximately 400 communities the amount of fluoride is more than twice optimum level.

III. Effects and Benefits

A. Appearance of Teeth[15,16]

Teeth exposed to an optimum or slightly higher level of fluoride frequently are clear white, shining, opaque, and without blemishes. When there is slightly more than optimum level for the individual, there may be white areas, such as bands or flecks, which can be seen professionally by drying the teeth and observing under a dental light. Without such close scrutiny, such spots may blend with the beauty of the overall appearance. Dental fluorosis associated with higher than optimum fluoride levels has been classified on page 264.

B. Dental Caries: Permanent Teeth

Continuous use of fluoridated water from birth results in an average of 60 to 70 percent fewer carious lesions. The effects are similar to those found in communities with optimum level natural fluoride in the water. Many more individuals are caries-free when there is fluoride in the water.

1. *Distribution.* Anterior teeth, particularly maxillary, have more protection from fluoride than posterior.[13] The anterior teeth are contacted by the drinking water as it passes into the mouth and fluoride is added to the enamel after eruption.

2. *Posteruption.* Although maximum benefits are derived when fluoridated water is consumed through the entire pre-eruptive period, there are also significant benefits to teeth which have erupted prior to exposure to fluoride.[17,18,19]

3. *Progression.* Not only are there fewer carious lesions, but the rate of decay is slowed. Caries progression is also reduced in the surfaces which receive fluoride for the first time after eruption.[20]

C. Dental Caries: Primary Teeth

With fluoridation from birth, there is reduced caries incidence in the primary teeth up to 50 percent.[17] For example, the children ages six to nine in Newburgh had five times as many primary canines and molars present and caries-free as the children of Kingston where there was no fluoride.[21]

D. Prenatal Fluoride

There has been no clear clinical evidence that prenatal fluoride ingestion (from drinking water or prescription) by the mother has an effect on the calcification of the baby's primary teeth.[22,23,24] A major portion of the calcification of primary teeth takes place after birth: the crowns of primary incisors are not fully completed until approximately three months, canines at nine months, and second molars at eleven months, average. The outermost layers of the enamel are formed last, so that fluoride ingested after birth has the most influence on the primary teeth.

E. **Tooth Loss**

Both primary and permanent tooth loss is much greater in teeth without fluoride[21] because of increased dental caries which progresses more rapidly.

F. **Malocclusion**

With fewer extractions, particularly less premature loss of primary molars, there is less malocclusion from local causes.[25]

G. **Adults**

When a person resides in a fluoride area throughout life, benefits continue. Examinations of Colorado Springs adults ages 20 to 44 who had used water with natural fluoride, showed 60 percent less caries experience than adults in fluoride-deficient Boulder. In Boulder, adults also had had three to four times as many permanent teeth extracted.[26] In a survey of adults in Rockford, Illinois (no fluoride), there were about seven times as many edentulous persons as there were in a comparable group in Aurora (natural fluoride).[27]

H. **Bone**

There is evidence that fluoride is important to the maintenance of normal bone and the improvement of calcium metabolism. Studies have shown that there are fewer bone fractures, and when they occur they heal more quickly; less osteoporosis, especially in women, and less calcification of the aorta, especially in men, when there is increased exposure to fluoride in the water over the

years.[28,29,30] Fluoride has been used to improve the bone in the treatment of osteoporosis.[31]

I. **Periodontal Diseases**

Favorable effects of fluoride previously mentioned have indirect effects on periodontal health. Improved bone density resulting from fluoride can affect the alveolar bone along with all bones and may have an effect on bone resorption and resistance to local factors.

Dental caries favors debris retention and therefore irritation to gingival tissues, particularly lesions adjacent to the gingival margin and proximal lesions which favor food impaction. With dental caries, tooth loss, and malocclusion decreased, a difference can be expected in the severity of periodontal conditions.

The incidence of periodontal diseases increases with age. With the use of fluorides, particularly fluoridation, fewer teeth are lost because of dental caries at younger ages. Therefore there is need for emphasis on periodontal disease prevention and control in communities with fluoride in the drinking water.

IV. Partial Defluoridation

As noted earlier, approximately 400 communities use water which contains more than twice optimal level fluoride. With excess fluoride, the water does not meet the requirements of the United States Public Health Service. Defluoridation can be accomplished by one of several chemical systems.[32]

The efficacy of the methods has been shown. The water supply in Britton, South Dakota, has been reduced from almost 7 ppm to 1.5 ppm since 1948, and in Bartlett, Texas, since 1952, from 8 ppm to 1.8 ppm. Examinations have shown a dramatic reduction in incidence of objectionable fluorosis in children born since defluoridation.[33],[34]

V. School Fluoridation

To bring the benefits of fluoridation to children living where there is no central water system, fluoridation of a school water supply has been shown to be a satisfactory method. Because of the intermittent use of the water, only part of each day for five days each week during the school year, the amount of fluoride added is increased over the usual one ppm. Although children are five or six years old before they go to school, definite benefits have been shown. The effect is about twice as great on late erupting teeth since they receive the benefit of systemic fluoride and topical exposure, whereas early erupting teeth have only topical benefits.[35]

After 12 years of fluoride at 5 ppm in the school drinking water of Elk Lake, Pennsylvania, children who had attended that school regularly had 39 percent fewer decayed, missing, and filled teeth than the control group. The greatest benefits were found on proximal tooth surfaces.[35]

The benefits increase with increased fluoride levels. Whereas in Elk Lake after four years at 5 ppm there was 23 percent benefit, in the schools of Seagrove, North Carolina, after four years with fluoride level at 6.3 ppm, there was a 30 percent decrease in decayed, missing, and filled teeth when compared with the control.[36]

VI. Discontinued Fluoridation

The control of dental caries by fluorides can be clearly shown in a community when fluoride is removed. For example, in Antigo, Wisconsin, the action of antifluoridationists in 1960 brought about the discontinuance of fluoridation which had been installed in 1949. Examinations in the years following revealed the marked drop in number of children who were caries-free, and the steep increases in caries rates. For example, from 1960 to 1966 there was a 67 percent decrease in the number of caries-free children in the second grade.[37] Fluoridation was reinstated in 1966 by popular demand.

VII. Economic Benefits

A. Cost of Fluoridation

In the United States costs after installation have been estimated to average between 7 and 14 cents per person per year. When the benefits are considered, and the fact that ALL children are reached, not just those whose parents make the effort to seek preventive professional care, there is little question about the need for fluoridation in all possible domestic water supplies.

No other method for the administration of fluorides has consistently shown equal benefits. All other methods require more professional time, more effort on the part of the individual, and/or more financial outlay.

B. Cost of Professional Care

1. *Influence of Fluoridation.* An example which has been duplicated in kind many times is that of Hartford, Connecticut. One of the preschool dental clinics was closed when it was no longer needed because of the significant decrease in dental caries since fluoridation was started in 1960.[38]

   By this and other testimonials, the real effects of fluoridation are evident. Individual, family, and community costs of dental care can be reduced markedly. In addition, the quantity of dental care, number of dental appointments, the extent of individual restorations, and the number of dental extractions are all reduced.

2. *Newburgh-Kingston Study.*[39] Newburgh, New York, and the control

city, Kingston (without fluoridation) have been used to demonstrate a specific program of dental care. After six years of dental clinic operation for the five- and six-year-old lifelong residents of the poorest socioeconomic areas of the cities, the cost for care of the children exposed to fluoridation has been shown to be less than half that required for the Kingston children.

At the initial examinations 41 percent of the Newburgh children were caries-free, whereas only 17 percent of the Kingston children were. Of the needed restorations, about 75 percent of those for the Kingston children were compound; in Newburgh only about 55 percent involved more than one surface. At the annual recall, the Kingston children consistently required more restorative services; the Newburgh children required only about one-half as many appointments. These findings have marked significance for all types of dental programs for all ages.

DIETARY SUPPLEMENTS

Approximately 23 percent of the population of the United States live in areas which do not have central water systems. Without fluoride in the drinking water, individuals and communities must resort to other means for making fluoride available. Other methods are not substitutes for fluoridation but are needed as follows:

A. For people who use a private water supply which does not have natural fluoride and which is not practical to fluoridate.

B. For those whose community water supply has not yet been fluoridated.

C. At the start of fluoridation, fluoride applications and other methods are used to protect the teeth of children too old to receive the full benefits from fluoridation.

D. As a supplement to fluoridation: multiple use of fluorides has been shown to provide additive benefits.

I. Foods

Certain foods contain fluoride but not enough to constitute a significant part of the day's need for caries prevention. Meat, eggs, vegetables, cereals, and fruits have very small but measurable amounts, while tea and fish have larger amounts.

Fluoridated salt has been used, particularly in Switzerland, and although reduced incidence of dental caries has been shown, effects comparable to fluoridation have not been attained. It has been estimated that by the use of salt as it is currently available (in Switzerland 90 mg. fluoride per kilogram of salt is specified by governmental regulation), the amount of fluoride ingested daily is about one-third to one-half that obtained from one ppm fluoridated water, when average amounts of water used by individuals are compared.[40,41]

Studies on the fluoridation of milk are limited.[40,42] There is evidence that the fluoride is utilized, although absorption from milk is slower than from water, an effect which may be related to the formation of insoluble calcium fluoride. With many milk plants as contrasted to one or a few central water systems, technical problems in the control of milk fluoridation could be very complicated. The use of fluoride in milk is not considered an acceptable alternate for water fluoridation.

II. Fluoride Supplements

A fluoride supplement can be administered as a pill, chewable tablet, lozenge, drop, or mouthwash for swallowing after rinsing. The supplement may be prescribed on an individual patient basis for daily use at home, or it may be administered to school classroom groups as part of a total public health program.

By chewing and rinsing a supplement before swallowing, there is dual action: first, locally on the tooth surface, and, second, systemically on teeth that have not erupted (figures 29–1 and 29–2, pages 422–423). After chewing, the mixture should be swished over and between the teeth for one minute in order that maximum benefit can be obtained. The maximum topical effect occurs on newly erupted teeth.

Studies using preschool children have shown caries incidence reduced by 50 to 80 percent in primary teeth. The benefit was greater for those children who started earlier and continued longer.[43] Studies in permanent teeth have been summarized to show a caries incidence reduction of 20 to 40 percent when the tablets were used over a two- to four-year period.[43,44]

For maximum possible effect, fluoride must be administered at least during the period of tooth development, from birth until 12 to 14 years of age or longer for the maturation of the crown of the third permanent molar.

A. Principles for Administration

The American Dental Association has classified a number of the proprietary fluoride preparations as *Accepted.** Prescriptions are advised when the fluoride concentration in the drinking water used by the child is known to be less than 0.7 ppm.†

1. Available forms
   a. *Tablets:* scored or unscored; may be swallowed, chewed, rinsed

*Consult *Accepted Dental Therapeutics* for current list of fluoride preparations. For a description of the American Dental Association classification of products see page 350.

†For list of communities and the amount of fluoride in the water supply, consult the local health department, the state department of dental health, or write for the current issue of *Fluoridation Census,* an N.I.H. Publication. Address: Division of Dental Health, United States Public Health Service, 8120 Woodmont Avenue, Bethesda, Maryland 20014.

and swallowed, crushed and dissolved in water or fruit juice, or dissolved slowly in the mouth as a lozenge. The resulting mix should be swished over and between the teeth for one minute.

   b. *Liquids:* dilution is prepared so that each drop contains the fluoride ion content specified on the label direction. The number of drops can be adjusted in accord with dentist's prescription and the fluoride level of the drinking water. They may be used as drops placed directly on the child's tongue, or mixed with water, milk, fruit juices, or other food, provided the liquid or food will be completely consumed.

   c. *Mouthrinse:* measured amount of rinse contains prescribed daily fluoride content for systemic use in accord with fluoride content of drinking water. The rinse is swished for at least one minute before swallowing.

2. Fluoride prescribed for daily use when there is no fluoride in the drinking water.[45]
   a. *Over three years:* 1.0 mg. (prescription: 2.2 mg. sodium fluoride. A 2.2 mg. tablet contains 1.0 mg. fluoride).
   b. *Between two and three years:* 0.5 mg. (one-half of a 2.2 mg. tablet).
   c. *Birth to two years:* dissolve a 2.2 mg. tablet in one quart of water, or purchase bottled 1.0 ppm fluoridated water for drinking and preparation of formula and other foods.

3. Fluoride prescribed is adjusted to the fluoride in the water system up to 0.7 ppm. Table 29–1 shows the amount of daily fluoride and the prescription of sodium fluoride pre-

scribed to provide the necessary amount at the different levels of fluoride in the drinking water.

4. Limitation on total prescription: no more than 264 mg. of sodium fluoride should be prescribed at one time, which is sufficient for four months when 2.2 mg. are used daily. The amount (264 mg.) is below the toxic or lethal doses and therefore eliminates the hazard of storing large amounts in the home.

5. Storage: tablets should be kept out of the reach of children.

6. Vitamins with fluoride
   a. Preparations are available in liquid and tablet form.
   b. The American Dental Association has not considered for acceptance vitamin fluoride combinations for several reasons: it is more difficult to adjust the prescribed fluoride to the amount already received through the water supply (table 29–1) since the preparation contains a fixed amount; because there is no evidence that the vitamins enhance the effectiveness of the fluoride; and because of unnecessary expense in buying

vitamins which are not needed or prescribed.[45]

B. **Group Administration**

Administration of fluoride supplements to groups of children as part of school health program has been shown to be beneficial.[46,47] They should be started early, when the child enters kindergarten. Supervised group administration can be carried out by school personnel and adult volunteers under the supervision of a dental hygienist.

There are several advantages in the use of tablet administration as part of school health program especially when compared with prescription on an individual basis. A minimum of professional service time is needed and no special effort is required by the individual or his parents. It is difficult undertaking to supervise use of a daily supplement until the child is 13 to 15 years of age.

C. **Role of Dental Hygienist**

1. Patient instruction: the dental hygienist in private practice participates in instruction, motivation and supervision for those patients who receive a prescription for fluoride tablets. When prescribed on an individual basis, problems arise in the continued administration of the tablets over the years of childhood, apparently even when parents are conscientious and highly motivated.

2. Patient recall: it is generally advisable to plan recall appointments at the time when the patient's prescription will be in need of renewing so that encouragement and supervision can be provided.

TOPICAL FLUORIDE APPLICATION

Topical application of fluoride preparations may frequently be an essential part

Table 29-1. Fluoride Prescription Adjustment to Fluoride in the Drinking Water

Fluoride Content Drinking Water	Adjusted Allowance	
PPM	SODIUM FLUORIDE PRESCRIPTION MG. PER DAY	DAILY FLUORIDE PROVIDED MG. PER DAY
0.0	2.2	1.0
0.2	1.8	0.8
0.4	1.3	0.6
0.6	0.9	0.4

(From American Dental Association, *Accepted Dental Therapeutics*)

of a total preventive program particularly when fluoridation is not available. Although a number of fluoride preparations have been tried and caries-preventive effects shown, those most generally used have been sodium fluoride, acidulated phosphate-fluoride, and stannous fluoride.

Research has continued since the early 1940s when Bibby[48] conducted the initial topical sodium fluoride study using Brockton, Massachusetts, school children and demonstrated better than one-third fewer new carious lesions at the end of a two-year study. Since then research has involved several fluoride compounds and a variety of preparations including solutions, gels, pastes, and dentifrices. These have been tried as agents to be applied professionally in the dental office, individually for home treatment, and for group preventive efforts such as in school dental health or the armed services preventive dentistry programs.

AGENTS FOR TOPICAL FLUORIDE APPLICATION

Benefits and characteristics of sodium fluoride, acidulated phosphate-fluoride, and stannous fluoride solutions will be described first. Directions for specific clinical procedures for topical application follow. Other modes for dispensing topical fluorides such as gels, sprays, rinses, brushing with solution, prophylaxis pastes, and dentifrices will then be considered.

I. Sodium Fluoride

The original applications by Bibby in 1942 utilized a 0.1 percent aqueous sodium fluoride solution applied for seven to eight minutes on teeth thoroughly cleaned by oral prophylaxis at four-month intervals.[48] Extensive studies by Knutson and others were sponsored by the United States Public Health Service in the 1940s. They were designed to determine the most effective concentration of sodium fluoride, the minimum time required for application, and procedural details.[49,50]

The effectiveness of sodium fluoride as a topical agent has been demonstrated in numerous studies. A 30 to 40 percent reduction in caries incidence can be expected in permanent teeth and 20 to 30 percent in primary teeth from a controlled, carefully-performed topical application. Greatest protection is afforded newly erupted teeth, which is true of all topical applications. Later research showed sodium fluoride less effective than acidulated phosphate-fluoride and stannous fluoride on the basis of one and two annual applications.[51]

A. **Solution**

Two percent aqueous sodium fluoride (neutral pH 7.0).

B. **Frequency of Application**

As originally planned a series of four applications, two days to a week apart, were given at intervals throughout childhood in accord with the tooth eruption pattern of the individual child so that teeth may receive protection as soon after eruption as possible. Ages 3, 7, 10, and 13 were considered average and used for applications in public health programs. In addition, a single application is recommended at four- to six-month intervals between the series of four in accord with routine dental and dental hygiene recall for the individual.

C. **Advantages**
1. Solution is relatively stable when kept in a polyethylene bottle.
2. Patient acceptance is favorable: solution tastes salty but is not objectionable.
3. No tooth staining or adverse gingival reactions occur.
4. Patient education: although the series of appointments required for

four treatments has been considered a disadvantage, it is a distinct advantage for instruction of the patient in plaque control procedures. A series of appointments is usually necessary for a patient to gain proficiency in the use of the toothbrush, and the fluoride appointment series gives the opportunity for continuing instruction and review. Toothbrushing practice precedes the fluoride application and thus serves to prepare the teeth by removing plaque and debris.

II. Acidulated Phosphate-Fluoride

For the first clinical study, reported in 1963, a 1.23 percent fluoride with orthophosphoric acid was used for a single annual four-minute application. In this research, caries incidence was reduced by 70 percent after two years.[52]

A succeeding study which resulted in an average of 50 percent fewer new carious lesions, showed that the caries-reducing effect was greater in the children with cleaner mouths. Those with inadequate personal daily care had only 44 percent reduction, whereas in the cleaner mouths there was 60 percent.[53] When acidulated phosphate-fluoride is compared with stannous fluoride, the acidulated phosphate-fluoride has proven more effective than, or at least equal to, stannous fluoride for caries inhibition.[51]

The use of acidulated phosphate-fluoride in the form of a gel is described on page 437. Laboratory studies using extracted teeth have shown that the amount of fluoride taken up by the enamel is the same whether the solution or the gel is applied, assuming the fluoride content, pH, and other factors are similar. Longer exposure and more treatments increase the fluoride concentration in the enamel.[54] In clinical research the gel and solution showed comparable effectiveness. Caries incidence was reduced 28 percent by solution and 24 percent by gel.[55]

A. Solution
A 1.23 percent sodium fluoride with 0.1 M orthophosphoric acid (pH between 3.0 and 3.5). Variations of this formula have been used.

B. Frequency of Application
At least twice annually, at recall appointments. More frequently will permit more fluoride uptake by the enamel, and therefore greater protection, which applies particularly to patients with rampant caries.

C. Advantages
1. Stable solution when kept in a polyethylene bottle.
2. No staining of the tooth structure.
3. Patient acceptance favorable: taste not objectionable.

III. Stannous Fluoride

The initial clinical study was reported in 1955.[56] Annually four applications of two percent stannous fluoride were made with a cotton applicator or by a four-minute spray. Under the conditions of the study, caries reductions were 59 percent and 65 percent respectively. Many studies have been conducted since and a variety of results obtained which have been summarized in the literature.[57]

A four percent solution has also been used,[58] and single application techniques with eight and ten percent.[59,60] The appeal of a single application to save appointment time led to generalized use of the eight percent solution as well as the ten percent which was shown to be beneficial for adult teeth.

A. Solutions and Frequency
1. The two- and four-percent solutions: used the same as two percent sodium fluoride with four applications spaced two days to a week apart repeated at three-year intervals in accord with the tooth erup-

tion pattern of the individual child to provide protection for new teeth soon after eruption.

2. The eight or ten percent solutions: single applications at four- or six-month intervals beginning at approximately age three.

B. **Preparation of Solution**[61,62]

A fresh solution of stannous fluoride must be used for each patient and prepared after the teeth are prepared, just prior to application. The solution quickly undergoes hydrolysis and oxidation to form stannous hydroxide and stannic ion, therefore decreasing in effectiveness.

1. Obtain from a pharmacist Lilly No. 0 gelatin capsules containing stannous fluoride powder: 0.2 Gm. for two percent; 0.4 Gm. for four percent; 0.8 Gm. for eight percent; and 1.0 Gm. for ten percent.

2. Keep capsules in a tightly sealed container.

3. Immediately before use add the contents of one capsule to 10.0 ml. distilled water and shake. Use a 25 ml. graduated cylinder for measuring the water and a 25 ml. polyethylene bottle for mixing the solution.

4. Do not add flavoring or coloring agents.

5. When contents have dissolved, transfer to a dappen dish and apply immediately to clean, dry, isolated teeth (pages 434–436).

6. Discard excess solution.

C. **Adverse Effects**

1. *Gingival Reactions.* The occasional reactions which occur range from a mild irritation with blanching to a severe reaction comparable to a chemical burn followed by sloughing.[63,64] They are reversible and the tissue returns to normal within a few days to a week. Severe reac-

tions have not generally been demonstrated except with higher concentrations and when the solution was applied to inflamed gingival tissues or tissues markedly irritated during polishing with a rubber cup (page 545).

2. *Pigmentation of Teeth.* Brown staining occurs primarily in areas of decalcification, dental caries, hypocalcification, pits, grooves, and margins of restorations.[63,65] The reaction causing the pigmentation results from the deposition of tin (stannous ion) probably in the form of tin sulfate. Tin phosphates are also formed and deposited on the enamel, which may retard the deposition of fluoride.[5]

D. **Precautions for Use**

1. Prevent gingival tissue reactions

   a. When a patient presents with moderate or severe gingivitis, begin toothbrushing and other plaque control instruction, complete the scaling with careful check for complete removal of local irritants, and postpone fluoride application until a future appointment when the tissue is healed.

   b. Other suggestions for tissue protection: use a rubber dam isolation technique, or coat the gingiva with lubricant (petrolatum) and use the 30-second application.[66,67] Many tissue reactions can also be prevented by using weaker solutions (two or four percent stannous fluoride).

2. Use a coverall to protect a patient's clothing in case the solution is inadvertently spilled. Stannous fluoride reacts to discolor certain materials.

3. Make necessary radiographs prior to stannous fluoride application to

avoid film contamination by stannous ions in the patient's mouth or on the fingers of the operator.[68] Once contaminated, the ions may remain on the fingers for several hours, even following routine handwashing. Cleaning with citric acid followed by thorough rinsing has been recommended for removing the stannous ions.[69]

4. Prevent clogging of the saliva ejector by running at least a cupful of water through after application on one side of the mouth, and again at the completion of the entire treatment.

5. Provide particular care for equipment which contacts the stannous fluoride solution: a grayish-white deposit collects when the solution is left for a short time. Sterilizing equipment and disinfecting solution can become contaminated if instruments and dishes are not thoroughly precleaned. Disposable dappen dishes are recommended.

E. **Disadvantages of Stannous Fluoride**
   1. Unstable solution: mixing fresh solution for each application is required.
   2. Patient acceptance limited: astringent quality and unpleasant taste.
   3. Staining of teeth (page 265).
   4. Gingival reactions.

CLINICAL PROCEDURES FOR TOPICAL FLUORIDE APPLICATIONS

I. Principles for Application

Maximum benefits derived from topical fluoride preparations can be expected in proportion to the care taken for a well-defined, exacting application procedure. Essentials include the factors listed here:

A. **Preparation of the Teeth**
   Prior to application, a decision must be made concerning the extent of preparation needed for the teeth of each patient. It is not necessary to polish the teeth before a topical fluoride application.[70] When teeth are polished with an abrasive agent such as pumice, as much as two to four microns of enamel surface is removed.[71] The surface layer of enamel has the greatest concentration of fluoride and is therefore more protective against dental caries than underlying layers.

It has been shown that dental caries prevention was comparable in two groups of children who received a sodium fluoride topical application which for one group was immediately preceded by a pumice cleaning.[72] In another research study, the fluoride content of the enamel was measured three days after a topical fluoride application on teeth which were brushed only and teeth that were pumiced. The fluoride content of the two groups was similar which means that the uptake of fluoride was not interrupted by the presence of pellicle left after toothbrushing.[73]

Therefore, a patient with clean teeth or one participating in a plaque control program should only brush with a commercial fluoride dentifrice and use dental floss to remove all possible dental plaque prior to topical application of fluoride. Appointments for scaling should be completed prior to the application. Only when polishing is required for stain removal should pumicing before a fluoride be needed.

When it is planned that polishing with a rubber cup will be done, a fluoride-containing prophylaxis paste should definitely be used. Although only a small amount of fluoride is added to the tooth from the paste, it has been suggested that the fluoride paste may replace the fluoride removed by the polishing abrasive.[71]

Solution

Exacting preparation and care of the solution in accord with its physical and chemical properties.

Isolation of Teeth

Drying of the teeth and isolation during the required length of time to permit fluoride to contact tooth surfaces without dilution or contamination by saliva.

Clock-timed Procedure

Continuous application to provide constant availability of fluoride ions for formation of fluorapatite.

Instructions for Patient

To avoid use of foods or liquids during at least 30 minutes following the application: permits fluoride an extended contact with tooth for additional benefit.

Repetition

Applications are made at intervals in accord with the eruption pattern and dental caries susceptibility of the individual. More frequent applications increase the fluoride content of the enamel. A minimum of two treatments annually should be recommended.

Armamentarium

Cotton roll holders of appropriate size.*

Cotton rolls of proper lengths attached to holders (see Section III, D and E following).

Cotton pellets (six to eight medium size) and cotton pliers. Cotton applicators may be used.

Dappen dish for fluoride solution.

Saliva ejector connected and water control adjusted.

*Garmer Cotton Roll Holders, Junior (#1) and Adult (#2). Garmer Company, Minneapolis, Minnesota.

F. Air tip connected to compressed air outlet.

G. Timer for four minutes (egg timer or a dark-room alarm).

H. Equipment for stannous fluoride solution (page 433).

III. Cotton Roll Preparation

A. **Prepare in Advance**

Autoclave cotton rolls on preprepared tray or in separate packages.

B. **Objectives**

To isolate the teeth in comfort for the patient and prevent absorption of the fluoride by the cotton rolls. For stannous fluoride, cotton rolls prevent the bitter-tasting solution from dispersing around the mouth. Cotton rolls that are too long are easily displaced by action of the tongue and cheek.

C. **Supply**
1. Use No. 2 cotton rolls except for small mouths or very shallow vestibules when a No. 1 may be fitted and maintained more effectively.
2. Bevel ends at 45 degrees to facilitate placement and retention in the mucobuccal fold and under the tongue.

D. **Lengths: Continuous Cotton Roll Technique**
1. *Facial* (5 to 6 inch cotton roll)
   a. Attach to facial prong of cotton roll holder.
   b. To extend (in the mucobuccal fold) from the mandibular labial frenum to the maxillary labial frenum.
2. *Lingual* (1¼ to 2 inch cotton roll)
   a. Attach to lingual prong of holder.
   b. To extend from canine area to just distal to the most posterior tooth.
   c. Extra cotton roll (1 to 1¼ inches): for most patients a short cotton roll is needed under the side of

the tongue (before the cotton roll holder is placed) for balance. The vestibule is more shallow than the floor of the mouth, which permits the cotton roll holder to tip toward the lingual if not supported by an extra cotton roll.

E. **Lengths: Discontinuous Cotton Roll Technique**
 1. *Indications.* The continuous method can only be used when retraction of the cotton roll from the distobuccal surfaces of the most posterior teeth can be assured during the application. Usually when second permanent molars (and always the third) have erupted, separate facial cotton rolls are needed for the maxillary and mandibular teeth.
 2. *Facial Maxillary* (3 inches)
   a. Will be finger-held.
   b. To extend from labial frenum to area distal to most posterior tooth and the opening to Stensen's duct.
 3. *Facial Mandibular* (3 inches)
   a. Attach to facial prong of holder.
   b. To extend from mandibular labial frenum to the distal of the most posterior tooth. Prevent dislodgment by activity of muscles of throat or cheeks by not extending the cotton roll over the retromolar area.
 4. *Lingual Mandibular.* Same as for continuous technique (D.2. previously).

IV. Patient Preparation

A. **Preparation of the Teeth** (see I.A. page 434).

B. **Patient Position**
   The patient should be positioned upright to prevent fluoride solution and excess saliva from passing into the throat.

V. Isolation Procedure

A. Place single cotton roll beneath th edge of the tongue.

B. Insert holder with attached cotto rolls over the mandibular teeth: adju to proper position.
 1. Lingual cotton roll is placed besid and under the lateral margin of th tongue but not so it presses th tongue down.
 2. Check that the cotton rolls a positioned to protect the oral ti sues from contact with the met holder.
 3. Hold the holder with left han while adjusting the chin clamp wit the right; fasten securely.

C. Insert saliva ejector gently in th region of the canine of the sid opposite the holder.

D. Adjust maxillary: the continuous co ton roll curves up, distal to the mo posterior tooth.
 1. Retract the cheek and twist th cotton roll slightly (toward th gingiva) as it is brought into pos tion in the mucobuccal fold.
 2. Adapt the end in position besid the labial frenum.

E. Hold maxillary section of the cotto roll with the index and middle finge (on the left side the thumb and inde finger are used). When the discontinu ous procedure is used, the maxillar facial cotton roll is held as describe here.
 1. Thumb is kept over or distal to th most posterior tooth (use the inde finger on the left) to assure access c molar surfaces to fluoride.
 2. Maintain retraction throughout ap plication.

F. Final check before application
 1. Cotton is not on the teeth.
 2. Oral tissues are protected fro metal parts of the holder.

3. Cotton rolls are not extended too far distally so they can be easily displaced.

4. Application Procedure

A. Dry teeth thoroughly with compressed air: maxillary first, then mandibular. Direct the air to each surface and proximal area as complete dryness contributes to the effectiveness of fluoride.

B. Apply fluoride solution quickly to moisten all teeth: mandibular teeth first, then maxillary.

C. Start the timer: patient may be instructed to do this so that retraction is not interrupted.

D. Maintain wet tooth surfaces by continuous application of the solution throughout the four-minute period.

E. Completion of application
   1. Remove saliva ejector.
   2. Release cotton roll holder clamp and remove holder with cotton rolls attached.
   3. Remove remaining cotton rolls with cotton pliers.

F. Proceed to opposite side of mouth. The patient does not rinse either between sides or at completion of both sides.

G. Instruct patient not to rinse, eat, drink, or brush the teeth for at least 30 minutes, preferably longer.

FLUORIDE GEL PREPARATIONS

To date, tests to determine the effectiveness of fluoride gel applied by tray or mouthpiece have varied in their findings, which may be related to the difference in procedures used during the research. By far the most significant research has been that in which custom-fitted polyvinyl mouthpieces were used to apply an acidulated phosphate-fluoride gel and a plain neutral sodium fluoride gel. Both contained 1.1 percent sodium fluoride. Research statistics showed dental caries prevention to be 75 percent for the neutral and 80 percent for the acidulated after supervised daily six-minute applications by the children for nearly two school years.[74] Two years after the final application, reexamination showed close to 70 percent retained effect.[75]

When the gel is self-applied in trays once or a few times per year, the caries prevention ranges from 25 to 45 percent fewer new carious lesions.[76-79] Stannous fluoride has been prepared in a water-free stable gel.[80] Its effectiveness when applied by toothbrush or rubber cup has been described.[81]

I. Principles for Application

Some of the same factors which influence the benefits obtained from use of a solution also apply to application of a gel (page 434). Additional factors which may influence results should be considered. A gel preparation may not disperse as readily as a solution does about the teeth. Tray selection may make a difference. Soft wax trays may not be firm enough to force the gel into the inaccessible but strategic pits, fissures, and proximal areas. It is also possible that in the warmth of the mouth, the wax softens and by becoming flexible permits salivary contamination or dilution. Such problems may not arise when custom-fitted polyvinyl trays are used.

II. Gel Content
   1. Fluoride 1.23 percent in 0.1 M orthophosphoric acid at pH 3.0 (same as the acidulated phosphate solution).
   2. Gelling agent: hydroxyethyl cellulose.
   3. Flavoring agent.

III. Modes for Application
   1. Cotton roll isolation procedure with application using cotton pellets and

cotton pliers (page 436). Other isolation procedures may also be used (page 442).

2. Trays: custom-fitted polyvinyl, or foam rubber preferable; wax trays with or without cotton lining also have been used.

IV. Procedure for Tray System

1. Preparation of Teeth (see I.A.).
2. Tray preparation
   a. Custom-fitted vinyl tray can be prepared for an individual patient and kept in a labeled box for use at continuing appointments.
   b. Wax tray: trimmed to the general size and contour of the mouth: check in the mouth for proper molding and length to cover distal surfaces of most-posterior teeth.
3. Place 3 to 5 drops of gel in the base of the tray and spread around. A thin layer is sufficient for a well-fitted tray. When excess gel is applied, it can be forced out from under the edge of the tray and may pass into the throat.

V. Application: Single Arch

1. Dry maxillary teeth: place tray over teeth and immediately insert saliva ejector.
2. Mold wax tray firmly around the teeth, starting over the occlusal and press horizontally to force the gel into the interproximal areas. A well-adapted tray can help exclude saliva.
3. Place a cotton roll over each side in the premolar area and request patient to close gently, without excess pressure, to hold the tray in position. The slight pressure can aid by forcing the gel into the pits, fissures and other inaccessible areas; with too much pressure on a soft wax tray, the sides of the tray may

spread, thus encouraging contami nation by saliva.

4. Start the timer: leave tray in posi tion for at least four minutes; si preferred.
5. Remove tray with cotton pliers.
6. Patient does not rinse.
7. Dry mandibular teeth and place th tray; mold carefully over the teeth as before, to press the gel betwee the teeth.
8. Insert saliva ejector and a cotton ro on each premolar-molar region be fore requesting patient to clos gently.
9. Procedure is timed as before, an tray removed. Wipe excess gel fro the teeth.
10. Instruct patient not to eat, drin rinse, or brush the teeth for at lea 30 minutes, preferably longer.

VI. Additional Technique Suggestions

1. Acidulated phosphate-fluoride ge are stable when kept in poly ethylene containers.
2. Relation to gingiva: an occasiona reaction may occur in the form of white color change within about 1 minutes after application. It can b wiped off, or if left untouched, wil disappear within an hour or two. N postoperative effects occur, and n subjective symptoms have bee reported. Suggestions for preven tion of a gingival reaction:
   a. Provide plaque control instruc tion and postpone applicatio when gingiva is inflamed. Th reaction rarely occurs excep when there is moderate to sever inflammation.
   b. Use minimum amount of gel an confine it as much as possible t the base of the tray. When a wa tray is used, hold with horizonta pressure to force small excesse

between the teeth rather than over the gingiva.

3. Use of a double-arch technique in which both trays are inserted and timed simultaneously is not recommended for routine use, particularly when soft wax trays are used because of difficulty of control and adaptation.

VII. Self Applied: Custom Tray

Fluoride gels (0.5 percent fluoride with a pH 4.5 to 7.0) may be used in a custom-made tray (mouthguard type which covers the cervical third) for home use on a daily or weekly basis.

A. Directions
1. Use toothbrush and floss: thoroughly remove all plaque.
2. Dry mouth by swallowing several times.
3. Apply a few drops or a small ribbon to the inside of each tray. Do not overload so that gel squeezes out excessively when applied.
4. Apply trays over the teeth. Close with pressure to hold them in place. The slight pressure will force the gel to the proximal areas.
5. Retain for four minutes.

B. Indications for Special Patients
Tray application on a daily basis is particularly applicable to patients with a high risk of dental caries. Examples are patients who have
1. Rampant caries.
2. Xerostomia.
3. Exposure to radiation therapy (page 622).
4. An overdenture (page 368).
5. Gingival recession and, therefore, are susceptible to cemental caries.

APPLICATION BY SPRAY

A spray technique has not been used extensively but reports have shown moderate effectiveness in prevention of dental caries. For examples, one study showed sodium fluoride (two percent) to be equally effective when applied by spray as by cotton applicator,[50] and in another study stannous fluoride (two percent) was somewhat more effective by spray than by cotton applicator.[56]

Without oral prophylaxis, an acidulated phosphate-fluoride solution was used as a spray three times spaced during each of three school years as a research study, but with implications useful in a school dental health program. There was reduction in new carious lesions, with greatest benefit to those children with cleaner mouths who practiced regular daily brushing.[82]

In another study, an acidulated phosphate-fluoride spray was applied during and following the use of a prophylaxis paste containing acidulated phosphate-fluoride.[83] Caries reductions from these procedures were not as great as from conventional topical fluoride application and generally should be considered a supplement rather than a substitute for more effective applications when made on an individual basis.

Based on these studies, for patients who do not or cannot cooperate by maintaining oral cleanliness even with repeated instruction, clinical procedures can be planned to include frequent applications by spray. The spray may also be used for rinsing during operative procedures.

FLUORIDE MOUTHWASH: RINSING AND TOOTHBRUSHING

Self-applied fluoride by use of a mouthrinse provides a practical and effective means for dental caries prevention and desensitization. A summary of research studies using various concentrations shows that reductions in dental caries incidence range from 20 to 50 percent.[84] The caries-preventing effects of fluoride solutions are related to frequency of use, whether daily, weekly, or fortnightly.

More frequent use has been shown to be more beneficial.

Rinsing is a more efficient method for fluoride use than professionally-applied techniques, and the benefits can be greater. It has definite advantages when applied in a school health preventive program since materials are not complicated or expensive, and it does not take children out of the classroom. Minimal instruction is needed for teachers and adult volunteers to carry out the classroom procedures. Overall supervision can be provided by dental hygienists.

On an individual basis, home use of a fluoride mouthrinse is convenient for all ages. Instructions to parents for supervision of children is provided by the dental hygienist as part of the dental hygiene treatment plan. When fluoride supplements are indicated, the rinse supplement, which is actively swished over the teeth before swallowing, may be easier for certain patients than use of a chewable tablet and contains the same amount of ingestible fluoride.[47]

I. Mouthrinses

A. Sodium Fluoride

1. Solutions and frequency
   a. Aqueous solution of sodium fluoride 0.2 percent, pH 7.0 (neutral), used weekly or once every two weeks.
   b. Aqueous solution of sodium fluoride 0.05 percent, pH 7.0 (neutral), used daily.
   c. Aqueous solution of acidulated phosphate sodium fluoride 0.02 percent, pH approximately 4.0, used daily.
2. Directions. For a child, 7 to 10 ml.; and for teen-age and adult, 10–15 ml.* should be swished vigorously for not less than one minute. Rinsing directions are on page 342.

B. Stannous Fluoride

Stannous fluoride mouthwashe with concentrations of 0.05 percer and 0.1 percent in a water-free glyc erin base have been studied in labora tory and clinical research. In one stud the 0.1 percent mouthwash was pre pared daily for use in a school pro gram.[85] Brown and yellow staining c plaque was observed in children wit inadequate personal daily plaque re moval techniques.

II. Brush With Solution

Brushing with a fluoride solution ha been shown to produce significant reduc tions in dental caries incidence. Periodi supervised brushing with sodiur fluoride, sodium monofluorophosphate and acidulated phosphate-fluoride ha demonstrated beneficial results. Thes have been summarized in the literature and included in *Suggested Readings* a the end of this chapter.

Despite a small increase in time an supervision, use of toothbrushing with th solution may be preferred over rinsin because of the importance of brushing t the removal of dental plaque. Brushin with fluoride combines efforts to preven both dental caries and periodontal dis eases.

FLUORIDE DENTIFRICES

The principal fluoride compounds cur rently utilized in dentifrices are stannou fluoride, sodium fluoride, and sodiur monofluorophosphate. A few of thes dentifrices have been accepted by th American Dental Association.[45]*

I. Benefits

Various reductions in caries incidenc have been shown by the reported researcl findings. Direct comparisons cannot b made between the studies because of th

*For description of American Dental Associatio classification, see page 350.

*One teaspoonful = 5 ml.

differences in research procedures. An overall average would probably fall in the range of 20 to 30 percent caries inhibition.

Greater benefits have been demonstrated for newly erupted teeth, a finding in keeping with the usual effect of topically applied fluoride. Added benefits have been shown for children who have used drinking water with fluoride at optimum level.[87] Reviews of the literature are available.[88,89]

Dentifrice Components

The first sodium fluoride dentifrice study did not show statistically significant caries reduction.[90] It has been demonstrated that other ingredients of a dentifrice must be compatible with the fluoride ions. When the abrasive agent contains calcium, fluoride and calcium can react, thus rendering the fluoride inactive.

Components of dentifrices in general are described on pages 344–346. Fluoride dentifrices are made with the basic essential ingredients, a compatible abrasive agent, and a source of fluoride ions. Specific formulae for the dentifrices approved by the American Dental Association are included in *Accepted Dental Therapeutics*.

1. Recommendation

A fluoride dentifrice should be recommended for all patients as part of the complete preventive program. Certain fluoride dentifrices may also have desensitizing properties (page 564).

Since stannous fluoride dentifrices stain teeth a light to moderate brown, they should not be recommended for use on exposed cementum.

FLUORIDE PROPHYLAXIS PASTES

Application of fluoride by pastes cannot be considered a substitute for conventional topical application on the basis of present-day research. While moderate caries-preventive effects have been demonstrated,[91,92] other studies have had minimal or no statistically significant results.[93,94] A bibliography of recent reports is included with the suggested readings at the end of the chapter.

Incompatibility of the fluoride agent with the abrasive or other paste ingredients has been a problem with certain combinations. It is not merely a question of adding a fluoride solution to a cleaning paste. When mixed, agents may react, and the effect of the fluoride can be neutralized or at least the shelf-life may be limited.

Another limitation on the potential of the paste preparations is that the abrasive generally removes a thin layer of enamel during polishing, which removes also the outer layer of fluoride, possibly as fast as it is added from the paste.[71,95,96] If fluoride is added at the same rate that it is removed, which is not known, it could be a good reason for using the paste, even though no additional benefits could be derived.[71] On the other hand, when certain compatible agents are used, isolation of the teeth for application of the paste and allowing the paste to remain in contact with the enamel for three to four minutes after the polishing action is completed, may permit uptake of fluoride by the enamel.[95]

In order for the dental hygienist to be able to evaluate fluoride preparations which become available on the market, a continuing review of the new research will be needed as additional studies are reported. Because the caries prevention which can be expected from the use of prophylaxis pastes is minimal, other means for applying fluoride must be used if the patient is to receive optimum protection by fluorides.

COMBINED FLUORIDE PROGRAM

Most patients can benefit from the use of more than one method for use of fluorides. When the preventive program is planned for an individual patient, the fluoride preparations and modes of application selected should provide the greatest possible protection against dental caries.

When self-administered methods are chosen, patient cooperation is a significant factor. For example, a daily application of fluoride gel in a custom-made tray may be ideal for a patient, but cooperation may be difficult to obtain even when the patient has well-meaning parents. A single daily chewable tablet or daily mouthrinse may not be as difficult for some patients.

Age and eruption pattern influence the method selected, as it is particularly important to apply fluorides as soon after eruption as possible. Recall appointments can be scheduled for frequent topical applications and for continuing instruction and motivation. All methods are supplemented by the use of a dentifrice with fluoride.

The effectiveness of various combinations of fluoride therapies has been measured. For example, in communities where there is fluoride in the drinking water, using other methods for caries prevention show added benefits. In one study[97] topical stannous fluoride (eight percent) applied annually for children who had used fluoridated water all their lives resulted in approximately 20 percent fewer new carious lesions. Since this percentage might represent only one cavity or less for many children in a fluoridated area, the practical significance of the use of topical applications could be questioned provided another means for prevention is available which would not require as much professional time as the topical applications.

In another study in a fluoridated area, use of a stannous fluoride prophylaxis paste, topical application of 8 percent solution, and the 0.4 percent dentifrice individually reduced caries incidence,

but the greatest benefit occurred with a three together.[98] Research in a nonfluor dated area demonstrated similar benef cial results by combining the paste solution, and dentifrice.[91]

The United States Navy's preventiv program utilized stannous fluoride com bination treatment by annual applicatio of prophylaxis paste followed by topica 10 percent solution in conjunction wit daily use of 0.4 percent dentifrice. In th reported research after two years, eac mode of fluoride influenced caries pre vention individually, but together the realized approximately 70 percent fewe new carious lesions.[92] One importan consideration which can be derived from the Navy studies is the significant benefit to young adults. Too often, preventio through the use of fluorides inappro priately is considered for children only.

TECHNICAL HINTS

I. Alternate Isolation Procedures for Topical Application

The procedure described on page 43 was for isolation of one-half of the denti tion at one time. Objectives are to con serve time but also to maintain as dry field as possible and to keep the fluorid solution from being absorbed by cotto rolls, or the saliva from contaminating o diluting the solution. Other system which may be applied include:

A. **Rubber Dam**[99]
  1. *Use.* For application of fluorid following operative procedures.
  2. *Preparation.* When the rubber dan has not been fitted to include th entire quadrant, additional hole may be made in the dam with a explorer.
  3. *Advantages*
     a. Better patient control, particu larly a small child or handi capped patient with specia problems.

b. Time saving: thoroughly dry teeth can be maintained. Particularly useful for general anesthesia or hospital patient.[66]
c. Stannous fluoride: the solution is confined and the patient does not experience the unpleasant taste.

B. **Single Quadrant**

Each quadrant can be done separately by holding the cotton rolls with the fingers. In a very small mouth it may be possible to hold a Number 1 continuous cotton roll around the entire maxillary arch to make the entire application in one timing. This can be particularly useful for a small child when cotton roll holders may not stay in place.

II. Appointment Planning

Because of the post-application ruling concerning no eating for at least one-half hour, avoid scheduling topical fluoride procedures just before the mealtime hours. This would be particularly important for patients on special diets, such as diabetics.

III. Fluoride Application Following Polishing of Restorations

Since abrasive stones and polishing agents remove a layer of surface enamel and since polishing procedures extend over the margins of the restoration, a topical application of fluoride can be particularly important (page 553). The removal of surface fluoride about the margin weakens the enamel and may render it more susceptible to dental caries if precautions are not taken.

FACTORS TO TEACH THE PATIENT

I. Personal Use of Fluorides

A. Purposes, action, and expected benefits relative to the specific forms of fluoride treatment which the patient will receive.

B. Specific instruction concerning self-applied techniques which will be performed at home. Prepared printed instruction materials can be especially useful.

C. Chewable tablets: avoid eating, drinking, or toothbrushing for one-half hour following use. The preferred time for use is after toothbrushing before going to bed.

D. Relate brushing technique to need for fluoride in dentifrice to reach all tooth surfaces.

II. Preparation for Topical Fluoride Application

When the teeth are free from plaque and the gingival tissue is firm and healthy, there is greater uptake of fluoride by the teeth and less possibility of a slight tissue reaction. When the gingiva is inflamed, the patient will need instruction in order to understand why the topical application is postponed until the tissue has healed.

III. Fluorides Are Part of the Total Preventive Program

Control of dietary sugars, particularly between-meal foods containing sucrose, and professional care are still necessary to supplement fluoride treatment for caries control.

IV. Recall

There is a need for continuing applications of topical agents. Frequent applications increase the fluoride content of the enamel and provide greater resistance to dental caries.

V. Fluoridation

In a nonfluoridated community, information concerning the significance of fluoridation to the entire community and its benefits and operation should be available and disseminated.

VI. Stannous Fluoride

When topical stannous fluoride preparations are used, the patient (or parent) should be informed about the possibility of tooth staining.

References

1. Brudevold, F., Gardner, D. E., and Smith, F. A.: The Distribution of Fluoride in Human Enamel, *J. Dent. Res.*, 35, 420, June, 1956.
2. Sicher, H. and Bhaskar, S. N., eds.: *Orban's Oral Histology and Embryology*, 7th ed. St. Louis, Mosby, 1972, pp. 67–88.
3. Permar, D.: *Oral Embryology and Microscopic Anatomy*, 5th ed. Philadelphia, Lea & Febiger, 1972, pp. 131–140.
4. Isaac, S., Brudevold, F., and Gardner, D. E.: The Relation of Fluoride in the Drinking Water to the Distribution of Fluoride in Enamel, *J. Dent. Res.*, 37, 318, April, 1958.
5. Brudevold, F., McCann, H. G., Nilsson, R., Richardson, B., and Coklica, V.: The Chemistry of Caries Inhibition Problems and Challenges in Topical Treatments, *J. Dent. Res.*, 46, 37, January-February, 1967.
6. Dawes, C., Jenkins, G. N., Hardwick, J. L., and Leach, S. A.: The Relation Between the Fluoride Concentrations in the Dental Plaque and in Drinking Water, *Br. Dent. J.*, 119, 164, August 17, 1965.
7. Jenkins, G. N., Edgar, W. M., and Ferguson, D. B.: The Distribution and Metabolic Effects of Human Plaque Fluorine, *Arch. Oral Biol.*, 14, 105, January, 1969.
8. Richards, L. F., Westmoreland, W. W., Tashiro, M., McKay, C. H., and Morrison, J. T.: Determining Optimum Fluoride Levels for Community Water Supplies in Relation to Temperature, *J. Am. Dent. Assoc.*, 74, 389, February, 1967.
9. McNeil, D. R.: *The Fight for Fluoridation.* New York, Oxford University Press, 1957, pp. 3–43.
10. Russell, A. L.: Epidemiology and the Rational Bases of Dental Public Health and Dental Practice, in Young, W. O. and Striffler, D. F.: *The Dentist, His Practice, and His Community*, 2nd ed. Philadelphia, Saunders, 1969, pp. 37–42.
11. McKay, F. S.: The Relation of Mottled Enamel to Caries, *J. Am. Dent. Assoc.*, 15, 1429, August, 1928.
12. Churchill, H. V.: Occurrence of Fluorides in Some Waters of United States, *J. Indust. & Engin. Chem.*, 23, 996, 1931.
13. Dean, H. T., Arnold, F. A., Jr., and Elvove, E.: Domestic Water and Dental Caries. V. Additional Studies of the Relation of Fluoride Domestic Waters to Dental Caries Experience in 4425 White Children, Aged 12 to 14 Years, of 13 Cities in 4 States, *Pub. Health Rep.*, 57, 1155, August 7, 1942.
14. *Natural Fluoride Content of Community Water Supplies*, 1969. United States Department of Health, Education, and Welfare Public Health Service, National Institutes of Health, Bethesda, Maryland.
15. Forrest, J. R.: Caries Incidence and Enamel Defects in Areas with Different Levels of Fluoride in the Drinking Water, *Br. Dent. J.*, 100, 195, April 17, 1956.
16. Diefenbach, V. L., Nevitt, G. A., and Frankel, J. M.: Fluoridation and the Appearance of Teeth, *J. Am. Dent. Assoc.*, 71, 1129, November, 1965.
17. Arnold, F. A., Dean, H. T., Jay, P., and Knutson, J. W.: Effect of Fluoridated Public Water Supplies on Dental Caries Prevalence Tenth Year of the Grand Rapids–Muskegon Study, *Pub. Health Rep.*, 71, 652, July, 1956.
18. Hayes, R. L., Littleton, N. W., and White, C. L.: Posteruptive Effects of Fluoridation on First Permanent Molars of Children in Grand Rapids, Michigan, *Am. J. Public Health*, 47, 192, February, 1957.
19. Russell, A. L. and Hamilton, P. M.: Dental Caries in Permanent First Molars after Eight Years of Fluoridation, *Arch. Oral Biol.*, 6, 50, July, 1961.
20. Backer Dirks, O., Houwink, B., and Kwant, G. W.: Some Special Features of the Caries Preventive Effect of Water Fluoridation, *Arch. Oral Biol.*, 4, 187, August, 1961.
21. Ast, D. B. and Fitzgerald, B.: Effectiveness of Water Fluoridation, *J. Am. Dent. Assoc.*, 65, 581, November, 1962.
22. Carlos, J. P., Gittelsohn, A. M., and Haddon, W., Jr.: Caries in Deciduous Teeth in Relation to Maternal Ingestion of Fluoride, *Pub. Health Rep.*, 77, 658, August, 1962.
23. Horowitz, H. S. and Heifetz, S. B.: Effects of Prenatal Exposure to Fluoridation on Dental Caries, *Pub. Health Rep.*, 82, 297, April, 1967.
24. Katz, S. and Muhler, J. C.: Prenatal and Postnatal Fluoride and Dental Caries Experience in Deciduous Teeth, *J. Am. Dent. Assoc.*, 76, 305, February, 1968.
25. Salzmann, J. A.: The Effects of Fluoride on the Prevalence of Malocclusion, *J. Am. Coll. Dent.*, 35, 82, January, 1968.
26. Russell, A. L. and Elvove, E.: Domestic Water and Dental Caries. VII. A Study of the Fluoride-Dental Caries Relationship in an Adult Population, *Pub. Health Rep.*, 66, 1389, October 26, 1951.
27. Englander, H. R. and Wallace, D. A.: Effects of Naturally Fluoridated Water on Dental Caries in Adults, *Pub. Health Rep.*, 77, 887, October, 1962.
28. Sognnaes, R. F.: Fluoride Protection of Bones and Teeth, *Science*, 150, 989, November 19, 1965.
29. Bernstein, D. S., Sadowsky, N., Hegsted, D. M., Guri, C. D., and Stare, F. J.: Prevalence of Osteoporosis in High- and Low-fluoride

Areas in North Dakota, *J. Am. Med. Assoc.*, *198*, 499, October 31, 1966.

30. Fluoride, Bony Structure, and Aortic Calcification, *Nutrition Rev.*, 25, 100, April, 1967.

31. Grøn, P., McCann, H. G., and Bernstein, D.: Effect of Fluoride on Human Osteoporotic Bone Mineral, *J. Bone & Joint Surg.*, *48A*, 892, July, 1966.

32. Maier, F. J.: *Manual of Water Fluoridation Practice*. New York, McGraw-Hill, 1963, pp. 209–213.

33. Horowitz, H. S., Maier, F. J., and Law, F. E.: Partial Defluoridation of a Community Water Supply and Dental Fluorosis, *Pub. Health Rep.*, 82, 965, November, 1967.

34. Horowitz, H. S. and Heifetz, S. B.: The Effect of Partial Defluoridation of a Water Supply on Dental Fluorosis—Final Results in Bartlett, Texas, After 17 Years, *Am. J. Public Health*, *62*, 767, June, 1972.

35. Horowitz, H. S.: School Fluoridation for the Prevention of Dental Caries, *Int. Dent. J.*, 23, 346, June, 1973.

36. Heifetz, S. B. and Horowitz, H. S.: Effect of School Water Fluoridation on Dental Caries: Interim Results in Seagrove, N.C. after Four Years, *J. Am. Dent. Assoc.*, 88, 352, February, 1974.

37. Lemke, C. W., Doherty, J. M., and Arra, M. C.: Controlled Fluoridation: The Dental Effects of Discontinuation in Antigo, Wisconsin, *J. Am. Dent. Assoc.*, 80, 782, April, 1970.

38. Children's Caries Reduced by Fluoridation; Hartford Closes Dental Clinic, *J. Am. Dent. Assoc.*, 67, 125, July, 1963.

39. Ast, D. B., Cons, N. C., Pollard, S. T., and Garfinkel, J.: Time and Cost Factors to Provide Regular Periodic Dental Care for Children in a Fluoridated and Nonfluoridated Area: Final Report, *J. Am. Dent. Assoc.*, 80, 770, April, 1970.

40. Mühlemann, H. R.: Dietary Fluoride and Dental Caries, *Int. Dent. J.*, 15, 209, June, 1965.

41. Mühlemann, H. R.: Fluoridated Domestic Salt: A Discussion of Dosage, *Int. Dent. J.*, 17, 10, March, 1967.

42. Rusoff, L. L., Konikoff, B. S., Frye, J. B., Johnston, J. E., and Frye, W. W.: Fluoride Addition to Milk and Its Effect on Dental Caries in School Children, *Am. J. Clin. Nutr.*, 11, 94, August, 1962.

43. Driscoll, W. S.: The Use of Fluoride Tablets for the Prevention of Dental Caries, in Forrester, D. J. and Schulz, E. M., eds.: *International Workshop on Fluorides and Dental Caries Reductions*. Baltimore, Maryland, 1974, pp. 25–111.

44. Stookey, G. K.: Fluoride Therapy, in Bernier, J. L. and Muhler, J. C., eds.: *Improving Dental Practice Through Preventive Measures*, 2nd ed. St. Louis, Mosby, 1970, pp. 96–110.

45. American Dental Association, Council on Dental Therapeutics: *Accepted Dental Therapeutics*, 36th ed. Chicago, American Dental Association, 1975, pp. 291–305.

46. Driscoll, W. S., Heifetz, S. B., and Korts, D. C.: Effect of Acidulated Phosphate-fluoride Chewable Tablets on Dental Caries in Schoolchildren: Results After 30 Months, *J. Am. Dent. Assoc.*, 89, 115, July, 1974.

47. Aasenden, R., DePaola, P. F., and Brudevold, F.: Effects of Daily Rinsing and Ingestion of Fluoride Solutions Upon Dental Caries and Enamel Fluoride, *Arch. Oral Biol.*, 17, 1705, December, 1972.

48. Bibby, B. G.: Use of Fluorine in the Prevention of Dental Caries. II. The Effects of Sodium Fluoride Applications, *J. Am. Dent. Assoc.*, 31, 317, March 1, 1944.

49. Knutson, J. W.: Sodium Fluoride Solutions: Technic for Application to the Teeth, *J. Am. Dent. Assoc.*, 36, 37, January, 1948.

50. Galagan, D. J. and Knutson, J. W.: The Effect of Topically Applied Fluorides on Dental Caries Experience. VI. Experiments with Sodium Fluoride and Calcium Chloride . . . Widely Spaced Applications . . . Use of Different Solution Concentrations, *Pub. Health Rep.*, 63, 1215, September 17, 1948.

51. Grøn, P. and DePaola, P. F.: Caries Prevention in the Dental Office, *Ala. J. Med. Sci.*, 5, 370, July, 1968.

52. Wellock, W. D. and Brudevold, F.: A Study of Acidulated Fluoride Solutions—II. The Caries Inhibiting Effect of Single Annual Topical Applications of an Acidic Fluoride and Phosphate Solution. A Two Year Experience, *Arch. Oral Biol.*, 8, 179, March-April, 1963.

53. Wellock, W. D., Maitland, A., and Brudevold, F.: Caries Increments, Tooth Discoloration, and State of Oral Hygiene in Children Given Single Annual Applications of Acid Phosphate-Fluoride and Stannous Fluoride, *Arch. Oral Biol.*, 10, 453, May-June, 1965.

54. Wei, S. H. Y.: Fluoride Uptake by Enamel from Topical Solutions and Gels: an *In Vitro* Study, *J. Dent. Child.*, 40, 299, July-August, 1973.

55. Horowitz, H. S. and Doyle, J.: The Effect on Dental Caries of Topically Applied Acidulated Phosphate-fluorides: Results After Three Years, *J. Am. Dent. Assoc.*, 82, 359, February, 1971.

56. Howell, C. L., Gish, C. W., Smiley, R. D., and Muhler, J. C.: Effect of Topically Applied Stannous Fluoride on Dental Caries Experience in Children, *J. Am. Dent. Assoc.*, 50, 14, January, 1955.

57. Stookey: op. cit., pp. 112–156.

58. McDonald, R. E. and Muhler, J. C.: Superiority of Topical Application of Stannous Fluoride on Primary Teeth, *J. Dent. Child.*, 24, 84, 2nd Quarter, 1957.

59. Gish, C. W., Howell, C. L., and Muhler, J. C.: A New Approach to the Topical Application of

Fluorides for the Reduction of Dental Caries in Children, *J. Dent. Res.*, 36, 784, October, 1957.

60. Muhler, J. C.: The Effect of a Single Topical Application of Stannous Fluoride on the Incidence of Dental Caries in Adults, *J. Dent. Res.*, 37, 415, June, 1958.

61. Muhler, J. C.: Topical Application of Stannous Fluoride, *J. Am. Dent. Assoc.*, 54, 352, March, 1957.

62. Dudding, N. J. and Muhler, J. C.: Technique of Application of Stannous Fluoride in a Compatible Prophylactic Paste and as a Topical Agent, *J. Dent. Child.*, 29, 219, 4th Quarter, 1962.

63. Muhler, J. C.: Effect on Gingiva and Occurrence of Pigmentation on Teeth Following the Topical Application of Stannous Fluoride or Stannous Chlorofluoride, *J. Periodont.*, 28, 281, October, 1957.

64. Swieterman, R. P., Muhler, J. C., and Swenson, H. M.: The Effect of Highly Concentrated Solutions of Stannous Fluoride on Human Gingival Tissue, *J. Periodont.*, 32, 131, April, 1961.

65. Hine, J. F., Swartz, M. L., and Phillips, R. W.: Staining of Resin and Silicate Restorations by Topically Applied Solutions of Stannous Fluoride, *J. Periodont.*, 28, 138, April, 1957.

66. McDonald, R. E.: Gingival Tissue Reaction to Topical Application of Stannous Fluoride for the General Anesthesia Patient, *J. Dent. Child.*, 31, 100, 2nd Quarter, 1964.

67. Mercer, V. and Muhler, J. C.: The Effect of a 30-second Topical SnF$_2$ Treatment on Dental Caries Reductions in Children, *J. Oral Thera. and Pharm.*, 1, 141, September, 1964.

68. Dahl, L. O. and Muhler, J. C.: The Effect of Microconcentrations of Stannous Fluoride Solutions on Dental X-ray Films, *J. Am. Dent. Assoc.*, 58, 24, February, 1959.

69. Yamane, G. M., Meskin, L. H., and Mehaffey, P.: Stannous Ion Contamination of Radiographic Films. Etiology and Prevention, *J. Am. Dent. Hyg. Assoc.*, 42, 147, 3rd Quarter, 1968.

70. Wei, S. H. Y.: The Potential Benefits To Be Derived from Topical Fluorides in Fluoridated Communities, in Forrester, D. J. and Schulz, E. M., eds.: *International Workshop on Fluorides and Dental Caries Reductions.* Baltimore, Maryland, 1974, pp. 193–196.

71. Vrbic, V., Brudevold, F., and McCann, H. G.: Acquisition of Fluoride by Enamel from Fluoride Pumice Pastes, *Helv. Odontol. Acta*, 11, 21, April, 1967.

72. Chrietzberg, J. E.: Toothbrushing as a Substitute for Quick Cleansing in the Topical Fluoride Technic, *J. Am. Dent. Assoc.*, 42, 435, April, 1951.

73. Tinanoff, N., Wei, S. H. Y., and Parkins, F. M.: Effect of a Pumice Prophylaxis on Fluoride Uptake in Tooth Enamel, *J. Am. Dent. Assoc.*, 88, 384, February, 1974.

74. Englander, H. R., Keyes, P. H., and Gestwic M.: Clinical Anticaries Effect of Repeat Topical Sodium Fluoride Applications Mouthpieces, *J. Am. Dent. Assoc.*, 75, 6: September, 1967.

75. Englander, H. R., Carlos, J. P., Senning, R. and Mellberg, J. R.: Residual Anticari Effect of Repeated Topical Sodium Fluori Applications by Mouthpieces, *J. Am. Der Assoc.*, 78, 783, April, 1969.

76. Bryan, E. T. and Williams, J. E.: The Cari static Effectiveness of a Phosphate-fluori Gel Administered Annually to School Ch dren: Final Results, *J. Public Health Den 30, 13, Winter, 1970.

77. Englander, H. R., Sherrill, L. T., Miller, B. (Carlos, J. P., Mellberg, J. R., and Senning, S.: Incremental Rates of Dental Caries Af Repeated Topical Sodium Fluoride Applic tions in Children with Lifelong Consum tion of Fluoridated Water, *J. Am. Der Assoc.*, 82, 354, February, 1971.

78. Horowitz, H. S. and Kau, M. C. W.: Retain Anticaries Protection from Topical Applied Acidulated Phosphate-fluoride: 3 and 36-month Post-treatment Effects, *J. Pre Dent.*, 1, 22, May-June, 1974.

79. Trubman, A. and Crellin, J. A.: Effect on Dent Caries of Self-application of Acidulate Phosphate Fluoride Paste and Gel, *J. Ar Dent. Assoc.*, 86, 153, January, 1973.

80. Shannon, I. L.: Preventive Dental Services the Veterans' Administration Hospital, *Public Health Dent.*, 30, 156, Summer, 197

81. Cowan, R. D. and Shannon, I. L.: Protectiv Effectiveness of a Stannous Fluoride Ge *Aust. Dent. J.*, 17, 293, August, 1972.

82. DePaola, P. F., Wellock, W. D., Maitland, A and Brudevold, F.: The Relationship Cariostasis, Oral Hygiene, and Past Cari Experience in Children Receiving Thre Sprays Annually with Acidulate Phosphate-fluoride: Three-year Results, *Am. Dent. Assoc.*, 77, 91, July, 1968.

83. DePaola, P. F.: Combined Use of a Sodiu Fluoride Prophylaxis Paste and a Spra Containing Acidulated Sodium Fluorid Solution, *J. Am. Dent. Assoc.*, 75, 140 December, 1967.

84. Torell, P. and Ericsson, Y.: The Potenti Benefits Derived from Fluoride Mout Rinses, in Forrester, D. J. and Schulz, E. M eds.: *International Workshop on Fluoride and Dental Caries Reductions.* Baltimor Maryland, 1974, pp. 114–176.

85. Radike, A. W., Gish, C. W., Peterson, J. K King, J. D., and Segreto, V. A.: Clinic Evaluation of Stannous Fluoride as a Anticaries Mouthrinse, *J. Am. Dent. Assoc 86, 404, February, 1973.

86. McConchie, J. M.: The Potential Benefits "Brush-in" Programmes as Regards Preven tion of Dental Caries, Dental Health Educ tion and Public Relations, in Forrester, D. .

and Schulz, E. M., eds.: *International Workshop on Fluorides and Dental Caries Reductions*. Baltimore, Maryland, 1974, pp. 273–277.

87. Gish, C. W. and Muhler, J. C.: Effectiveness of a SnF_2-$Ca_2P_2O_7$ Dentifrice on Dental Caries in Children Whose Teeth Calcified in a Natural Fluoride Area. II. Results at the End of 24 Months, *J. Am. Dent. Assoc.*, 73, 853, October, 1966.

88. Heifetz, S. B. and Horowitz, H. S.: Fluoride Dentifrices, in Newbrun, E., ed.: *Fluorides and Dental Caries*. Springfield, Charles C Thomas, 1972, pp. 22–33.

89. Duckworth, R.: Fluoride Dentifrices. A Review of Clinical Trials in the United Kingdom, *Br. Dent. J.*, 124, 505, June 4, 1968.

90. Bibby, B. G.: A Test of the Effect of Fluoride-containing Dentifrices on Dental Caries, *J. Dent. Res.*, 24, 297, December, 1945.

91. Bixler, D. and Muhler, J. C.: Effect on Dental Caries in Children in a Nonfluoride Area of Combined Use of Three Agents Containing Stannous Fluoride: A Prophylactic Paste, a Solution, and a Dentifrice. II. Results at the End of 24 and 36 Months, *J. Am. Dent. Assoc.*, 72, 392, February, 1966.

92. Scola, F. P. and Ostrom, C. A.: Clinical Evaluation of Stannous Fluoride When Used as a Constituent of a Compatible Prophylactic Paste, as a Topical Solution, and in a Dentifrice in Naval Personnel. II. Report of Findings After Two Years, *J. Am. Dent. Assoc.*, 77, 594, September, 1968.

93. Horowitz, H. S. and Lucye, H. S.: A Clinical Study of Stannous Fluoride in a Prophylaxis Paste and as a Solution. *J. Oral Thera. and Pharm.*, 3, 17, July, 1966.

94. Peterson, J. K., Horowitz, H. S., Jordan, W. A., and Pugnier, V.: Effectiveness of an Acidulated Phosphate Fluoride-pumice Prophylactic Paste: A Two-year Report, *J. Dent. Res.*, 48, 346, May-June, 1969.

95. Mellberg, J. R. and Nicholson, C. R.: In Vitro Evaluation of an Acidulated Phosphate Fluoride Prophylaxis Paste, *Arch. Oral Biol.*, 13, 1223, October, 1968.

96. Zuniga, M. A. and Caldwell, R. C.: The Effect of Fluoride-containing Prophylaxis Pastes on Normal and "White-spot" Enamel, *J. Dent. Child.*, 36, 345, September-October, 1969.

97. Horowitz, H. S. and Heifetz, S. B.: Evaluation of Topical Applications of Stannous Fluoride to Teeth of Children Born and Reared in a Fluoridated Community: Final Report, *J. Dent. Child.*, 36, 355, September-October, 1969.

98. Gish, C. W. and Muhler, J. C.: Effect on Dental Caries in Children in a Fluoride Area of: Combined Use of Three Agents Containing Stannous Fluoride: A Prophylactic Paste, a Solution and a Dentifrice, *J. Am. Dent. Assoc.*, 70, 914, April, 1965.

99. Spedding, R. H.: Three Efficient Technics of Applying a Topical Fluoride Solution, *Dent. Clin. North Am.*, p. 499, July, 1965.

Suggested Readings

Aasenden, R.: Post-eruptive Changes in the Fluoride Concentrations of Human Tooth Surface Enamel, *Arch. Oral Biol.*, 20, 359, May/June, 1975.

Buonocore, M. G. and Ripa, L. W.: Pharmacologic and Therapeutic Aspects of Fluoride, *J. Prev. Dent.*, 1, 12, November-December, 1974.

Bushee, E. J., Grissom, D. K., and Smith, D. R.: An Analysis of Various Fluoride Prophylaxis Products for Free Fluoride Ion Concentrations, *J. Dent. Child.*, 38, 279, July-August, 1971.

Going, R. E., Loehman, R. E., and Chan, M. S.: Mouthguard Materials: Their Physical and Mechanical Properties, *J. Am. Dent. Assoc.*, 89, 132, July, 1974.

Horowitz, H. S.: A Review of Systemic and Topical Fluorides for the Prevention of Dental Caries, *Community Dent. Oral Epidemiol.*, 1, 104, No. 1, 1973.

Horowitz, H. S.: Fluoride: Research on Clinical and Public Health Applications, *J. Am. Dent. Assoc.*, 87, 1013, October, 1973 (Special Issue).

Jenkins, G. N.: Theories on the Mode of Action of Fluoride in Reducing Dental Decay, *J. Dent. Res.*, 42, 444, January-February, 1963 (Supplement).

Katz, S., McDonald, J. L., and Stookey, G. K.: *Preventive Dentistry in Action*. Upper Montclair, N.J., D. C. P. Publishing, 1972, pp. 150-188.

Keyes, P. and Englander, H. R.: Fluoride Therapy in the Treatment of Dentomicrobial Plaque Diseases, *J. Am. Soc. Prev. Dent.*, 5, 16, January-February, 1975.

Newbrun, E., ed.: *Fluorides and Dental Caries*. Springfield, Charles C Thomas, 1972, 132 pp.

Fluoridation

Aasenden, R., Allukian, M., Brudevold, F., and Wellock, W. D.: An *In Vivo* Study on Enamel Fluoride in Children Living in a Fluoridated and in a Nonfluoridated Area, *Arch. Oral Biol.*, 16, 1399, December, 1971.

Bernhardt, M. E.: Fluoridation International, *J. Am. Dent. Assoc.*, 80, 731, April, 1970.

Denby, G. C. and Hollis, M. J.: The Effect of Fluoridation on a Dental Public Health Programme, *New Zeal. Dent. J.*, 62, 32, January, 1966.

Doherty, N. and Powell, E.: Effects of Age and Years of Exposure on the Economic Benefits of Fluoridation, *J. Dent. Res.*, 53, 912, July-August, 1974.

Douglas, B. L., Wallace, D. A., Lerner, M., and Coppersmith, S. B.: Impact of Water Fluoridation on Dental Practice and Dental Manpower, *J. Am. Dent. Assoc.*, 84, 355, February, 1972.

Forrest, J. R.: The Effectiveness of Fluoridation in Europe: A Review, *Br. Dent. J.*, 123, 269, September 19, 1967.

Fuller, J. F.: Cost-benefit and Cost-effectiveness Analysis, *New Zeal. Dent. J.*, 70, 282, October, 1974.

Horowitz, H. S., Law, F. E., and Pritzker, T.: Effect of School Water Fluoridation on Dental Caries, St. Thomas, V. I., *Pub. Health Rep.*, 80, 381, May, 1965.

Horowitz, H. S., Heifetz, S. B., and Law, F. E.: Effect of School Water Fluoridation on Dental Caries: Final Results in Elk Lake, Pa., After 12 Years, *J. Am. Dent. Assoc.*, 84, 832, April, 1972.

Knutson, J. W.: Water Fluoridation After 25 Years, *J. Am. Dent. Assoc.*, 80, 765, April, 1970.

Künzel, W.: The Cost and Economic Consequences of Water Fluoridation, *Caries Res.*, 8, 28, Supplement No. 1, 1974.

United States Department of Health, Education, and Welfare, Public Health Service: *A Guide to Reading on Fluoridation*. Public Health Service Publication No. 1680, Superintendent of Documents, United States Government Printing Office, Washington, D.C., 1967, 11 pp.

Fluoride Tablets

Aasenden, R. and Peebles, T. C.: Effects of Fluoride Supplementation from Birth on Human Deciduous and Permanent Teeth, *Arch. Oral Biol.*, 19, 321, April, 1974.

Arnold, F. A., McClure, F. J., and White, C. L.: Sodium Fluoride Tablets for Children, *Dent. Prog.*, 1, 8, October, 1960.

DePaola, P. F. and Lax, M.: The Caries-inhibiting Effect of Acidulated Phosphate-fluoride Chewable Tablets: A Two-year Double-blind Study, *J. Am. Dent. Assoc.*, 76, 554, March, 1968.

Hennon, D. K., Stookey, G. K., and Muhler, J. C.: The Clinical Anticariogenic Effectiveness of Supplementary Fluoride-vitamin Preparations—Results at the End of Four Years, *J. Dent. Child.*, 34, 439, November, 1967.

Topical Application

Aasenden, R., Brudevold, F., and Richardson, B.: Clearance of Fluoride from the Mouth after Topical Treatment or the Use of a Fluoride Mouthrinse, *Arch. Oral Biol.*, 13, 625, June, 1968.

Cartwright, H. V., Lindahl, R. L., and Bawden, J. W.: Clinical Findings on the Effectiveness of Stannous Fluoride and Acid Phosphate Fluoride as Caries Reducing Agents in Children, *J. Dent. Child.*, 35, 36, January, 1968.

DePaola, P. F.: A Review of Clinical Trials Utilizing Acidulated Phosphate-fluoride Topical Agents, *J. Am. Coll. Dent.*, 35, 22, January, 1968.

Fanning, E. A., Gotjamanos, T., Vowles, N. J., and Van Der Wielen, I.: The Effects of Fluoride Dentifrices on the Incidence and Distribution of Stained Tooth Surfaces in Children, *Arch. Oral Biol.*, 13, 467, April, 1968.

Forrester, D. J. and Auger, M. F.: A Review of Currently Available Topical Fluoride Agents, *J. Dent. Child.*, 38, 272, July-August, 1971.

Heifetz, S. B., Horowitz, H. S., and Driscoll, W. S Utilization of Fluorides in Areas Lacking Centra Water Supplies, *J. Can. Dent. Assoc.*, 40, 13 February, 1974.

Horowitz, H. S. and Chamberlin, S. R.: Pigmentatio of Teeth Following Topical Applications o Stannous Fluoride in a Nonfluoridated Area, *Public Health Dent.*, 31, 32, Winter, 1971.

Horowitz, H. S. and Heifetz, S. B.: The Curren Status of Topical Fluorides in Preventive Denti try, *J. Am. Dent. Assoc.*, 81, 166, July, 1970.

Wei, S. H. Y.: The Potential Benefits to be Derive from Topical Fluorides in Fluoridated Com munities, in Forrester, D. J. and Schulz, E. M eds.: *International Workshop on Fluorides an Dental Caries Reductions.* Baltimore, Marylan 1974, pp. 179-240.

Williams, H. J., Shannon, I. L., and Stevens, F. D The Treatment of Intact Root Surfaces wit Combinations of Fluoride, *J. Am. Soc. Pre Dent.*, 4, 40, July-August, 1974.

Xhonga, F. A. and Sognnaes, R. F.: Dental Erosio Progress of Erosion Measured Clinically Afte Various Fluoride Applications, *J. Am. Den Assoc.*, 87, 1223, November, 1973.

Rinse and Brush with Solution

American Dental Association, Council on Denta Therapeutics: Council Classifies Fluoride Mout rinses, *J. Am. Dent. Assoc.*, 91, 1250, Decembe 1975.

Berggren, H.: Topical Fluorides (Including Den frices), *Int. Dent. J.*, 17, 40, March, 1967.

Berggren, H. and Welander, E.: Supervised Toot brushing with a Sodium Fluoride Solution 5,000 Swedish School Children, *Acta Odon Scand.*, 18, 209, No. 3, 1960.

Birkeland, J. M.: Intra- and Interindividual Observ tions on Fluoride Ion Activity and Retaine Fluoride with Sodium Fluoride Mouth Rinse *Caries Res.*, 7, 39, No. 1, 1973.

Brams, N. U.: Preventive Dentistry in the Scandin vian School Dental Health Service, *Int. Dent. J* 17, 384, June, 1967.

Bullen, D. C. T., McCombie, F., and Hole, L. W Two Year Effect of Supervised Toothbrushin with an Acidulated Fluoride-phosphate Solutio *J. Can. Dent. Assoc.*, 32, 89, February, 1966.

Conchie, J. M., McCombie, F., and Hole, L. W Three Years of Supervised Toothbrushing with Fluoride-phosphate Solution, *J. Public Healt Dent.*, 29, 11, Winter, 1969.

Craig, J. W.: Sodium Fluoride Mouth Rinsing, *Den Health*, 7, 48, July-September, 1968.

Dunn, B. W. and Shannon, I. L.: The Topic Application of Stannous Fluoride in the Unite States Air Force, *J. Oral Thera. and Pharm.*, 4, 3 July, 1967.

Finn, S. B., Moller, P., Jamison, H., Regattieri, L and Manson-Hing, L.: The Clinical Cariostat Effectiveness of Two Concentrations of Acidu lated Phosphate-fluoride Mouthwash, *J. An Dent. Assoc.*, 90, 398, February, 1975.

Forsman, B.: The Caries-Preventing Effect of Mouthrinsing with 0.025% Sodium Fluoride Solution in Swedish Children, *Community Dent. Oral Epidemiol.*, 2, 58, No. 2, 1974.

Frankl, S. N., Fleisch, S., and Diodati, R. R.: The Topical Anticariogenic Effect of Daily Rinsing with an Acidulated Phosphate Fluoride Solution, *J. Am. Dent. Assoc.*, 85, 882, October, 1972.

Gallagher, S. J., Glasgow, I., and Caldwell, R.: Self-application of Fluoride by Rinsing, *J. Public Health Dent.*, 34, 13, Winter, 1974.

Goaz, P. W., McElwaine, L. P., Biswell, H. A., and White, W. E.: Anticariogenic Effect of a Sodium Monofluorophosphate Solution in Children after 21 Months of Use, *J. Dent. Res.*, 45, 286, March-April, 1966.

Heifetz, S. B., Driscoll, W. S., and Creighton, W. E.: The Effect on Dental Caries of Weekly Rinsing with a Neutral Sodium Fluoride or an Acidulated Phosphate-fluoride Mouthwash, *J. Am. Dent. Assoc.*, 87, 364, August, 1973.

Heifetz, S. B., Horowitz, H. S., and Driscoll, W. S.: Two-year Evaluation of a Self-administered Procedure for the Topical Application of Acidulated Phosphate-fluoride: Final Report, *J. Public Health Dent.*, 30, 7, Winter, 1970.

Horowitz, H. S.: The Prevention of Dental Caries by Mouthrinsing with Solutions of Neutral Sodium Fluoride, *Int. Dent. J.*, 23, 585, December, 1973.

Horowitz, H. S., Creighton, W. E., and McClendon, B. J.: The Effect on Human Dental Caries of Weekly Oral Rinsing with a Sodium Fluoride Mouthwash: A Final Report, *Arch. Oral Biol.*, 16, 609, June, 1971.

Horowitz, H. S., Heifetz, S. B., McClendon, B. J., Viegas, A. R., Guimaraes, L. O. C., and Lopes, E. S.: Evaluation of Self-administered Prophylaxis and Supervised Toothbrushing with Acidulated Phosphate Fluoride, *Caries Res.*, 8, 39, No. 1, 1974.

Koch, G.: Effect of Sodium Fluoride in Dentifrice and Mouthwash on Incidence of Dental Caries in Schoolchildren, *Odontol. Revy*, Supplement 12, 1967, 125 pp.

Marthaler, T. M., König, K. G., and Mühlemann, H. R.: The Effect of a Fluoride Gel Used for Supervised Toothbrushing 15 or 30 Times per Year, *Helv. Odontol. Acta*, 14, 67, October, 1970.

Rugg-Gunn, A. J., Holloway, P. J., and Davies, T. G. H.: Caries Prevention by Daily Fluoride Mouthrinsing, *Br. Dent. J.*, 135, 353, October 16, 1973.

Torell, P. and Ericsson, Y.: Two-year Clinical Tests with Different Methods of Local Caries-preventive Fluorine Application in Swedish School-children, *Acta Odont. Scand.*, 23, 287, June, 1965.

Weisz, W. S.: Reduction of Dental Caries Through Use of a Sodium Fluoride Mouthwash, *J. Am. Dent. Assoc.*, 60, 438, April, 1960.

Dentifrices

Aasenden, R.: Fluoride Levels of Human Surface Enamel After the Use of Fluoride Dentifrices, *Arch. Oral Biol.*, 18, 133, January, 1973.

Lind, O. P., Möller, I. J., von der Fehr, F. R., and Larsen, M. J.: Caries-preventive Effect of a Dentifrice Containing 2% Sodium Monofluorophosphate in a Natural Fluoride Area in Denmark, *Community Dent. Oral Epidemiol.*, 2, 104, No. 3, 1974.

Reed, M. W.: Clinical Evaluation of Three Concentrations of Sodium Fluoride in Dentifrices, *J. Am. Dent. Assoc.*, 87, 1401, December, 1973.

Zacherl, W. A.: Clinical Evaluation of Neutral Sodium Fluoride, Stannous Fluoride, Sodium Monofluorophosphate and Acidulated Fluoride-phosphate Dentifrices, *J. Can. Dent. Assoc.*, 38, 35, January, 1972.

Prophylaxis Pastes

DePaola, P. F. and Mellberg, J. R.: Caries Experience and Fluoride Uptake in Children Receiving Semiannual Prophylaxes with an Acidulated Phosphate Fluoride Paste, *J. Am. Dent. Assoc.*, 87, 155, July, 1973.

Gish, C. W., Mercer, V. H., Stookey, G. K., and Dahl, L. O.: Self-application of a Fluoride as a Community Preventive Measure: Rationale, Procedures, and Three-year Results, *J. Am. Dent. Assoc.*, 90, 388, February, 1975.

Peterson, J. K., Horowitz, H. S., Jordan, W. A., and Pugnier, V.: Effectiveness of an Acidulated Phosphate Fluoride-pumice Prophylactic Paste: A Two-year Report, *J. Dent. Res.*, 48, 346, May-June, 1969.

Scola, F. P.: Self-preparation Stannous Fluoride Prophylactic Technique in Preventive Dentistry: Report after Two Years, *J. Am. Dent. Assoc.*, 81, 1369, December, 1970.

Stearns, R. I.: Incorporation of Fluoride by Human Enamel: III. *In Vivo* Effects of Nonfluoride and Fluoride Prophylactic Pastes and APF Gels, *J. Dent. Res.*, 52, 30, January-February, 1973.

Amine Fluorides

DePaola, P. F., Bookstein, F., Foley, S., and Bakhos, J.: The Effect of High-concentration F Mouthrinses on Dental Caries in Children, *I. A. D. R. Program and Abstracts of Papers*, No. L311, February, 1975, p. L78.

Dolan, M. M., Kavanagh, B. J., and Yankell, S.L.: Artificial Plaque Prevention with Organic Fluorides, *J. Periodont.*, 43, 561, September, 1972.

Marthaler, T. H.: Caries Inhibition After Seven Years of Unsupervised Use of Amine Fluoride Dentifrices, *Br. Dent. J.*, 124, 510, June 4, 1968.

Marthaler, T. M.: Caries-inhibition by an Amine Fluoride Dentifrice. Results after 6 Years in Children with Low Caries Activity, *Helv. Odontol. Acta*, 18, Supplement 8, 35, April, 1974.

Shern, R., Swing, K. W., and Crawford, J. J.: Prevention of Plaque Formation by Organic Fluorides, *J. Oral Med.*, 25, 93, July-September, 1970.

Shern, R. J., Rundell, B. B., and Defever, C. J.: Effects of An Amine Fluoride Mouthrinse on the Formation and Microbial Content of Plaque, *Helv. Odontol. Acta, 18,* Supplement 8, 57, April, 1974.

Shern, R. J., Duany, L. F., Senning, R. S., and Zinner, D. D.: Clinical Study of an Amine Fluoride Gel and Acidulated Phosphate Fluoride Gel, *A. A. D. R. Program and Abstracts of Papers,* No. 290, February, 1975, p. 117.

Silvera, R. S.: Salivary Fluoride Levels after Mouthrinsing with Inorganic Fluoride and Amine Fluoride, *Helv. Odontol. Acta, 18,* Supplement 8, 79, April, 1974.

Chapter **30**

Sealants

As part of a complete preventive program, the use of pit and fissure sealants may be indicated for selected patients. Since fluorides protect smooth tooth surfaces more than occlusal surfaces, a method to reduce the incidence of occlusal dental caries is needed. Research studies have shown that the incidence of occlusal caries can be reduced as much as 65 to 90 percent by the application of an adhesive sealant to the occlusal surfaces of caries-free molars and premolars.[1-4]

I. Definition and Action

A pit and fissure resin sealant is an organic polymer which bonds to the enamel surface mainly by mechanical retention. It acts as a physical barrier to prevent oral bacteria and their nutrients from collecting within a pit or fissure and creating the acid environment essential to the initiation of dental caries.

Currently the sealants in clinical use incorporate bisphenol A and glycidyl methacrylate (Bis-G-MA). The technique of application and mode of polymerization differ among available commercial products. Research studies have been conducted to test various potential sealant materials. A list of the reports and review articles is provided in the *Suggested Readings* at the end of this chapter.

II. Selection of Teeth for Sealant Application

All caries-free pits and fissures are not necessarily indicated for sealant application. When evaluation is made and teeth for sealant are chosen selectively, consideration is given the patient's overall caries susceptibility, existing restorations and carious lesions, occlusal anatomy, as well as the other preventive measures used for and by the patient.[5]

Factors to be considered are as follows:

A. Sealants are indicated for occlusal pits and fissures, buccal pits, and cingulum pits of teeth with no dental caries in the surfaces to be treated.

B. Application should be made as soon as possible following eruption. When there is a delay, caries may start, and the surface no longer can be considered for sealant. When possible, sealant can be applied before full eruption, provided there is no tissue flap over the occlusal to interfere with application procedures.

C. Overall caries susceptibility is significant. When there are current carious lesions and previous restorations, newly erupted teeth should be treated with sealants promptly.

D. Sealant is not indicated when there are proximal carious lesions of the same tooth. When the proximal caries is restored, tooth preparation will involve the occlusal surface, and the sealant would be removed.

E. Teeth with deep, narrow pits and fissures are indicated more than when the pits and fissures are shallow and well-coalesced. The latter are less likely to become carious.

F. The age of the patient may have particular significance. However, when teeth have been erupted several years and have not become carious, it should not necessarily follow that they are less susceptible indefinitely. Habits may change. For example, application of a sealant to caries-free occlusal surfaces during early teenage years when caries rates are high may prove to be very important to the individual.

G. Other preventive measures which are being used for and by the patient are necessary. Sealant application should be part of a complete prevention program, not an isolated procedure. As an isolated procedure, there can be patient (and parent) misunderstanding of the selected area of prevention which this measure represents. Other surfaces and other teeth need other methods of preventive protection.

III. Detection of Pit and Fissure Caries

When selecting a tooth for which a sealant application may be indicated, recognition of a gross carious lesion when the tooth structure is clearly broken down and discolored is not difficult. The more difficult lesions to discriminate are those which are small and do not have classic observable characteristics.

Criteria which have been defined for the determination of pit and fissure lesions of facial, occlusal and lingual surfaces are:[6]

A. Area is carious when the explorer "catches" or resists removal after the insertion into a pit or fissure with moderate to firm pressure and when this is accompanied by one or more of the following signs of caries:
  1. A softness at the base of the area.
  2. Opacity adjacent to the pit or fissure as evidence of undermining or demineralization.
  3. Softened enamel adjacent to the pit or fissure which may be scraped away with an explorer.

B. Area is carious if there is loss of the normal translucency of the enamel, adjacent to a pit, which is in contrast to the surrounding tooth structure. The condition is considered to be reliable evidence of undermining. In some of these cases, the explorer may not catch or penetrate the pit.

IV. Application

The manufacturer's directions must be followed carefully for each specific product. Although the basic techniques are similar, there are characteristic steps unique to each product.

General directions are described here in sequence, with brief explanations of the purposes of each step. The main steps are cleaning and drying the tooth surfaces, conditioning (enamel etching), applying the sealant, and polymerization. The success of treatment is dependent to a large degree on precision in the techniques of application.

A. **Clean the Tooth Surface**
  1. Purposes
     a. Remove deposits and debris completely.

b. Permit the chemicals of the sealant procedures to have maximum contact with the enamel surface.

2. Cleaning agent: fine pumice and water. It is important that there be no oil present. Commercial polishing pastes frequently contain ingredients with glycerin or oil, such as flavoring agents.

3. Apply with rubber cup and bristle brush. "Jab" the bristle ends into the pits and fissures in the attempt to remove as much of the bacterial debris as possible.

4. Rinse. Use water only, not mouthwash.

5. Use a fine Number 23 explorer to loosen debris and pumice from the pits and fissures. Rinse thoroughly.

B. **Isolate the Tooth**
1. Purposes
   a. Keep the tooth clean and dry for optimal action and bonding of the sealant.
   b. Eliminate possible contact of saliva and moisture from the breath.
   c. Keep the materials fom contacting the oral tissues, being swallowed accidentally, or being unpleasant to the patient because of flavor.
2. Rubber dam.
   a. Rubber dam application is the method of choice because the most complete isolation is obtained.[7]
   b. It is essential when profuse saliva flow and overactive tongue and oral muscles make retraction and consistent maintenance of a dry, clean field impossible.
   c. Combined treatment should be planned. When a quadrant will have a rubber dam and anesthesia for restoration of other teeth, teeth indicated for sealant may be treated.

d. Rubber dam is not possible when
   (1) Without anesthesia, application of the clamp could not be tolerated by the patient.
   (2) Teeth are not fully erupted and may not hold the rubber dam clamp.

3. Cotton rolls. When rubber dam is not feasible, cotton roll holders are placed, and saliva ejector positioned. Cotton roll isolation procedures are described on pages 435–436.

C. **Dry the Tooth**
1. Purposes
   a. Prepare the tooth for the conditioner.
   b. Prevent dilution and contamination of the conditioner.
2. Use only dry, clean air. Many syringes, particularly the multipurpose types, emit a combination of air and water spray. Some syringes may emit oil.
   a. Clear the air by releasing the spray into a sink before directing it onto the tooth.
   b. Test the air for water content by blowing on the back of the hand or on a mirror surface.

D. **Apply Conditioner for Enamel Etching**
1. Purposes. To increase the adherence of the sealant, the conditioner is used to
   a. Create surface irregularities to increase the area for retention.
   b. Increase the size of the microspaces between prisms so they are accessible to the adhesive.
2. Conditioner used: phosphoric acid. When a 37 percent solution is used, it is applied for one minute; a 50 percent solution is applied for 30 to 60 seconds. The most retentive conditions have been shown to be created when 30 to 37 percent phosphoric acid is used.[8]

3. Rinse with water spray. Suction water out. When cotton roll isolation technique is used, prevent contact of the saliva with the etched enamel.
4. Examine the surface. The etched surface should be a dull, chalky white. When it is not, repeat the application of the conditioner. Primary teeth or older permanent teeth may require a repeat application.

E. **Rinse Thoroughly with Water Spray. Suction the Fluid.**
1. Purposes.
   a. Remove excess acid and complexes formed from the action of the minerals of the tooth and the acid.
   b. Prevent saliva on the etched surface which will reduce the bonding strength of the sealant by depositing the salivary constituents on the surface.
2. Change the cotton rolls immediately and quickly when a rubber dam is not used. Prevent contact of tongue, cheeks, or saliva while changing the cotton rolls.

F. **Dry the Tooth Thoroughly Again**
1. Purposes
   a. Prepare the tooth for the sealant application.
   b. Prevent moisture from reducing the affinity of the adhesive for the enamel surface and preventing penetration of the adhesive into the microspaces created by etching.
2. Dry the tooth thoroughly for 10 to 15 seconds. Use only clean, dry air (see C. above).

G. **Apply the Sealant**
   There are two general types of preparations in current use: one is polymerized by chemical means (benzoyl peroxide) and the other by ul-

traviolet light activating a two percent benzoin methyl ether catalyst. Only general instructions are provided here. The manufacturer's instructions should be followed for specific applications.
1. Chemical polymerization. For the preparation of Concise Enamel Bond, the catalyst and the universal sealant are mixed on a pad and applied to the tooth with a small disposable sponge. It should be clocked for two minutes setting time.[9]
2. Ultraviolet light. Nuva-Seal initiator and sealant are applied to the tooth, and the ultraviolet light, which must be activated five to eight minutes before use, is directed over the sealant. Care must be taken that each portion of the sealant receives the light for 30 clocked seconds. When the light is moved around, or from tooth to tooth when a series of teeth are receiving sealant, polymerization may not be complete in all areas, and the sealant will fail.[10]
   There have been reported reversible cases of eye damage from use of the Nuva-Light. Modifications to the light have solved this problem. It is essential however that each Nuva-Light be checked to determine whether the modifications have been made.
3. Other products: Johnson and Johnson *Adaptic Acid-etch Bonding Agent;* Lee Pharmaceutical *Epoxylite 9075;* Kerr *Pit and Fissure Sealant;* Bosworth *Enamel Bond System.*

H. **Rinse**
1. Examine the surfaces for complete coverage. An explorer will move smoothly over the shiny surface.
2. Remove cotton rolls or rubber dam.

V. Penetration of Sealant

The penetration of a sealant depends on the configuration of the pit or fissure, the presence of deposits and debris within the pit or fissure, and the properties of the sealant itself.[11]

A. Pit and Fissure Anatomy

A review of the anatomy of pits and fissures may be helpful in understanding the effects of sealants in the prevention of dental caries. The shape and depth of pits and fissures vary considerably even within one tooth. There are long narrow pits and grooves which reach to, or nearly to, the dentinoenamel junction. Others are wide V-shaped or narrow V-shaped, while still others may have a long constricted form with a bulbous terminal portion (figure 30–1). The pit or fissure may take a wavy course so that it does not lead directly from the outer surface to the dentinoenamel junction.

B. Contents of a Pit or Fissure

A pit or fissure contains dental plaque, pellicle, debris, and sometimes relatively intact remnants of tooth development.[11]

C. Effect of Cleaning

When a tooth is cleaned and the conditioner is applied, it is not possible to clean out the narrow, long fissures, nor for the conditioner to reach the deeper portions. Retained cleaning material can block the sealant from filling the fissure. It can also become mixed with the sealant.

D. Amount of Penetration

Wide V and shallow fissures are more apt to be filled by sealant (figure 30–2B). Although ideally the sealant should penetrate to the bottom of a pit or fissure, this is frequently impossible because of the debris. Microscopic examination of pits and fissures after

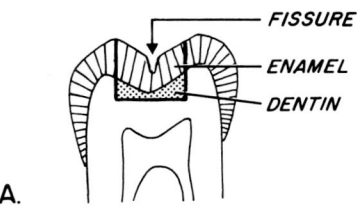

A.

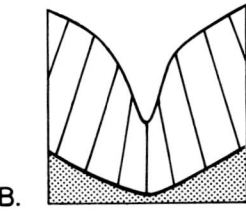

B.

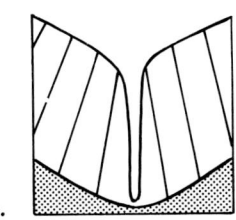

C.

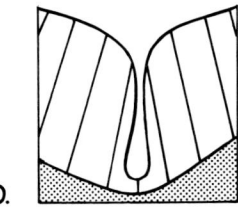

D.

Figure 30–1. Occlusal fissures. Drawings made from microscopic slides to show variations in the shape and depth of fissures. **A.** Tooth showing section enlarged for B, C, and D. **B.** Wide V-shaped fissure. **C.** Long narrow groove which reaches nearly to the dentinoenamel junction. **D.** Long constricted form with a bulbous terminal portion.

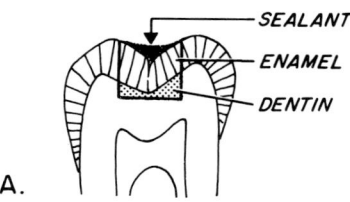

A.

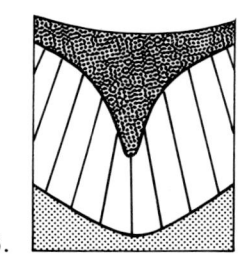

B.

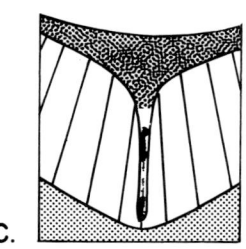

C.

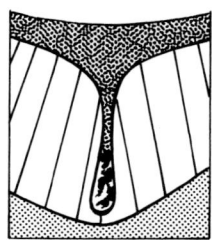

D.

Figure 30–2. Pit and fissure sealant in fissures. Drawings made from microscopic slides to show extent of a fissure filled by sealant. **A.** Tooth showing section enlarged for B, C, and D. **B.** Sealant fills wide V-shaped fissure. **C.** and **D.** Partially filled fissures due to narrow constriction of the groove and blockage by trapped debris.

sealant application has shown that the sealant does not penetrate to the bottom because residual debris, cleaning agents, and trapped air prevent passage of the material (figure 30–2C and D).

E. Caries Prevention

Although access of sealant to the bottom of a fissure or pit is limited, caries prevention by sealants is high.[1-3] The sealant closes the opening to the pit or fissure, and there is no access for additional microorganisms, nutrients (sucrose in particular), and oxygen for aerobic bacteria. The number of viable organisms decreases with time.[12]

VI. Fluoride and Sealant

An original objective in the development of sealants for preventive dentistry was to provide a seal following the topical application of fluoride. Following a topical application without sealant, the loss of fluoride from enamel during the first few days is relatively great. When a sealant was used, considerably more fluoride was retained by the enamel and caries prevention was increased.[13] The sealant used was cyanoacrylate, and although it wore off after a few days, the main purpose had been accomplished.

The development of sealant for mechanical blocking of pits and fissures has not been related to fluoride retention specifically. However, the greatest caries prevention from this type of sealant is obtained when the enamel has had the benefit of fluoride.

A. Topical Application in Conjunction with Sealant

When fluoride is used, it must be applied before the conditioner or after the sealant. It should not be applied between because the bond strength is reduced between the sealant and the etched enamel surface.[14]

B. Combined Preventive Program

Sealants must be considered a part of a total preventive program. While sealant is applicable for certain occlusal surfaces, fluoride applications and other fluoride sources for self-administration are still necessary for all other surfaces.

VII. Retention and Replacement

Complete retention after two years has been shown to range from 54 to 100 per cent.[1-3,15] In one group at the end of the second year, 73 percent had complete retention, 11 percent had partial retention, and 16 percent had no visible retained sealant.[2] Although surface sealant may be lost, sealant in the pits and fissures and that which penetrated into the microspaces of the enamel still remains and provides protection.[16]

A. Factors Which Influence Retention Time

1. Precision of technique. Each step in the preparation of the tooth and the application of the sealant must be carefully performed. It is generally believed that improper technique is the major cause of early loss of sealant from the tooth surface.

2. Any contact of the etched enamel surface either by saliva, water, or any other contaminant before application of the sealant will markedly decrease the effectiveness of the sealant.

3. Abrasion through use, and wear factors such as bruxism, an abrasive dentifrice, and a hard toothbrush, could also influence the removal of sealant from inclined planes.

B. Reexamination.
At each recall, or at least every six months, the sealant should be inspected for deficiencies which may have developed.

C. Replacement.
Consult the manufacturer's instructions. Tooth preparation is the same as for an original application. Re-etching the tooth surface is always essential.

FACTORS TO TEACH THE PATIENT

I. Sealants as a part of a total preventive program. There should be a clear understanding of the teeth and surfaces involved.

II. What a sealant is and why such a meticulous application procedure is required.

III. What can be expected from a sealant: how long it will last, how it prevents dental caries.

IV. Preventive measures for other tooth surfaces. Sealants are not substitutes for other preventive measures including limitations of dietary sucrose, fluorides, and plaque control.

V. Need for examination of the sealant periodically with replacement when indicated.

References

1. Buonocore, M. G.: Caries Prevention in Pits and Fissures Sealed with an Adhesive Resin Polymerized by Ultraviolet Light: A Two-year Study of a Single Adhesive Application, *J. Am. Dent. Assoc.*, 82, 1090, May, 1971.
2. Horowitz, H. S., Heifetz, S. B., and McCune, R. J.: The Effectiveness of an Adhesive Sealant in Preventing Occlusal Caries: Findings After Two Years in Kalispell, Montana, *J. Am. Dent. Assoc.*, 89, 885, October, 1974.
3. Rock, W. P.: Fissure Sealants, Further Results of Clinical Trials, *Br. Dent. J.*, 136, 317, April 16, 1974.
4. Ripa, L. W. and Cole, W. W.: Occlusal Sealing and Caries Prevention: Results 12 Months After a Single Application of Adhesive Resin, *J. Dent. Res.*, 49, 171, January, 1970.
5. Ripa, L. W.: Occlusal Sealing: Rationale of the Technique and Historical Review, *J. Am. Soc. Prev. Dent.*, 3, 32, January-February, 1973.
6. Radike, A. W.: Criteria for Diagnosis of Dental Caries, in American Dental Association, Council on Dental Research and Council on Dental Therapeutics: *Clinical Testing of Cariostatic Agents.* Chicago, American Dental Association, 1968, pp. 87–88.
7. Buonocore, M. G.: Sealants: Questions and Answers, *J. Am. Soc. Prev. Dent.*, 3, 44, January-February, 1973.
8. Silverstone, L. M.: Fissure Sealants. Laboratory Studies, *Caries Res.*, 8, 2, No. 1, 1974.

9. 3M Company, Dental Products, 2501 Hudson, St. Paul, Minnesota 55119.

10. L. D. Caulk Company, P. O. Box 359, Milford, Delaware 19963.

11. Taylor, C. L. and Gwinnett, A. J.: A Study of the Penetration of Sealants into Pits and Fissures, *J. Am. Dent. Assoc.*, *87*, *1181*, November, 1973.

12. Handelman, S. L., Buonocore, M. G., and Schoute, P. C.: Progress Report on the Effect of a Fissure Sealant on Bacteria in Dental Caries, *J. Am. Dent. Assoc.*, *87*, 1189, November, 1973.

13. Dogon, I. L., VanLeeuwen, M., and Kirklin, M.: *In vivo* Studies on the "Sealing" of Fluoride in Teeth: Two Year Clinical Results, *I.A.D.R. Program and Abstracts of Papers*, No. 211, March, 1971, p. 105.

14. Gwinnett, A. J.: The Sequence of Topical Fluoride and Occlusal Sealant Applications, *J. Am. Soc. Prev. Dent.*, *3*, 54, July-August, 1973.

15. Hinding, J. H. and Buonocore, M. G.: The Effects of Varying the Application Protocol on the Retention of Pit and Fissure Sealant: A Two-year Clinical Study, *J. Am. Dent Assoc.*, *89*, 127, July, 1974.

16. Buonocore, M. G.: Pit and Fissure Sealing, *Dent. Clin. North Am.*, *19*, 367, April, 1975.

Suggested Readings

American Dental Association, Council on Dental Materials and Devices: *Guide to Dental Materials and Devices*, 7th ed. Chicago, American Dental Association, 1974–1975, pp. 116–117, 273–274.

Arana, E. M.: Clinical Observations of Enamel After Acid-etch Procedure, *J. Am. Dent. Assoc.*, *89*, 1102, November, 1974.

Buonocore, M. G.: Adhesive Sealing of Pits and Fissures for Caries Prevention, with Use of Ultraviolet Light, *J. Am. Dent. Assoc.*, *80*, 324, February, 1970.

Buonocore, M. G.: Adhesives in the Prevention of Caries, *J. Am. Dent. Assoc.*, *87*, 1000, October, 1973, (Special Issue).

Cueto, E. I. and Buonocore, M. G.: Sealing of Pits and Fissures with an Adhesive Resin: Its Use in Caries Prevention, *J. Am. Dent. Assoc.*, *75*, 121, July, 1967.

Graves, R. C. and Burt, B. A.: The Pattern of the Carious Attack in Children as a Consideration in the Use of Fissure Sealants, *J. Prev. Dent.*, *2*, 28, May-June, 1975.

Gwinnett, A. J.: The Bonding of Sealants to Enamel, *J. Am. Soc. Prev. Dent.*, *3*, 21, January-February, 1973.

Hinding, J.: Extended Cariostasis Following Loss of Pit and Fissure Sealant from Human Teeth, *J. Dent. Child.*, *41*, 201, May-June, 1974.

Katz, S., McDonald, J. L., and Stookey, G. K.: *Preventive Dentistry in Action.* Upper Montclair, N.J., D. C. P. Publishing, 1972, pp. 268–275.

Martinez, C. R.: Sealants—How Effective Are They? in Goldman, H. M., Gilmore, H. W., Irby, W. B., and Olsen, N. H.: *Current Therapy in Dentistry*, Vol. 5. St. Louis, Mosby, 1974, pp. 545–554.

Merrill, S. A., Leinfelder K. F., Oldenburg, T. R., and Taylor, D. F.: Methods of Evaluating Pit and Fissure Sealants, *J. Dent. Child.*, *42*, 43, March-April, 1975.

Pugnier, V. A.: Cyanoacrylate Resins in Caries Prevention: A Two-year Study, *J. Am. Dent. Assoc.*, *84*, 829, April, 1972.

Roydhouse, R. H.: Prevention of Occlusal Fissure Caries by Use of a Sealant; A Pilot Study, *J. Dent. Child.*, *35*, 253, May, 1968.

Rudolph, J. J., Phillips, R. W., and Swartz, M. L.: *In vitro* Assessment of Microleakage of Pit and Fissure Sealants, *J. Prosthet. Dent.*, *32*, 62, July, 1974.

Ryge, G. and Baskin, P.: The Future of Pit and Fissure Sealants, *J. Am. Soc. Prev. Dent.*, *3*, 54, January-February, 1973.

Silverstone, L. M., Saxton, C. A., Dogon, I. L., and Fejerskov, O.: Variation in the Pattern of Acid Etching of Human Dental Enamel Examined by Scanning Electron Microscopy, *Caries Res.*, *9*, 373, No. 5, 1975.

Rubber Dam Application

Bell, B. H. and Grainger, D. A.: *Basic Operative Dentistry Procedures*, 2nd ed. Philadelphia, Lea & Febiger, 1971, pp. 18–21.

Bell, R., Solomon, E., and Randell, S.: Application of Rubber Dam by the Dental Assistant, *Dent. Assist.*, *43*, 20, November, 1974.

Castano, F. A. and Alden, B. A., eds.: *Handbook of Expanded Dental Auxiliary Practice.* Philadelphia, Lippincott, 1973, pp. 68–73.

Cosgrove, D. J.: Rubber Dam in Routine Dentistry, *Dent. Assist.*, *39*, 12, January, 1970.

Cunningham, P. R., Osborne, J. W., and Kaye, L. A.: *Controlling the Operative Field by Use of the Rubber Dam.* Buffalo, State University of New York, 1969.

Park, V. R., Ashman, J. R., and Shelly, G. J.: *A Textbook for Dental Assistants*, 2nd ed. Philadelphia, Saunders, 1975, pp. 355–357, 403–404.

Simon, W. J.: *Clinical Dental Assisting.* Hagerstown, Md., Medical Department, Harper & Row, 1973, pp. 170–175.

V

Instrumentation

INTRODUCTION

Instrumentation for scaling, root planing, gingival curettage, polishing of the teeth and restorations, and postoperative care is included in Part V. Postoperative procedures for dressing placement and removal, suture removal, and treatment of hypersensitive teeth are outlined. Immediate evaluation of techniques and their effects, short-term follow-up, and recall and maintenance evaluation are described.

In the sequence of patient treatment, introduction to preventive measures is first, before professional instrumentation. The first objective of treatment is to create an environment in which the tissues can return to health. The patient's self-care on a daily basis is essential to keep the teeth and gingival tissues free from disease caused by microorganisms. Professional instrumentation makes a limited contribution to arresting the progression of disease without daily plaque control measures by the patient.

I. Oral Prophylaxis: Definition

The term *oral prophylaxis* means those specific treatment procedures aimed at removing local irritants to the gingiva and smoothing and polishing the tooth surfaces. A smooth tooth surface resists the retention of dental deposits. The oral prophylaxis performed with these objectives is truly a *preventive periodontal treatment procedure.*[1]

There is a definite need for clarification and new terminology for the various services performed under the title "oral prophylaxis." Through common usage an oral prophylaxis has taken on a variety of meanings.

Since *prophylaxis* means *prevention of disease,* then *oral prophylaxis,* as the *prevention of oral disease,* would include such preventive procedures as restoring individual teeth, replacing missing teeth, adjusting the occlusion, correction of faulty proximal contacts, and many other procedures the basic purposes of which are preventive.[2] Unfortunately the term oral prophylaxis also is sometimes applied to mean a superficial five to 10-minute polishing of the enamel surfaces which appear above the gingival margin.

II. Preventive Periodontal Treatment Procedure

In the development of a meaningful concept of the oral prophylaxis upon which the techniques and anticipated outcomes described in this book could be based, the acceptable definition could only be one based on the preventive aspects of periodontal diseases. Such treatment procedures must include the *complete* removal of all calculus, and the smoothing of the surfaces of the clinical crown, which is that part of the tooth above the junctional epithelium. Instrumentation performed in this manner can expect to contribute to the accomplishment of the objectives listed below.

III. Objectives of Instrumentation

Specific objectives for each type of instrumentation are included in the chapter which describes the details of technique. General objectives are that dental hygiene instrumentation

A. Aids in the prevention and control of gingival and periodontal diseases by removal of local irritants.

B. Comprises the total gingival treatment needed for certain patients with uncomplicated disease, and the initial preparatory phase of treatment for others with more advanced disease.

C. Assists in the maintenance phase of care.

D. Aids the patient in obtaining, so that he may maintain, oral cleanliness.

E. Assists in instructing the patient in the appearance and feeling of a

thoroughly clean mouth as an aid in motivating him to develop adequate habits of personal oral care.

F. Improves oral esthetics.

G. Introduces the child patient to dental office procedures.

H. Prepares the teeth for application of caries preventive agents.

I. Prepares the teeth and gingiva for dental operations including those performed by the restorative dentist, prosthodontist, orthodontist, pedodontist, and oral surgeon.

IV. Appointment Sequence

At this time information about the dental hygiene treatment plan, particularly pages 294–299, should be studied.

The patient history should be carefully reviewed and preappointment preparation such as premedication checked. The oral tissues are reexamined for orientation in a first appointment and evaluated for the effects of previous treatment when at a succeeding appointment. Instruction is provided as needed and as designated by the treatment plan. Instrumentation, with explanation to the patient for complete patient understanding and cooperation, can then be carried out.

References

1. *World Workshop in Periodontics.* Ann Arbor, University of Michigan, 1966, p. 450.
2. Bunting, R. W.: *Oral Hygiene*, 3rd ed. Philadelphia, Lea & Febiger, 1957, p. 233.

Chapter 31

Principles for Instrumentation

Instrumentation begins with the identification of the various types of instruments for specific services to be performed, and knowledge of the parts of those instruments. Then, to put the instruments into action to accomplish a particular task, requirements are a correct grasp, finger rest, application, adaptation, angulation, and stroke.

A study of oral and dental anatomy and histology necessarily accompanies techniques. Development of a thorough, efficient, and safe procedure depends on an understanding of the characteristics of the teeth and periodontal tissues being influenced.

Knowledge of the specific morphology and topography of each tooth and the relationship to the other teeth in the permanent, mixed, and primary dentitions, is essential to the understanding and use of the instruments. Recognition of the characteristic signs of health and disease of the periodontal tissues provides the basis for application of instruments for treatment.

The dental hygienist's work requires a high degree of skill in the care and use of the fine instruments. Skill is dependent on knowledge and understanding for, as it has been said, "it is the operator who accomplishes the task, not the instrument."[1]

INSTRUMENT IDENTIFICATION

I. Recognition of Instruments

The instruments needed for examination and evaluation were described in Chapter 12, page 183, and instruments for scaling, planing, and gingival curettage are described in Chapter 32, page 473. Other instruments needed for various services may be found with other chapters.

Each dental hygienist must learn to recognize the specific instruments by sight and to distinguish each at a glance by the profile of the instrument on the sterile tray. It is important to be able to designate their names and numbers, and to associate them promptly with the various phases of instrumentation. Such spot identification contributes to neatness of tray arrangement and efficiency of operation through prompt selection of the proper instrument for the service to be performed.

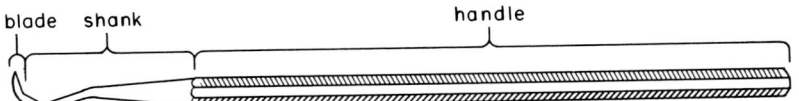

Figure 31–1. Scaler to illustrate the parts of an instrument. The working end of the scaler is the blade.

II. Instrument Parts

There are three major parts: the working end, the shank, and the handle or shaft. The relationship of these parts is illustrated by the scaler in figure 31–1.

A. Working End

The working end refers to that part used to carry out the purpose and function of the instrument. Each working end is unique to the particular instrument.

1. Sharp instruments. The working end of a sharp instrument is called a *blade*. The parts of a sharp blade are the
    a. Cutting edge: a line where two surfaces meet. For example the facial surface and the lateral surfaces meet to form the sharp cutting edge of a sickle (figures 32–1 and 32–2, page 474) or a curet (figure 32–5, page 477).
    b. Lateral surfaces: the lateral surfaces meet or are continuous (as in the curved curet) to form the back of the instrument.

2. Non-sharp instruments. The working end of a non-sharp instrument is a dull blade, or a *nib*. Although the term nib is primarily applied to instruments for restorative dentistry such as a condenser or burnisher, it may also apply to non-sharp ends such as the wood point at the end of the porte polisher (page 557) and the rubber cup of the prophylaxis angle (page 544).

B. Shank

1. Connects the working end with the handle.

2. May be angled, curved, or straight; the more restricted the access to an area, the greater number of shank angles are usually required. Anterior teeth are more accessible; therefore straight-shanked instruments can be used. Posterior teeth need angled-shank instruments, particularly for proximal surfaces.

C. Handle

1. Double-ended instruments have paired (mirror image) or complementary working ends attached to one handle. Single-ended instruments have one working end.

2. Cone socket handles are separable from the shank and working end and permit instrument exchanges and replacements.

INSTRUMENT USE

I. Instrument Grasp

Stability is essential for effective, controlled action of an instrument. The correct use depends on maintaining *control* of the movement of the instrument through use of an effective *grasp* and the establishment and maintenance of an appropriate, firm, fulcrum *finger rest*.

A. Functions of the Instrument Grasp

The manner in which the instrument is held influences the entire procedure. A rigid grasp in which the instrument is gripped tightly, lessens the tactile sensitivity and hence the effectiveness of instrumentation. The appropriate grasp is firm, displays the confidence of the operator in the work being done, and provides the following effects:

1. Increased fingertip tactile sensitivity.
2. Positive control of the instrument with flexibility of motion.
3. Decreased hazard of trauma to the dental and periodontal tissues, which results in less postoperative discomfort for the patient.
4. Prevention of fatigue to operator's fingers, hand, and arm.

B. **Types**
   1. *Modified Pen Grasp.*
      a. Description. The modified pen grasp is a three-finger grasp with the tips of the thumb, index finger, and middle (second) finger all in contact with the instrument. The ring finger is the finger rest. The instrument is held by the thumb and index finger at the junction of the shank and handle, with the middle (second) finger placed on the shank to hold and guide the movement (figure 31–2).
      b. The shank of the instrument is held against the pad of the middle finger. The instrument is not held across the nail or the side of the middle finger as in a pen grasp usually used for writing (figure 31–3). The specific position of the middle finger is extremely important to instrument control in preventing the instrument from slipping during manipulation.
   2. *Palm Grasp*
      a. Description. The handle of the instrument is held in the palm by cupped index, middle, ring, and little fingers. Thumb is free to serve as fulcrum (figure 31–4).
      b. Limitations of use. Instruments for scaling, planing, and gingival curettage are not used with a palm grasp. The possible excep-

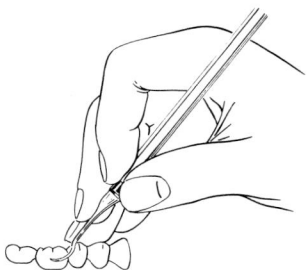

Figure 31–2.   Instrument grasp and finger rest. In the *modified pen grasp* as shown, the instrument is held by the thumb and index finger near the junction of the handle and shank, with the middle finger placed on the shank to control and guide the movement. The finger rest is maintained by the ring and little fingers on a firm tooth surface near the area of operation.

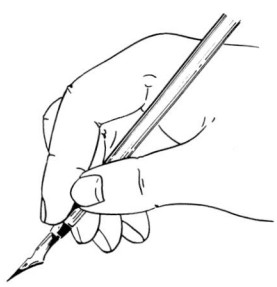

Figure 31–3.   Pen grasp. For writing, a pen is frequently held with the side of the pen handle against the side of the middle finger. Compare this with figure 31–2 which shows a modified pen grasp as used during instrumentation.

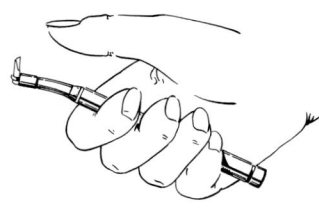

Figure 31–4.   Palm grasp. Instrument handle is held in the palm by cupped index, middle, ring, and little fingers. Thumb is free and serves as the finger rest.

tion is the chisel when it is used to remove gross calculus by a push stroke (page 476). The palm grasp limits operation in that there is less tactile sensitivity and less flexibility of movement.

   c. Examples of uses
     (1) Air syringe
     (2) Rubber dam clamp holder
     (3) Handpiece grasp for instrument sharpening (figure 32–15, page 489)
     (4) Porte polisher for facial surfaces.

II. Fulcrum: Finger Rest

A fulcrum must always be used when instruments are applied to the teeth.

A. Definition
1. The support, or point of rest, on which a lever turns in moving a body.
2. The support, or point of finger rest on the tooth surface, on which the hand turns in moving an instrument.

B. Objectives
An effective, well-established fulcrum is essential to the following:
1. Stability for controlled action of the instrument.
2. Prevention of injury to the patient's oral tissues which can result from irregular pressure and uncontrolled movement.
3. Comfort for the patient; confidence in operator's ability which results from the feeling of securely applied instruments.

C. Digits Used for Fulcrum
1. Modified pen grasp
   a. Ring finger. Little finger is held close beside ring finger (figure 31–2).
   b. Supplementary: pad of middle finger rests lightly on incisal or

occlusal surface of tooth being scaled or polished: ring finger maintains regular fulcrum position and middle finger maintains its grasp on instrument.
   c. Fingers are slightly curved for support.
2. Palm grasp: thumb.

D. Location of Fulcrum
1. *Purposes for Selection*
   a. For convenience to area of operation.
   b. For ease in adaptation of instrument, maintenance of effective grasp, and application of correct angulation of the instrument to the tooth.
   c. For stability and control of instrument during the strokes.
2. *Principles*
   a. Maintain rest on firm solid tooth or teeth. The patient's chin, lips, and cheeks are mobile and flexible and therefore unreliable for stability.
   b. Where possible, the rest should be on the same arch, maxillary or mandibular, as the instrumentation; also where possible, in the same quadrant.
   c. The first choice for a rest is usually the tooth adjacent to the one where the instruments are to be applied.

E. Variations of Fulcrum
1. Need for variation
A basic fulcrum location cannot always be used or may require supplementation. Variations may be used only after conventional fulcrum positioning has been tried and shown ineffective. Repeated attempts to vary fulcrum rests are inefficient and time-consuming.
   a. A patient's facial musculature, oral anatomic features, dental anatomy, or a physical handicap

affecting the oral cavity indirectly may interfere with customary positioning for instrumentation.

b. Tenacious calculus in difficult-access areas may not be displaced and root surfaces planed by the usual procedures. Greater support and pressure to the instrument are required.

2. General categories of variations[2,3]

When the problem in instrumentation seems to be related to space and accessibility, the height and position of the patient's oral cavity should be checked as well as a possible change in operator's working position. When a variation in finger rest is used, apply basic rules for stability and control and avoid rests on movable tissues. Three types of variations are suggested here: a substitute, supplementary, or a reinforced finger rest. Descriptions are given for the right-handed operator.

a. *Substitute*

(1) Missing teeth where finger rest is usually applied. For an edentulous area a cotton roll or gauze sponge may be packed into the area to provide a solid dry rest area. Otherwise a rest across the dental arch or in the opposite arch may provide stability.

(2) Mobile teeth, or teeth with inadequate bony support (as shown by radiographs), should be either avoided as finger rests or used only with minimal pressure for brief periods. Not only would the rest on a mobile tooth be unstable, but pressure, movement, and undue stress on the tooth could traumatize and tear the periodontal ligament fibers.

(3) Index finger of left hand may be placed in the vestibule over a cotton roll. The usual finger rest can be placed on that. This aids retraction and visibility, particularly in the mouth of a small child.

b. *Supplemental*

(1) Third (middle) finger, which is the support finger on the shank of the instrument (modified pen grasp), can be rested on the incisal or occlusal beside the ring finger rest. Unless its grasp on the instrument is maintained, this position cannot strengthen or supplement the fulcrum, but rather can weaken it.

(2) Index finger of left hand placed on the occlusal of teeth adjacent to working area, and ring finger fulcrum is applied to the left index finger. This supplement or support is especially applicable for the maxillary right lingual area, but only when the patient's head can be turned for adequate direct vision. Such supplements are not useful for distal surfaces where the mouth mirror is essential for vision.

c. *Reinforced*

(1) In this type, a support is placed between the instrument handle and the working end to provide additional strength and force, particularly for hard tenacious calculus in pockets. Greater control of the instrument can result and, when applied correctly, reduce the danger of instrument breakage. A definite rest for both hands is needed.

(2) Index finger of left hand can be rested on the tooth adjacent to the one being scaled (or on the tooth being scaled if there is no danger of stabbing the finger should the instrument slip). The ring finger (right hand) applies the fulcrum to the left index finger. The thumb of the left hand is placed on the instrument shank (or handle) for a reinforcement.

F. **Touch or Pressure Applied to Fulcrum**

The fulcrum finger maintains a firm hold with moderate pressure to balance the action of the instrument being applied. Excessive pressure on the fulcrum rest can result in decreased stability for the controlled action of the instrument as well as fatigue in the operator's fingers and hand.

1. Mandibular fulcrums: heavy pressure on the movable mandible can cause fatigue and discomfort for the patient.
2. Maxillary fulcrums: since the maxilla is stationary, fulcrums on maxillary teeth should be used whenever possible for maxillary instrumentation to provide greater stability during instrumentation as well as comfort for the patient.

III. Adaptation

With an appropriate grasp and finger rest, the instrument is next ready for application. The working end of the instrument is adapted to the surface of the tooth or tissue where instrumentation is to take place. *Adaptation* refers to the relationship between the instrument and the surface of the tooth or soft tissue.

A. **Relation to Tooth Morphology**

Adaptation of instruments and tooth and soft tissue morphology are closely related. Adaptation depends on a knowledge of oral anatomy and morphology. The adaptation of the instrument is of significance because of the completeness of service, as well as of the potential damage to the teeth and gingival tissue. Improperly adapted instruments can damage the tooth surface or remove excess tooth substance.

Areas where instrument adaptation is most difficult and which require more attention, time, and careful application of skill, include the following:[4]

1. Line angles. All line angles require that the instrument be rolled between the fingers to turn the working end as the instrument is activated. At each change of direction around a line angle, the instrument must be turned to keep it adapted to the surface.
2. Convex and rounded surfaces, particularly of narrow roots.
3. Cervical area where the root is constricted.
4. Proximal root surfaces which may be concave and may have longitudinal grooves and open furcations. The same features may be on facial and lingual surfaces and present nearly an equally difficult problem.

B. **Characteristics of a Well-adapted Instrument**

1. The working end of the instrument is correctly positioned for the task to be accomplished. For example, when scaling, the angle formed by the facial surface of the instrument and the tooth surface is crucial. Angulation is described below.
2. As much as possible of the working end of the instrument is used. The instrument is adapted for maximum usefulness of the working end. For example, this may be two to three

millimeters of the end of a curet when on a "flat" surface, whereas at a convex surface of a narrow root, less than two millimeters may be adaptable.

3. It will not harm the tissue being worked on or the surrounding or adjacent tissues.
4. It will not damage or break the instrument itself.
5. The working end is applied so that it fits closely to the surface; it is applied to conform to the contour of the surface.
6. As the instrument is activated, it can be adjusted to changes required by variations in the surface topography.

IV. Angulation

A factor closely related to, and directly influencing, instrument adaptation is angulation. Angulation refers to the angle formed by a working end of an instrument with the surface to which the instrument is applied. Each instrument is applied to a surface in a specific manner for optimum operation.

A. **Probe.** The usual adaptation of a probe is to maintain the side of the working tip on the tooth, with the long axis of the working end close to parallel with the tooth surface (page 189). As used for a bleeding index, the tip is placed inside the pocket wall and pressed slightly on the wall as the probe is moved in a horizontal direction around the tooth (figure 19–1, page 279).

B. **Explorer.** An explorer is held with the tip at a right angle to the occlusal surface when detecting occlusal pit or fissure caries, but on other surfaces the side of the tip is kept on the tooth at all times. The angle is five degrees or less.

C. **Scalers and Curets.** For scaling and root planing, they are adapted to the tooth surface at an angulation which permits effective calculus removal and planing. An angle less than 90 degrees but not less than 45 degrees is effective. For gingival curettage, the angle is made with the soft tissue wall of the inside of the pocket and also is less than 90 degrees but more than 45. Angulation for a scaler or curet means the angle formed by the face of the instrument with the surface of the tooth or soft tissue. This is further described on page 521 with figure 34–1.

V. Stroke

A. **Definition.** A stroke is a single unbroken movement made by an instrument. It is the action of an instrument in the performance of the task for which it was designed.

B. **Characteristics***
1. Types
   a. *Pull.* Example: scaler removing calculus.
   b. *Push.* Example: exploratory stroke when a curet is being positioned.
   c. *Combined push and pull.* Example: explorer in a walking stroke, which is moving the instrument up and down with equal pressure on the surface.
   d. *Walking stroke.* Example: probe is moved up and down, touching the bottom of the sulcus with each down stroke (figure 12–6, page 191).
2. Directions
   a. *Vertical:* strokes parallel with the long axis of a tooth.
   b. *Horizontal:* strokes perpendicular with the long axis of a tooth. They are sometimes called circumferential, which should not

*Description of strokes for each instrument is included in the respective chapters. The probe is described on pages 191, 279; the explorer, page 200; scalers and curets, pages 503 and 505–506; curettage, page 521; handpiece, page 546.

be interpreted to mean that a stroke can be made to go around a tooth or large segment of a tooth. A horizontal stroke necessarily must be a short stroke because of the constant changes in the topography.

    c. *Diagonal or oblique:* stroke which is diagonal to the long axis of the tooth.

    d. *Circular:* stroke used with a porte polisher. A small one-to-two mm. diameter circular stroke is used with pressure, for example to apply desensitizing paste (page 565).

C. **Factors Which Influence Selection of Stroke**
1. Size, contour, and position of gingiva.
2. Surface and section of surface where the instrument is used.
3. Depth of sulcus or pocket.
4. Size and shape of instrument used.

D. **Nature of Stroke**
1. Motion for a stroke is generated by a unified action of the shoulder, arm, wrist, and hand.
2. The grasp of a scaler or curet is light while the working end is positioned for the stroke and then the instrument is held more firmly during movement. An explorer and a probe should be held lightly for tactile sensitivity at all times.
3. During a stroke the whole hand pivots or rotates around the fulcrum.
4. The length of the stroke is limited by the action of the entire arm.
5. The stroke is short, controlled, decisive, and directed to protect the tissues from trauma.

E. **Touch and Pressure**
1. Explorers and probe: a light touch for maximum degree of tactile sensitivity.
2. Scalers and curets: a light but secure touch without pressure for the exploratory stroke used in preparation for calculus removal or root planing (page 505), then a definite controlled pressure for deposit removal during the working stroke.
3. Porte polisher: firm, secure, even pressure during the polishing stroke. A circular stroke may be used and when the instrument is applied near the gingival margin, the stroke is lightened during that part of the circle which is directed toward the gingiva.
4. Prophylaxis angle: the rubber cup is applied with light pressure in short but firm strokes.

VI. **Visibility and Accessibility**
A. **Effects of Adequate Vision and Accessibility**
1. Instrumentation will be more thorough with minimum trauma to the oral tissues.
2. Length of time required will be lessened, accompanied by less fatigue for patient and dental hygienist.
3. Patient cooperation will be increased because of shortened operating time and less discomfort.

B. **Components**
1. Patient and operator positions (pages 48–53).
2. Efficient use of direct or reflected (by mouth mirror) illumination for each tooth surface.
3. Adequate yet gentle retraction of lips, cheeks, and tongue with consideration for the patient's comfort and operator's convenience.

VII. **Thoroughness of Procedure**
    During treatment, each particle of deposit and stain must be removed from the tooth surfaces. A firm technique with a painstaking approach will achieve both

he complete removal of deposits and omfort for the patient. Since time is nvolved, a happy medium is possible vith time minimized, yet the patient's issues treated with maximum respect.

"Roughness, under the guise of increased diligence, should not be confused vith thoroughness."[5] Roughness is generally associated with carelessness, and either has any place in dental hygiene rocedures. Possible effects of roughness re:

1. Infliction of unnecessary pain during operation.
2. Prolonged postoperative discomfort.
3. Production of excessive bleeding and debris which hinder the efficiency of the operator.
4. Production of tissue lacerations which retard healing.
5. Gouging of tooth surfaces which may produce postoperative sensitivity.
6. Forcing of infected material into the deeper periodontal tissues which can lead to postoperative infection.

DEXTERITY DEVELOPMENT FOR THE USE OF INSTRUMENTS

This section is included particularly for he beginning dental hygiene student and or the graduate dental hygienist who plans to return to practice after a period of retirement. A primary objective when earning or reviewing techniques for nstrumentation is to develop the ability o hold instruments correctly while employing them for use.

However generally dexterous a person may be, the use of new or unusual nstruments requires different procedures or coordination. Control is essential, and guided strength contributes to control.

Proficiency during techniques comes rom repeated correct use of the instruments. Exercise for the fingers, hands, and arms supplement experience. Directed exercises are needed for both hands, separately and together. To facilitate the development of dexterity, certain exercises have been selected to supplement other types of practice such as the use of instruments on a manikin. A regular period of time each day during the training period should be set aside for exercises.

I. Squeezing a Ball

A. **Purposes**
1. To develop general muscles of hand and arm.
2. To develop strength and control for use of palm grasp.

B. **Tennis Ball**
1. Hold ball in palm of hand, grip with thumb and all fingers.
2. Tighten and release grip at regular intervals.
3. One hand rests while other is holding the ball.

C. **Chip Blower**
1. Hold bulb in palm of hand, grip with middle, ring, and little finger.
2. Use thumb and index finger to maintain nozzle in stationary position such as that required when directing air on the teeth.
3. Rest one hand while other is exercising the chip blower.

II. Stretching a Rubber Band

A. **Purposes**
1. To strengthen fingers and hand muscles.
2. To develop control of finger movements.
3. To develop ability to separate ring and middle fingers, while keeping ring and little fingers together and index and middle fingers together to simulate application of a finger rest.

B. **Rubber Band on Finger Joints**
   1. Place rubber band at joint between first phalanx and second phalanx.
   2. Stretch band by separating middle and ring fingers.
   3. Place rubber band at joint between second phalanx and third phalanx and proceed as before.
   4. Place rubber bands on both hands and do exercises together.
   5. Use rubber bands of smaller size as strength and control increase.

C. **Rubber Band on Finger Joints with Use of Fulcrum**
   1. Place rubber band on joint between first phalanx and second phalanx.
   2. Establish fulcrum finger (ring finger) on tabletop with little finger closely adjacent to it; elbow and forearm free as they are during instrumentation. Stretch band by separating middle and ring fingers.
   3. Touch thumb and index and middle fingers to simulate a modified pen grasp for instrument. Stretch band by separating middle and ring fingers.
   4. Variations.
      a. Hold instrument in modified pen grasp while doing the exercise.
      b. Do writing exercise with rubber band in place.
   5. Rest one hand while other is being exercised.

III. Writing

A. **Purposes**
   1. To develop correct instrument modified pen grasp.
   2. To propel instrument without moving fingers.
   3. To practice use of instruments when mouth mirror is required.
   4. To develop control and precision.

B. **Circles and Vertical Lines**
   1. Hold long, well-sharpened, wooden lead pencil with modified pen grasp.
   2. Establish fulcrum finger (ring finger) on tabletop; forearm and elbow free.
   3. Inscribe counterclockwise small circles and vertical lines on paper, rapidly and lightly at first, slowly and with more pressure later.
   4. Accomplish writing by activation of the hand by the upper arm, without flexing or extending the thumb and fingers holding the pencil.
   5. Practice each hand separately at first, then use pencil in each hand at the same time, alternating writing action to simulate adaptation of, first, the mirror and then the explorer or scaler.

C. **Using Mouth Mirror**
   1. Hold mouth mirror with modified pen grasp in left hand close to pencil while practicing writing exercises (III B) through the mirror. Reverse hands.
   2. Using engineer's graph paper and modified pen grasp with fulcrum as described earlier, follow the lines of the small squares while looking in mirror held with opposite hand.

D. **Everyday Penmanship**
   1. Use modified pen grasp whenever possible for writing.
   2. Practice word writing with the left hand (with the right hand for left-handed person) to increase dexterity for handling mouth mirror.

IV. Mouth Mirror, Cotton Pliers, and Explorer

A. **Purposes**
   1. To develop ability to turn mouth mirror at various angles.
   2. To develop dexterity in holding objects with cotton pliers while operating.
   3. To establish desired grasp of explorer to assure maximum touch sensitivity.

B. **Mouth Mirror**
1. Holding mouth mirror with modified pen grasp, ring finger on tabletop as fulcrum finger with little finger closely adjacent to it, elbow and forearm free.
2. Practice turning mirror with fingers, adjusting as to the several surfaces of the tooth.
3. Hold a small object in opposite hand for viewing in mirror.
4. Practice crossing the mirror over fulcrum finger as in position for retracting lower lip with fulcrum finger while viewing lingual surfaces of mandibular anterior teeth in mouth mirror.

C. **Cotton Pliers**
1. Make small tight cotton pellets with thumb and index and middle fingers of each hand; then make one in each hand simultaneously.
2. Hold cotton pliers with modified pen grasp and establish fulcrum finger on tabletop; elbow and forearm free.
3. Practice picking up cotton pellets.
   a. Use in wiping motion on tabletop or other object.
   b. Move to different area to release pellet.

D. **Explorer**
1. Hold explorer with modified pen grasp and establish fulcrum finger on tabletop with upper arm and forearm free.
2. Use extracted teeth to feel with explorer tip until a light grasp permits maximum security of grasp and maximum sense of touch. Extracted teeth can provide a contrast

between exploring enamel, cementum, calculus, or other rough area of tooth surface (page 181).

TECHNICAL HINTS

A. Time spent on exercises should be sufficient in any one period to cause moderate (but never severe) strain and fatigue of hand muscles.

B. To relax the muscles of the hands during a practice session, wash hands in warm water.

References

1. Goldman, H. M. and Cohen, D. W.: *Periodontal Therapy*, 4th ed. St. Louis, Mosby, 1968, p. 389.
2. Pattison, A. M. and Behrens, J.: *Dental Hygiene: The Detection and Removal of Calculus.* Reston, Virginia, Reston Publishing, 1973, pp. 112, 247.
3. Pederson, J.: *Variations in Fulcrum* (mimeographed). Albuquerque, University of New Mexico, Dental Hygiene Program, 1974.
4. Terwilliger, D. and Schwindt, S.: *Instrument Adaptation as Related to Tooth Root Morphology.* Ann Arbor, School of Dentistry, University of Michigan, 1975, 80 pp.
5. Glickman, I.: *Clinical Periodontology*, 3rd ed. Philadelphia, Saunders, 1964, p. 496.

Suggested Readings

Barton, R. E., Sockwell, C. L., and Taylor, D. F.: Cutting Instruments; Patient and Operator Positions, in Sturdevant, C. M., Barton, R. E., and Brauer, J. C., eds.: *The Art and Science of Operative Dentistry.* New York, Blakiston Division, McGraw-Hill, 1968, pp. 117–121.

Hard, D.: Oral Prophylaxis, in Bunting, R. W.: *Oral Hygiene*, 3rd ed. Philadelphia, Lea & Febiger, 1957, pp. 249–258.

Hirschfeld, L.: Subgingival Curettage in Periodontal Treatment, *J. Am. Dent. Assoc.*, 44, 301, March, 1952.

Lieberman, N. W.: Your Best Dental Instrument, Your Hands: Exercises to Reduce Muscle Fatigue, *Dent. Surv.*, 49, 56, April, 1973.

Tondrowski, V. E.: Preclinical Procedures for the Dental Hygiene Student, *J. Dent. Educ.*, 20, 321, November, 1956.

Chapter 32

Instruments and Sharpening

Knowledge and understanding of the purpose and use of each instrument and the development of dexterity in the effective manipulation of the instruments are basic to clinical dental hygiene practice. The clinical results obtained for the patient depend in part on the proficiency and thoroughness with which the instrumentation is accomplished. The main purpose of instrumentation is to create an environment about the teeth in which the tissues can heal and be maintained in health.

Each instrument is designed for a specific application during calculus removal and root planing. When an instrument is intended for submarginal use, the design should be such that the gingival tissue surrounding the working area will not be damaged. The five general categories of instruments for scaling and root planing are the sickle, hoe, chisel, curet, and file. The characteristics and functional purposes of each type will be described in the sections following.

Instruments are made of carbon steel, stainless steel, or stainless steel with tungsten carbide blades. Carbide steel is harder than stainless and will maintain sharpness longer, but when unprotected and not given careful postoperative care, it can become discolored from corrosion; stainless steel on the other hand will usually maintain its bright shiny appearance. The tungsten carbide instruments retain their sharpness for long periods.

When an instrument is to be used for the first time, it is advisable to examine the blade and cutting edge under a magnifying glass. A clear understanding of the relationship of the cutting edge or edges to the other parts of the instrument is essential for correct angulation during instrumentation and for positioning on the sharpening stone so that the original form can be preserved during sharpening.

I. Sickle Scaler

By definition a sickle is curved. However, there are variations in the shapes of sickle scalers and in some forms the blade and cutting edges are straight. When reference is made to the instrument with a curved or straight blade, the types have frequently been called "curved sickle" or "straight sickle."

Straight and curved sickles may be further classified as straight or modified (contra-angled) with reference to the angulation of the shank as it relates to the instrument handle and the blade. In this grouping, straight sickles are generally single, whereas modified are generally paired for adaptation from both facial and lingual aspects. Paired instruments may be made on separate handles or double-ended.

To the new student, classification as "curved" or "straight" and "straight" or "modified" may seem confusing. However, in general use, when reference is made to the various instruments, it may be more convenient to call the individual instrument by its trade name or number.

A. **Curved Sickle Scaler**
1. Two cutting edges on a curved blade (figure 32–1).
2. Facial or inner surface between the cutting edges is flat in cross section and curved lengthwise.
3. The facial surface converges with the two lateral surfaces to form the tip of the scaler which is a sharp point.
4. Cross section of the blade: some are triangular (figure 32–1 B); others are trapezoidal.
5. Internal angles of 70 to 80 degrees are formed where the lateral sur-

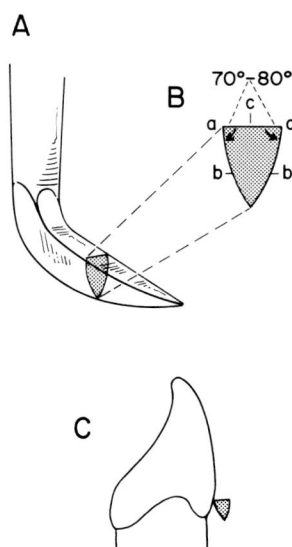

Figure 32–2. Straight sickle scaler. **A.** The two straight cutting edges meet at the pointed end. **B.** Cross section shows lateral surfaces (b and b) and facial surface (c). Cutting edges (a and a) are formed where the lateral surfaces meet the facial surface. **C.** The blade is applied to the tooth for scaling so that the facial surface is at an angle of less than 90 degrees with the tooth surface but not less than 45 degrees.

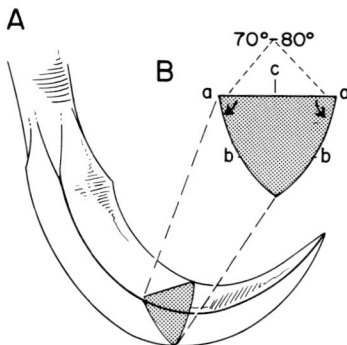

Figure 32–1. Curved sickle scaler. **A.** The curved blade terminates in a point. **B.** Cross section shows the two lateral surfaces (b and b) and the facial surface (c). The two cutting edges (a and a) are formed where the lateral surfaces meet the facial surface at a 70 to 80 degree angle.

faces (b and b in figure 32–1 B) meet the facial surface (c) at the cutting edges (a and a).

B. **Straight Sickle**
1. Two cutting edges on a straight blade (figure 32–2).
2. Facial surface between the cutting edges is flat.
3. The facial surface converges with the two lateral surfaces to form the tip of the scaler which is a sharp point.
4. Cross section of the blade: triangular (figure 32–2 B).
5. Internal angles of 70 to 80 degrees are formed where the lateral surfaces (b and b in figure 32–2 B) meet the facial surface (c) at the cutting edges (a and a).

C. **Angulation of the Shank**
1. Both curved and straight bladed sickles are available with angulated or straight shanks.
2. *Straight.* Single instrument in which the relationships of the shank, blade, and handle are in a flat plane; adaptable primarily for anterior teeth, although may be used for scaling premolars when the lips and cheeks permit retraction for correct angulation.
3. *Modified or Contra-Angle.* Paired instruments which are mirror images of each other to provide access to the proximal surfaces of posterior teeth; one adapts from the buccal and the other from the lingual.

D. **Purposes and Uses of Sickle Scalers**
1. Principally for the *removal of supramarginal calculus.*
2. May be useful for removal of gross calculus which is slightly below the gingival margin when the calculus is continuous with the supramarginal calculus and when the gingival tissue is spongy and flexible to permit easy insertion of the instrument.
3. Contraindications for use of sickle scalers submarginally:
   a. Cause undue trauma to the gingival tissue because of the large size, thickness, and length of the blade.
   b. Pointed tip and straight cutting edges cannot be adapted to the curved tooth surfaces: there is greater possibility for grooving or scratching the cemental surface.
   c. Tactile sensitivity decreased with larger, heavier blades.
4. Small sickle scalers, such as the Jaquettes, can be useful for fine supramarginal deposits in the contact areas and between overlapping teeth.

E. **Application**
1. Angulation: blade is applied to the tooth so that the inner or facial surface of the scaler is at an angle of less than 90 degrees with the tooth surface but not less than 45 degrees (figure 32–2C).
2. Stroke: pull stroke only for this type of blade.

II. **Hoe Scaler**

A. **Characteristics**
1. Single, straight cutting edge (figure 32–3).
2. Blade turned at a 99- to 100-degree angle to the shank.
3. Cutting edge beveled at a 45-degree angle to the end of the blade (figure 32–3B).
4. Shank: variously angulated for adaptation of cutting edges to accessible tooth surfaces; some are paired.

B. **Purposes and Uses**
1. Removes supramarginal calculus, particularly large, accessible tenacious pieces.

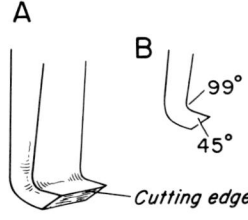
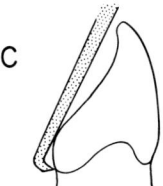

Figure 32–3. Hoe scaler. **A.** The hoe has a single cutting edge. **B.** The blade is turned at an angle of 99 degrees to the shank, and the cutting edge is beveled at a 45-degree angle. **C.** Adaptation to the tooth for removal of calculus is with a two-point contact when possible.

2. May be useful to remove gross calculus two to three millimeters below the gingival margin provided the tissue is spongy and flexible and is easily displaced.
3. Contraindications for use submarginally
    a. Insertion of the thick-bladed instrument into the sulcus causes distension of the pocket wall.
    b. Lack of adaptability of the wide straight cutting edge to the curved root surface.
    c. Difficulty of use without gouging the cemental surface.
    d. Lack of sensitivity because of the bulk of the instrument and the marked angulation of the shanks of some hoes.
    e. Cannot reach the bottom of the pocket without stretching and possibly tearing the gingival pocket wall unnecessarily because of the size and shape of the blade.

C. **Application**
    1. With full width of the cutting edge in contact with the tooth surface and, when possible, a two-point contact with the tooth during the positioning and activation to stabilize the instrument. Two-point contact means contact of the cutting edge and the side of the shank with the tooth (figure 32–3 C).
    2. Positioning of the shank : parallel to or nearly parallel to the long axis of the tooth.
    3. Hoes are not generally applied to proximal surfaces except the surface adjacent to an edentulous area.
    4. Stroke: pull stroke toward occlusal or incisal.

III. Chisel Scaler

A. **Characteristics**
    1. Single straight cutting edge (figure 32–4).

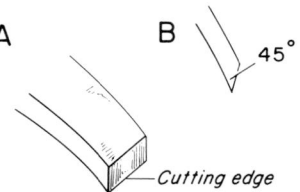

Figure 32–4. Chisel scaler. **A.** The chisel has a single cutting edge, and the blade is continuous with the slightly curved shank. **B.** There is a 45-degree bevel at the cutting edge.

2. Blade is continuous with a slightly curved shank.
3. End of blade is flat and beveled at 45 degrees (figure 32–4 B).

B. **Purposes and Uses**
    1. Remove supramarginal calculus from exposed proximal surfaces of anterior teeth where interdental gingiva is missing.
    2. Well-suited for quick dislodgment of heavy calculus from the proximal areas of mandibular anterior teeth. When the calculus on the lingual forms a continuous bridge across several teeth, the chisel can be pushed horizontally from the labial to break up the large masses of calculus.
    3. Useful for proximal surfaces of premolars when flexibility of the lips and cheeks permits retraction for proper positioning of the cutting edge.

C. **Application**
    1. Full width of cutting edge should be applied, as the sharp corners can nick and groove the tooth surface.
    2. Stroke: horizontal only, from labial to lingual on proximal surfaces of anterior, particularly mandibular teeth.

IV. Curet

A. **Characteristics**
    1. Two cutting edges on a curved, spoon-shaped blade (figure 32–5 A);

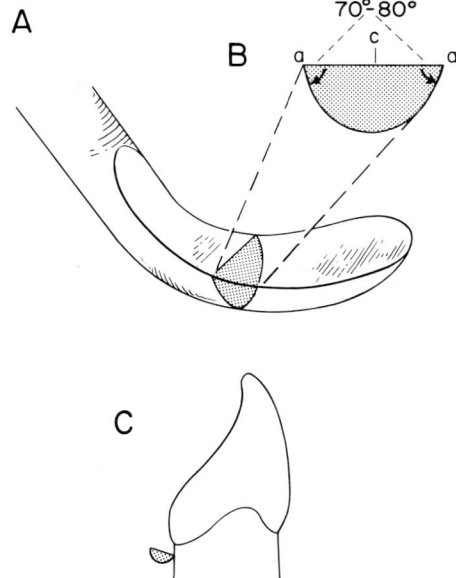

A

B

70°–80°
c
a   a

C

Figure 32–5. Curet. **A.** The two cutting edges are on the curved, spoon-shaped blade. **B.** Cross section is a half circle in shape, with the facial surface (c) between the two cutting edges (a and a). **C.** The blade is applied to the tooth so that the facial surface is at less than a 90-degree but not less than a 45-degree angle with the tooth surface.

one cutting edge has a greater curvature than the other. The two cutting edges curve around to meet at the toe. In reality, a curet has one continuous cutting edge because the two sides are united without interruption by the rounded toe.
2. Facial or inner surface between the cutting edge is flat in cross section (figure 32–5 B) and curved lengthwise.
3. Back or undersurface is rounded. Lateral aspects of the undersurface converge with the facial surface and terminate in a rounded end.
4. Cross section of the blade is shaped like a half circle (figure 32–5 B).
5. Internal angles of 70 to 80 degrees are formed where the lateral surfaces meet the facial surface (c) at

the cutting edges (a and a in figure 32–5 B).
6. Shank: shank, blade, and handle may be in a relatively flat plane for curets primarily adaptable to anterior teeth. For posterior teeth the shank is contra-angled for access to proximal surfaces.
7. Instruments are paired.

B. **Purposes and Uses**
1. Standard instrument for submarginal scaling and root planing (see also page 504).
2. Removal of fine supramarginal calculus close to the gingival margin: the rounded instrument is best adapted to the cervical area.
3. Curettage of the lining of the gingival wall of the sulcus or pocket.

C. **Application**
1. Angulation: blade is applied to the tooth so that the inner or facial surface is at an angle less than 90 degrees but not less than 45 degrees with the tooth surface (figure 32–5 C).
2. Curets are paired, mirror images of each other, with various angles of the shanks for access to all surfaces of all teeth. Curets for posterior use have greater curvatures of the shank.
3. Larger curets are used for submarginal scaling in the coronal portion of the sulcus or pocket; smaller curets are for fine scaling and root planing.
4. The design of the curet allows easy entrance into the sulcus and the curved blade with rounded end permits access to the base of the sulcus. The slender shank permits entrance to the sulcus with a minimum of tissue distention.
5. Stroke: pull stroke only; applied in vertical, horizontal, or oblique directions.

V. File

A. Characteristics
1. Multiple cutting edges lined up as a series of miniature hoes on a round, oval, or rectangular base (figure 32–6 A).
2. The multiple blades are at a 90- or 105-degree angle with the shank (figure 32–6 B).
3. Shanks are variously angulated, similar to the hoes; some are paired instruments, others single.
4. Reduced tactile sensitivity because of the size and shape; files are wide, flat, and bulky.

B. Purposes and Uses
In general, the file can be considered a supplementary instrument rather than the definitive instrument for routine use during scaling and root planing by the dental hygienist.

While never used by some dentists, the file is used by others for one or more of the following purposes:
1. Removal of calculus (accomplished by crushing or fragmentation).
2. Smoothing tooth surfaces: smoothing the tooth at the cementoenamel junction.
3. Root planing, primarily the exposed root surface following periodontal surgery.

4. Smoothing down overextended or rough amalgam restorations, particularly on proximal surfaces or in the cervical area.

C. Application
1. The entire working surface is placed flat against the area to be treated.
2. Adaptation to the curved tooth surfaces is difficult. In certain relationships the file has only a tangential contact.
3. Pressure applied permits the cutting edges to grasp the surface.
4. Two-point contact is applied when possible: the shank is placed against the contour of the crown.
5. Stroke: pull only.
6. When the file is used to assist in root planing, it is advisable to follow the file with a curet, since research has shown that a greater degree of smoothness can be attained.[1,2]

SPECIFICATIONS FOR INSTRUMENTS FOR SCALING AND ROOT PLANING

I. Basic Qualities[3,4]

Each instrument is designed for a specific purpose and is intended to be used for the purpose for which it was designed. Characteristics of instruments which influence their usefulness are listed below. An instrument should:

A. Be effective and efficient for calculus removal and smoothing tooth surfaces with the least possible trauma to the gingival tissue or the tooth surface.

B. Provide comfort to the operator without causing fatigue or muscle cramp.
   1. Light weight. Hollow handles usually have a comfortable wide diameter, and are light weight.
   2. Grasp: diameter and surface texture of the handle appropriate for prolonged use.

A

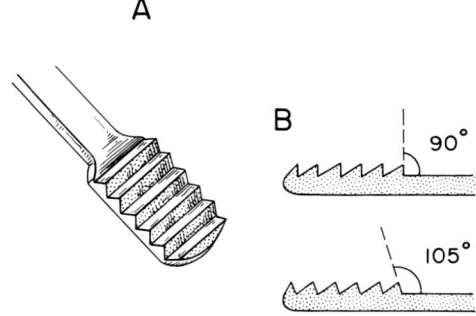

B

90°

105°

Figure 32–6. Periodontal file. **A.** A file has multiple cutting edges. **B.** Files are designed with each multiple blade at a 90- or 105-degree angle with the shank.

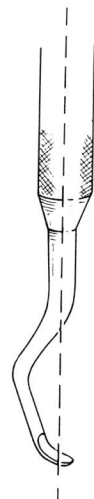

Figure 32–7. Instrument balance. The cutting edges should be centered over the long axis of the handle.

C. Permit maximum use of tactile sensitivity. Large, bulky instruments do not assist in transferring surface irregularities to the fingertips.

D. Have balance.
1. The blade should be centered in line with the long axis of the handle (figure 32–7).
2. The distance from the cutting edge (working part) of the blade to the junction of the shank and handle (where the instrument is held) should not be greater than 35 to 40 mm. (1½ inches). Too short a distance may limit the action; too long, may make the instrument unbalanced.

E. Have a blade of a size in keeping with:
1. Tooth anatomy; root curvatures.
2. Location and extent of calculus deposits.
3. Anatomy of the gingival sulcus.

F. Be easy to care for when cleaning, sterilizing, sharpening.

II. Sharp Cutting Edges

Instruments must be sharp if scaling and root planing are to be completed efficiently with minimal trauma to the tissues. With the instrument blade maintained with its original contour and cutting edges sharp, the following may be expected in contrast with the use of dull instruments:

A. Greater precision of operation, improved quality of results, with less operating time involved.

B. Increased tactile sensitivity during instrumentation: a sharp instrument does not have to be gripped as firmly as a dull one.

C. Greater control of the instrument with lighter grasp possible, less pressure required on the tooth being scaled or planed, and decreased pressure on the finger rest.

D. Fewer strokes required.

E. Less possibility of burnishing the calculus rather than removing it.

F. Prevention of unnecessary trauma to gingival tissues, and therefore less discomfort experienced by the patient.

G. Decreased possibility of nicking, grooving, or scratching the tooth surfaces.

H. Less fatigue for the dental hygienist.

INSTRUMENT SHARPENING

Objectives for techniques of sharpening emphasize the *conservation of instrument blades* and the *preservation of their original shape*. Instruments designed for a particular purpose should continue to be used in the manner in which they were designed and not be distorted by inaccurate sharpening techniques.

Sharpening procedures are not easy to learn and require skill and patience to accomplish. It is no doubt true that more instruments are worn out from sharpening than from use,[5] which applies especially during the period of learning to sharpen.

This chapter describes sharpening procedures for the sickle, hoe, chisel, curet, and explorer using various sharpening stones and devices. The principles of sharpening which are outlined and illustrated here may be applied to various types of sharpening stones and instruments which may be encountered.

I. Sharpening Stones

A. Materials and Their Sources

1. *Natural Abrasive Stones.* Quarried from mineral deposits, the hard Arkansas oilstone is used for dental instruments because of its fine abrasive particle size.
2. *Artificial Materials*
   a. Hard, nonmetallic substances impregnated with aluminum oxide, silicon carbide, or diamond particles; these are larger and coarser than particles of the Arkansas stone. Examples: Ruby stone, carborundum stones, and the diamond hone.
   b. Solid aluminum oxide. Example: moonstone.[6]
   c. Steel alloys: metals which are harder than most dental instrument steel and therefore capable of sharpening the instrument. Example: tungsten carbide steel used in the Neivert Whittler.

B. Categories

Sharpening stones as they are manufactured for use may be classified into two general groups: the ones for manual (unmounted) sharpening, and those for motor-driven (mandrel-mounted) sharpening. Examples of procedures using both unmounted and mounted stones are supplied in this chapter.

1. *Unmounted*
   a. Stationary flat stones: rectangular stones with square or rounded edges, or with one side grooved for the special adaptation of curved blades.
   b. Hand stones: cylindrical (tapered or straight) or rectangular with rounded edges.
   c. Other types: sharpening devices such as the Neivert Whittler (page 487) or the diamond hone.[7]
2. *Mandrel-Mounted.* Cylindrical (straight or tapered) small stones of various diameters designed to fit the various sizes of instrument blades.

II. Facilities for Sharpening

The work area where instrument sharpening is accomplished should be arranged for convenience and comfort. Because sharpening is an everyday event, it needs to be planned so that available time can be utilized effectively without inconveniences.

A. Place

A definite place should be arranged where materials for sharpening can be kept together, and work can be done from a seated position.

B. Lighting

A permanently fixed light which can be concentrated over the work area is needed; light must be shaded to protect the eyes.

C. Working Surface

The working surface should be firm and stationary. The bracket table or cervical tray is undesirable because of lack of stability.

D. Equipment

An adequate assortment of stones and the materials for their maintenance and cleanliness, magnifying glass, and other incidental materials related to specific procedures should be available.

III. Dynamics of Sharpening

A. Sharpening Stone Surface

The sharpening stone acts as an abrasive to reshape a dulled blade by grinding the surface until the cutting edge is restored. The surface of the stone is made up of masses of minute crystals which are the abrasive particles that accomplish the grinding of the instrument. A smaller particle size or a finer grain, as it is generally called, abrades or reduces more slowly and produces a finer cutting edge.

B. Cutting Edge

The cutting edge is the *line* formed where two surfaces of a blade meet at an angle. The edge is a line and therefore has length but no thickness. The edge becomes dull by pressing it against a hard surface (the tooth) or it may be nicked when it is drawn over a rough surface. When the edge is dull, it is rounded and therefore has thickness. The object in sharpening is to reshape the cutting edge to a line.

C. Sharpening

Sharpening is accomplished by grinding the surface or surfaces which form the cutting edge.

IV. Tests for Instrument Sharpness

A. Visual

1. Examine the cutting edge under adequate light, preferably with a magnifying glass.
2. Since the sharp cutting edge is a fine *line*, it will not reflect light.
3. The dull cutting edge presents a rounded, shiny *surface*, which reflects light.

B. Plastic Testing Stick[8]

1. Use a basic plastic or acrylic ¼ inch rod, 3 inches long: the hardness and texture approximate a fingernail.
2. Apply the instrument blade to the plastic stick at the correct angle for scaling; press lightly but firmly.
3. The sharp cutting edge will engage or grip the plastic and move with resistance if an attempt is made to draw the cutting edge over the surface.
4. The dull cutting edge will not catch without undue pressure, and will slide easily over the surface of the stick.
5. Test each area along an entire cutting edge since, during use, the edge is not uniformly dulled.

C. Fingernail Test

1. This test works similarly to the plastic testing stick: when the sharp cutting edge is applied to the nail at the appropriate angle, it will engage or grip the nail. The dulled instrument will not catch without undue pressure.
2. Although the fingernail test has been rather widely used over the years, it is not recommended for sanitary and esthetic reasons.

V. Some Basic Principles

A. Objectives

1. To produce a sharp cutting edge.
2. To preserve the original shape of the blade.

B. Care of Instruments

1. Sharpen at first sign of dullness: when instruments become grossly dulled, recontouring wastes the instrument and it is difficult to restore the original contour and still have a strong blade.
2. Do not sharpen unclean instruments: a contaminated sharpening stone can become a means for transfer of infectious agents.
3. After sharpening, instruments are

scrubbed to remove oil and metal shavings and then prepared for autoclaving.

4. Handle instruments carefully to preserve sharpness.

C. **Preparation of Stone**
1. Arkansas stone. Spread on a thin layer of clean light oil. Excess oil obscures view of cutting edge. Petroleum jelly on swab, or water, may be used on sterilized stone at the dental chair. The lubricant
   a. Facilitates movement of the instrument blade over the stone and prevents scratching.
   b. Keeps the metallic particles removed during sharpening in suspension and so helps prevent clogging of the pores of the stone (glazing).
   c. Protects and preserves the stone from drying.
2. Artificial stone. Follow the manufacturer's directions.

D. **Sharpening**
1. Select the sharpening method and sharpening stone or device consistent with the size and shape of the instrument being treated.
2. Before starting to sharpen, analyze the cutting edge and establish the proper angle between the stone and the blade surface; maintain the angle through the firm grasp, secure finger rest, moderate pressure, short stroke, and other features of the technique appropriate to the individual instrument.
3. Maintain control so that the entire surface is reduced evenly: care must be taken not to create a new bevel at the cutting edge.
4. Prevent grooving of the sharpening stone by varying the areas for instrument placement while sharpening. Resurfacing procedure is described on page 491.

D. **After Sharpening**
   Gently hone or burnish the non-beveled surface adjacent to the cutting edge.
1. Honing: by definition, a *hone* is a sharpening stone and *honing* means sharpening. In common usage, honing has been applied to the process whereby the "bur" or "wire edge" is removed from the side of the cutting edge which was not reduced.
2. During sharpening some of the metal particles removed during grinding remain attached to the edge of the instrument and create the wire edge. If left, it is possible for the tiny particles to be removed when the instrument is applied to the tooth surface during treatment.
3. By sharpening into, toward, or against the cutting edge, the production of a wire edge will be minimized.
4. Method for removal: Using an even and light pressure, pass a flat Arkansas stone along the non-beveled side of the cutting edge. One or two strokes is usually sufficient. If heavy pressure is applied, the bevel of the cutting edge can be altered.

SHARPENING CURETS AND SICKLES

Sharpening both the lateral and facial surfaces will preserve the original contour of the blade. For both curets and sickles the internal angle at the cutting edge is 70 to 80 degrees (figures 32–1 and 32–5). To preserve this angle, sharpening stones must be placed and activated carefully.

Manual sharpening procedures are the methods of choice in order that the blade not be reduced unnecessarily by the rapid-cutting mounted stone and the shape not be altered because of less control by the operator. Techniques in this section show the use of a flat stone for manual sharpening of lateral surfaces.

When sharpening lateral surfaces, the flat stone may be used in one of two ways: the stone may be moved while the instrument is stationary, or the stone may be stationary and the instrument moved over it.

MOVING FLAT STONE: STATIONARY INSTRUMENT

The side of the cutting edge formed by the lateral surface is reduced by this method. The technique described applies to both curets and sickles. Because the sickle is pointed and the curet is round on the toe end, there is a variation in the adaptation of the sharpening stone to that portion of the blade.

I. **Prepare the Stone** as described on page 482.

II. **Examine the Cutting Edge to Be Sharpened:** test for sharpness to determine specific areas which are dull.

III. **Stabilize the Instrument**

A. Grasp the instrument in a palm grasp and hold the hand against the edge of a solid workbench or table under adequate light (figure 32–8 A). The instrument should be low enough so that the operator will have no difficulty in seeing the cutting edges and the angle formed by the instrument and the sharpening stone.

B. Turn the facial surface of the instrument up and parallel with the floor.

IV. **Apply Sharpening Stone**

A. Apply the stone in a vertical position to the lateral surface at the heel of the cutting edge. Figure 32–8 B shows the position for one side of the blade, and figure 32–8 C shows the position for the other side.

B. Adjust the angle at which the stone is held to maintain the internal 70 to 80 degrees of the blade. The angle on the outside, between the instrument and

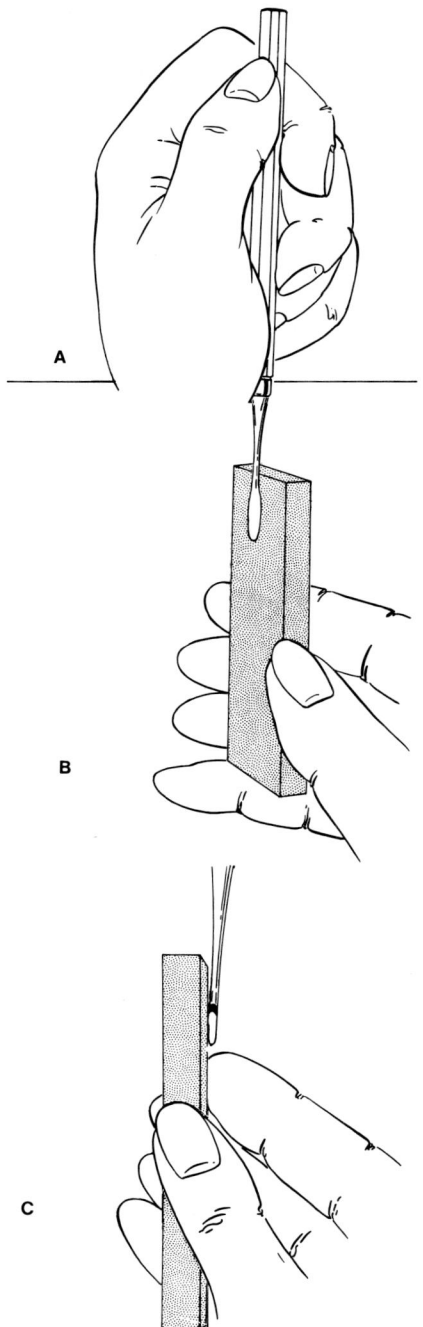

Figure 32–8. Sharpening a curet or scaler using a moving flat stone. **A.** Hold instrument with a firm grasp while stabilizing the hand on the edge of a stationary table or bench. **B.** Stone is angled with the facial surface of the instrument at 100 to 110 degrees (figure 32–9) to maintain the internal angle of the blade at 70 to 80 degrees. **C.** Stone reversed to sharpen opposite cutting edge.

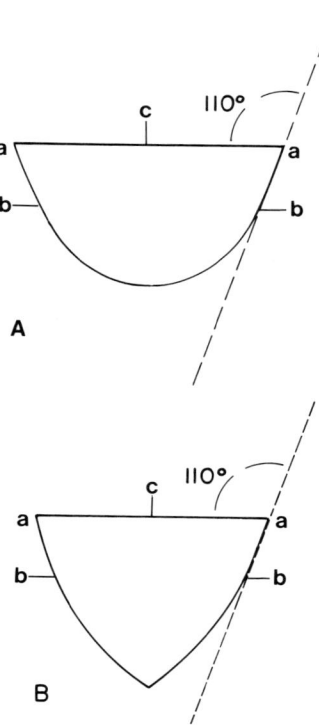

A

B

Figure 32–9. Angulation for sharpening. Cross sections of curet (A) and sickle scaler (B) to show correct angulation of the blade with the flat sharpening stone (broken line) when reducing the lateral surface (b). Angle shown on diagram between facial surface (c) and the stone at the cutting edge (a) will be 100 to 110 degrees to maintain an internal angle of 70 to 80 degrees.

the stone, will be 100 to 110 degrees (figure 32–9 A and B).

V. Activate the Sharpening Stone

A. Keep the stone in contact with the blade and at the proper angle throughout the procedure.

B. Move the stone up and down with short rhythmical strokes about one-half to one-quarter inch high. Put more pressure on the down stroke.

C. Follow the cutting edge from heel to toe, applying several strokes to each millimeter.

D. Do not change the angle of the stone with the facial surface of the instru-

ment: when the angle is varied, an irregularity will be ground into the cutting edge.

E. Keep the wrist straight and use the whole arm to standardize the stroke and the adaptation of the stone to the instrument.

F. Variation at the toe-end
1. Sickle: the stone is held straight as it nears the pointed tip.
2. Curet: adapt the stone's position so that sharpening continues around the round toe. The same angle between the stone and the facial surface is maintained.

G. Finish with a down stroke.

VI. Test for sharpness and determine whether to repeat the first side before starting the second.

STATIONARY FLAT STONE: MOVING INSTRUMENT

I. Sickle Scaler

A. Prepare the stone (page 482) and place the stone flat on a firm table or bench top under adequate light. Do not tilt the stone while sharpening.

B. Examine cutting edges to be sharpened: test for sharpness.

C. Hold the instrument with a firm pen grasp using thumb, index, and middle (second) finger to prevent the instrument from rotating or changing angles during sharpening (figure 32–10 B).

D. Establish finger rest on side of stone using ring and little fingers.

E. Stabilize stone with fingers of opposite hand.

F. Apply cutting edge to be sharpened to the stone: maintain 70 to 80 degree internal angle of the instrument (figure 32–9 B).

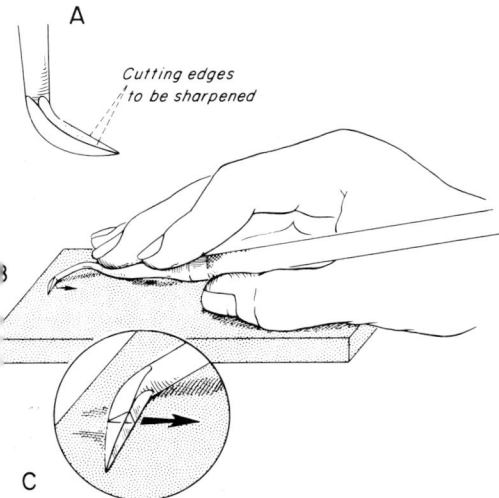

A

Cutting edges
to be sharpened

C

igure 32–10.   Sharpening the straight sickle scaler. **A.** The cutting edges to be sharpened. **B.** With a modified pen grasp and a finger rest firmly established on the side of the stone, the scaler is positioned for sharpening. **C.** The full length of the cutting edge is applied when possible and maintained on the stone. Arrows indicate direction of the sharpening stroke.

G. Apply moderate to light but firm pressure while instrument is in motion: heavy pressure can reduce control of instrument, cause scratching of the stone, and produce an unfavorable bevel at the cutting edge.

H. Use a short, slow stroke to maintain the exact relation of the cutting edge to the stone.
   1. Direction: pull blade forward, toward the cutting edge.
   2. All fingers move with the arm as a unit.
   3. Release pressure from stone and slide whole unit back to repeat the stroke.

I. Test for sharpness after one or two strokes: repeat as needed for ideal sharpness.

J. Turn instrument and proceed to sharpen other lateral surface: when instrument placement is awkward for

the modified contra-angled sickle, use a narrow side of the Arkansas stone.

K. Sharpening the facial surface of a straight blade*
   1. Position the surface over a side of the flat stone with the tip pointed down.
   2. Apply entire facial surface flat against the stone.
   3. With firmly established finger rest, apply moderate to light but firm pressure for a short slow stroke while the exact relation of the flat facial surface is maintained on the stone.

II. Curet

A. Prepare the stone (page 482) and place it flat on a steady work bench or table.

B. Examine the cutting edges to be sharpened: test for sharpness.

C. Hold the instrument in a modified pen grasp and establish a secure finger rest (figure 32–11 B).

D. Apply the cutting edge to the stone. An angle of 110 degrees is formed by stone and facial surface.
   1. Since the curet is curved, only a small section of the cutting edge can be applied at one time.
   2. Sharpening is performed in a *series* of applications of the cutting edge to the stone, each overlapping the previous, as the instrument is turned and drawn steadily along the stone.
   3. The portion of the cutting edge nearest the shank is applied first (figure 32–11 C, a).

E. Apply moderate to light but firm pressure while the instrument is activated.

*Facial surface of a curved sickle is sharpened with a hand sharpening cone (page 486) or the Nievert Whittler (page 487).

A

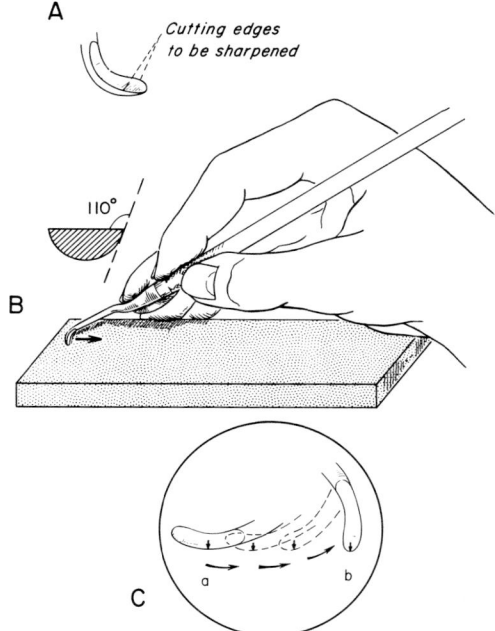

Cutting edges
to be sharpened

110°

B

C

Figure 32–11.   Sharpening a curet on a flat stone. **A.** Cutting edges to be sharpened. **B.** Position of the blade on the stone at the beginning of the stroke. With the finger rest stabilized on the edge of the stone, the cutting edge is maintained at the proper angulation (110 degrees) as the instrument is drawn along the stone with an even moderate pressure. **C.** To show the movement of the blade, the arrows indicate each portion of the cutting edge being sharpened as the blade is turned on the stone from the beginning (a) to the completion of the stroke (b) at the center of the rounded end of the curet. The instrument is turned over and the opposite cutting edge is sharpened.

F. Use a slow steady stroke to maintain control and to assure that each portion of the cutting edge receives equal treatment.

G. Move the blade forward into the cutting edge; turn the instrument continuously until the center of the round end of the blade is reached (figure 32–11 C, b).

H. Test for sharpness along the entire cutting edge; reapply to stone as necessary for ideal sharpness.

I. Turn the instrument to sharpen the second cutting edge. Overlap at the center of the round tip.

J. Methods for sharpening the facial aspect: Use the hand sharpening cone (below) or the Neivert Whittler (page 487).

HAND SHARPENING CONE

I. Description

A. **Types**
   Hand stones are cylindrical (tapered or straight) Arkansas cones; or rectangular with rounded edges and tapered carborundum stones.

B. **Uses**
   1. Arkansas: tapered cone is recommended for curved cutting edges of sickles and curets.
   2. Carborundum: coarser grain is useful for preliminary shaping or sharpening of excessively dulled instruments; it is followed by use of a finer stone to refine the cutting edge.

II. Sharpening Procedure

A. **Preparation of Stone** (page 482).

B. **Position**
   1. Hand-held instrument: hold in left hand across palm with fingers and thumb grasping firmly; direct blade toward self with face of the blade up.
   2. For additional support: place instrument over the edge of a firm hard block and maintain rigidly (figure 32–12).
   3. Stabilize arms between the wrist and elbows on the edge of a solid table or bench top.
   4. Tapered cone: with a firm grasp of the sharpening cone, position the appropriate diameter of the cone to fit the curvature of the surface to be sharpened; apply the stone straight

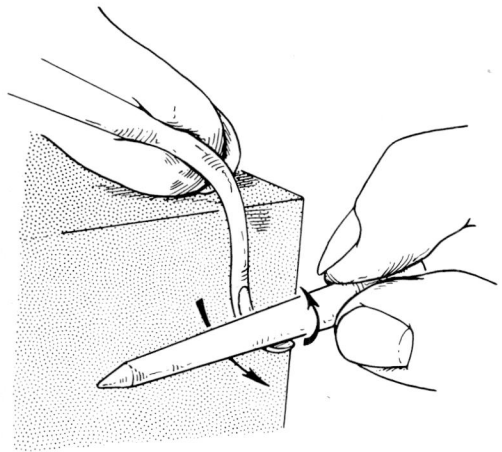

Figure 32–12.   Hand sharpening cone. A cylindrical stone is applied to a curet. The instrument is stabilized over a firm block and the stone is positioned at the appropriate diameter to fit the curvature of the surface to be sharpened. An even pressure is applied across the facial surface of the instrument so that both cutting edges will be sharpened evenly.

across the facial surface so that an even pressure can be applied to both cutting edges simultaneously to produce an evenly sharpened instrument (figure 32–12).

C. **Motion**
1. Rotate stone counterclockwise over the instrument with even, firm pressure.
2. Continue rotation of stone upward (as in a circle) when approaching the end of the curet to prevent tapering off and reshaping the curvature of the tip. (Figure 32–15B illustrates this for the mounted stone. The same principle applies to the hand operated instrument.)
3. A horizontal stroke may be used. The instrument is maintained stationary as described above, and the stone is moved back and forth across the facial surface. Care must be taken to maintain the stone straight across so that an even

pressure is applied simultaneously to both cutting edges.

D. **Test for sharpness** after a few applications; repeat as necessary to obtain ideal sharpness.

THE NEIVERT WHITTLER

I. Description
A. **Working End**
    The working end consists of five sharpening edges and a rounded burnishing edge of tungsten carbide.

B. **Handle**
    The handle is made of stainless steel; it is bulky and hexagonal for comfortable grasping (figure 32–13).

II. Uses
A. Manufacturer's instructions describe sharpening straight and curved blades: dental instruments, scissors, knives.

B. Particularly useful for facial surfaces of curved scalers and curets.

C. Honing: the outer rounded edge is designed for honing (burnishing).

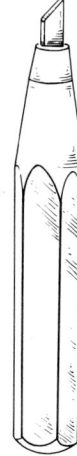

Figure 32–13.   The Neivert Whittler. The drawing is approximately one-half the instrument's size.

III. Sharpening Procedure

A. Position

Stability and control are most important.

1. Hold instrument to be sharpened firmly in the left hand, across palm, grasping with all fingers and the thumb, with the surface to be sharpened turned toward self. The instrument can also be stabilized over the edge of a firm, hard surface as shown for the cone in figure 32–12.
2. Stabilize arms between the wrists and the elbows on the edge of a solid table or bench top.
3. Whittler is held in a palm grasp with thumb under handle adjacent to the working end and at the same time the thumb rest is applied beneath the instrument blade on the left hand (figure 32–14 A).

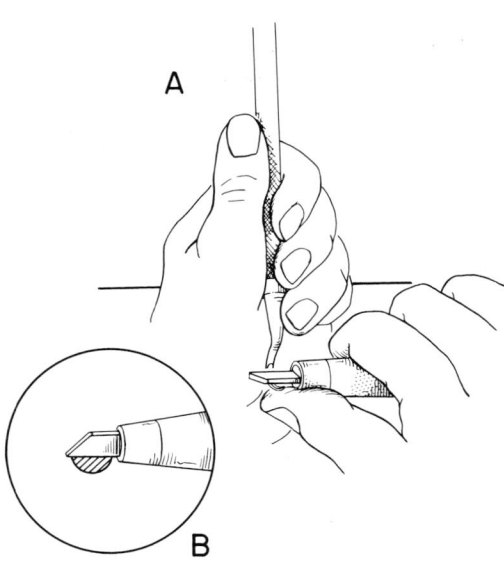

Figure 32–14. Sharpening a curet with a Neivert Whittler. **A.** The instrument to be sharpened is stabilized in the left hand, while the sharpener is grasped in a palm grasp with the thumb rest close to the instrument to be sharpened. **B.** The blade of the sharpener is placed and maintained straight across the facial surface of the curet to produce evenly sharpened cutting edges.

4. Working end: apply to the curvature of the surface to be sharpened straight across so that even pressure can be applied to both cutting edges and an evenly sharpened instrument will result (figure 32–14 B).

B. Motion

1. Draw the Whittler edge across the length of the facial surface with a moderate, even pressure.
2. As the end is approached, continue in an upward motion to prevent tapering off and reshaping curvature of the tip.

C. Test for sharpness after a few applications.

D. Burnish (hone) lateral surfaces of blade next to cutting edges.

MANDREL MOUNTED STONES

I. Description

A. Types

1. Arkansas: fine grain for finished sharpening.
2. Ruby stone: coarser grain especially useful for recontouring excessively dull instrument; when used for routine sharpening, it should be applied conservatively.

B. Shapes

The stones are cylindrical with flat end or cone-shape.

C. Use

1. Applicable to most cutting edges: various sizes and grains of stones are selectively utilized.
2. Reshaping: coarse-grained Ruby stone is especially useful for this.
3. Artificial stones may be autoclaved and are used with water, therefore they are useful for sharpening sterile instruments and for use during the patient's appointment

I. Sharpening Procedure

A. Select a sharpening stone with a diameter appropriate to fit the blade of the instrument to be sharpened.

B. Apply oil to Arkansas stone; dip Ruby stone in water and repeat at intervals during sharpening to aid in reducing heat production.

C. **Position**
1. Hold instrument to be sharpened in a palm grasp with blade face up.
2. Hold handpiece in other hand using a palm grasp with the thumb securely placed against the thumb of the hand holding the instrument (figure 32–15).
3. Stabilize arms between wrists and elbows on the edge of a solid table or bench top.
4. Apply stone to surface to be sharpened straight across so that light even pressure can be applied to both cutting edges simultaneously and an evenly sharpened instrument will result.

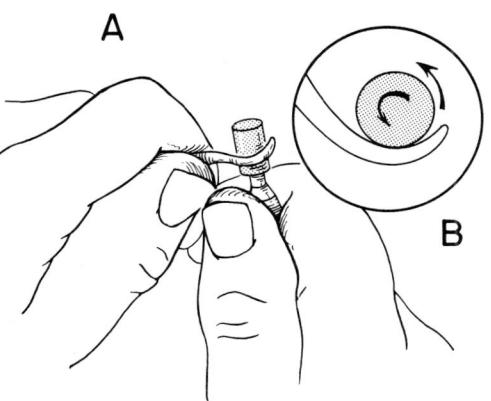

igure 32–15. Sharpening with a mandrel mounted stone. **A.** A stone with a diameter appropriate for the curved blade to be sharpened is positioned across the facial surface for even sharpening of the cutting edges. Hands and arms are stabilized for precision and control. **B.** With low speed to minimize heat production, the rotating stone is passed along the instrument surface. Near the end of the blade the stone is moved upward to prevent flattening off the instrument end.

D. **Motion**
1. *Use Low Speed*
   a. To minimize heat production (alteration of the temper of the steel can result with repeated use).
   b. To allow complete control of position of sharpening stone on blade.
2. *Apply Light Pressure.* To prevent undue reduction of instrument, yet heavy enough so that surface will be smooth.
3. Pass the rotating stone upward when approaching the end of the blade to prevent tapering off and reshaping the tip.

E. **Test for Sharpness**
   Test for sharpness after one or two applications; repeat when necessary.

F. **Hone** the lateral borders of the cutting edges.

III. Disadvantages of Motor-Driven Sharpening

A. Inconsistent results because of variations in speed and difficulty of stabilization of instrument and sharpening stone.

B. Excess reduction of instrument during shorter period of use; less conservation of instruments than by manual methods.

C. Frictional heat may affect the temper of the steel.

SHARPENING THE HOE SCALER

Characteristics of the hoe scaler are described on page 475. The hoe has only one surface to be ground. Since placement of the small surface on the Arkansas stone is difficult to visualize, use of a magnifying glass can be particularly helpful.

I. Examine Surface To Be Ground (figure 32–16A); test for sharpness.

A

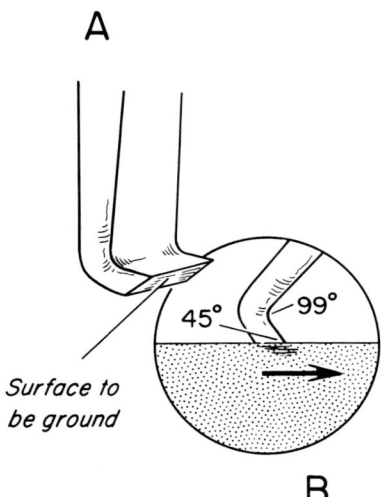

45°   99°

Surface to
be ground

B

Figure 32–16. Sharpening the hoe scaler. **A.** Surface to be ground. **B.** Hoe adapted to the surface of a flat stone at the proper angle to maintain the original bevel of 45 degrees. Arrow indicates direction of the sharpening stroke, which is toward the cutting edge.

II. Sharpening Procedure

A. Hold instrument in modified pen grasp; establish finger rest on the stone.
B. Apply the surface to be ground to the stone in correct relationship to maintain the 45-degree bevel (figure 32–16B).
C. With moderate, steady pressure, pull the instrument toward the cutting edge a short distance, letting the whole hand move with the arm as a unit.
D. Release pressure and slide the instrument back; repeat.
E. Test for sharpness and reapply as needed for ideal sharpness.
F. Hone the undersurface of the blade adjacent to the cutting edge.

III. Round Corners

Corners should be rounded at each end of the cutting edge.
A. Purpose: to prevent laceration of soft tissue or grooving of tooth surface.

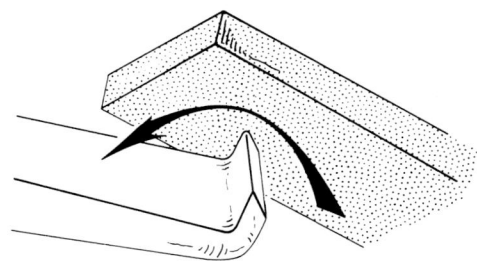

Figure 32–17. Round the sharp corners of the hoe scaler. A flat stone is rubbed over the instrument with a gentle rolling motion.

B. Hold instrument in left hand with corners of cutting edge directed inward.
C. With sharpening stone in right hand, rub the surface of the stone across each corner with a gentle rolling motion (figure 32–17); two or three applications are usually sufficient.

SHARPENING THE CHISEL SCALER

Sharpening procedures for the chisel are similar to those for the hoe. Again, the surface is small, the angulation difficult to visualize, and the use of a magnifying glass recommended. Review the characteristics of the chisel scaler on page 476.

I. Examine Surface To Be Ground

(figure 32–18A); test for sharpness.

II. Sharpening Procedure

A. Hold instrument with a modified pen grasp, establish finger rest, and apply the surface to be ground to the stone in the correct relationship to maintain the 45-degree bevel (figure 32–18B).
B. With moderate, steady pressure, push the instrument forward, toward the cutting edge, without changing the relationship with the stone.
C. After two or three applications, test for sharpness and reapply as necessary for an ideal cutting edge.
D. Hone the nonbeveled surface.

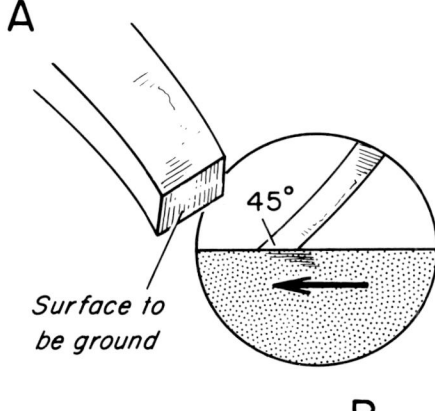

A

45°

Surface to
be ground

B

Figure 32–18. Sharpening the chisel scaler. **A.** Surface to be ground. **B.** The chisel is adapted to the surface of a flat stone at the appropriate angle to maintain the original bevel of 45 degrees. Arrow indicates direction of the sharpening stroke, which is toward the cutting edge.

III. Round Corners

Round the corners at each end of the cutting edge. In a manner similar to that shown in figure 32–17 for the hoe scaler, rub the surface of the flat stone across each corner of the chisel with a gentle, even, rolling motion. Two or three applications are usually sufficient.

SHARPENING EXPLORERS

I. Tests for Sharpness

A. **Visual**

When examined under concentrated light, a dull explorer tip will appear rounded; the tip may reflect light.

B. **Plastic Testing Stick**

A sharp explorer will grip the plastic on light pressure and move with resistance when pulled over the surface; a dull explorer will not catch and will slide.

II. Recontour

Small-nosed pliers can be used to straighten a bent tip.

III. Sharpening Procedure

A. Prepare unmounted flat stone.

B. Instrument is held with a modified pen grasp; finger rest established on side of stone.

C. Placement and movement of the tip over the stone resembles somewhat the procedure for the curet on the unmounted stone (figure 32–11, page 486).
1. Place side of tip on stone at approximately 15- to 20-degree angle of stone with shank of explorer.
2. As tip is moved over the surface, the handle is rotated so that even pressure can be applied to each part of the tip.

CARE OF SHARPENING STONES

I. Flat Arkansas Stone

A. **Post-sharpening Procedures**
1. Routinely wipe off used oil and rub with clean oil to remove particles left after sharpening.
2. Clean with ammonia, gasoline, or kerosene and rub until stone is free from discoloration.
3. Stone may be sterilized by autoclave or hot oil.
4. Spread a thin layer of oil over all surfaces after sterilization and before storage.

B. **Resurface Stone**
1. Stone may become "glazed" by metal particles from instruments being ground constantly into the surface.
2. Rub the stone over emery paper placed on a flat solid surface.

C. **Storage**
1. Fold a gauze sponge to fit inside the cover of the box containing the stone; moisten the gauze with oil to aid in keeping the stone from drying.

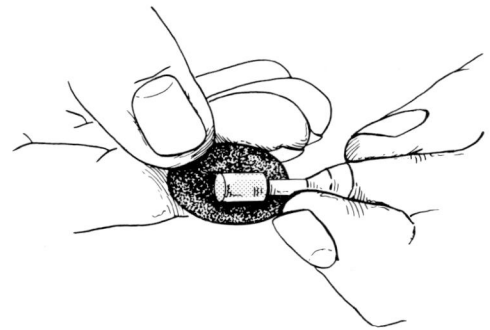

Figure 32-19. Care of the mounted Ruby stone. A Joe Dandy disk is used to maintain a smooth surface without grooves.

2. Keep box covered to protect stone from drying, dust, and breakage.

II. Mounted Stones

A. Arkansas Mounted Stones
Same basic procedures as for the flat stone.

B. Ruby Stone
1. Clean by scrubbing with soap and water.
2. Maintain an ungrooved surface: frequently apply the stone to a Joe Dandy disk (figure 32-19). A sandpaper disk is too flexible for this purpose.
3. Sterilize by autoclave: store in autoclave bag.

C. Manufacturer's Directions should be followed for all stones.

TECHNICAL HINTS

I. Prevent unnecessary dulling of instruments by applying the following suggestions:
   A. When handling instruments for cleaning, sterilizing, or other reason, keep blades from hooking, bumping, or pressing against each other as cutting edges become dull from contact with hard surfaces. Thinner instruments such as explorers and probes are subject to bending and breaking.
   B. Boiling water disinfection will dull instruments (pages 32-33).
   C. During instrumentation, utilize instruments at the appropriate angulation to the teeth; avoid pressing instrument against hard surface of metallic restorations.
   D. Use of a tray system for sterilization and management of instruments can aid greatly in maintaining instruments separately.

II. Discard instruments that have been reduced so much from frequent sharpening that even moderate to slight pressure will flex the blade. There is danger of a tip breaking off in the sulcus or between the teeth during instrumentation.

III. Sharpening of files has not been included in this chapter for several reasons. Since sharpening files is a difficult procedure because of the several parallel cutting edges, the amount of time consumed in sharpening with limited promise of effective results, may not be justified. The dental hygienist who is expected to sharpen them can obtain a jeweler's tang file for the purpose. Use of a professional sharpening service or return of the files to the manufacturer for sharpening is highly recommended.

References

1. Barnes, J. E. and Schaffer, E. M.: Subgingival Root Planing: A Comparison Using Files, Hoes, and Curettes, *J. Periodont.*, 31, 300, September, 1960.
2. Green, E. and Ramfjord, S. P.: Tooth Roughness After Subgingival Root Planing, *J. Periodont.*, 37, 396, September-October, 1966.
3. Orban, B. and Manella, V. B.: A Macroscopic and Microscopic Study of Instruments Designed for Root Planing, *J. Periodont.*, 27, 120, April, 1956.
4. Grant, D. A., Stern, I. B., and Everett, F. G.: *Orban's Periodontics*, 4th ed. St. Louis, Mosby, 1972, pp. 372-374.
5. Halik, F. J.: The Role of Subgingival Curettage in Periodontal Therapy, *Dent. Clin. North Am.*, 13, 19, January, 1969.

6. W. R. Case & Sons Cutlery Company, Bradford, Pennsylvania 16701.
7. Graitcer, D. L.: New Sharpening Technic for Cutting Instruments, *Dent. Surv.*, *36*, 1307, October, 1960.
8. Hu-Friedy Manufacturing Company, 3118–36 N. Rockwell Street, Chicago, Illinois 60618.
9. Green, E. and Seyer, P. C.: *Sharpening Curets and Sickle Scalers*. Berkeley, California, Praxis Pub., 1972, 40 pp.

Suggested Readings

Allen, D. L., McFall, W. T., and Hunter, G. C.: *Periodontics for the Dental Hygienist*, 2nd ed. Philadelphia, Lea & Febiger, 1974, pp. 117–121, 144–145.
Barton, R. E., Sockwell, C. L., and Taylor, D. F.: Cutting Instruments; Patient and Operator Positions, in Sturdevant, C. M., Barton, R. E., and Brauer, J. C., eds: *The Art and Science of Operative Dentistry*. New York, Blakiston Division, McGraw-Hill, 1968, pp. 121–126.
Foss, C. L. and Orban, T. R.: Sharpening Periodontal Instruments, *J. Periodont.*, *27*, 135, April, 1956.
Glickman, I.: *Clinical Periodontology*, 4th ed. Philadelphia, Saunders, 1972, pp. 610–619.
Goldman, H. M. and Cohen, D. W.: *Periodontal Therapy*, 5th ed. St. Louis, Mosby, 1973, pp. 386–391.
Hall, W. B.: Oral Prophylaxis, in Steele, P. F., ed.: *Dimensions of Dental Hygiene*, 2nd ed. Philadelphia, Lea & Febiger, 1975, pp. 157–168, 189–196.
Instructions for Sharpening Dental Instruments, Chicago, Hu-Friedy Manufacturing Company.
Swenson, H. M.: The Sharpening of Prophylactic Instruments, *J. Am. Dent. Hyg. Assoc.*, *31*, 6, January, 1957.

Chapter 33

Scaling and Planing

Complete submarginal scaling, root planing, and gingival curettage are specific procedures in the treatment of inflammatory gingival and periodontal diseases. Scaling to remove calculus, root planing to produce a smooth and glassy tooth surface, and curettage to remove the diseased sulcular epithelial lining and underlying inflamed connective tissue are all directed toward an ultimate goal of pocket elimination and tissue health.

The success of treatment is dependent on the control of dental plaque. Therefore, instruction and supervision in plaque control procedures precedes, continues simultaneously with, and follows instrumentation for treatment.

To be effective, scaling and planing must be thorough. When calculus is left on the teeth and surfaces are not smooth, gingival irritation and inflammation can persist because plaque collects more readily on rough surfaces.

Efficient application of techniques and the thoroughness of the services performed are directly influenced by the procedures of examination and evaluation. The patient's history, oral inspection, radiographic survey, study casts, charting, and all other findings of the initial examination and evaluation prior to treatment planning now become the guides to treatment.

Development of ability, skill, and efficiency in the successful removal of calculus through positive scaling procedures requires more than the development of dexterity for applying instruments to the tooth surfaces. In these refined and exacting techniques the dental hygienist must apply knowledge of the anatomic, histologic, and physiologic characteristics of the teeth and gingival tissues to the fullest advantage of the patient.

I. Definitions

A. Scaling

Scaling is the basic procedure by which calculus is removed from the surfaces of the teeth. Scaling is divided into supramarginal and submarginal scaling depending on the location of the calculus in relation to the gingival margin (figure 33–2, page 501).

B. Root Planing

Root planing is the process by which the surfaces of the roots are made

495

smooth by the removal of residual fine calculus and diseased cementum. When the root surface is exposed following gingival recession or surgery, root planing is performed supramarginally, otherwise it is a submarginal procedure.*

II. Purposes

A few longitudinal studies have shown the important relationship between combined oral prophylaxis and supervised patient care. These studies demonstrated that, with periodic thorough scaling and root planing and controlled self-care by the patient, with instruction and review, various effects were produced. Benefits included reduced incidence of gingivitis, control of the quantity of calculus deposition, slower migration of the junctional epithelium, and generally cleaner mouths than observed in subjects of control groups who did not have such meticulous care.[1-4]

Scaling and planing will have limited temporary effects without self-care by the patient on a daily basis, without removal of other plaque retention factors such as overhanging margins, and without follow-up on other required dental and periodontal treatment. Plaque forms promptly, and calculus recurs within a few days in certain mouths.

The complete removal of calculus and planing to provide a smooth surface will contribute to the following:

A. Creation of an environment in which the gingival tissues can heal and inflammation can be resolved.
   1. Shrinkage of previously enlarged, spongy tissue.
   2. Reduction of pocket depth.
   3. Cessation of bleeding on provocation.

*Root planing is sometimes called root curettage. In this book the term curettage is reserved for curettage of the soft tissues. Gingival curettage is the process by which the diseased tissue lining the gingival sulcus or pocket wall is removed (page 519).

B. Regeneration of gingival tissues.
   1. Restoration of normal color, size, contour, consistency, and surface texture (table 11–1, page 172).
   2. Adaptation of the gingival tissue to the tooth surface.

C. Initial preparation (tissue conditioning) prior to complicated and advanced periodontal therapy.[5]
   1. Reduction in etiologic and predisposing factors.
   2. Permit reevaluation: surgery may be lessened or confined to specific areas.
   3. Decreases time required during a surgical procedure. Root planing would have to be completed before healing could take place.

D. Remove diseased cementum.

E. Increased effectiveness of plaque control measures.

F. Delayed reformation of calculus deposits since bacterial plaque and calculus retention is less on a smooth than a rough surface.

G. Removal of subsequent calculus deposits is easier because calculus is less firmly attached to a smooth surface than to a rough one (page 254).

PREPARATION FOR INSTRUMENTATION

I. Bacteremia Following Instrumentation

A bacteremia means the presence of bacteria in the blood. A transient bacteremia may occur after any type of oral surgery, periodontal treatment, scaling, and oral prophylaxis.[6-8]

A. **Factors Affecting Incidence**

   The incidence of bacteremia has been directly related to the degree of trauma inflicted during surgery or instrumentation[9] and especially related to the severity of the periodontal condition which was present at the time of instrumentation.[10,11] In one study[11] patients with clinically healthy gingiva had a 21.6 percent incidence of bacteremia, those with gingivitis 29.0 percent, and those with periodontitis 51.2 percent following scaling and root planing. No difference in incidence of bacteremia was found associated with ultrasonic or manual instrumentation.[12]

B. Precautions

1. Premedication. Certain patients who require premedication for prevention of bacteremia are listed on page 71. Although transient and of no known clinical significance in most instances, prophylactic antibiotic premedication must be planned in advance of an appointment for certain specially susceptible patients. The importance of obtaining a patient history and applying information from the history before instrumentation cannot be overemphasized.

2. Antiseptic mouthrinse. The routine use of an antiseptic mouthrinse such as one containing povidoneiodine (Betadine) is recommended. Significant reductions in oral surfaces bacteria and post-surgery bacteremia have been shown (pages 42–43).[13,14]

II. Examination

A. Use of Patient Records

The preliminary observations made during the preparation of the diagnostic workup provide basic information for planning procedures and indicating the number of appointments needed. A more specific inspection is required to conduct the treatment:

1. To determine exact location of calculus deposits.
2. To select instruments to be used.
3. To recognize irregularities of tooth surfaces, restorations, or other problem areas.
4. During instrumentation: to avoid unnecessary repetition and make each phase of the operation meaningful.
5. At expected completion of procedures: to assure complete removal of deposits.

B. Use of Radiographs

The radiographic survey can be a useful adjunct during scaling procedures and should always be available on a viewbox during appointments. Radiographic findings were outlined on pages 202–205. Limitations relative to the appearance of calculus in the radiograph were described. Overhanging restorations, carious lesions, and other factors which may interfere with scaling and planing or which should be treated as areas of plaque retention must be noted.

C. Supramarginal Examination

1. *Visual:* Gross and moderate deposits and surface irregularities can be seen readily. Fine, unstained, white or yellowish calculus is frequently invisible when wet with saliva. Dry calculus is seen more readily than wet calculus. Procedures for calculus detection were described on page 252.

2. *Tactile Method:* The enamel surface is smooth; when an explorer is passed over, it slides freely, smoothly, and quietly. Calculus deposits are rough: the explorer does not slide freely but meets with resistance, and produces a scratchy sound.

D. Submarginal Examination

1. *Anatomy of the submarginal area:* A pocket is a diseased sulcus. A pocket has an inner wall which is the tooth surface and an outer wall which is covered on the inside by

the sulcular epithelium. The base or bottom of the pocket is the junctional epithelium. The types of pockets were described on page 176. Total treatment is dependent on the type of pocket and the characteristics of the gingival tissue of the pocket wall.

2. *Direct visual inspection*
   a. Clinical appearance of the gingival tissues which reveals or is highly suggestive of the presence of submarginal calculus:
      (1) Gingival tissue which is soft, spongy, nonresilient, bluish-red, with enlargement of the marginal gingiva, a rolled edge which tends to be separated from the tooth surface, and with a smooth shiny surface on which stippling is indistinct or missing.
      (2) Dark-colored submarginal calculus may sometimes be seen as a dark area beneath relatively translucent marginal gingiva.

   (3) Follow-up evaluation on week after scaling: the tissu appearance can be helpful i detecting remaining parti cles of calculus. Healin with tissue shrinkage wil have occurred generall throughout, and only thos areas of gingiva which cove remaining calculus wil maintain the bluish-re color, enlargement, an other characteristics men tioned above.

   b. Direct examination for submar ginal calculus:
      (1) When there are submargina deposits under soft, spong tissue, the lining of th pocket wall may be loose an resilient and can be sepa rated or stretched away fron the tooth surface.
      (2) Procedure: apply compresse air gently to the gingiva margin, deflect the tissu and look into the sulcus o pocket. Submarginal cal

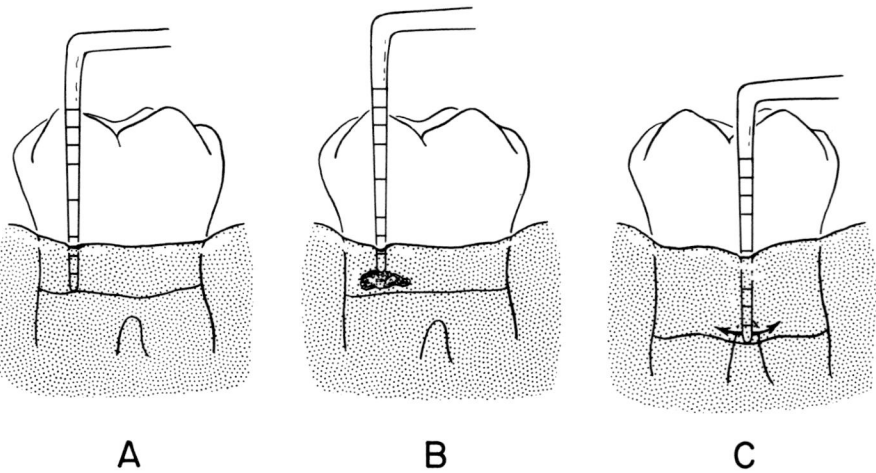

A   B   C

Figure 33–1.   Submarginal examination with a periodontal probe. **A.** Probe is inserted to the bottom of th pocket until the resistance of the soft tissue attachment is felt. **B.** As the probe passes over the root surfac it may be intercepted by a hard mass of calculus. **C.** The probe is used to examine root topography: her the probe is in a furcation area.

culus deposits which may be seen are generally dark brown or other dark color.

3. *Tactile examination: periodontal probe.* The pocket depths recorded for the periodontal charting prepared during the initial patient examination can be used as a guide for submarginal scaling. Additional circumferential probing may be necessary for a complete definition of the working area. Probing techniques are described on pages 188–192.

   a. Detection of irregularities of the tooth surface: various irregularities are listed on page 181. For example, as the probe passes over the tooth surface, it may be intercepted by a hard mass of calculus (figure 33–1 B). The calculus may be localized, or it may extend as a band around the entire tooth.

   b. Topography of the tooth surface: many grooves, curves, and furrow-like variations are found which can complicate instrumentation. When there is increased pocket depth, the anatomical features of the roots become evident. For example, the groove and the furcation between the roots of a mandibular molar can be probed (figure 33–1 C). Application of the curets into the furcation area for calculus removal and root planing is difficult and challenging. Such areas must also be examined with the explorer.

4. *Tactile examination: explorer*

   a. Purposes. The submarginal explorer No. 17 is used to determine the texture and character of the tooth surface and to distinguish by tactile means the cause and nature of surface roughness.

   b. Use. The explorer is the instrument of evaluation: before scaling and root planing the extent and nature of the calculus deposits are evaluated and treatment procedures are planned; progress and completion of techniques are also evaluated until the tooth surface is smooth to the critical touch of the explorer.

PROCEDURE FOR SCALING

I. Clinical Approach

Criteria for determination of sequence were described in detail and an example of a treatment plan was presented on pages 298–299. In general, treatment is started where the disease condition is most involved to allow for a longer healing period.

The specific order for instrumentation varies with the severity of the case. Prerequisite to any selected procedure is the use of an efficient routine to minimize time.

With respect to the use of individual instruments, one time-saver is to apply one instrument to all tooth surfaces where it is applicable within a quadrant or area being treated, followed by the next instrument; this minimizes transfer to and from the tray.

A. **Advantages of a Systematic Procedure**

   1. Insures thoroughness in the completion of treatment.
   2. Demonstrates ease and smoothness of operation.
   3. Increases efficiency through repeated routine.
   4. Decreases operating time.
   5. Increases patient comfort.
   6. Increases patient's confidence in the operator.

B. **Overall System**

   1. *Complete a Selected Area.* Scale one quadrant (or selected group of

teeth) thoroughly before moving on to the next rather than move from area to area.

2. *Single Appointment.* When it is expected that scaling can be completed in a single appointment, it may be advisable to remove gross supramarginal deposits throughout the entire dentition by manual or ultrasonic techniques and then return to concentrate on the finer scaling for each area. At the follow-up appointment one week later, when the response to treatment is observed, some additional localized scaling may be indicated.

3. *Planned Multiple Appointments.* When there is generalized supra- and submarginal calculus and extensive scaling and root planing to be done, a series of appointments must be planned as outlined on page 299.

   a. Initial appointment: a generalized scaling may be performed by manual, ultrasonic, or combined techniques.

   (1) Initial scaling should be as thorough as possible for the appointed time: generalized removal of gross deposits randomly without a directed effort to remove as much calculus as possible may do more harm than good.

   (2) Calculus roughened by partial removal may be a source of greater irritation to the gingiva because of its ability to hold new plaque, as well as sharp edges which provide mechanical trauma. The tissues may have been adjusted to the shape and surface texture of the original deposit.

   (3) During personal oral care the gingival pocket wall may be pressed by the toothbrush against the roughened calculus. The continuing source of irritation prevents healing in the tissue and may even cause an acute inflammation.

   b. Quadrant scaling and root planing appointments.

   (1) Scheduled at one week intervals to permit progressive healing.

   (2) Local anesthesia for each quadrant is frequently indicated.

   (3) Plaque control procedures can be reviewed and supplemented before scaling at each appointment.

II. Calculus Removal

Calculus is removed by systematic scaling from tooth to tooth and section by section of the calculus deposit on each tooth surface. Each scaling stroke overlaps the previous one as the scaler is positioned progressively along the area of the deposit.

A. Location of Instrumentation

Removal of calculus relates to the mode of attachment (page 254). Calculus removal from enamel is different from calculus removal and surface planing required for cementum. The nature of the strokes required varies for different parts of a tooth surface.

Figure 33–2 illustrates the location of instrumentation on the tooth surface. The type of pocket, the position of the margin of the free gingiva, and the level of attachment of the junctional epithelium all determine the location of instrumentation and instrument selection for that instrumentation.

B. Steps

Scaling is not a shaving process in which layers are removed. Such a

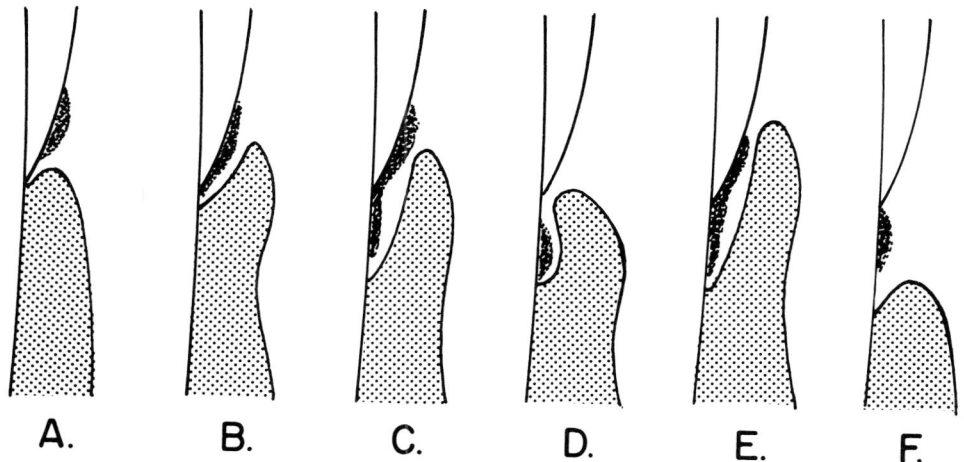

A.   B.   C.   D.   E.   F.

Figure 33–2. Factors influencing instrumentation. Shown are varying conditions encountered which require different approaches. **A.** Supramarginal calculus on enamel. **B.** Gingival pocket with both supra- and submarginal calculus, **C.** Periodontal pocket with both supra- and submarginal calculus, **D.** Periodontal pocket with submarginal calculus on cementum only, **E.** Periodontal pocket with submarginal calculus on both enamel and cementum, and **F.** Calculus on cementum over gingival recession.

procedure tends to make the surface of the calculus smooth and sometimes indistinguishable from the tooth surface, since the oldest calculus, that next to the tooth surface, is the hardest calculus.

In scaling, large pieces of calculus may fracture off first, and then the steps for calculus removal described in subsequent sections of this chapter can be applied to the fine, hard deposits close to the tooth surface. The sharp scaler or curet grips the calculus at its margin and cuts into the calculus at the tooth surface level. Removal takes place as the instrument is pulled along, the attachment is undermined, and after several strokes the tooth surface is free of calculus.

There are five fundamental steps in the application of an instrument for calculus removal and root planing. In the sections following, the steps are described in detail for supramarginal instrumentation and then followed by additional adaptations required for submarginal instrumentation. The five steps are:

1. Grasp of instrument.
2. Establishment of finger rest.
3. Exploratory stroke: position the cutting edge of the blade.
4. Working stroke: activate the instrument.
5. Completion of stroke: prepare for the next.

SUPRAMARGINAL SCALING

I. Instruments

A. Sickle, Hoe, Chisel

These instruments are designed for supramarginal instrumentation. They are sometimes used to remove gross calculus which is a millimeter or two below the gingival margin provided the tissue of the gingival pocket wall is loose and the instrument can be inserted without force.

B. Curet

A curet is used primarily for submarginal instrumentation but is recommended for supramarginal scaling and planing in instances such as the following:

1. When a curved, rounded instrument is particularly adaptable for removing fine, hard deposits near the gingival margin.
2. When gingival recession has caused exposure of cementum and root planing techniques are required.

II. Steps for Calculus Removal

A. Grasp of Instrument

1. Apply modified pen grasp (figure 31–2, page 463).
2. Use a light grasp while instrument is positioned and at the completion of the stroke; tighten grasp during the working stroke.

B. Establish the Finger Rest

1. Use ring and little fingers on firm tooth or teeth for the major rest; apply supplementary rests for increased stability when indicated (page 464).
2. The fulcrum where the finger rest is applied must be dry for stability. Plaque and saliva make the tooth surface slippery. Use a folded gauze sponge in the vestibular area with a corner over the fulcrum rest tooth; dry with compressed air or wipe with cotton, maintain retraction, and repeat the drying as needed for continued instrument control.
3. Finger rests are applied on the tooth adjacent to the one being scaled, or as close as possible and convenient. Long stretches between the rest and the point of instrument application can decrease control.
4. Use light but firm pressure on the finger rest while the instrument is being positioned and at the end of the stroke.
5. During the working stroke, the pressure on the fulcrum increases

slightly to balance the pressure of the instrument on the tooth being scaled.

C. Position the Cutting Edge of the Blade

1. Exploratory stroke: the exploratory stroke is a preliminary stroke in which the blade is applied lightly over the calculus until the base of the deposit is located, and then the blade is positioned for the working stroke. Use of the exploratory stroke has greatest application in the submarginal area when preparation for scaling is difficult because of invisibility (page 505). It also has particular use during supramarginal instrumentation of the proximal surfaces.
2. Angulation of the blade.
   a. *Sickle Scaler.* Blade is applied beneath the calculus deposit so that the inner or facial surface is at an angle of less than 90 degrees (but not less than 45 degrees) with the tooth surface (figure 32–2, page 474).
   b. *Hoe Scaler.* With the full width of the cutting edge in contact with the tooth, and with the shank adapted closely to the side of the tooth or with the shank in contact with the crown of the tooth (figure 32–3, page 475).
   c. *Chisel Scaler.* With the full width of the cutting edge in contact with the tooth, and with the shank adapted closely to the tooth, in position for scaling from labial to lingual.
   d. *Curet.* At an angle of less than 90 degrees (but not less than 45 degrees) between the tooth surface and the facial surface of the blade (figure 32–5, page 477).
3. Hold the cutting edge firmly against the tooth surface in preparation for activating the instrument.

D. **Activate the Instrument: Working Stroke**
  1. *Tighten the grasp;* move the instrument firmly and deliberately.
  2. *Maintain the cutting edge* evenly on the tooth surface during the stroke.
  3. *Direction of strokes*
     a. Vertical pull strokes are used for scalers and hoes; horizontal and oblique strokes may be used when away from the cervical region near the gingival margin.
     b. Vertical, horizontal, and oblique strokes may be used for the curet.
     c. Horizontal push strokes only are used for the chisel from labial to lingual at right angles with the long axis of anterior teeth.
  4. *Pressure of the instrument* on tooth surface: when the instrument is sharp, the minimum pressure applied will allow the cutting edge to grip the tooth surface; a balance of pressure is maintained between the pressure of the instrument, the grasp of the instrument, and the pressure on the finger rest.
  5. *Control of motion:* without independent finger movement, the hand, wrist, and arm act as a continuum to activate the instrument (pages 467–468).
  6. *Length of stroke:* short
     a. Short stroke permits accommodation of the cutting edge to changes in the topography of the tooth surface.
     b. Short stroke assists in maintaining *control* and *precision*.
     c. Stroke is confined to the area of the deposit on the tooth surface. The area in the vicinity of the cementoenamel junction where the majority of the deposits are located is called the *instrumentation zone*.[15] Extending the instrument up the side of the tooth in unnecessarily long strokes is time-consuming, dulls the instrument, and decreases control by and concentration of the operator.

E. **Completion of Stroke**
  1. Hold instrument in place momentarily, maintain the finger rest, lighten the grasp on the instrument and then return the instrument to position for a repeat stroke.
  2. Repeat strokes until surface is smooth.

F. **Continuation of Procedure**
  1. Move instrument laterally on the tooth surface to adjacent undisturbed deposit; maintain the same finger rest.
  2. Overlap strokes to insure complete removal of deposit.
  3. Repeat strokes until the tooth surface has been completely scaled.
  4. Inspect surface with explorer assisted by compressed air and repeat as needed to produce a smooth, glass-like surface.

SUBMARGINAL INSTRUMENTATION

Dexterity, deliberateness, and diligence are key words in submarginal area techniques. The principal objective is to remove the calculus and to plane the root surface with a minimum of trauma to the gingival tissue. Procedures are guided by the recognized need for removal of all calculus and the production of a very smooth surface which will resist the formation of plaque and calculus to assure maximum tissue response for oral health.

Root planing follows calculus removal to provide a smooth surface. It is a continuation of submarginal scaling and an integral part of it. Not all root planing is submarginal because when root surfaces are exposed as a result of recession or periodontal surgery for pocket elimination, the cemental surface is supramarginal (figure 33–2 F).

I. Comparison with Supramarginal Instrumentation

Although the basic techniques described previously for removal of supramarginal calculus are applied in the submarginal area, techniques are complicated by several factors, notably the following:

A. **Accessibility**

Instrumentation is necessary in areas where access is difficult.

B. **Invisible Working Area**

Techniques are almost entirely dependent on tactile sensitivity which must be acute in order to locate and remove minute roughnesses of the tooth surface.

C. **Calculus Attachment**

Attachment to the cementum is more tenacious than to the enamel. On the cementum, calculus attaches to minute irregularities by penetration into the cementum, or by attachment into areas of cemental resorption, which makes removal difficult. Attachment to the enamel, the site of most supramarginal scaling, is primarily by means of the acquired pellicle or cuticle (page 254).

D. **Morphology of Calculus**

Submarginal calculus is irregularly deposited and occurs in nodular, ledge or ring-like, smooth veneer, and other forms (table 16–1, page 251).

E. **Variations in Root Surface Topography**

Although many variations can be expected as part of the normal tooth anatomy, others are unusual variations which complicate scaling primarily because of their invisibility (page 181).

F. **Variations in Depth of Pockets**

Pockets must be measured about each tooth as variations in depth can occur on a single surface; instruments must be adapted to reach the bottom of the pocket around the entire periphery of each tooth.

G. **Gingival Wall**

The gingival wall is close to the tooth surface with only a narrow area for manipulation of instruments. The width of the pocket varies; it narrows down at the base next to the junctional epithelium.

II. Instrument Selection: Curets

As mentioned previously, gross calculus which is just below the gingival margin may be removed during supramarginal scaling provided the tissue is loose and resilient enough to permit easy access by the instruments without having to force them into the sulcus. The ultrasonic scaler may also be used to remove gross submarginal deposits (page 509).

Deeper in the pocket and close to the root surface, the curets are the instruments of choice for a number of reasons, including:

A. Fine, thin instruments permit increased tactile sensitivity which bulkier instruments cannot. Increased sensitivity is essential to thoroughness in areas with limited accessibility and visibility.

B. Root planing with curets produces smoother surfaces than planing with other instruments.[16–19]

C. The curved, narrow, fine curets with rounded ends can be adapted to the anatomic features of the submarginal area with less trauma to the tooth surface and the gingival tissue. Supramarginal sickles, hoes, and chisels have sharp points or corners and are thick, bulky, and straight.

D. The sulcus or pocket narrows in the deeper area close to the junctional epithelium. The smallest, smoothest instruments are best applied to this narrow area to prevent the need for excess stretching of the gingival wall which can cause a splitting of the junctional epithelium from the tooth.

E. Because of the rounded end, a horizontal stroke can be used conservatively. The length of the horizontal stroke would depend on variations in pocket depth. When used in position for a vertical stroke, the round back of the curet can be placed against the bottom of the pocket.

III. Submarginal Procedures

The surface to be scaled must first be examined with probe and explorer to define the area and the calculus, as described on pages 498–499. Then, the same basic five steps for calculus removal are followed as for supramarginal scaling with variations listed below.

To remove heavier submarginal calculus, first, a larger, stronger curet is used for convenience and efficiency. The smaller, delicate curets should be reserved and kept sharp for fine scaling and root planing, particularly in the narrow depths of the pocket.

A. **Grasp of Instrument**
   The modified pen grasp is used. The grasp is lightened as increased tactile sense is needed for refinement of the root surface with continued scaling.

B. **Establish the Finger Rest**
   1. Definite finger rest on dry, firm tooth structure as close to the tooth being treated as possible and convenient.
   2. Complete control is essential.

C. **Position the Cutting Edge of the Blade**
   1. Position the blade on the tooth surface near the gingival margin where the instrument will be inserted for submarginal scaling.

a. Hold at the appropriate angulation for scaling, that is, with the facial surface of the blade at less than a 90-degree angle with the tooth surface (figure 32–5, page 477; and figure 34–1B, page 521).
   b. The facial surface of the blade will be facing toward the incisal or occlusal for a vertical stroke and tipped slightly for an oblique stroke; for a horizontal stroke, the curved tip of the blade is directed toward the apex.
   c. Note the relationship of the handle, fulcrum, grasp, blade, and tooth so that after insertion the blade may be promptly repositioned for calculus removal.
2. *Exploratory Stroke**
   a. Direct the tip of the curet gingivally; maintain contact with the tooth surface.
   b. With light grasp, insert the curet gently under the gingival margin (figure 33–3A).
   c. Keep the instrument tip in light contact with the tooth or calculus surface. The blade is closed toward the tooth surface and held at an angle of zero degrees during the exploratory stroke (figure 33–3B).
   d. Pass the instrument over the surface of the deposit to the base of the sulcus until tension of the soft tissue attachment is felt.
   e. Adjust the blade to the correct angulation with the tooth surface (as determined before insertion) just below the calculus deposit (figure 33–3C).

*The exploratory stroke is sometimes referred to as the preliminary or preparatory stroke. When the term "exploratory" is used, it should be distinguished from the meaning of the word as it applies to the use of an explorer. The curet is not used as an explorer, and the calculus has been identified previously by using an explorer.

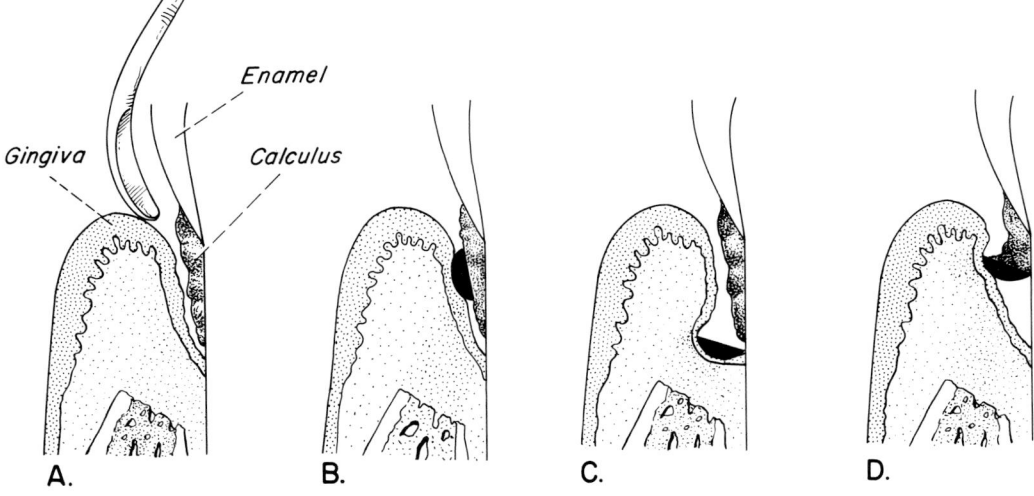

Figure 33–3. Submarginal scaling and planing. **A.** The curet is gently inserted under the gingival margin
B. With an exploratory stroke the blade is passed over the surface of the tooth or calculus. Note zero degree
angle of the face of the curet with the calculus. **C.** The curet is lowered to the base of the pocket until the
tension of the soft tissue is felt, and then it is positioned at less than 90 degrees for scaling. **D.** The blade is
moved along the root surface in a scaling stroke to remove calculus, or a planing stroke to smooth the
surface.

f. Utilize as much of the cutting
edge of the blade as possible in
accord with the anatomical contour of the tooth.

D. **Activate the Instrument: Working
Stroke**
1. *Tighten the grasp* and move the
instrument firmly and deliberately
(figure 33–3 D).
2. *Maintain the cutting edge* evenly
on the tooth surface during the
stroke and at the completion of the
stroke.
3. *Direction of Strokes*
   a. Vertical, oblique, or horizontal
   strokes may be applied.
   b. All strokes are limited in length
   by the constant adjustment needed
   to conform with the curved tooth
   surfaces and the varying depths
   of the sulcus or pocket around
   the tooth.
   c. Horizontal strokes cannot be
   applied to the bottom of the
   sulcus or pocket except where

the probe measurements show
the depth is uniform; otherwise
the curet would be dragged into
the junctional epithelium at the
higher areas.
d. Not recommended: push-pull
type strokes are not used submarginally as these would tend
to push particles deep into the
sulcus and into the soft tissue.
4. *Pressure of Instrument.* A balance
of pressure between the pressure of
the instrument, the grasp of the
instrument, and the finger rest must
be maintained. Undue pressure
decreases control and lessens tactile sensitivity.
5. *Control of Motion.* Without independent finger movement, the
hand, wrist, and arm act as a
continuum to activate the instrument.
6. *Length of Stroke*
   a. Short decisive strokes, the
   length dependent on the height

of the deposit (instrumentation zone, page 503).

b. Within the confines of the pocket to prevent the need for repeated removal and reinsertion of the instrument which is not only time consuming but means that the instrument must pass over the more sensitive areas for the patient (the necks of the teeth and the gingival margin).

7. *Calculus Removal.* Calculus should not be shaved off in layers, but when possible the whole thickness should be moved in one piece. By shaving, a thin coating of calculus may be left which may be smooth and indiscernible from the tooth surface, yet be a nucleus for new plaque and calculus formation.

8. *Completion of Stroke.* Maintain finger rest, lighten grasp, repeat exploratory stroke within the sulcus. Reposition for a repeat or adjacent stroke. Several strokes are generally required for each area.

E. **Plane the Root Surface**

The technique for planing is basically the same as for scaling. Instrument control, application of the cutting edge, directions for strokes, and other principles are not essentially different. What is different is the ultimate perfection of resulting smoothness attained because of the high degree of tactile sensitivity involved and the precise instrumentation.

Specific differences in technique are related to touch and pressure. A lighter grasp must be used to increase tactile sensitivity. Since increased pressure is not needed, a lighter shaving-like stroke can be used for smoothing or finishing the root surface.

1. *Check the sharpness of the curets.* Generally curets dulled during

scaling should be resharpened or laid aside and a freshly sharpened set used for root planing.

2. *Strokes*
   a. Apply light pressure for maximum sensitivity to minute irregularities of the surface.
   b. Use short, even strokes which systematically overlap and cross over each other. As the surface becomes smoother, longer strokes will help to remove small lines left by shorter strokes.
   c. Directions: Vertical, then oblique, then, when applicable at levels away from the junctional epithelium, horizontal.
   d. Number of strokes: Many strokes are needed, sometimes as many as 30 or 40 may be applied before a section of the root surface feels glassy smooth and hard.
   e. Adaptation of instrument: Careful application is necessary to adapt the curet to the morphological features of the roots. The convex rounded surfaces, the constricted cervical area, the concavities and grooves of proximal surfaces, and furcations all require precise adaptation (page 466).
   f. As planing nears completion, there is a gradual change in the sound of the instrument on the root surface. At the completion, the instrument can be nearly as quiet as it would be on polished enamel.

3. Examine with a submarginal explorer to establish completion of instrumentation.

F. **Irrigate All Sulci or Pockets**

This should be done thoroughly with warm water to remove any particles of cementum or calculus. Research has shown that bits of calculus, debris, or microorganisms can be implanted into the underlying tissue.[20-22]

EFFECTS OF SCALING AND PLANING

An evaluation of instrumentation may be made immediately after completion by exploring to ascertain that the tooth surfaces are smooth and hard. The real evaluation, the true test of successful treatment, cannot be made until approximately one week when the response of the gingival tissue will be apparent.

I. Effect on Gingiva

A. Coincidental Curettage

Without intentional curettage during scaling and root planing, there is some debridement (coincidental curettage) of the lining of the sulcus or pocket.[20-22] This effect was noted particularly in the deeper aspects where the pocket narrows toward the junctional epithelium. The partial curettage which occurs is due to the outer or unused cutting edge of the curet even though a less than 90-degree angulation of the facial surface of the blade to the tooth surface is maintained.

The junctional epithelium may be partially removed, depending on the severity of the inflammation, the size of the instrument, and the amount of trauma inflicted by the operator. Partial curettage may be considered beneficial. The objectives of curettage are described on pages 519–520.

B. Healing

With scaling, planing, and plaque control, the adjacent gingival tissue heals by resolution of the inflammation. Edema recedes, necrotic cells are cleared away, and the tissue regenerates.

Healing has been shown to start with beginning epithelial regeneration within two days of scaling; new epithelial attachment has been demonstrated by five days, and complete regeneration by approximately two weeks.[22-24] Healing time is generally related to the severity of the periodontal inflammation at the start of treatment.

C. Effect of Partial Scaling

When even a small amount of submarginal calculus is left on a tooth surface, an area of inflammation will persist. At examination on the subsequent appointment some tissue shrinkage may have occurred, but the remaining deposit must be removed for complete resolution.

When large or small deposits are left after incomplete scaling particularly in a deep pocket, an acute periodontal abscess may form. A periodontal abscess will result in pain, swelling, tooth sensitivity, and various symptoms.[25] Such abscesses can be prevented by completing calculus removal and planing. Only as many teeth as can be completed in a given appointment should be undertaken. Other teeth should be left untouched except for plaque control instruction.

II. Effect on Tooth Surface

Research has shown that following careful submarginal scaling, some calculus frequently may remain. During root planing, the residual calculus is removed and, to obtain a smooth and hard root surface, the cementum is partly or wholly removed, the amount varying from surface to surface.[16,26,27] It is necessary to remove cementum because the surface, exposed after recession of the junctional epithelium during pocket formation, is rough, soft, and diseased. If it was not smoothed, the roughness would serve as a nidus for additional plaque bacteria and subsequently additional calculus.

Teeth which had been scaled were

studied by electronmicroscopy.[27] The tooth surfaces which were under calculus were less mineralized than exposed root surfaces. An exchange of minerals occurs between the saliva and the tooth. Following exposure for three to four weeks after scaling, some surfaces became hypermineralized while others became decalcified and carious. Knowledge of the processes involved in the surface changes can aid in the prevention of cemental caries, erosion, hypersensitivity, and calculus. Fluoride-containing dentifrice and mouthrinse should be routinely recommended following root planing when there is exposed cementum.

USE OF ULTRASONICS

Ultrasonic instrumentation is an adjunct to manual scaling but not a substitute. Because of the ease of removal of tooth deposits by ultrasonic techniques, the application is most effective with patients having gross stains, calculus, and debris.

Root planing is not accomplished by ultrasonic instruments and must be completed by curets.[28] The ultrasonic method, therefore, is principally for treatment when deposits are gross but is not applicable for preventive scaling measures when small deposits are removed at frequent recall appointments.

Histological studies have shown postoperative healing following ultrasonic instrumentation to be at least as satisfactory and in some instances more satisfactory than hand scaling.[29,30]

Research on the effects on the tooth surface has shown that when there is an undesirable surface alteration following ultrasonic instrumentation it can be associated with the power setting, the pressure of the tip on the tooth, or a tip that is not blunt. The appearance of the affected surface may be granular or stippled.[31-34]

It has been pointed out that if the energy output is low, the hand pressure light, and the tip of the instrument broad and polished where it touches the tooth, presumably there would be no effect on the tooth surface, at least not within a reasonable number of applications.[31] While the instrument tip is on calculus the tooth surface is unaffected, which brings out several operational factors. The tooth surface should be examined with an explorer frequently during operation so that excessive application of the instrument to the tooth structure can be avoided. It is also important that minimal instrument application be made when there are small discrete calculus deposits or thin stains to be removed.

In addition to the removal of heavy deposits and stains, ultrasonics may be used in a variety of ways including the removal of overhanging restorations and in periodontal curettage and surgery. In orthodontics, ultrasonic instrumentation has been found effective for scaling prior to fitting and cementing appliances, and for the removal of excess cement after initial cementation and when appliances are removed.[35] Reference to the ultrasonic cleaning unit for instruments has been made on page 20.

I. Mode of Action[31,36]

The ultrasonic unit consists of an electric generator, a handpiece assembly, a set of interchangeable prophylaxis inserts, and a foot control. The ultrasonic principle is based on the use of very high frequency sound waves.

A. The ultrasonic machine converts high frequency electrical energy into mechanical energy in the form of rapid vibrations.

B. The instrument tip vibrations vary for different models, but may be, for example, 25,000 cycles per second with an amplitude of 1/1000 cm. The vibratory action fractures the deposit and causes it to be removed from the tooth.

C. Ultrasonic waves are dissipated in the form of heat. The heat is reduced by keeping the handpiece cooled internally and the working end cooled by a constant flow of water which is expelled through a metal tube or by means of an internal flow through the working end.

D. Effects of water: the atomized water forms minute vacuum bubbles which collapse with release of tremendous local pressure; the effect is cleansing to the area. Since it is necessary to have the instrument in contact with the deposit on the tooth surface if the deposit is to be removed, the bubbling cavitational action of the water has little if any actual influence on deposit removal.

II. Technique for Use[31,36–38]

A. **Preparation of Prophylaxis Inserts**
  1. Tune according to manufacturer's specifications.
  2. Use lowest power setting at which the calculus will be loosened.
  3. Instrument tips must be dull: if sharp they would nick and gouge the tooth surface.

B. **Preparation of Patient**
  1. Review patient history; ultrasonic is contraindicated for patient with a pacemaker.[39]
  2. Have the patient use an antiseptic mouth rinse for 30 seconds prior to ultrasonic scaling to lower the oral bacterial count and hence lower the bacterial count of the aerosols produced (pages 27–28).
  3. Use coverall and towel.
  4. Topical anesthetic may be applied to allay gingival sensitivity.

C. **Aspiration of Water**
  Use an evacuator or effective saliva ejector.

D. **Instrumentation**
  1. Use modified pen grasp for handpiece and apply fulcrum to appropriate, convenient tooth surfaces to stabilize the instrument and permit systematic coverage of tooth surfaces being scaled.
  2. Application of working end: parallel to long axis of the tooth or at no more than a 15-degree angle to tooth surface. Adaptation to variations in tooth topography and morphology is difficult but necessary. To maintain a less than 15-degree angle in all positions takes practice and concentration.
  3. Stroke
    a. Keep the tip in motion at all times.
    b. Check to be sure that the water reaches the operating area.
    c. Brush lightly over the deposit moving in a vertical or diagonal direction: six strokes usually suffice. Pressure removes tooth structure.
    d. Move instrument with smooth, light, constant and overlapping strokes.
    e. Increased number of strokes will not damage the tooth surface provided the instrument is blunt, the tip is not held perpendicular to the long axis of the tooth, and no positive pressure is used.
    f. Instrument tends to bind when inserted interproximally, and the excess pressure stops the vibration. Remove and reactivate the instrument.
  4. Complete one tooth before starting another.
  5. Release foot pedal switch at regular intervals to aid in water control; stop to evaluate the tooth surfaces with an explorer periodically.
  6. Complete procedure with manual instruments.

a. Check submarginal areas with a submarginal explorer Number 17.
b. Remove remaining submarginal deposits and plane the surface smooth with curets.

E. **Care of Prophylaxis Inserts**
   1. Autoclave.
   2. Handle with care to avoid damage to working ends or internal mechanisms.

III. Advantages and Limitations

A. **Advantages**
   1. Calculus removal and tooth debridement may be accomplished with less effort than manual. More time can be devoted to thorough, careful root planing.
   2. Effective for preparation for periodontal surgery.
   3. Requires minimum tissue manipulation for hypersensitive tissues (as in acute necrotizing ulcerative gingivitis).
   4. Water jet cleanses the field of operation.
   5. Patient may experience less pain during instrumentation, and less postoperative discomfort can be expected.
   6. Operating time is reduced for removal of heavy stains and calculus.

B. **Limitations**
   1. Contraindicated for use on young, growing tissues, therefore it should not be used on children.
   2. Lack of tactile perception during instrumentation.
   3. Impeded visibility during operation; indirect vision with water-sprayed mouth mirror presents problems.
   4. Will not complete the entire procedure: access to all areas is not possible, and fine submarginal calculus is not removed.

5. Patient and operator have discomfort and inconvenience of spraying or dripping of water.

USE OF A TOPICAL ANESTHETIC

A topical anesthetic is a drug applied to the mucous membrane to produce a loss of sensation. A topical anesthetic can be used with a degree of success for short-duration desensitization of the gingiva. As a soft tissue anesthetic, a topical agent does not influence sensations in the teeth and, therefore, is not a substitute for local anesthetic administered by injection.

Pain reaction varies from person to person and even in the same person depending on emotional state and degree of fatigue. A person with a low reaction to pain, who is hyporeactive, is said to have a *high pain threshold.* When there is a high reaction, the person is hyperreactive and has a *low pain threshold.* In addition to emotional state and fatigue, other factors which influence pain threshold are age, sex, fear, and apprehension. Older individuals have a tendency to have a higher pain threshold than younger, males higher than females, but in fear or apprehension there will be a lowered pain threshold.[40]

I. Indications for Use

A local anesthetic should be used in dental hygiene practice when indicated by the patient's pain threshold or by evidence of fear and apprehension. Although primarily a local anesthetic would be indicated for deep submarginal scaling, root planing, and curettage, it may be indicated for any degree of severity of condition.

Pain threshold can usually be detected during initial examination. A patient who hyperreacts to gentle, careful probing, may indeed have a low pain threshold, and a note should be made on the record to indicate possible need for anesthesia.

A topical anesthetic can be used for

many dental hygiene and dental services including the following:

A. Prior to injection for local anesthesia.

B. Prevention of gagging in radiographic techniques and impression making.

C. Relief of pain from localized diseased areas.

D. During instrumentation for probing, exploring, scaling, and sometimes root planing and gingival curettage. When root planing and curettage are deep and generalized, a local anesthetic is usually indicated.

E. Suture removal.

F. Dressing replacement after removal of the initial dressing. When pressure is needed for adaptation of the dressing, a topical application provides relief (pages 530–531).

II. Action of the Topical Anesthetic

The purpose is to desensitize the mucous membrane by anesthetizing the terminal nerve endings. A superficial anesthesia is produced which is related to the amount of absorption of the drug by the tissue. The absorption varies with the thickness of the stratified squamous epithelial covering and the degree of keratinization. The skin and lips are very resistant; the attached gingiva and cheek and palatal mucosa absorb drugs slowly; whereas the tissues without keratinization absorb more readily.

III. Requirements of an Adequate Topical Anesthetic

A. Produces effective lasting anesthesia.

B. Is miscible and stable in vehicle used.

C. Anesthetizing agent readily released from the preparation when applied.

D. Is nonirritating to the tissues.

E. Does not induce hypersensitivity reactions or other toxic effect at the concentration required for anesthesia.

F. Does not delay healing.

G. Can be readily washed off with water.

IV. Preparations Used: Characteristics

A number of preparations have been used in the form of gels, ointments, solutions, troches, or powders. The American Dental Association, Council on Dental Therapeutics evaluates and classifies topical anesthetics.[41]

Examples of anesthetics used in topical preparations are benzocaine, lidocaine (Xylocaine), chlorobutanol, and nupercaine.[41-43] Products containing butacaine, cocaine, and tetracaine should be avoided or used cautiously because of known toxic reactions. General properties and characteristics of preparations of anesthetics for surface use are listed below.

A. Oils, alcohols, or glycols are used as the vehicle since most of the anesthetizing substances are only slightly soluble in water.

B. Most topical anesthetics are prepared in fairly concentrated form to allow for the resistance of the thick epithelial covering and viscid coating of saliva on the tissues.

C. The drugs are absorbed slowly due to their slight solubility and the resistance of the mucous membrane.

D. Alcohols or glycols in concentrated solutions may be irritating to the sensitive mucous membranes and therefore are inferior vehicles (percent of alcohol or glycol should not be greater than 10 percent).

E. Pastes or ointments are more effective than liquids but may be considered more difficult to apply.

F. Carbowaxes used as vehicles for topical anesthetics are somewhat hygroscopic, so that the jar in which the ointment is kept should be closed tightly.

G. Pressurized spray preparations need to be used with caution since it is difficult to control the amount of material expelled and to limit the area of application. Inhalation of the fine spray into the lungs can produce a toxic reaction. When the liquid flows into the throat (as may be possible with application of any type of preparation), coughing may be initiated.

V. Technique for Application of a Topical Anesthetic

A. Consult history and other records for pertinent information concerning a patient's previous experiences with anesthetics.

B. Explain purpose and anticipated effect to the patient.

C. Dry area with gauze sponge or cotton roll. Compressed air may be used with consideration for sensitive tissues.

D. Application
  1. Ointment
     a. Use of a syringe: prepare a B.D. 18 gauge Yale needle by bending the last ¼ to ½ inch to an angle of 50 to 60 degrees with the long axis of the needle (use orthodontic pliers for bending). Sterilize the needle and attach it to 3 cc. B.D. Yale syringe. The syringe is filled with five percent Xylocaine ointment, reassembled, and warmed slightly under hot tap water to permit flow through the needle. Application around and into the sulcus is facilitated.[44]
     b. Apply with a cotton pellet and rub into the proximal area. This method is less exact than the use of the syringe.
  2. Liquid: apply directly over the dry tissues with a cotton swab or pellet.

E. Wait briefly for anesthetic to take effect before proceeding.

TECHNICAL HINTS

I. Summary: Methods to Minimize Patient Discomfort

A. **Tissue Sensitivity**
  1. Gingival tissue: use topical anesthetic and/or local anesthetic as needed.
  2. Exposed cementum or dentin: apply desensitizing agent (pages 564–566).
  3. Protect lips and corners of mouth from irritation during instrumentation by application of petrolatum, cocoa butter, or other appropriate lubricant.
  4. Use only warm water or mouthwash for rinsing.

B. **Preventive Instrumentation**
  1. Use appropriate instrument, applied at the correct angulation, for each tooth surface.
  2. Curets applied to base of sulcus or pocket must be small to prevent undue stretching of gingival wall and hence unnecessary detachment of the junctional epithelium.
  3. Instruments must be sharp, but the cementum can be scratched if sharp curets are not applied correctly and discriminately.
  4. Maintain control of instrument at all times through effective grasp, appropriate finger rest, and correctly applied strokes to prevent accidental trauma to gingival tissue.
  5. Apply minimum effective pressure on finger rest and of instrument on tooth to prevent patient from developing tired muscles and an overstretched temporomandibular joint.
  6. Finger rests on soft tissue give the patient a feeling of more pressure than finger rests on the teeth and consequently may give the impression that the dental hygienist is heavy-handed.

C. **Postoperative Care** (pages 570–572)
1. Massage of gingival tissue at completion of instrumentation can be soothing and restful for the patient.
2. An antiseptic may be applied or the patient requested to rinse with mouthwash to decrease initial discomfort.
3. Provide instruction for personal care, such as rinsing with warm salt water and other appropriate measures for post-appointment follow-up.

II. Maintenance of a Clear Field

A. Use saliva ejector and evacuator as needed.
B. Use of rolled gauze sponge or cotton rolls.
1. A gauze sponge rolled the long dimension and placed in the mucobuccal fold beneath teeth being treated can assist by:
   a. Retracting the cheek or lip.
   b. Keeping teeth dry for secure finger rest.
   c. Drying the individual area for better vision.
2. Aid in retraction of tongue and keeping field free from saliva by placing cotton roll under tongue.
C. Maintenance of clear field and/or control of bleeding.
1. Application of pressure with cotton roll or pellet.
2. Application of three percent hydrogen peroxide with cotton pellet, followed by patient rinsing and/or dry pellet applied with pressure.
3. Use of compressed air to deflect tissue and remove debris.

III. Broken Instrument

The procedure to follow when an instrument blade tip breaks in the patient's mouth during operation should be in accord with the dentist's own policy. Therefore, it is recommended that this be discussed before an accident happens so that the procedure can be clarified.

The principal objective in the location of a broken instrument tip is *to know positively that the tip has been removed.* With this in mind, rinsing, use of suction or compressed air, or other procedures which could cause the removal of the tip unknowingly would be out of order. A general procedure is suggested here.

A. Cease operation, retain retraction without moving the patient's head unnecessarily, and isolate with gauze or cotton roll.
B. Do not alarm patient by describing the accident.
C. Examine the immediate field of operation, the floor of the mouth, and the mucobuccal fold. Blot the gingival tissue dry with a cotton roll and examine around the tooth.
D. Apply transilluminator or mouth light when available.
E. The gingival sulcus can be gently examined using a curet in a spooning-like stroke, but with care not to push the tip into the base of the sulcus (should the tip be there).
F. Consult the dentist for assistance in accord with previously discussed policy.
G. When tip is not removed by any means mentioned thus far, make periapical and bite-wing radiographs of the area.

IV. Applications for Scaling Principles

A. Removal of excess cement following cementation of orthodontic bands.
B. Removal of pieces of periodontal dressings that adhere to the teeth when a dressing is removed (page 530).

V. Protection of the Dental Hygienist

Wear rimmed glasses for protection from bits of calculus or debris which could accidentally get into the eyes (figure 4–3, page 39). Calculus and debris are highly contaminated. Aerosols from the ultrasonic water spray contain large numbers of organisms and can be collected from the air of the room 35 minutes after scaling has ceased.[45]

FACTORS TO TEACH THE PATIENT

I. The nature, occurrence, and etiology of calculus.

II. The importance of the complete removal of calculus to the health of the oral tissues in the prevention of periodontal diseases.

III. Relationship of the accumulation of deposits to the patient's personal oral hygiene procedures.

IV. Basic reasons for need and advantages of more than one appointment to complete the scaling and root planing.

V. Needed frequency of recall appointments in relation to oral health.

References

1. Lightner, L. M., O'Leary, T. J., Jividen, G. J., Crump, P. P., and Drake, R. B.: Preventive Periodontic Treatment Procedures: Results After One Year, *J. Am. Dent. Assoc.*, 76, 1043, May, 1968.
2. Lovdal, A., Arno, A., Schei, O., and Waerhaug, J.: Combined Effect of Subgingival Scaling and Controlled Oral Hygiene on the Incidence of Gingivitis, *Acta Odontol. Scand.*, 19, 537, December, 1961.
3. Suomi, J. D., Greene, J. C., Vermillion, J. R., Chang, J. J., and Leatherwood, E. C.: The Effect of Controlled Oral Hygiene Procedures on the Progression of Periodontal Disease in Adults: Results After Two Years, *J. Periodont.*, 40, 416, July, 1969.
4. Ramfjord, S. P., Nissle, R. R., Shick, R. A., and Cooper, H.: Subgingival Curettage Versus Surgical Elimination of Periodontal Pockets, *J. Periodont.*, 39, 167, May, 1968.
5. Miller, G. M. and Cohen, D. W.: Role of Initial Preparation of the Mouth in Periodontal Therapy, in Goldman, H. M. and Cohen, D. W.: *Periodontal Therapy*, 5th ed. St. Louis, Mosby, 1973, pp. 372–379, 875.
6. De Leo, A. A., Schoenknecht, M. D., Anderson, M. W., and Peterson, J. C.: The Incidence of Bacteremia Following Oral Prophylaxis on Pediatric Patients, *Oral Surg.*, 37, 36, January, 1974.
7. Korn, N. A. and Schaffer, E. M.: Comparison of the Postoperative Bacteremias Induced Following Different Periodontal Procedures, *J. Periodont.*, 33, 226, July, 1962.
8. Royer, R., Gaines, R., and Kruger, G.: Bacteremia Following Exodontia, Prophylaxis, and Gingivectomy, *J. Dent. Res.*, 43, 877, September-October, 1964 (Supplement).
9. Bender, I. B., Seltzer, S., Tashman, S., and Meloff, G.: Dental Procedures in Patients with Rheumatic Heart Disease, *Oral Surg.*, 16, 466, April, 1963.
10. Winslow, M. B. and Kobernick, S. D.: Bacteremia after Prophylaxis, *J. Am. Dent. Assoc.*, 61, 69, July, 1960.
11. Connor, H. D., Haberman, S., Collings, C. K., and Winford, T. E.: Bacteremias Following Periodontal Scaling in Patients with Healthy Appearing Gingiva, *J. Periodont.*, 38, 466, November-December, 1967.
12. Bandt, C. L., Korn, N. A., and Schaffer, E. M.: Bacteremias from Ultrasonic and Hand Instrumentation, *J. Periodont.*, 35, 214, May-June, 1964.
13. Randall, E. and Brenman, H. S.: Local Degerming with Povidone-Iodine. I. Prior to Dental Prophylaxis, *J. Periodont.*, 45, 866, December, 1974.
14. Brenman, H. S. and Randall, E.: Local Degerming with Povidone-Iodine. II. Prior to Gingivectomy, *J. Periodont.*, 45, 870, December, 1974.
15. Glickman, I.: *Clinical Periodontology*, 4th ed. Philadelphia, Saunders, 1972, pp. 624–625.
16. Schaffer, E. M.: Histological Results of Root Curettage of Human Teeth, *J. Periodont.*, 27, 296, October, 1956.
17. Barnes, J. E. and Schaffer, E. M.: Subgingival Root Planing: A Comparison Using Files, Hoes and Curettes, *J. Periodont.*, 31, 300, September, 1960.
18. Green, E. and Ramfjord, S. P.: Tooth Roughness After Subgingival Root Planing, *J. Periodont.*, 37, 396, September-October, 1966.
19. Kerry, G. J.: Roughness of Root Surfaces After Use of Ultrasonic Instruments and Hand Curettes, *J. Periodont.*, 38, 340, July-August, 1967.
20. Ramfjord, S. and Kiester, G.: The Gingival Sulcus and the Periodontal Pocket Immediately Following Scaling of Teeth, *J. Periodont.*, 25, 167, July, 1954.
21. Moskow, B. S.: Response of the Gingival Sulcus to Instrumentation: A Histological Investigation. I. The Scaling Procedure, *J. Periodont.*, 33, 282, July, 1962.
22. Schaffer, E. M., Stende, G., and King, D.: Healing of Periodontal Pocket Tissues Following Ultrasonic Scaling and Hand Planing, *J. Periodont.*, 35, 140, March-April, 1964.
23. O'Bannon, J. Y.: The Gingival Tissues Before and After Scaling the Teeth, *J. Periodont.*, 35, 69, January-February, 1964.

24. Stone, S., Ramfjord, S. P., and Waldron, J.: Scaling and Gingival Curettage. A Radioautographic Study, *J. Periodont.*, 37, 415, September-October, 1966.

25. Glickman: op. cit., pp. 243–245.

26. Orban, B. and Manella, V. B.: A Macroscopic and Microscopic Study of Instruments Designed for Root Planing, *J. Periodont.*, 27, 120, April, 1956.

27. Selvig, K. A.: Biological Changes at the Tooth-saliva Interface in Periodontal Disease, *J. Dent. Res.*, 48, 846, September-October, 1969 (Supplement).

28. Stende, G. W. and Schaffer, E. M.: A Comparison of Ultrasonic and Hand Scaling, *J. Periodont.*, 32, 312, October, 1961.

29. Bhaskar, S. N., Grower, M. F., and Cutright, D. E.: Gingival Healing After Hand and Ultrasonic Scaling—Biochemical and Histologic Analysis, *J. Periodont.*, 43, 31, January, 1972.

30. Donzé, Y., Krüger, J., Ketterl, W., and Rateitschak, K. H.: Treatment of Gingivitis with Cavitron or Hand Instruments: A Comparative Study, *Helv. Odontol. Acta*, 17, 31, April, 1973.

31. Clark, S. M.: The Ultrasonic Dental Unit: A Guide for the Clinical Application of Ultrasonics in Dentistry and in Dental Hygiene, *J. Periodont.*, 40, 621, November, 1969.

32. Stewart, J. L., Briggs, R. L., Drisko, R. R., and Jamison, H. C.: Relative Calculus and Tooth Structure Loss with Use of Power-driven Scaling Instruments, *J. Am. Dent. Assoc.*, 83, 840, October, 1971.

33. Moskow, B. S. and Bressman, E.: Cemental Response to Ultrasonic and Hand Instrumentation, *J. Am. Dent. Assoc.*, 68, 698, May, 1964.

34. Belting, C. M. and Spjut, P. J.: Effects of High-speed Periodontal Instruments on the Root Surface During Subgingival Calculus Removal, *J. Am. Dent. Assoc.*, 69, 578, November, 1964.

35. Jarabek, J. R.: The Cavitron—An Auxiliary in Clinical Orthodontics, *Ill. Dent. J.*, 30, 604, September, 1961.

36. Ewen, S. and Glickstein, C.: *Ultrasonic Therapy in Periodontics.* Springfield, Illinois, Charles C Thomas, 1968, pp. 12–45.

37. Schaffer, E. M.: Objective Evaluation of Ultrasonic Versus Hand Instrumentation in Periodontics, *Dent. Clin. North Am.*, p. 165, March, 1964.

38. Jacobson, L.: Ultrasonic Scaling, *Aust. Dent. J.*, 19, 379, December, 1974.

39. Ore, D. E. and Shriner, W. A.: Doctor: Don't Shut Off That Pacemaker, *Chicago Dent. Soc. Rev.*, pp. 22–23, August, 1974.

40. Bennett, C. R.: *Monheim's Local Anesthesia and Pain Control in Dental Practice*, 5th ed. St. Louis, Mosby, 1974, pp. 8–10.

41. American Dental Association, Council on Dental Therapeutics: *Accepted Dental Therapeutics*, 36th ed. Chicago, American Dental Association, 1975, pp. 104–108.

42. Bennett: op. cit., pp. 149–153.

43. Kutscher, A. H., Zegarelli, E. V., Hyman, G. A., McLean, P., and Kutscher, H. W., eds.: *Pharmacology for the Dental Hygienist.* Philadelphia, Lea & Febiger, 1967, pp. 86–87, 323–324.

44. Holder, T. D.: Use of 5% Xylocaine as an Adjunct in Curettage and Root Planing Procedures, *J. Oreg. Dent. Assoc.*, 37, 9, June, 1968.

45. Larato, D. C.: Effect of an Ultrasonic Scaler on Bacterial Counts in Air, *J. Periodont.*, 38, 550, November-December, 1967.

Suggested Readings

American Dental Association, Council on Dental Materials and Devices: *Guide to Dental Materials and Devices*, 7th ed. Chicago, American Dental Association, 1974–1975, pp. 155–157.

Bellini, H. T. and Johansen, J. R.: Average Time Required for Scaling and Surgery in Periodontal Therapy, *Acta Odontol. Scand.*, 31, 283, No. 5, 1973.

Bodecker, C. F.: Difficulty of Completely Removing Subgingival Calculus, *J. Am. Dent. Assoc.*, 30, 703, May, 1943.

Burke, S. W. and Green, E.: Effectiveness of Periodontal Files, *J. Periodont.*, 41, 39, January, 1970.

Frisch, J., Levin, M. P., and Bhaskar, S. N.: Calculus Removal. Effectiveness of Scaling, *J. South. Calif. Dent. Assoc.*, 38, 36, January, 1970.

Goldman, H. M. and Cohen, D. W.: *Periodontal Therapy*, 5th ed. St. Louis, Mosby, 1973, pp. 358, 398–399, 608–609.

Green, E.: Root Planing with Dull and Sharp Curettes, *J. Periodont.*, 39, 348, November, 1968.

Hirschfeld, L.: Subgingival Curettage in Periodontal Treatment, *J. Am. Dent. Assoc.*, 44, 301, March, 1952.

Parr, R. W., John, R., and Ratcliff, P. A.: *Tooth Preparation.* Berkeley, California, Praxis Pub., 1974, 52 pp.

Pattison, A. M. and Behrens, J.: *Dental Hygiene: The Detection and Removal of Calculus.* Reston, Virginia, Reston Publishing, 1973, pp. 161–241.

Stahl, S. S.: The Nature of Healthy and Diseased Root Surfaces, *J. Periodont.*, 46, 156, March, 1975.

Ultrasonics

Clark, S. M., Grupe, H. E., and Mahler, D. B.: The Effect of Ultrasonic Instrumentation on Root Surfaces, *J. Periodont.*, 39, 135, May, 1968.

Green, G. H. and Sanderson, A. D.: Ultrasonics and Periodontal Therapy—A Review of Clinical and Biologic Effects, *J. Periodont.*, 36, 232, May-June, 1965.

Haggerty, P. C.: Ultrasonics: A Practice-building, Work-saving Adjunct to the Practice of Periodontics, *Dent. Clin. North Am.*, 13, 33, January, 1969.

Johnston, L. E. and DeMarco, T. J.: The Clinical Effectiveness of a New Prophylaxis Device, *J. Periodont.*, 45, 222, April, 1974.

Jones, S. J., Lozdan, J., and Boyde, A.: Tooth Surfaces Treated *in Situ* with Periodontal Instruments, *Br. Dent. J., 132*, 57, January 18, 1972.

Nadler, H.: Ultrasonics in Periodontics, *Periodont. Abstr., 13*, 165, December, 1965.

Pameijer, C. H., Stallard, R. E., and Hiep, N.: Surface Characteristics of Teeth Following Periodontal Instrumentation: A Scanning Electron Microscope Study, *J. Periodont., 43*, 628, October, 1972.

Suppipat, N.: Ultrasonics in Periodontics, *J. Clin. Periodont., 1*, 206, No. 4, 1974.

Wilkinson, R. F. and Maybury, J. E.: Scanning Electron Microscopy of the Root Surface Following Instrumentation, *J. Periodont., 44*, 559, September, 1973.

Williams, G. H., Pollok, N. L., Shay, D. E., and Barr, C. E.: Laminar Air Purge of Microorganisms in Dental Aerosols: Prophylactic Procedures with an Ultrasonic Scaler, *J. Dent. Res., 49*, 1498, November-December, 1970.

Woodruff, H. C., Levin, M. P., and Brady, J. M.: The Effects of Two Ultrasonic Instruments on Root Surfaces, *J. Periodont., 46*, 119, February, 1975.

Anesthesia

Alling, C. C. and Christopher, A.: Status Report on Dental Anesthetic Needles and Syringes, *J. Am. Dent. Assoc., 89*, 1171, November, 1974.

Giddon, D. B., Quadland, M., Rachwall, P. C., Springer, J., and Tursky, B.: Development of a Method for Comparing Topical Anesthetics in Different Application and Dosage Forms, *J. Oral Thera. and Pharm., 4*, 270, January, 1968.

Gurney, B. F.: Chemotherapy in Dental Practice. Topical Anesthetics: Oil Soluble, *Dent. Dig., 72*, 513, November, 1966.

Gurney, B. F.: Chemotherapy in Dental Practice. Topical Anesthetics: Water Soluble, *Dent. Dig., 72*, 558, December, 1966.

Tolas, A. G.: Medical Problems Which Influence Choice of Anesthetic, *Dent. Clin. North Am., 17*, 211, April, 1973.

Chapter 34

Gingival Curettage

Gingival curettage is a planned systematic procedure to remove the diseased sulcular epithelial lining and underlying inflamed connective tissue of a gingival or periodontal pocket. It contributes to the treatment of pockets and may be the definitive treatment by which a pocket can be eliminated. It also may be part of the preparatory or initial phase of treatment which leads to reevaluation for determining the more complex periodontal therapy required.

Coincidental curettage which occurs as a result of the movement of the inactive side of a curet blade along the pocket wall during scaling and root planing, was described in Chapter 33, page 508. Coincidental curettage also may occur following ultrasonic scaling.[1] As described here, curettage is a specific, deliberate procedure with clear objectives, and a definite part of the patient's treatment plan. Root planing is completed first, and is a necessary prerequisite to curettage. When curettage is performed with an ultrasonic instrument, root planing with hand curets is also required.

In health, the lining of the sulcus is nonkeratinized stratified squamous epithelium. In disease, the pocket wall is characterized by degenerative changes in the sulcular epithelium with partial destruction, ulceration with exposure of the underlying connective tissue, and suppuration (cells and fluid) from the inflamed connective tissue. Soft, spongy enlargement is related to edema and local circulatory stasis, whereas hard, firm enlargement is due to long-standing chronic inflammation with fibrosis in the connective tissue.

I. Purposes

A. **Overall Objectives.** As a part of the treatment for the restoration of gingival health, with effective plaque control, curettage can contribute to
   1. Reduction or elimination of inflammation.
   2. Reduction or eradication of gingival or periodontal pockets.

B. **Specific Objectives.** Removal of the inflamed, ulcerated soft tissue of the pocket wall can
   1. Allow inflammation to subside by establishing drainage for edema and hyperemia.

2. Cause shrinkage of the free gingiva, and hence reduce pocket depth.
3. Promote fibrosis and healing.
4. Permit replacement of the diseased pocket lining with newly formed connective tissue and sulcular epithelium which can be maintained in health.
5. Strengthen the attachment of the junctional epithelium to the tooth surface. Although a slight area of reattachment may be possible, and has been observed in research,[2] it is not considered a predictable result.

II.   Indications for Gingival Curettage

A. Gingival tissue with a soft, spongy consistency, and other signs of inflammation (table 11-1, page 172).
B. Pockets that are relatively shallow.
C. Persistence of hyperemia, edema, and pocket depth after complete scaling and root planing.
D. Deep pockets which cannot be expected to shrink enough for elimination, but curettage may be used to reduce inflammation and pocket depth for maintenance in a patient who cannot have surgery for other health reasons or may be required to postpone surgery.
E. Presurgical tissue preparation to lessen inflammation and make the tissue more fibrotic for surgical management.

III.   Contraindications for Gingival Curettage

A. Gingival tissue with a firm, fibrous consistency contains fibrotic, collagenous elements which do not permit shrinkage of a pocket wall. Pocket elimination, therefore, cannot be an objective.
B. Except for presurgical tissue preparation, curettage is not indicated for mucogingival involvement, frenal attachments, infrabony pockets, or other complications which require specific surgical procedures.

IV.   Treatment Sequence

A. **Relation to Scaling and Root Planing**
   Curettage is performed after scaling and planing. For certain patients it is done immediately after, in the same appointment, whereas for others it is postponed a few weeks to observe the tissue changes following scaling and root planing. At that time, if healing is adequate and the tissues have responded favorably, curettage may not be indicated. Other patients may have only localized, isolated areas which need curettage and those may be done at the time of the root planing or later.

B. **Appointment Plan**
   At an appointment treatment is confined to one or possibly two quadrants. However, the plan for treatment depends on the severity of the condition, depth of pockets, and whether treatment is localized or generalized. The extent of treatment is also influenced by the use of anesthesia, whether topical application is adequate, or local anesthetic is to be administered.
   The treatment plan outlined on page 299 is illustrative of the steps needed. With local anesthetic and the use of periodontal dressings, several appointments are needed in a series over several weeks for continuing evaluation.

V.   Treatment Procedures

A. **Preparation of the Patient**
   1. Instruction in personal care. When plaque is not yet under control, additional help must be provided the patient because after curettage, healing is dependent on plaque removal on a daily basis.

2. Complete scaling and planing. When part or all is performed on the same day as curettage, the pockets must be carefully irrigated, using suction to remove particles of calculus, cementum, and other debris so they cannot be forced into the tissue during curettage.

3. Anesthesia for pain control. Topical anesthetic may be sufficient for some patients and some areas, particularly when the pockets are shallow. The anesthetic may be applied to a group of teeth, and then curets dipped in the agent and carried into the sulcus for additional benefit.

4. Careful probing and examination of each pocket is needed to define the depth and working area.

B. Instruments

Only precisely sharp fine curets are used. Instruments used for curettage are best kept separate from others used for scaling and planing, to preserve their sharpness, and have them ready for use. When scaling and planing immediately precede curettage, the same instruments should not be used.

C. Instrumentation

1. *Use modified pen grasp* and lead with the fulcrum finger to the rest near the area of operation.

2. *Position the blade* on the tooth surface over the pocket to be treated.

   a. Hold blade in correct position with cutting edge on tooth. Angulation will be greater than 90 degrees with the tooth surface in order that a less than 90 degree angle will be applied to the sulcular epithelium.

   b. The blade is open, that is, both cutting edges can be seen. When the curet is in correct position for scaling or planing, only the rounded back of the blade can be

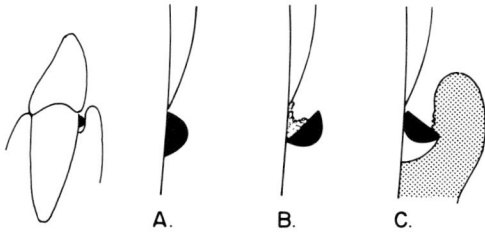

Figure 34–1. Angulation of a curet during instrumentation. **A.** Enlargement of pocket area diagrammed on left showing a cross section of the blade of a curet in black, angulated at zero degrees with the tooth surface as used for an exploratory or insertion stroke. **B.** Blade angulated for scaling and root planing at less than 90 degrees but greater than 45 degrees. **C.** Blade angulated with the gingival wall of the pocket for gingival curettage at the correct angle which is greater than 45 degrees but less than 90 degrees.

seen. A comparison of angulation during scaling and curettage is shown in figure 34–1.

   c. With the curet in position at the gingival margin, note the relation of the handle, fulcrum, grasp, and angulation of the face of the curet with the tooth, so that, after insertion, the blade can be properly repositioned at the bottom of the pocket.

3. *Insertion of curet into sulcus*

   a. Direct the toe of the blade toward the gingival margin, and open the blade more so that it can be slipped under the margin without trauma.

   b. Slide the curet to the bottom of the sulcus; use toe-end to determine bottom of the pocket. Tension of the soft tissue will be felt.

   c. Reposition the blade to the correct angulation for curettage (figure 34–2).

4. *Strokes.*

   a. Vertical and oblique strokes are used near the bottom of the pocket; horizontal strokes may be used nearer the top.

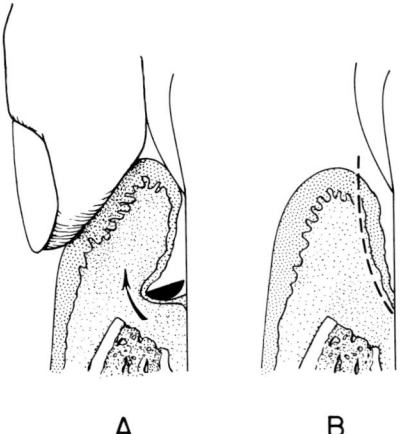

A   B

Figure 34–2. Gingival curettage. **A.** Curet positioned at the bottom of the pocket with the cutting edge toward the gingival wall. Pressure can be applied with a thumb or finger to the outside of the pocket for support while the curet is activated. **B.** The objective of curettage is to remove the lining of the pocket so that new healthy tissue can replace the old.

b. Support the pocket wall. Apply finger of non-working hand to outside of the pocket wall to offset pressure applied by the instrument on the inner surface. For treatment of an interdental papilla, apply pressure against the adjacent tooth.

c. Number of strokes. Only a few are needed when the curet is sharp. The number of strokes may vary from as few as two or three to 12 or 15. An experienced sense of touch can be developed to distinguish the soft mushy granulation tissue from the underlying firm connective tissue.

d. Removal of diseased tissue. The debris and soft particles of pocket lining are brought out of the sulcus to be removed by evacuation.

5. *Proceed systematically around each tooth,* overlapping from the lingual and facial at the proximal.

D. **Irrigation.** Debris removal by irrigation is important to aid healing.

E. **Tissue Adaptation and Hemostasis.** Press the area with gauze to adapt the gingival margins to the tooth. All bleeding should be stopped by pressure applied on the tissues for a short while. Although a blood clot is essential to healing, excess pressure from a large clot can permit the gingival tissue to heal away from the tooth. Physiologic form is an objective of healing.

F. **Apply Periodontal Dressing.** The objectives of the dressing are described on page 525. A dressing is needed particularly when there is tissue separation from the teeth, and when pressure of the dressing can aid in molding the tissue to heal in a physiologic form. The dressing usually is left in place for one week before removal.

VI. Postoperative Care

A. **Postoperative Instructions**
1. Dressing placed: Printed instructions are advisable. Suggestions for care following dressing placement may be found on page 528 (table 35–1).
2. Without dressing:
   a. Plaque removal is very important. Use soft (.006" filament diameter) toothbrush with rounded ends. Definite plaque removal but care not to traumatize the healing tissue is necessary.
   b. Rinse with warm weak saline solution (pages 348, 572).

B. **Follow-up**
1. Dressing removal in approximately one week. Specific plaque removal instructions given.
2. Tooth sensitivity. Advise the patient that most sensitivity is transient. Toothbrushing with a fluoride dentifrice and using a fluoride

mouthrinse daily can be most effective. Desensitizing agents can be applied to persistent spots (page 564).

3. Polishing. Polishing is not usually advised immediately following dressing removal because the healing has not been completed and abrasive in a newly forming sulcus can be an irritant. Instruction for daily complete plaque removal by the patient is necessary to prevent re-infection.

II. Healing

A. Effects of Instrumentation

Removal of the sulcular lining and underlying inflamed connective tissue creates a surgical wound. Healing follows the usual pattern with epithelialization and collagenation and resolution of inflammation in the connective tissue. The effects are as follows:

1. Shrinkage of the gingival walls with fluid drainage.
2. Reepithelialization with coverage of the exposed connective tissue.
3. Formation of new connective tissue beneath the new epithelial lining of the sulcus and attachment.
4. Return to normal circulation.

B. Steps in Healing[3]

1. Formation of a blood clot immediately after curettage. The clot fills the pocket area which is adapted against the tooth by pressure and a dressing.
2. Initial tissue reaction of inflammation as with any wound.
3. Proliferation of fibroblasts and new vessels to form granulation tissue.
4. Epithelial cells arise from the epithelium at the margin of the gingiva. The epithelium migrates in and over the granulation tissue. This begins by 24 hours following the curettage.
5. New epithelium covers the sulcus

lining within five to six days, and the new junctional epithelium is formed by five days.

6. Connective tissue healing proceeds and is well organized by two weeks.
7. Keratinization of oral (outer) epithelium may be observed by two weeks; reaches normal thickness by 28 to 40 days.

C. Interferences with Healing

1. Residual and newly formed calculus. Repeated root planing is frequently necessary.
2. Plaque and other local irritants. Meticulous self-care must be supervised over several weeks following curettage.
3. Systemic factors may be involved when healing delay cannot be otherwise accounted for, but local factors must be rechecked first.

D. Clinical Appearance of the Healed Tissue

When healing is complete, the usual signs of healthy gingiva should be evident. Those were outlined in table 11-1 on page 172. There should be minimal probe measurement in the sulcus, the sulcus should be free from bleeding on probing, stippling is apparent, and the color, size, shape, and other characteristics normal.

FACTORS TO TEACH THE PATIENT

I. Why pockets need to be treated; how curettage contributes to pocket reduction or elimination.
II. Reasons for periodontal dressing placement.
III. Postoperative care with and without a dressing. Care of teeth and gingiva not involved in the curettage.
IV. Relationship of plaque and plaque control to healing.
V. Desensitization using proper toothbrushing technique applied to cervical areas, and a fluoride dentifrice and rinse.

References

1. Schaffer, E. M., Stende, G., and King, D.: Healing of Periodontal Pocket Tissues Following Ultrasonic Scaling and Hand Planing, *J. Periodont.*, 35, 140, March-April, 1964.
2. Ramfjord, S. P., Nissle, R. R., Shick, R. A., and Cooper, H.: Subgingival Curettage Versus Surgical Elimination of Periodontal Pockets, *J. Periodont.*, 39, 167, May, 1968.
3. Goldman, H. M. and Cohen, D. W.: *Periodontal Therapy*, 5th ed. St. Louis, Mosby, 1973, pp. 903–907.

Suggested Readings

Bohannan, H. M. and Saxe, S. R.: Periodontics in General Practice, in Morris, A. L. and Bohannan, H. M., eds.: *The Dental Specialties in General Practice*. Philadelphia, Saunders, 1969, pp. 301–304.

Chace, R.: Subgingival Curettage in Periodontal Therapy, *J. Periodont.*, 45, 107, February, 1974.

Glickman, I.: *Clinical Periodontology*, 4th ed. Philadelphia, Saunders, 1972, pp. 623–631.

Grant, D. A., Stern, I. B., and Everett, F. G.: *Orban's Periodontics*, 4th ed. St. Louis, Mosby, 1972, pp. 436–445.

Kon, S., Novaes, A. B., Ruben, M. P., and Goldman, H. M.: Visualization of Microvascularization of the Healing Periodontal Wound. II. Curettage, *J. Periodont.*, 40, 96, February, 1969.

Moskow, B. S.: Response of the Gingival Sulcus to Instrumentation: A Histological Investigation. 2. Gingival Curettage, *J. Periodont.*, 35, 112, March-April, 1964.

Oshrain, H. I., Salkind, A., and Mandel, I. D.: Bacteriologic Studies of Periodontal Pockets Ten Minutes After Curettage, *J. Periodont.*, 43, 685, November, 1972.

Ratcliff, P. A.: Periodontal Therapy—Review of Literature. Section VI in *World Workshop in Periodontics*. Ann Arbor, American Academy of Periodontology and University of Michigan, 1966, pp. 291–298.

Ratcliff, P. A.: An Analysis of Repair Systems in Periodontal Therapy, *Periodont. Abstr.*, 14, 57, June, 1966.

Ratcliff, P. A. and Oliver, G. V.: Periodontics, in Steele, P. F., ed.: *Dimensions of Dental Hygiene*, 2nd ed. Philadelphia, Lea & Febiger, 1975, pp. 338–344, 373–375.

Stahl, S. S., Weiner, J. M., Benjamin, S., and Yamada, L.: Soft Tissue Healing Following Curettage and Root Planing, *J. Periodont.*, 42, 678, November, 1971.

Stone, S., Ramfjord, S. P., and Waldron, J.: Scaling and Gingival Curettage. A Radioautographic Study, *J. Periodont.*, 37, 415, September-October, 1966.

Tandy, R. B.: Gingival Curettage, Literature Review, *Periodont. Abstr.*, 18, 100, June, 1970.

Curettage by Ultrasonics

Goldman, H. M.: Curettage by Ultrasonic Instrument, *Oral Surg.*, 13, 43, January, 1960.

Nadler, H.: Removal of Crevicular Epithelium by Ultrasonic Curettes, *J. Periodont.*, 33, 220, July, 1962.

Sanderson, A. D.: Gingival Curettage by Hand and Ultrasonic Instruments: A Histologic Comparison, *J. Periodont.*, 37, 279, July-August, 1966.

Chapter 35

Periodontal Dressings

A dressing is a material applied for protecting a wound and favoring its healing. A periodontal dressing is usually placed over the surgical wound following periodontal surgery and is frequently indicated after gingival curettage.

I. Purposes and Uses

A. Protect the surgical wound from injury to encourage healing, reduce chances of infection, and prevent secondary bleeding.

B. Aid in shaping or molding the newly formed tissues; aid in holding a flap in place or immobilizing a graft.

C. Provide patient comfort during the healing period by isolating the wound from external irritations and injuries.

II. Types of Dressings

Dressings are usually classified in two groups: eugenol-containing and those without eugenol. Healing has been shown by research to progress at about the same rate under either dressing, so selection by the dentist can be based on such factors as firmness of the material, durability, con-

sistency, ease of manipulation, or personal preference.

A. **Eugenol-containing**
1. Basic ingredients.
   a. Powder: zinc oxide, powdered rosin and tannic acid. Some formulae include other substances such as asbestos fibers and zinc acetate or stearate.
   b. Liquid: eugenol with an oil such as peanut or cottonseed, and thymol.
2. Examples: well-known dressings are Ward's (Wonderpack), Periodontal Dressing Powder and Liquid ("PPC"), and Kirkland. Formulae for the last two are given below as examples of the ingredients and their proportions.[1]

   a. Kirkland Periodontal Pack
      Powder: Each 100 Grams contains
Zinc oxide	40.00 Gm.
Rosin	40.00 Gm.
Tannic acid	20.00 Gm.

      Liquid: Each 100 milliliters contains
Eugenol	46.5 ml.
Peanut oil	46.5 ml.
Rosin	7.7 Gm.

b. Periodontal Dressing Powder and Liquid ("PPC")

Powder: Each 100 Grams contains

Zinc oxide	42.9 Gm.
Powdered rosin	38.1 Gm.
Tannic acid	9.5 Gm.
Kaolin	2.4 Gm.
Mica	7.1 Gm.

Liquid: Each 100 milliliters contains

Eugenol	98.0 ml.
Thymol	2.0 Gm.
Color	

B. Non-eugenol-containing

Eugenol has an unpleasant sharp taste and can be irritating to the mucous membrane. Over the years, in search for a substitute for eugenol, other formulae have been developed. Other ingredients such as antibiotics which would provide bacteriostatic effects have been tried.

1. Hydrogenated Fat Dressing.[2] The powder contains zinc oxide and rosin powder to which may be added bacitracin. The powder is mixed with an ointment containing zinc oxide with hydrogenated fat. It is mixed to a putty-like consistency and may be stored by wrapping in foil and refrigerating.

2. Coe-Pak. Prepared by mixing pastes from two tubes: one containing metallic oxides with a fungicide, and the other non-ionizing carboxylic acids with a germicide-fungicide. It sets within a few minutes and cannot be prepared in advance.

   When it is desirable to have a firmer dressing, some zinc oxide powder (a eugenol-containing dressing powder) can be added to the Coe-Pak during mixing.

III. Clinical Application: Eugenol-Containing Dressing

A. Mixing

1. Mix powder and liquid on a paper mixing pad, incorporating the powder gradually to form a thick past Use a metal spatula or woode tongue depressor.

2. Knead additional powder into th paste with the fingers until th consistency is firm and thick, b not sticky. (Orange solvent will a in cleaning the hands afterward but wearing rubber gloves is re ommended.)

3. Divide the mass into quantitie appropriate for application to quadrant or other specific are Wrap pieces in foil or waxed pap for storage in freezer.

B. Application

1. Roll the mixed dressing into round strip.

2. Inspect area to be sure bleeding ha stopped.

3. Quadrant application: apply co tinuous (one strip) from lingual t facial; or two strips may be used t cover a quadrant, the first to exten from the distal of the most posteri tooth over the facial surfaces, an the second to overlap the first on th distal and extend along the lingual

4. Moisten the fingers with water dip the fingers in dressing powde to prevent sticking during applica tion.

5. Press at the interproximal areas t gain retention and provide com plete coverage for the treatmen area. Adapt with a plastic instru ment.

6. Edentulous areas can usually b filled to make the dressing continu ous between the teeth unless to great a gap exists.

7. Muscle trim (border mold) th cheeks, lips, and tongue to preven movement or dislodgment of th dressing.

8. Check frena for freedom of move ment.

a. Lingual: request patient to touch palate with tip of tongue.

b. Buccal: retract cheek up and out over maxillary premolars and out from mandibular premolars.

c. Anterior: retract upper lip up and out over maxillary central incisors and retract lower lip out and up for mandibular midline frenum.

d. Adjust dressing by rolling and folding back the border, unless there is gross excess which should be removed.

9. Check the occlusion: the dressing should extend only to the height of the contour of the teeth and should not be in contact during closure.

10. Variation for open interproximal embrasures with missing papillae and recession: use small sections of dressing to mold into wedge shapes to press interproximally from facial and from lingual. It is very important that the proximal gingiva be completely and firmly covered. A strip of dressing can then be added facially and lingually for complete coverage.

IV. Clinical Application: Non-Eugenol Dressing (Coe-Pak)

A. **Mixing**

1. Place equal lengths of material from each tube beside each other (but not touching) on the mixing pad. Prepare only the amount needed which can be readily estimated after a few experiences.

2. Since working time is relatively brief, prepare the patient by stabilizing the head and placing a gauze sponge over the area which will receive the dressing. Request the patient to close.

3. Mix the two pastes together quickly until the colors are blended and neither color is perceptible separately. Mix over a small area, not across width of pad.

4. When mixing is complete, gather the material together with the spatula (or tongue depressor) and place on the edge of a tongue depressor. Promptly wipe a metal spatula clean.

B. **Application**

1. After one minute, touch the mixture with a finger coated with petroleum jelly. As soon as the mixture feels warm, it usually can be managed and should be placed promptly. Coat the fingers with petroleum jelly.

2. Roll the dressing into a strip the approximate length and thickness needed for the specific area. Application of excess material should be avoided since removal of the excess is unnecessarily time-consuming and awkward.

3. Apply in a continuous piece: for a quadrant, place center of the roll at the posterior surface of the most posterior tooth and bring around to facial and lingual. Press the dressing at the interproximal areas (lingual and facial can be done simultaneously).

4. Mold the dressing into place to the height of contour, and border mold to prevent displacement by the tongue, cheeks, lips. Check frena (III.B.8).

5. Check the occlusion: patient may feel the excess, or teeth prints will show the location. When excess dressing is removed, use a cutting motion with a plastic instrument or scaler. Do not pull on a section of the dressing as the whole dressing is very cohesive and can be dislodged in one piece.

V. Characteristics of a Well-Placed Dressing

Dressings must be placed in keeping with biologic principles which will contribute to healing and yet be tolerated by the patient. A satisfactory dressing has the following characteristics:

A. Is secure and rigid. A movable dressing is an irritant and can promote hemorrhage.

B. Has as little bulk as possible, yet bulky enough to give strength.

C. Is locked mechanically interdentally and cannot be displaced by action of tongue, cheek, or lips.

D. Covers all of the surgical wound without unnecessary over-extension.

E. Fills interdental area to cover the surgerized area and discourage food retention.

VI. Patient Dismissal and Instructions

A. Patient must not be dismissed until bleeding or oozing from under dressing has ceased.

B. Written instructions are more effective than verbal. Table 35–1 lists items for which instructions should be given a patient who has a periodontal dressing. Printed instructions can be prepared from these items. Other instructions for the patient after general oral surgery or tooth removal may be found on page 614.

VII. Dressing Removal

During healing, epithelium will cover a wound in six days and complete restoration of epithelium and connective tissue can be expected by 21 days. The dressing may be left in place from seven to ten days as predetermined by the dentist.

Table 35-1. Instructions for Postoperative Care

Factor	Instructions to Patient	Purpose of Instruction
Information about the Dressing	Dressing to protect the surgery and to help it heal. Do not disturb it; keep it on until the next appointment.	Understanding and cooperation by the patient
Care During the First Few Hours	Dressing will not be hard for a few hours. Do not eat anything which requires chewing. Use only cool liquids. Keep quiet; get rest.	Dressing must harden and be undisturbed.
Discomfort After the Anesthesia Wears Off	Take two aspirin or similar preparation. When a prescription is given, the instructions may be reviewed.	Pain control
Ice Pack or Cold Compress	Use as directed only. Apply every 30 minutes for 15 minutes, or 30 minutes on and 30 minutes off.	Prevent swelling from edema
Bleeding	Slight temporary bleeding within the first few hours is not unusual. Prevent disturbing the healing. Persistent or excessive bleeding should be reported to the dentist for treatment as indicated.	Alleviate patient alarm over small amount of bleeding, but assure patient of help as needed.

Table 35-1.   Continued

Factor	Instructions to Patient	Purpose of Instruction
Dressing Care and Retention	Avoid pressing the dressing with the tongue or trying to clean under it. Small particles may chip off during the week. No problem unless the sharp edge bothers the tongue or the dressing seems to have loosened. Call the dentist if the whole dressing or a large portion of it falls off before the fifth day. It should be replaced. If after the fifth day, call for an early replacement appointment when area is unusually sensitive. Otherwise rinse with saline solution and cover the area with white petrolatum.	Dressing needed for wound protection. Epithelium covers wound by fifth day in normal healing.
Smoking	Do not smoke	Heat and smoke irritate the gingiva and delay healing.
Rinsing	Do not rinse on the day of the surgery. Second day: use saline solution made with one-half teaspoon (measured) in one-half glass of warm water every two to three hours. Third and subsequent days: use the saline solution or a pleasant tasting mouthwash diluted one-third mouthwash to two-thirds water.	Might disturb clot. Saline may aid healing. Pleasant flavored mouthwash may reduce mouth odors from debris on the dressing.
Toothbrushing and Flossing	Use better-than-usual brushing and flossing on unoperated areas. Brush occlusal surface over dressing. Use soft brush with water carefully on surface of dressing to clean off debris and film. Brush the tongue.	Plaque control Oral sanitation Odor and taste control Reduce numbers of oral microorganisms.
Eating	Highly nutritious food is needed during healing. Check the Basic 4. Use soft-textured diet. Omit foods that are highly seasoned, spicy, hot. Avoid sticky, crunchy or coarse foods that could break the dressing.	Healing Protect the dressing from breakage or displacement.
Mastication	Avoid foods that require excessive chewing. Use ground meat, or cut meat into small pieces. Chew only on unoperated side. Take small bite-sized pieces at a time.	Dressing protection

When the dressing breaks or falls off before the appointed time for removal, it usually should be replaced rather than patched because the remaining segment is generally loose.

A. **Patient Examination**
1. Question patient and record postoperative effects or discomfort. When part or all of the dressing was broken off, record its duration.
2. Examine mucosa about the dressing, and record appearance.

B. **Procedure for Removal**
1. Insert a large scaler, hoe, or plastic instrument under the border of the dressing (coronal or apical border or both); apply lateral pressure.
2. Watch for sutures that may be caught in the dressing. They may need to be cut for release. Use principles for suture removal as on page 533.
3. Remove pieces of dressing gently with cotton pliers to avoid scratching the thin epithelial covering of the healing tissue with the rough edges of dressing.
4. Observe tissue condition and record appearance. Note any deviations from normal healing as expected in the length of time since the treatment.
5. Use a scaler for removal of pieces attached to tooth surfaces; use curet for particles near the gingival margin. Some root planing may be indicated, and all calculus and roughness should be eliminated to prevent plaque retention.
6. Syringe with a gentle stream of *warm* water, and provide *warm* diluted mouth wash for the patient's comfort.

C. **Plaque Control follow-up is essential after dressing removal.**
1. Use a soft brush (.006″ filaments) on treated area with careful attention to plaque removal at the gingival margin. Use usual methods for all other areas of the mouth.
2. Increase intensity of care on the treated area each day, with a return to complete procedures by three or four days.
3. Rinse with warm mild saline solution, forcing the liquid between the teeth, to encourage healing.
4. When teeth are sensitive, a fluoride dentifrice containing monofluorophosphate should be used (page 564).

D. **Follow-up**
Return for observation of complete healing in one week to one month depending on the individual patient's progress and total treatment plan.

VIII. Dressing Replacement

A. **Indications**
1. Dressing broken or displaced before time for removal.
2. A second dressing for an extended period of time is frequently indicated and depends on the
   a. Extent of the surgery and degree of periodontal disease involvement.
   b. Need for additional healing period for certain types of surgery such as graft or reattachment.

B. **Choice of Dressing for Replacement**
Coe-Pak is frequently used as replacement dressing because of its smooth texture and ease of application. It can be applied while it is soft and pliable, thus diminishing the amount of pressure needed to adapt the dressing material proximally for retention and tissue coverage. Without undue pressure during application the patient suffers less discomfort and the chances of initiating bleeding are

diminished. Use a topical anesthetic to prevent patient discomfort.

SUTURE REMOVAL

A suture is a strand or fiber used to unite parts of the body. Sutures are necessary in many oral operations wherever a surgical wound must be closed, a flap positioned, or tissue grafted.

Purposes of Sutures

A. Maintain the sutured tissues until healing is great enough to provide the tissues with sufficient strength to undergo normal physiologic activity.

B. By holding and stabilizing the replaced and readapted tissue, sutures contribute to the following:
1. Maintaining the clot during the initial healing period.
2. Reducing the size of the wound, therefore lessening the time required for healing.
3. Protecting the area from foreign debris and trauma.

Types of Sutures and Needles

Sutures are classified as absorbable and nonabsorbable. Absorbable sutures are digested by body tissue fluids and enzymes, carried away by phagocytic action, and with the normal healing process are replaced by scar tissue. In medical surgery, absorbable sutures can be used internally. Nonabsorbable sutures are made of inert materials and, when used on the surface, are removed after five to ten days as indicated by the type of surgery.

A. **Absorbable Sutures**
1. Surgical gut. Prepared from the submucosa of sheep intestines, and prepared for use as plain or chrome.
   a. Plain. Processed, sterilized, and tested.
   b. Chrome. Special treatment of the suture material with chromic acid to control and lengthen the absorption time.

2. Polyglycolic acid (PGA). Synthetic material which tends to produce a milder tissue reaction than surgical gut or nonabsorbable materials and inhibits bacterial growth.[3,4]

B. **Nonabsorbable Sutures**
1. Surgical silk, black twisted or braided. Most widely used, particularly in oral surgery.
2. Surgical cotton and linen.
3. Wire: tantalum, silver, stainless steel, vitallium.
4. Synthetic fibers: polyester (example: Dupont Mersilene), nylon, Dermalon, orlon.

C. **Characteristics**
1. Braided, twisted, plain. Braiding provides more retention, but the suture is more permeable to bacteria.
2. Monofilament or multifilament. Monofilament gives less tissue reaction, but multifilament gives better retention.
3. Sizes. Described from 0 to 8–0. For example, 4–0 silk is frequently used in periodontal surgery.

D. **Needles**
Many types of suturing needles are available, and their use and selection are based on the patient's needs and the dentist's preference. The three basic characteristics of suture needles are as follows:
1. Shape of needle: straight, half-circle, 3/8 circle, half-curved.
2. Cross-sectional shape: round or triangular (has cutting edge). The tip may be a taper point or a trocar (triangular) point.
3. Eye.
   a. Regular eye: eye may be round or square, or a French spring eye which grips suture material.
   b. Atraumatic: No eye. The needle and an end of the suture material are swaged. The suture and needle are a continuous unit.

III. Suturing Techniques

Many different patterns of suturing are used. A dental hygienist who will be removing sutures as part of postoperative patient care needs to become familiar with the methods preferred by the dentist-surgeon. Assisting and observing at the time of surgery can be especially educational. When the patient is one for whom the hygienist participated in the initial preparation, knowledge of the surgical procedures used adds to the continuity of treatment.

At the time of surgery the number and type or description of the sutures placed should be recorded in the patient's record. At the time of removal the information is necessary, since, during healing, sutures may become loosened, misplaced, or sometimes covered with tissue. All sutures should be accounted for at the time of removal.

General types frequently used in the oral cavity are described here briefly to introduce terminology and to help orient the dental hygienist to the various sutures which may be encountered during removal. At the end of this chapter, the *Suggested Readings* include references which provide descriptions of suturing.

A. **Interrupted**

Each stitch is taken and tied separately.

B. **Continuous**

A series of stitches tied at one or both ends. Examples of sutures that may be applied in a series are the sling or suspension, and the blanket.

C. **Circumferential**

A term applied to a suture which encircles a tooth for suspension and retention of a flap.

D. **Blanket**

Each stitch is brought over a loop of the preceding one, thus forming a series of loops on one side of the incision and a series of stitches on the incision. It is also called a continuous lock. It is used for approximation of the gingival margins after alveolectomy.

E. **Sling or Suspension**

When a flap is only on one side facial or lingual, the sutures are passed through the interdental papilla through the proximal, around the tooth, and then into the adjacent papilla. The suture is adjusted so that the flap can be positioned for correct healing.

F. **Interdental**

Where there are lingual and facial flaps, interdental ligation joins the two by passing the suture through each interdental area. Coverage for the interdental area can be accomplished by coapting the edges of the papillae.

IV. Procedure for Removal

When a dressing has been placed over sutures, the steps here will overlap with Section VII, Dressing Removal, page 528. A suture can become caught in dressing material and may need to be cut and removed while the dressing is being removed. The same principles for removal are to be observed.

A. **Armamentarium for Suture Removal**

Mouth mirror
Cotton pliers
Curved sharp scissors with pointed tip (suture scissors)
Gauze sponge
Topical anesthetic; Gel or ointment preferred, since an aerosol could be traumatic to tender healing tissue.
Topical antiseptic
Cotton pellets
Saliva ejector tip

B. **Patient Examination**

1. Observe healing tissue about the suture(s).
2. Record any deviations of color, size, shape of the tissue, adaptation of flap, or coaptation of an incision healing by first intention.

C. **Preparation of the Patient**
1. Debridement of area: after the patient rinses, other debris particles may be removed using a cotton tipped applicator, a cotton pellet dipped in three percent peroxide, followed by another rinse by the patient, or wiping gently with a gauze sponge.
2. Place and adjust saliva ejector.
3. Retract and pat area with gauze sponge to remove surface moisture.
4. Swab area with topical antiseptic.
5. Apply topical anesthetic. Maintain retraction to prevent dilution.

D. **Retraction**
Three hands are really needed: one for retraction, one for cotton pliers to hold and remove the suture, and one for cutting the suture. When an assistant is not available, a cotton roll placed in the vestibule may provide enough retraction along with the finger rest and little finger of the left hand holding the cotton pliers.

E. **Steps for Removal**
As described here and illustrated in figure 35–1, removal is for a single interrupted suture. The same principles apply for the ends and each segment of a continuous suture, wherever septic suture material could pass through the soft tissue.
1. Grasp the suture knot with the cotton plier held in the left hand. Draw the suture gently up about two millimeters and hold with slight tension. A finger rest is needed for control.
2. Insert tip of sharp scissors under the suture, slightly depress the tissue with the back of the scissor blade, and cut the suture in the part that was previously buried in the tissue.
3. With left hand, hold knot end up and pull gently to allow suture to come out through the side opposite from where it was cut. This pre-

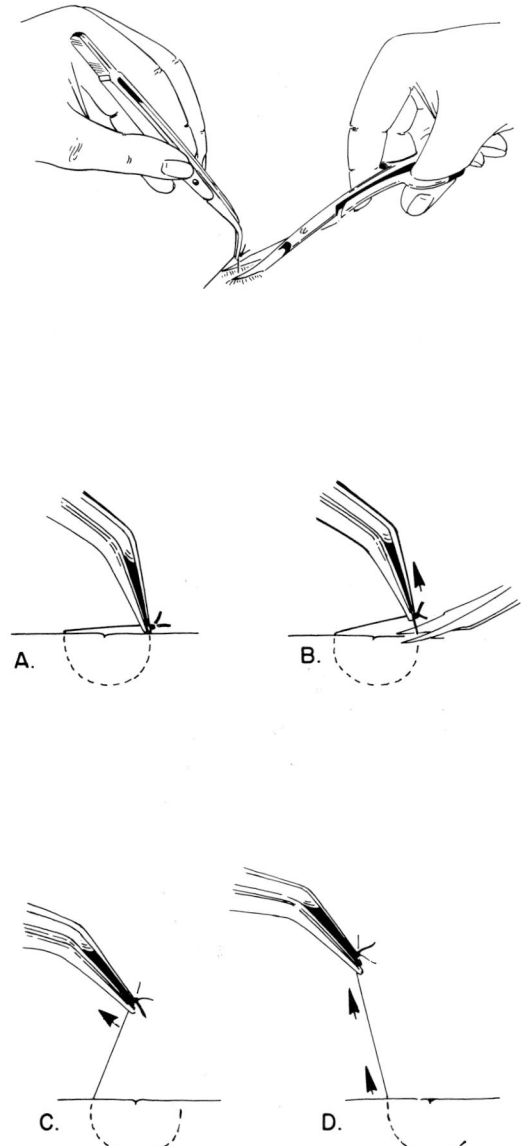

Figure 35–1. Suture removal. **A.** Suture grasped by cotton pliers near entrance into tissue. **B.** Suture pulled up gently while scissor is inserted close to tissue. Suture is cut in the part previously buried in the tissue. **C.** Suture held up for vertical removal. **D.** Suture pulled gently to pass the suture out on the side opposite from the cut. The object is to prevent the external part of the suture from passing through the tissue and introducing infection.

vents any part of the external segment of the suture to pass through
the tissue and introduce infection.
4. Withdraw gently and steadily.
5. Discard the suture and proceed to
remove the next suture.
6. Count total sutures and confirm
with the patient's record of the
surgical procedures of the previous
appointment.
7. Apply gauze sponge with slight
pressure on bleeding spots.
8. Request dentist to observe the area.
9. Request patient to close on the
sponge while dressing is readied
(when a dressing replacement is
indicated).
F. **Precautions**
   In summary of the points brought
   out in the above description, precautions are as follows:
   1. Count sutures; record number
   placed and number removed.
   2. Record all observations of the tissues by dentist and hygienist, and
   note any adverse reactions or bleeding problems. Record comments
   made by the patient.
   3. Sutures should not be left longer
   than five to ten days at the outset.
   Special arrangements for removal
   need to be made for the patient who
   cannot return for a scheduled appointment.
   4. Take care when removing a
   periodontal dressing to prevent
   ripping out a suture that may have
   become imbedded in the dressing.
   5. Provide proper post-appointment
   instructions for the patient.

TECHNICAL HINTS

I. Sutures placed without a dressing
may have a crust over them at the
time of removal. Apply mineral oil,
and in a short time the crust will
soften and can be wiped away. To
remove the suture with the crust can

cause unnecessary discomfort for the
patient.
II. Adaptation and retention of a dressing can be improved when the
dressing is covered with a well
adapted adhesive periodontal foi
when this is in accord with the
dentist's philosophy. Place the foi
over the lingual, occlusal and facia
but do not cover the margins in orde
to prevent irritating the mucosa.

FACTORS TO TEACH THE PATIENT

I. Care of the mouth during the perioc
of treatment while wearing dress
ings. See table 35–1.
II. Maintenance and follow-up care
after treatment is formally over.

References

1. American Dental Association, Council on Der
tal Therapeutics: *Accepted Dental Therapeu
tics*, 36th ed. Chicago, American Denta
Association, 1975, pp. 237–238.
2. Baer, P. N., Sumner, C. F., and Miller, G
Periodontal Dressings, *Dent. Clin. Nortl
Am., 13*, 181, January, 1969.
3. Wallace, W. R., Maxwell, G. R., and Cavalaris, C
J.: Comparison of Polyglycolic Acid Suture t
Black Silk, Chromic, and Plain Catgut i
Human Oral Tissues, *J. Oral Surg., 28*, 739
October, 1970.
4. Lilly, G. E., Osbon, D. B., Hutchinson, R. A., an
Heflich, R. H.: Clinical and Bacteriologi
Aspects of Polyglycolic Acid Sutures, *J. Ora
Surg., 31*, 103, February, 1973.

Suggested Readings

Castano, F. A. and Alden, B. A., eds.: *Handbook o
Expanded Dental Auxiliary Practice*. Philadel
phia, Lippincott, 1973, pp. 156–158.
DeRenzis, F. A. and Hildebrand, C. N.: Improvec
Technique for Periodontal Dressing Retention,*J
Periodont., 43*, 104, February, 1972.
Ewen, S. J.: Periodontal Uses of a Tissue Adhesive,*J
Periodont., 38*, 138, March-April, 1967.
Forrest, J. O.: The Use of Cyanoacrylates i
Periodontal Surgery,*J. Periodont., 45*, 225, April
1974.
Frisch, J. and Bhaskar, S. N.: Tissue Response t
Eugenol-Containing Periodontal Dressings, *J
Periodont., 38*, 402, September-October, 1967.
Glickman, I.: *Clinical Periodontology*, 4th ed
Philadelphia, Saunders, 1972, pp. 653–660, 719-
725.
Goldman, H. M. and Cohen, D. W.: *Periodonta
Therapy*, 5th ed. St. Louis, Mosby, 1973, pp
634–636.

Grant, D. A., Stern, I. B., and Everett, F. G.: *Orban's Periodontics*, 4th ed. St. Louis, Mosby, 1972, pp. 429–434, 476–482.

Kutscher, A. H., Zegarelli, E. V., Hyman, G. A., McLean, P., and Kutscher, H. W., eds.: *Pharmacology for the Dental Hygienist*. Philadelphia, Lea & Febiger, 1967, pp. 250–252.

Levin, M. P., Bhaskar, S. N., and Frisch, J.: Use of Sutures and Periodontal Dressings Following Surgical Procedures, in Ward, H. L., ed.: *A Periodontal Point of View*. Springfield, Charles C Thomas, 1973, pp. 347–358.

Molnar, E. J.: Coe-pak and TEM-coe, *CAL.*, *33*, 8, January, 1971.

Poulsom, R. C.: An Anaphylactoid Reaction to Periodontal Surgical Dressing: Report of Case, *J. Am. Dent. Assoc.*, *89*, 895, October, 1974.

Sutures

Archer, W. H.: *Oral Surgery*, 4th ed. Philadelphia, Saunders, 1966, pp. 64–65.

Berry, E. C. and Kohn, M. L.: *Introduction to Operating-room Technique*, 3rd ed. New York, Blakiston Division, McGraw-Hill, 1966, pp. 89–95.

Dahlberg, W. H.: Incisions and Suturing: Some Basic Considerations About Each in Periodontal Flap Surgery, *Dent. Clin. North Am.*, p. 149, January, 1969.

Ginsberg, F., Brunner, L. S., and Cantlin, V. L.: *A Manual of Operating Room Technology*. Philadelphia, Lippincott, 1966, pp. 72–73.

Kruger, G. O., ed.: *Textbook of Oral Surgery*, 4th ed. St. Louis, Mosby, 1974, pp. 6–11.

Kuba, S. K., Hoag, P. M., and Rosenfeld, L. D.: A Model for the Demonstration of Suturing Technics, *J. Periodont.*, *43*, 573, September, 1972.

Lilly, G. E.: Reaction of Oral Tissues to Suture Materials, *Oral Surg.*, *26*, 128, July, 1968.

Lilly, G. E., Armstrong, J. H., Salem, J. E., and Cutcher, J. L.: Reaction of Oral Tissues to Suture Materials, Part II, *Oral Surg.*, *26*, 592, October, 1968.

Lilly, G. E., Cutcher, J. L., Jones, J. C., and Armstrong, J. H.: Reaction of Oral Tissues to Suture Materials. IV., *Oral Surg.*, *33*, 152, January, 1972.

Lilly, G. E., Salem, J. E., Armstrong, J. H., and Cutcher, J. L.: Reaction of Oral Tissues to Suture Materials. Part III, *Oral Surg.*, *28*, 432, September, 1969.

Malamed, E. H.: Technique of Suturing Flaps in Periodontal Surgery, *Periodontics*, *1*, 207, September-October, 1963.

Morris, M. L.: Suturing Techniques in Periodontal Surgery, *Periodontics*, *3*, 84, March-April, 1965.

Prichard, J. F.: *Advanced Periodontal Disease, Surgical and Prosthetic Management*, 2nd ed. Philadelphia, Saunders, 1972, pp. 340–352.

Thoma, K. H.: *Oral Surgery*, 5th ed. St. Louis, Mosby, 1969, p. 98.

Weinstein, I. R. and Malkin, M.: Suturing Techniques, in Douglas, B. L., ed.: *Introduction to Hospital Dentistry*, 2nd ed. St. Louis, Mosby, 1970, pp. 75–89.

Chapter 36

Introduction to Polishing

After treatment by scaling, root planing, and other periodontal therapy, the teeth are evaluated for polishing. Polishing is a selective procedure and not every patient needs to have the teeth polished, especially on a routine basis.

When the evaluation is made, several factors must be taken into consideration. The first is that tooth structure is removed when teeth are polished since an abrasive is a major constituent of polishing agents. This factor has particular significance for children because the surface of young, newly erupted teeth is less mineralized. It is also an important consideration for the conscientious patient of any age whose teeth may be polished several times each year on regular recall appointments.

A second factor is that, despite the belief that a smooth tooth surface is more resistant to the reformation of deposits, pellicle, plaque, and calculus do recur. Except for the minority group of patients who practice superior plaque control, the deposits may return quite promptly. Effects of polishing as a preventive measure for gingival disease or dental caries have not been proven.

Appearance is important to patients. Unsightly stains will need removal for the new patient initially. As much of the heavy stain as possible should be removed while scaling, since the amount of enamel removed by scaling is negligible when compared with that removed by polishing. The heat produced by a polishing cup applied long enough to remove heavy stain could have adverse effects. In areas where root surfaces are planed, all stain will have been removed before polishing would be necessary. When planing is completed, the surface should be smooth and glassy. The need for further polishing of the root surface can be evaluated, but because cementum and dentin are easily abraded, polishing should be avoided whenever possible.

I. Objectives

The objectives need clarification since polishing has been a routine procedure in many dental offices and clinics.

Polishing is for the removal of stains. Calculus is removed by scaling and planing, not by polishing. Soft deposits, pellicle, dental plaque, materia alba, and debris are removed by toothbrushing and other self-care devices. The patient must understand that pellicle can form as soon as 20 minutes after polishing, and that plaque thick enough to be seen when a disclosing agent is used, will be present by 12 to 24 hours if not interrupted by toothbrushing. Limited professional time available, therefore, must not be used for such a short-lasting service unless there is a valid reason.

Reasons for polishing may be summarized as follows:

A. Remove extrinsic stains not otherwise removed by toothbrushing and scaling. This is for esthetic purposes, since stains are not known to be harmful to teeth or gingiva.

B. Prepare the teeth for application of caries preventive agents, notably sealants (page 452) and topical fluoride solutions and gels (page 434). New research has shown the topical fluoride to be of the same effectiveness whether the teeth were polished or not.[1]

C. Create a smooth tooth surface to produce the following effects:
1. Resist colonization of microorganisms so that deposits accumulate at a slower rate.
2. Help the instructed patient to obtain more effective results from self-care procedures.
3. Show the patient the appearance and feeling of a clean mouth to motivate him to practice adequate self-care.

D. Polish restorative materials. Polished amalgam resists tarnish and corrosion, increases the life of the restoration, and prevents rough edges from causing irritation or trapping plaque (page 551).

II. Effects of Polishing on Tooth Structure

Polishing must be performed carefully to avoid excessive loss of tooth structure and prevent damage to the gingival margin. Potential effects on the epithelium when polishing instruments contact the gingival margin forcefully are described on page 545. Research has shown the following with respect to the tooth surfaces:

A. A coarse abrasive can create a rougher tooth surface than before polishing. Grooves and scratches can be observed when examined under the microscope.[2,3]

B. A pumice–water slurry removed as much as four microns of fluoride-rich surface enamel during a 30-second prophylaxis.[4]

C. White spot areas of decalcification should be avoided during polishing because it has been shown that almost three times more surface enamel is lost over white spots than over intact enamel.[5]

D. Abrasion of dentin is five to six times greater than of enamel.[6] Conservative polishing procedures for the root surface and the area of the cementoenamel junction are indicated. Polishing is not usually needed, as stated above, when root planing leaves a smooth, glassy surface. When polishing of the root surface is performed, the finest grade abrasive should be used, and manual polishing is recommended.

CLEANING AND POLISHING AGENTS

Abrasive agents are applied with polishing instruments to remove dental stains and plaque. Abrasives selected should produce smooth tooth surfaces but not remove tooth structure unnecessarily, abrade gingival epithelium, or produce excessive frictional heat.

I. Definitions

A. Abrasive

A material composed of particles of sufficient hardness and sharpness to cut or scratch a softer material when drawn across its surface.

B. **Abrasion**

The wearing away of surface material by friction. Marked or severe abrasion would be destructive to a tooth surface.[7]

C. **Polishing**

The production, especially by friction, of a smooth, glossy, mirror-like surface that reflects light.[7] A very fine agent is used for polishing after a coarser agent is used for cleaning.

II. Factors Affecting Abrasive Action

During polishing, sharp edges of abrasive particles are moved along the surface of a material, abrading it by producing microscopic scratches or grooves. The rate of abrasion, or speed with which structural material is removed from the surface being polished, is governed by characteristics of the abrasive particles as well as by the manner in which they are applied.

A. **Characteristics of Abrasive Particles**[7]
1. *Shape:* Irregularly shaped particles with sharp edges produce deeper grooves and thus abrade faster than rounded particles with dull edges.
2. *Hardness:* Particles must be harder than the surface to be abraded; harder particles abrade faster.
3. *Body Strength:* Particles that fracture into smaller sharp-edged particles during use are more abrasive than those that wear down with use and become dull and rounded.
4. *Attrition Resistance:* Effective abrasive particles do not dull or become impregnated in the surface being abraded; particles with greater attrition resistance abrade faster.
5. *Particle Size (Grit)*
   a. The larger the particles the more abrasive they are with less polishing ability. Finer abrasive particles achieve a glossier finish.

b. Grades

Abrasive and polishing agents are graded from coarse to fine based on the size of the holes in a standard sieve through which they will pass. The finer abrasives are called powders or flours and are graded in order of increasing fineness as F, FF, FFF, etc. Particles imbedded in papers are graded 0, 00, 000, etc.

B. **Method of Application of Abrasives**
1. *Quantity Applied:* The more particles applied per unit time, the faster the rate of abrasion.
   a. Particles suspended in water or other vehicles are present in quantities proportional to the thickness of the paste. These vehicles act as lubricants to reduce the amount of frictional heat produced.
   b. Dry powders or flours represent the greatest quantity that can be applied per unit time. Frictional heat produced is proportional to the rate of abrasion, therefore the use of *dry agents* is *contraindicated* for polishing natural teeth because of the potential danger of thermal injury to the dental pulp.
2. *Speed of Application:* The greater the speed of application, the faster the rate of abrasion.
   a. With increased speed of application, pressure must be reduced.
   b. *Rapid abrasion* is *contraindicated* because it increases frictional heat.
3. *Pressure of Application:* The heavier the pressure applied, the faster the rate of abrasion.
   a. Particles to which pressure is applied produce deep grooves at first, but fracture according to their impact strength. With sufficient pressure, the particles may disintegrate.

b. *Heavy pressure* is *contraindicated* because it increases frictional heat.

4. *Summary*

a. Use wet agents.

b. Apply a rubber polishing cup using slow speed (page 545).

c. Use a quick, light touch.

III. Abrasive Agents[7,8]

The abrasives listed below are examples of commonly used agents. Some are available in several grades, and the specific use varies with the grade. For example, while a superfine grade might be used for polishing enamel surfaces and metallic restorations, a coarser grade would be for laboratory purposes only.

Abrasives for use daily in a dentifrice must necessarily be of a finer grade than for professional polishing accomplished a few times each year. Dentifrice abrasives are described on page 345.

A. **Silex (silicon dioxide)**

1. XXX silex: fairly abrasive.

2. Super-fine silex: can be used for stain removal from enamel.

B. **Pumice**

Powdered pumice is of volcanic origin and consists chiefly of complex silicates of aluminum, potassium, and sodium. The specifications for particle size are listed in the *National Formulary*[9] as follow:

1. Pumice flour or Superfine pumice: least abrasive, and may be used to remove stains from enamel.

2. Fine pumice: mildly abrasive.

3. Coarse pumice: not for use on natural teeth.

C. **Zirconium Silicate**

A cleaning and polishing agent. During use for cleaning a tooth surface, its rough irregular crystals lose their projections. The enamel then becomes polished to a high luster.[10]

D. **Recrystallized Kaolinite**

A cleaning and polishing agent. It has small, hard particles which give a high glossy finish without causing abrasive scratches or grooves.[11]

E. **Calcium Carbonate (whiting, calcite, chalk)**

There are various grades used for different polishing techniques.

F. **Tin Oxide (putty powder, stannic oxide)**

Polishing agent for teeth and metallic restorations.

G. **Emery (corundum)**

Not used directly on the enamel, except as it is made into strips or disks.

1. Aluminum oxide (alumina): the pure form of emery.

2. Levigated alumina: extremely fine particles of aluminum oxide which may be used for polishing metals but are destructive to tooth surfaces.

H. **Tripoli**

A mild abrasive and polishing agent.

I. **Rouge (jeweler's rouge)**

Iron oxide, a fine red powder sometimes impregnated on paper disks. It is useful for polishing gold and precious metal alloys in the laboratory.

IV. Preparation of Abrasives

Agents used for polishing the natural teeth and restorations are mixed with water or other lubricant to facilitate particle movement across the tooth surface and to reduce frictional heat. A quantity of polishing paste can be prepared in advance and kept in a closed jar. Glycerin added can help as a spreading factor and to prevent splashing during application of the polishing cup.

A. **Preparation of Single Quantity**

1. Place water or flavored mouthwash in a dappen dish. Some agents require a specific amount of water.

2. Add the dry agent to saturation and stir.

B. **Consistency:** moist as possible, but transportable between dappen dish and the teeth.

C. **Two Separate Dappen Dishes and Rubber Cups** are used when a cleaning abrasive is used first and followed by a polishing agent.

V. Commercial Preparations

Numerous dental prophylactic cleaning and polishing preparations are available. Some of these have been studied for their relative abrasive effect on enamel and dentin, and their cleaning properties.[6]

A. **Constituents**

Most commercially prepared polishing pastes contain an abrasive, water, a humectant, a binder, and agents for sweetening, flavoring, and color.[12,13] Proportions and purposes of each constituent with examples are as follows:

1. *Abrasive* 50–60%, main ingredient. Examples: pumice, silicon dioxide, zirconium silicate
2. *Water* 10–20%, solvent, and to provide desired consistency.
3. *Humectant* 20–25%, moisture-retainer, stabilize the ingredients. Examples: glycerin, sorbitol
4. *Binder* 1.5–2.0%, prevent separation, non-splatter. Examples: agar-agar, sodium silicate powder
5. *Sweetener,* artificial, non-cariogenic.
6. *Flavoring,* coloring agents.

B. **Packaging**

Commercial preparations are in the forms of pastes, powders, or tablets. Some are available in measured amounts contained in small plastic or other individual packets which contribute to the cleanliness and sterility of the procedure.

C. **Selection**

1. General. Selection of a preparation has been based on its qualities of abrasiveness, consistency for convenient use, or flavor for patient pleasure.
2. Surface fluoride replacement.[13] The use of an abrasive on the tooth surface removes the outer layer of enamel which contains the highest concentration of fluoride (figure 29–2, page 423). Fluoride in a polishing paste is intended to provide fluoride to replace that lost while polishing.

   A number of laboratory and clinical studies have been conducted to determine the effectiveness of incorporating fluoride into prophylactic pastes. Stannous fluoride and acidulated phosphate fluoride have been used primarily. Abrasives have included silex (silicon dioxide), lava pumice, flour of pumice, or zirconium silicate (Zircate).[6]

   Problems in the development of an effective paste are incompatibilities between the fluoride and the abrasive or other components of polishing pastes. Additional information and a bibliography of current references is included in the chapter on fluorides (page 441).

TECHNICAL HINTS

I. Polishing agent used before sealant application should not contain glycerin or agent with oil (page 453).

II. Polishing agent with zirconium silicate used before making radiographs may leave a residue which will appear opaque in the radiographs (page 140).[14]

FACTORS TO TEACH THE PATIENT

I. Stains and deposits removed by polishing will return promptly if plaque control is not carried out faithfully.

II. Polishing agents employed in the dental office are too abrasive for routine daily home use.

References

1. Tinanoff, N., Wei., S. H. Y., and Parkins, F. M.: Effect of a Pumice Prophylaxis on Fluoride Uptake in Tooth Enamel, *J. Am. Dent. Assoc.*, 88, 384, February, 1974.
2. Brasch, S. V., Lazarou, J., Van Abbé, N. J., and Forrest, J. O.: The Assessment of Dentifrice Abrasivity in vivo, *Br. Dent. J.*, 127, 119, August 5, 1969.
3. Jefferies, R. W.: Polishing Dental Enamel, *New Zeal. Dent. J.*, 69, 167, July, 1973.
4. Vrbic, V., Brudevold, F., and McCann, H. G.: Acquisition of Fluoride by Enamel from Fluoride Pumice Pastes, *Helv. Odontol. Acta*, 11, 21, April, 1967.
5. Zuniga, M. A. and Caldwell, R. C.: The Effect of Fluoride-containing Prophylaxis Pastes on Normal and "White-spot" Enamel, *J. Dent. Child.*, 55, 345, September-October, 1969.
6. Whitehurst, V. E., Stookey, G. K., and Muhler, J. C.: Studies Concerning the Cleaning, Polishing, and Therapeutic Properties of Commercial Prophylactic Pastes, *J. Oral Thera. and Pharm.*, 4, 181, November, 1967.
7. Phillips, R. W.: *Skinner's Science of Dental Materials*, 7th ed. Philadelphia, Saunders, 1973, pp. 623–630.
8. Kutscher, A. H., Zegarelli, E. V., Hyman, G. A., McLean, P., and Kutscher, H. W., eds.: *Pharmacology for the Dental Hygienist.* Philadelphia, Lea & Febiger, 1967, pp. 234–235.
9. American Pharmaceutical Association: *National Formulary XIII*. Washington, D.C., American Pharmaceutical Association, 1970, p. 611.
10. Muhler, J. C. and Stookey, G. K.: The Development of an Improved ZrSiO$_4$ Prophylactic Paste, *J. Periodont.*, 41, 290, May, 1970.
11. Stoll, F. A. and Werner, A. R.: Clinical Observations of a New Polishing Agent for Dental Prophylaxis, *J. Am. Dent. Hyg. Assoc.*, 37, 79, 2nd Quarter, 1963.
12. Jefopoulos, T.: *Dentifrices, 1970*. Park Ridge, N.J., Noyes Data Corporation, 1970, pp. 142–150.
13. Katz, S., McDonald, J. L., and Stookey, G. K.: *Preventive Dentistry in Action*, Upper Montclair, N.J., D. C. P. Publishing, 1972, pp. 189–194.
14. Manson-Hing, L. R.: Radiopaque Prophy Cleaner, *Oral Surg.*, 27, 758, June, 1969.

Suggested Readings

Brooks, E. B. and Voigt, J. P.: Particle Configuration of Prophylaxis Pastes as Observed by Scanning Electron Microscopy, *J. Periodont.*, 45, 23, January, 1974.
Craig, R. G., O'Brien, W. J., and Powers, J. M.: *Dental Materials. Properties and Manipulation.* St. Louis, Mosby, 1975, pp. 84–98.
Handleman, S. L. and Hess, C.: Effect of Dental Prophylaxis on Tooth–surface Flora, *J. Dent. Res.*, 49, 340, March-April, 1970.
Phillips, R. W.: *Elements of Dental Materials for Dental Hygienists and Assistants*, 2nd ed. Philadelphia, Saunders, 1971, pp. 265–271.
Zampa, S. T. and Green, E.: Effect of Polishing Agents on Root Roughness, *J. Periodont.*, 43, 125, February, 1972.

Chapter 37

Polishing Procedures

As described on page 537, polishing is a selective procedure. After scaling and other periodontal treatment, evaluation is made, and polishing of teeth and restorations may be needed, particularly when there are unsightly stains.

I. Preparation for Polishing

In preparation for polishing, a review should be made of pertinent information on stains (page 259), pellicle and plaque (page 235), fluoride in the surface enamel (page 423), and abrasives (page 538). Preparation of the patient includes plaque control and complete scaling and planing.

A. Plaque Control

Polishing should be withheld until the patient's plaque removal on a daily basis is adequate in order that the deposition of stains can be controlled. When a patient is informed of the relationship between self-care and the recurrence of stains, cooperation may be obtained. When a stain such as black line stain (page 261) returns even in a clean mouth, polishing frequency should be limited and, with each polishing, topical fluoride applied.

B. Scaling

As much stain as possible should be removed during scaling of the enamel, and all stain can be removed during root planing, since most of the stain will be located within the necrotic cementum.

II. Instruments

Both motor-driven and manual instruments may be useful when polishing. All polishing instruments should be used with discretion and in a manner requiring minimal abrasion of the tooth surface. Since tooth structure is removed when an abrasive is used on the enamel and still more when used on dentin or cementum, only a mild abrasive agent is appropriate.

Motor-driven implements and floss and polishing strips will be outlined first, followed by procedures for cleaning a removable denture and polishing amalgam restorations. In the next chapter hand polishing with a porte polisher will be described.

THE INSTRUMENTS

I. Handpiece

An instrument used to hold rotary instruments in the dental unit. It is connected by an arm, cable, belt, or tube to the source of power. Rotary instruments have been classified according to their rotational speeds designated by revolutions per minute (r.p.m.) as low speed, intermediate or high speed, and ultra or super speed.[1]

A. Low Speed or Conventional

Typical range under 10,000 r.p.m. Lowest speeds are used for polishing teeth.

B. High Speed or Intermediate

Between 10,000 and 100,000 r.p.m. Some high speed handpieces can be adjusted to speeds from zero to their capacity which makes it possible to use them with the proper attachments, for tooth polishing.

C. Ultra or Super Speed

Over 100,000 r.p.m.

II. Prophylaxis Angle

Contra or right-angle attachment for the handpiece to which polishing devices (rubber cup, bristle brush) are attached.

A. Characteristics

There are many types of prophylaxis angles available. They are generally made of stainless steel and may have hard chrome, carbon steel, or brass bearings. A few types are reversible in their action.

B. Service Life

The length of time which a prophylaxis angle is serviceable is related in part to the quality of materials used and the manner of construction. Primarily, however, *the length of life is directly proportional to the care provided in cleaning and lubricating after each use.* The care and sterilization of the prophylaxis angle are described on pages 16–17.

III. Prophylaxis Angle Attachments

A. Rubber Polishing Cups

1. Types
   a. Slip-on: with ribbed cup to aid in holding polishing agent.
   b. Slip-on: with bristles inside cup.
   c. Threaded (screw type): with plain ribbed cup or flange (webbed) type.
2. Materials
   a. Natural rubber: more resilient and will not stain the teeth.
   b. Synthetic: stiffer than natural rubber; white cups must be used since synthetic black may stain the teeth.

B. Bristle Brushes

1. Types
   a. For prophylaxis angle: slip-on or screw type.
   b. For handpiece: mandrel mounted.
2. Materials: nylon or natural bristles.

IV. Uses for Attachments

A. Handpiece With Straight Mandrel

1. Dixon bristle brush (Type C, soft) for polishing removable dentures (page 550).
2. Mounted stone for sharpening instruments (page 489).
3. Rubber cup on mandrel for polishing labial surfaces of anterior teeth.

B. Prophylaxis Angle With Rubber Cup or Brush

1. Rubber cup for removal of stains from the tooth surfaces and to polish restorations.
2. Brush
   a. For removing stains from deep pits and fissures and enamel surfaces away from gingival margin. A brush is not recommended for use on exposed cementum or dentin. They are easily grooved by such an instrument.
   b. For preliminary polishing of amalgam restorations.

USE OF THE PROPHYLAXIS ANGLE

I. Effects on Tissues: Precautions

The use of motor-driven instruments can provide the patient with discomfort if care and consideration for the oral tissues are not exercised to prevent unnecessary trauma.

Awareness of the potential tissue damage which may result is important. Tactile sensitivity of the operator while using a thick, bulky handpiece is diminished and unnecessary pressure may be applied inadvertently. Frictional heat may cause pain or discomfort.

A. **Tooth Structure**

Some loss of tooth structure occurs during polishing when an abrasive agent is used. Research on the effects on tooth structure was reviewed on page 538.

The greater the speed of application of a polishing agent, the faster the rate of abrasion (page 539). Therefore the speed at which the handpiece is operated should be at a low r.p.m.

B. **Epithelium**

Trauma to the gingival tissue can result from too high a speed, extended application of the rubber cup, and use of an abrasive polishing agent. In one study[2] a rubber cup with pumice rotated for two minutes caused a total removal of the epithelium just inside the crest. Complete healing from such a wound would be expected in 8 to 14 days.

II. Prophylaxis Angle Technique

As with all oral procedures, a systematic order of polishing should be followed. A variety of skills must be learned in using and caring for the equipment.

A. **Instrument Grasp:** Modified pen (page 463)
1. Hold middle finger as near working end of prophylaxis angle as possible to guide and support the handpiece. Use only the cushion of the middle finger, not the side of the first knuckle.
2. Methods of relieving awkwardness in use of large handpiece.
   a. Use firm grasp to give support.
   b. Rest handpiece handle in the V between index finger and thumb when consistent with other positioning for accessibility to the field of operation.
   c. Adjust height of motor arm to relieve weight in hand.

B. **Finger Rest** (page 464)
1. Establish firmly on tooth structure.
2. Use a wide fulcrum area when practical to aid in the balance of the large instrument. Example: place cushion of fulcrum finger across occlusal surfaces of premolars while polishing the molars.
3. Avoid use of mobile teeth as finger rests.

C. **Speed of Motor**
1. Use slowest available speed to minimize frictional heat.
2. Adjust r.p.m. by changing the position of the rheostat foot pedal.

D. **Use of Rheostat Pedal**
1. Adjust screw clamps on top of rheostat to provide freedom for pedal movement so that motor will stop immediately upon release of foot pressure (all rheostats do not have such an attachment).
2. Apply steady pressure with foot to produce an even, slow speed.
3. When seated during operation: keep sole of foot which activates rheostat pedal flat on the floor. Use toe to activate rheostat pedal.
4. When standing: keep body weight distributed evenly on both feet. Use toe to activate rheostat pedal.

E. **Preparation of Polishing Agent**
1. Agent is mixed as wet as possible but not so wet that it cannot be

carried conveniently in the rubber cup from the dappen dish to the teeth (pages 540–541).

2. Wetness aids in alleviating the frictional heat produced.

F. **Stroke and Procedure**
   1. *Rubber Cup*
      a. Observe where polishing is needed to prevent unnecessary rubber cup application.
      b. Distribute polishing agent over group of tooth surfaces to be polished.
      c. Fill rubber cup with polishing agent, establish finger rest, and bring rubber cup almost in contact with tooth surface before starting motor.
      d. Using slowest r.p.m., apply revolving cup lightly to tooth surface for two or three seconds.
      e. Move cup to adjacent area on tooth surface as in a patting action.
      f. Move cup from tooth to tooth, frequently replenishing supply of polishing agent.
      g. Turn handpiece to adapt rubber cup to fit each surface of the tooth, including proximal surfaces and gingival surfaces of fixed partial dentures.
      h. When two polishing agents of different abrasiveness are to be applied, use a separate rubber cup for each.
      i. Discard a rubber cup as it becomes less firm and before it wears on the edges.
   2. *Bristle Brush:* Use of a bristle brush should be avoided unless absolutely necessary. Lacerations of the gingiva and grooves and scratches in tooth structure, particularly roots, may result.
      a. Soak stiff brush in hot water to soften bristles.

      b. Distribute polishing agent over occlusal surfaces of teeth to be polished.
      c. Place fingers of left hand in a position which will both retract and protect cheek and tongue from the revolving brush.
      d. Establish a firm finger rest and bring brush almost in contact with the tooth before starting motor.
      e. Using slowest r.p.m., apply revolving brush lightly to the occlusal surface only, avoiding contact of bristles with soft tissues.
      f. Use a short stroke in a brushing motion, following the inclined planes of the cusps.
      g. Move from tooth to tooth to prevent generation of excessive frictional heat. Replenish supply of polishing agent frequently.

G. **Irrigate Teeth and Interdental Areas** thoroughly several times with water from the syringe to remove abrasive particles. The rotary movement of the rubber cup or bristle brush tends to force the abrasive into the gingival sulci, which may be a source of irritation to the soft tissues.

POLISHING PROXIMAL SURFACES

Considerable care must be exercised in the use of floss, tape, and polishing strips. Understanding the anatomy of the interdental papillae and their relationship to the contact areas and proximal surfaces of the teeth is prerequisite to the prevention of tissue damage. Inadequate contacts between teeth provide potential areas of food impaction and therefore contribute to periodontal disease. These contacts should be charted for consideration by the dentist during treatment planning.

As much polishing as possible of accessible proximal surfaces is accomplished during the use of the rubber cup in the prophylaxis angle. This is followed by the use of dental tape with polishing agent when necessary. Polishing strips are used only in selected instances when all other techniques fail to remove a stain.

The use of dental floss or tape for dental plaque control on proximal tooth surfaces is an essential part of self-care by the patient. This is described on pages 332–336.

I. Dental Tape and Floss

A. Description

Floss and tape are made of spun silk or nylon thread and are available unwaxed or coated with wax. The wax covering affords some protection for the tissues, facilitates the movement of the floss or tape, prevents excessive absorption of moisture, and assists in the prevention of shredding.

Unwaxed dental floss is considered particularly useful in the preparation of teeth for a topical fluoride application. When waxed floss is used for this purpose there is the possibility of wax remaining on small areas of the tooth surface, thus preventing uniform contact of fluoride with the enamel.

Tape is flat and has relatively sharp edges whereas floss is round. Either floss or tape may injure the tissue when used incorrectly or carelessly.

B. Uses
1. *Tape for Polishing*
   a. Proximal tooth surfaces.
   b. Gingival surface of fixed partial denture.
2. *Floss for Removing*
   a. Debris and food particles. Patient instruction and review at beginning of appointment prepares the teeth for scaling.
   b. Particles of polishing agents at completion of polishing procedures.
      (1) From interproximal areas and gingival sulci.

(2) From gingival surface of fixed partial dentures.
3. Retained abrasive particles after use of polishing strips.

C. Technique for Dental Floss and Tape

Techniques for tape and floss application are described on page 332 and illustrated in figures 23–1, 23–2, and 23–3. The same principles apply whether the patient or the operator is using the floss. Finger rests must be used to prevent snapping through contact areas.

1. *Polishing with Dental Tape.* Polishing agent is applied to the tooth, and the tape is moved gently back and forth over the area where stain was observed.
2. *Polishing Gingival Surface of a Fixed Partial Denture.* A floss threader is used to position the floss or tape over the gingival surface. Floss threaders are described and illustrated on page 357. Polishing agent is applied under the pontic, and the floss or tape moved back and forth.
3. *Floss after Polishing.* Particles of abrasive agent should be removed by irrigation and by using a clean length of floss applied in the usual manner.
4. *Rinse and Irrigate.* Irrigate with water spray syringe to clean out all abrasive agent.

II. Polishing Strips

A. Description

Polishing strips are also known as linen abrasive strips or finishing strips. They are thin, flexible, tape-shaped, and are available in four widths—extra narrow, narrow, medium, and wide. They are made of linen or plastic with one smooth side and the other which serves as a carrier for abrasive agents bonded to the side. They are available in extra fine, fine, medium, or coarse grit. *Only extra narrow or narrow strips with fine grit are suggested for stain removal and then only with discretion.*

B. **Use**
   1. *For Stain Removal on Proximal Surfaces of Anterior Teeth:* When other polishing techniques are unsuccessful.
   2. *Precautions for Use*
      a. Edge of strip is sharp and may cut gingival tissue or lip.
      b. Rough working side of strip is capable of removing tooth structure and may make nicks or grooves, particularly in the cementum.
      c. Polishing with polishing strip should be limited to enamel surfaces.

C. **Technique for Polishing Strip**
   1. *Grasp and Finger Rest*
      A strip no longer than six inches is most conveniently applied. The grasp and fulcrum must be well controlled. Protection of the lip by retraction with the thumb and index finger holding the strip is mandatory.
   2. *Positioning*
      a. Direct the abrasive side of strip toward the proximal surface to be polished as the strip is worked slowly and gently between the teeth with a slightly sawing motion. Bring strip just through the contact area. If the strip breaks, immediately use floss to remove particles of abrasive.
      b. When a space is clearly visible through an interproximal area and the interdental papilla is missing, a narrow polishing strip may be threaded through. Prepare strip by cutting the end on the diagonal to facilitate threading.

   3. *Polishing*
      a. Press abrasive side of strip against tooth. Draw back and forth in a ⅛ inch arc two or three times, rocking on the established fulcrum.
      b. Remove strip and insert for adjacent proximal surface. Do not attempt to turn the strip while it is in the interdental area.
   4. *Use Dental Floss*
      Follow each application of polishing strips with dental floss to remove abrasive particles.

CLEANING THE REMOVABLE DENTURE

A complete patient service includes the scaling and polishing of all natural teeth and their replacements. Complete and partial dentures may accumulate calculus, soft deposits, and stains which may affect the adaptation of the dentures in the mouth as well as afford a source of irritation to adjacent mucous membranes. The parts of a complete denture are illustrated in figure 24–8, page 362, and the parts of a partial in figure 24–11, page 369.

A learning experience in the proper care of the dentures can be provided for the patient while the dentures are cleaned professionally. Specific instruction for the patient is described on pages 363–370.

I. Objectives
A. Aids in preserving the natural teeth associated with a removable partial denture.
B. Removes calculus, soft deposits, and stains, thereby smoothing the surfaces of the denture.
C. Improves the appearance of the denture.
D. Gives the patient a feeling of complete oral cleanliness.
E. Emphasizes to the patient the importance of routine personal and professional care of the denture.

II. Removal of Denture

Generally the patient removes his denture himself. The dental hygienist will have occasion to remove dentures for certain patients, particularly those who may be handicapped or helpless (page 585), or as a first aid measure (page 725). Although denture removal may be complicated by anatomical features of the individual mouth, a general procedure is outlined here. The procedure should be reviewed with the dentist in order to follow a preferred technique.

A. **Wear Rubber Gloves.** When the patient is known to have, or is suspected of having, a communicable disease, or when a generally septic condition exists in the oral cavity, rubber gloves should be worn.

B. **Complete Maxillary Denture**
1. Grasp the denture firmly with the thumb on the facial surface at the height of the border of the denture under the lip and the index finger on the palatal surface.
2. With the other hand, elevate the lip to expose the border of the denture to break the seal.
3. Remove the denture gently in a downward and forward direction.
4. If the retention of the denture cannot be overcome by elevation of the lip, request the able patient to blow into his mouth with his lips closed. This generally will break the seal.

C. **Complete Mandibular Denture**
1. Grasp the denture firmly on the facial surface with the thumb and the lingual with the index finger.
2. With the other hand, retract the lower lip forward and remove the denture gently.

D. **Partial Denture with Clasps.** Exert an even pressure on both sides of the denture simultaneously, as the clasps are lifted over their abutment teeth.

Usually the line of insertion and removal of a partial denture is designed and constructed for an even, vertical removal.

III. Care of Dentures During Intra-Oral Procedures

A. Provide a cleansing tissue when requesting the patient to remove or insert his denture.

B. Receive removable denture in a paper cup or container with fitted cover.

C. Wear rubber gloves and wash the denture with surgical soap.

D. Immerse in antiseptic solution.

E. Place container in a safe place away from working area to minimize hazard of breakage.

IV. Procedure for Cleaning

Ultrasonic cleaning is the procedure of choice for the safety of the denture, for the preservation of the surface finish, to eliminate the possibility of scratching the denture surface through the use of scalers, polishing agents or other devices, and for the time saved. When ultrasonic equipment is not available, manual and motor-driven instruments must be used.

A. **Ultrasonic**
1. Principles and procedures have been described on pages 20–21.
2. Use the solution designated for stain and calculus removal and follow the manufacturer's directions specifically.
3. Rinse thoroughly and scrub free of solution and loosened debris with a moderately stiff brush before returning the denture to the patient. Brushes reserved for this purpose should be autoclaved.

B. **Manual and Motor-driven**
1. *Remove calculus* by careful scaling. Care must be taken not to scratch the denture.

2. *Method for holding denture;* grasp firmly and securely in the palm of the left hand (figure 24–9, page 365). Avoid excessive pressure on a partial denture bar or clasps to prevent bending.

3. *Polish only the external polished surface* of a denture: abrasive applied to the internal impression surface could affect the fit of the denture.

4. *Polishing at the dental chair*
   a. With a conventional dental chair, polishing over the cuspidor (lined with a towel) is sometimes convenient. Focus the dental light over the work area.
   b. Polish nonmetal parts with a mounted brush (Dixon C softened in warm water) using very wet superfine pumice or other appropriate abrasive. The finger rest is maintained on the denture.
   c. Polish metal parts lightly with a rubber polishing cup. A fine polishing agent should be used to prevent scratching of the metal.

5. *Polishing on the dental lathe in the laboratory*
   a. Prevention of cross contamination in the laboratory[3]
      (1) Wear a mask and safety glasses while working over a lathe.
      (2) Use autoclaved rag wheel and pumice.
      (3) Soak the prosthesis in an antiseptic solution for 15 minutes before returning it to the patient. The solution should be fresh for each patient, since cold solutions do not sterilize.
   b. Use a wet rag wheel with fine wet abrasive for nonmetal parts, and whiting or tin oxide on a separate rag wheel for the metal parts other than clasps. Keep denture and polishing agent wet at all times.
   c. Hold the denture in a two-handed grip. Cover the clasps and denture teeth with fingers to prevent abrasive from scratching the teeth and the clasps from hooking into the rag wheel. The clasps are cleaned later with the wood point in the porte polisher.
   d. Run the lathe at low speed and apply denture carefully. Constantly change the surface applied to the rag wheel to prevent excess frictional heat.

6. *Rinse the denture thoroughly* under warm (never hot) running water.
   a. Line the sink with a towel, or fill half-full with water to avoid breakage in case the denture is dropped.
   b. Brush the internal impression surface of the denture using a mild soap or a detergent; rinse thoroughly.

7. *Evaluate* the cleanliness of the denture: examine under bright light and apply compressed air stream to detect calculus or dental plaque.

8. *Disinfect*, rinse and return the denture to the patient on a paper towel. The denture should be wet for comfortable insertion.

POLISHING AMALGAM RESTORATIONS

Polishing a previously placed "old" amalgam restoration does not differ from polishing a new restoration except that the old one may have more marginal irregularities due to dimensional changes over the years, and therefore require more preliminary smoothing. The extent of procedures for a new restoration depends on the carving at the time the restoration was placed. The neatly and carefully carved restoration which fulfills the normal anatomic requirements will require very little smoothing of margins and surfaces before the finishing polish. A study of amalgam and its properties should preface learning to polish.[4,5]

Principles, procedures, and precautions are presented here for basic understanding. There are in practice nearly as many choices and combinations of specific instruments and materials for finishing and polishing amalgam restorations as there are operators who participate in this phase of patient service.

I. Purposes for Polishing

Purposes are related to tarnish and corrosion of the surface of the amalgam restoration. *Tarnish* is a surface discoloration, principally a sulfide, which is usually caused by foods and oral uncleanliness. It can occur on a properly polished restoration but not as thick and fast.

Corrosion is an actual chemical deterioration of the metal which usually begins as a tarnish and is caused by environmental factors such as air, moisture, acid or alkaline solutions, and other chemicals.[6] Smoothly polished amalgam resists corrosion. The corrosion may be carried into the dentinal tubules and the entire area around the restoration may appear bluish-black.

Polishing to a smooth, glossy finish contributes to the following:

A. Provides a smooth tooth surface which resists the retention of deposits.

B. Prevents irritation to the gingival tissue from the bacterial plaque which accumulates readily on rough surfaces.

C. Makes it easier for the patient to maintain oral cleanliness.

D. Helps to prevent recurrent dental caries.

E. Resists amalgam tarnish and corrosion.

F. Improves the appearance of the restoration.

G. Increases the length of service of the restoration.

II. Objectives

The finished restoration will have the following characteristics:

A. All margins will be smooth so that no margin is detectable when explored.
1. No deficient margins exist.
2. No overhanging margins can be detected.

B. Normal anatomical tooth form will be preserved.

C. The surface of the restoration is smooth, lustrous, glossy, and free from visible scratches.

III. Principles for Polishing

A. Wait at least 48 hours after amalgam has been placed and carved before polishing.[7] Amalgam must be completely "set."

B. Avoid heating the restoration by excess pressure, speed, or length of contact of instrument. This can alter the chemical structure, draw mercury to the surface, and change the physical properties of the material.
1. Use wet polishing agent and light intermittent contact of motor-driven polishing instruments.
2. Avoid dry polishing powders and disks. Dry materials increase the surface temperature.
3. Avoid rubber appliances such as rubber polishing or finishing points. They produce high temperatures. Rubber polishing cups should always be separated from the tooth by a moist abrasive mixture.

C. Use care not to obliterate the dental anatomy carved in the restoration.

D. Use secure finger rest and adequate retraction to protect soft oral tissues.

E. Avoid the contact area. It was formed by the smooth, polished matrix band and usually requires no further smoothing. The area may be polished during the final polishing as directed by the dentist. Even then, a small amount of amalgam removed may destroy the firm contact or alter its contour.

F. Do not isolate routinely with cotton rolls.
   1. Revolving polishing instruments catch the cotton rolls.
   2. Repeated need for rinsing to clear away excess polishing agent for vision would necessitate use of considerable time in changing cotton rolls.

G. The abrasive agent can clog a saliva ejector if one is used. Clearing the saliva ejector after operation is essential.

IV. Procedure for Polishing

A. **Removal of Irregularities in the Surface of the Amalgam**
   1. *Occlusal surface*
      a. Use mounted fine-grained flame- or pear-shaped green stones and finishing burs. Select size of finishing bur which will adapt to the main contours of the restoration and the grooves. When the bur is too large the depth of the grooves may remain untouched and the anatomy may be obliterated. When the bur is too small, it may nick enamel edges.
      b. Directions for use of a stone or bur on the margin
         (1) Slow speed; minimum pressure.
         (2) Constant motion; cooled.
         (3) Rotate stone from enamel to metal, or at right angles to it.

   2. *Proximal surface*
      a. Facial and lingual margins
         (1) Use waterproof ½ or ⅜ inch fine cuttle disks, in a straight or contra-angle handpiece depending on accessibility.
         (2) Apply disk with a light, intermittent stroke with constant motion, and low speed. The object is to minimize heat.
         (3) Do not extend the disk to a position near the contact, as a deficiency can be created.
      b. Gingival margin
         (1) Explore to check for roughness. If the matrix was properly adapted, there should be no need for removal of any gross excess amalgam. Although a file or knife could be used, it is better not to take the chance of roughening the area, creating a deficiency, or flattening a concavity unless absolutely necessary.
         (2) A fine, narrow or medium-wide polishing strip may be threaded through the embrasure when slight smoothing is indicated. Do not insert a strip by way of the occlusal since the contact could be destroyed. A strip would not adapt for the mesial of a maxillary first premolar or other convex surface.
   3. Explore all margins to check continuity and lack of interruption between the restoration and the enamel.

B. **Polishing**
   1. Agents. Use as mild an abrasive as possible.
      a. Flour of pumice and zirconium silicate have been used in water

or glycerin, but milder abrasives leave fewer scratches.

b. When a coarse polishing agent is employed, it is usually recommended that a final high gloss be produced using tin oxide in water or alcohol.

c. Use rubber polishing cup kept moist with sufficient polishing mixture.

2. Precaution. Do not overpolish. Excessive attempts to produce a glossy surface may subject the tooth and restoration to more heat than is compatible with patient comfort and the properties of the restorative material. Overpolishing, even with a fine abrasive, can alter the anatomy of the restoration.

3. Have patient rinse thoroughly to remove abrasive particles.

C. **Fluoride Application**

The use of abrasive stones and polishing agents at the margin of a restoration removes the surface enamel and, with it, the concentration of fluoride which is protective against dental caries.

1. Commercial, prepared polishing paste. A prepared paste containing fluoride may restore in part the lost fluoride (page 441), and can be used during the polishing procedure.

2. Topical Application. After polishing, a topical application should be made, followed by periodic applications at succeeding recall appointments. Self-application on a daily basis, using a mouth rinse, custom tray, or chewable tablet, may also be recommended (pages 441–442).

Overhanging Amalgam Restoration

A finished restoration follows the normal contours of the tooth. All junctions are smooth so that when an explorer is passed over the margin it is continuous with the tooth structure.

Defects in a restoration include a deficiency at the margin and an excess of restorative material which overhangs the margin. Another type of defective restoration is one with overcontouring of the total restoration so that the contact area is extended and the embrasure is narrowed and shortened. An example of an overcontoured crown is shown in figure 25–1C on page 374.

When a margin is deficient, a new restoration must be made to replace the old one. An attempt to even off the junction between the tooth and a deficient margin would require removal of an excess amount of tooth structure.

Excess amalgam overhanging at a margin can sometimes be removed and the area polished adequately for continued service of the restoration. A very gross overhang would be impractical to remove, so that replacement of the restoration would be indicated.

A. **Identification**

1. *Radiographic.* A proximal restoration with excess amalgam may not show its true extent or may not show at all because of superimposition in a radiograph.

2. *Exploration.* All restorations should be explored around their entire margins particularly the proximal where a Class II is not directly visible clinically.

B. **Causes of Irregularities of Margins**

1. Improperly adapted matrix band which permitted a ledge of amalgam to collect when the material was being packed.

2. Amalgam contraction or expansion after insertion.

3. Faulty manipulation of materials at the time of insertion: too high mercury content at the margin weakens the margin and leaves it susceptible to fracture.

4. Improper finishing and polishing of a new restoration.
5. Marginal corrosion causing deterioration and fracture of the margin.
6. Undermining of a margin by recurrent dental caries.

C. **Effects of Overhangs; Reasons for Removal**
1. Retention of plaque which contributes to periodontal disease and dental caries.
2. Creates problems of self-care.
   a. Irregular margin catches and tears dental floss.
   b. Area under the ledge of the overhang, particularly a proximal overhang, is inaccessible to a toothbrush and other devices.
3. Rough margin serves as a mechanical irritant to tongue and cheek.
4. Debris retention contributes to a general lack of oral sanitation and to halitosis from breakdown products of food.

D. **Removal of Proximal Amalgam Overhanging Restoration**
1. *Objective:* to remove excess amalgam so the junction between the amalgam and the enamel is smooth when explored with a fine explorer tip.
2. *Instruments*
   Removal of excess amalgam on the occlusal and facial and lingual portions of the proximal would require the same instruments and procedures as described in IV above for a new restoration. In addition, to remove the proximal portion which is under the contact area, the following instruments may be applied:
   a. Files. Care must be taken not to groove and scratch the tooth surface, particularly cementum. Files are described on page 478.
   b. Scalers. Only a strong scaler should be used, and only when

there is a small overhang. A scaler tip could be easily broken if applied with much force. It should also be remembered that using a metal cutting edge on metal (the amalgam) will dull the instrument rapidly.
   c. Ultrasonic scaler. A special tip attachment is available for the removal of excess amalgam.
   d. Rotary instruments. A finishing bur, green stone, or diamond stone may be used.
   e. Finishing strips. After the amalgam has been removed, a fine grit strip may be used, provided it can be threaded through the embrasure. It should not be inserted through the contact because of reducing the amalgam and changing the contour of the contact area.
3. *Technique suggestions*
   a. Wear glasses for protection from flying bits and from aerosols created by rotary and ultrasonic instruments.
   b. Retract carefully to protect the patient's cheek, tongue, and lips.
   c. Avoid letting particles of amalgam fall into the depths of the sulcus.
      (1) Use suction for clearing the debris promptly.
      (2) Use strokes that do not push the particles into the sulcus, that is, strokes that are perpendicular with the long axis of the tooth.

TECHNICAL HINTS

I. Maintain several prophylaxis angles in practice to facilitate use during successive appointments. When this is done, care of the prophylaxis angles should be accomplished as soon as possible after use: within a few hours at the most.

II. Test staining potential of a black synthetic rubber cup by using it as an eraser on white paper. If black appears, the teeth can be stained.

III. Prevent rheostat from sliding on highly polished floor by placing one or two drops of carbon tetrachloride under the rheostat.

IV. Wear eyeglasses and mask for protection from flying material and aerosols when using handpiece, prophylaxis angle, and dental lathe.

V. Protect patient's lips and intraoral soft tissues during the use of floss, tape, finishing strips, and polishing disks.

FACTORS TO TEACH THE PATIENT

I. How plaques and stains form on the natural teeth and their replacements and why too frequent polishing in the dental office is not advisable. When adequate self-care is carried out, polishing is not necessary.

II. The need for adapting toothbrushing and flossing techniques to cleanse abutment teeth.

III. The importance of having inadequate contact areas restored rather than using floss repeatedly to alleviate the discomforts of food impaction.

IV. The importance of regular cleansing of dentures with special attention to clasps.

V. How to handle and cleanse a denture.

References

1. American Dental Association, Council on Dental Materials and Devices, Peyton, F. A.: Status Report on Dental Operating Handpieces, *J. Am. Dent. Assoc.*, 89, 1162, November, 1974.
2. Löe, H.: Reactions of Marginal Periodontal Tissues to Restorative Procedures, *Int. Dent. J.*, 18, 759, December, 1968.
3. Katberg, J. W.: Cross-contamination via the Prosthodontic Laboratory, *J. Prosthet. Dent.*, 32, 412, October, 1974.
4. Phillips, R. W.: *Elements of Dental Materials for Dental Hygienists and Assistants*, 2nd ed. Philadelphia, Saunders, 1971, pp. 145–168.
5. Peyton, F. A. and Craig, R. G., eds.: *Restorative Dental Materials*, 4th ed. St. Louis, Mosby, 1971, pp 358–397.
6. Phillips: op. cit., pp. 138–144.
7. Phillips: op. cit., p. 165.

Suggested Readings

Goldman, H. M. and Cohen, D. W.: *Periodontal Therapy*, 5th ed. St. Louis, Mosby, 1973, pp. 397–398.

Larato, D. C.: Disinfection of Pumice, *J. Prosthet. Dent.*, 18, 534, December, 1967.

Nicholson, R. J., Stark, M. M., and Scott, H. E.: Calculus and Stain Removal from Acrylic Resin Dentures, *J. Prosthet. Dent.*, 20, 326, October, 1968.

Sockwell, C. L.: Dental Handpieces and Rotary Cutting Instruments, *Dent. Clin. North Am.*, 15, 219, January, 1971.

Walsh, R. F. and Ames, M. I.: Reinforcing the Aseptic Chain in Hospital Dental Practice, *J. Hosp. Dent. Pract.*, 6, 57, April, 1972.

Polishing Amalgam

American Dental Association, Council on Dental Materials and Devices: *Guide to Dental Materials and Devices*, 7th ed. Chicago, American Dental Association, 1974–1975, pp. 19–35.

Charbeneau, G. T.: A Suggested Technic for Polishing Amalgam Restorations, *J. Mich. Dent. Assoc.*, 47, 320, November, 1965.

Craig, R. G., O'Brien, W. J., and Powers, J. M.: *Dental Materials. Properties and Manipulation.* St. Louis, Mosby, 1975, pp. 70–83.

Ford, M. A.: Polishing Restorations, *Dent. Health*, 11, 49, Autumn, 1972.

Grajower, R., Kaufman E., and Rajstein, J.: Temperature in the Pulp Chamber During Polishing of Amalgam Restorations, *J. Dent. Res.*, 53, 1189, September-October, 1974.

Howard, W. W.: *Atlas of Operative Dentistry*, St. Louis, Mosby, 1968, pp. 60–62.

Phillips, R. W.: *Skinner's Science of Dental Materials*, 7th ed. Philadelphia, Saunders, 1973, pp. 316–365.

Singelyn, T. E.: Polishing Amalgam Restorations, *J. Am. Dent. Hyg. Assoc.*, 41, 81, 2nd Quarter, 1967.

Simon, W. J.: *Clinical Dental Assisting.* Hagerstown, Maryland, Harper & Row, 1973, pp. 239–242, 262–263.

Strickland, W. D.: Amalgam Restorations for Class I Cavity Preparations, in Sturdevant, C. M., Barton, R. E., and Brauer, J. C., eds.: *The Art and Science of Operative Dentistry.* New York, Blakiston Division, McGraw-Hill, 1968, pp. 225–227, 258–259, 276–277.

Swedlow, D. B., Kopel, H. M., Grenoble, D. E., and Katz, J. L.: Dental Amalgam Polishing with Discs as Observed by Scanning Electron Microscopy, *J. Prosthet. Dent.*, 27, 536, May, 1972.

Tidmarsh, B. G. and Gavin, J. B.: Finishing Amalgam Restorations—A Scanning Electron Microscope Study, *New Zeal. Dent. J.*, 69, 175, July, 1973.

Tocchini, J. J., ed.: *Restorative Dentistry*. New York, Blakiston Division, McGraw-Hill, 1967, pp. 347–352.

Weitman, R. T. and Eames, W. B.: Plaque Accumulation on Composite Surfaces After Various Finishing Procedures, *J. Am. Dent. Assoc.*, 91, 101, July, 1975.

Chapter 38

The Porte Polisher with Wood Point

The porte polisher is a prophylactic hand instrument constructed to hold a wood polishing point at a contra-angle. A comparison of the porte polisher and the prophylaxis angle is made in table 38–1.

Hand polishing is accomplished by pressure of the wood point on the tooth surfaces as a moist abrasive is applied. The firm, carefully directed, rhythmic strokes impart a vigorous massage to the periodontal tissues. This is considered beneficial to the periodontal ligament since the periodontal fibers serve as a cushion for the slight movement of the tooth which occurs as the pressure of the instrument is applied. Fones described the beneficial effects to the gingival margin.[1] He suggested that the slight bumping of the wood point on the tissue causes a light pressure and release which has a massaging effect in producing a stimulation of the peripheral circulation.

I. Purposes and Uses

The entire polishing procedure may be accomplished with the porte polisher although this is unusual in routine practice because of the time factor. Patients can be very appreciative of smooth, quiet,

hand polishing. With certain patients, under particular circumstances and for selected procedures, porte polishing is specifically indicated. Functions, purposes, and uses are suggested here.

A. Removes stains, films, and dental plaque from the natural and restored surfaces of the teeth.

B. Provides a high, smooth polish which may help the tooth surfaces to resist deposit accumulation.

C. Effectively polishes cervical areas of teeth which are hypersensitive to the heat produced by even a slowly revolving rubber polishing cup. A superfine, unflavored abrasive mixed with water only is appreciated by these patients.

D. Adapts to tooth surfaces which are inaccessible to the prophylaxis angle, such as the following:
   1. Exposed proximal surfaces of the teeth of patients who have undergone periodontal surgery.
   2. Lingual surfaces of lingually inclined mandibular molars, or distal surfaces of maxillary third permanent molars.

Table 38-1.   Comparison of the Porte Polisher and the Prophylaxis Angle

Characteristic	Porte Polisher	Prophylaxis Angle
Massaging effect	Provided for gingival margin and periodontal ligament	No effect
Protection of gingiva	Easy by use of slow, even strokes	Difficult because of speed at which rubber cup is moving
Danger of abrading enamel and cementum	Minimized	Greater because of faster speed and decreased sense of touch
Stain removal	Removes all stains	Time saved in the removal of gross stains but steady application of rubber cup could produce more heat than the patient could tolerate
Polish	High	Superficial cleaning
Heat	None	Much heat produced
Accessibility to tooth surface	Readily adapted to all surfaces	Limited because of size and weight of handpiece
Operator's sense of touch	Greater control of instrument is possible because sense of touch is present	Sense of touch is decreased because of weight and size of handpiece
Comfort to patient	Increased because of quietness and lack of discomfort from heat	Decreased because of noise, vibration, and heat produced
Comfort to operator	Light instrument, less tiring to trained hands	Heavy instrument is tiring to hold
Polishing agent	Less damage because of fewer strokes	Only very fine grain powder should be used; must be applied very wet
Portability	Is portable, therefore useful at any time (for example, bedridden patient)	Useful only in dental office, or with portable motor, with electricity
Care of instrument	Simple to sterilize	More time required for cleaning, oiling, sterilizing

E. Method of choice for application of certain desensitizing agents for exposed cementum and dentin (page 565).

F. Useful for the bedridden patient when portable motor-driven equipment is not available (pages 581–584).

G. Helpful for orientation of small children, handicapped, or other patients apprehensive of motor-driven equipment.

II. Characteristics of a Porte Polisher

Several types of porte polishers are available for use. Practical features which influence selection are suggested below.

A. Can be taken apart conveniently for cleaning and sterilization.

B. Will not rust or discolor when given ordinary care.

C. Has convenient adjustment for attachment of wood points of various widths.

D. Is light weight for comfort of operator during use.

E. Has handle of diameter convenient to type of instrument grasp required.

F. Has handle with a finish which resists slipping in the hand during operation.

III. Selection and Preparation of Wood Points

Although several kinds of wood including cedar, maple, and hard pine have been used for polishing points, orangewood is preferred because it is hard enough to withstand pressure without fraying readily, yet porous enough to hold polishing agents. Ready-made wood points are available commercially in standard sizes and shapes.

A supply of wood points of routinely used sizes and shapes should be cut, sterilized, and stored in a sterile container in advance of patient appointments. Wood points also can be included on a preprepared tray (page 23).

A. **Length**
   1. Short
      a. To maintain rigidity of wood.
      b. To prevent unnecessary retraction of cheek and tongue.
   2. Long enough to gain access to tooth surfaces without interference of shank of the porte polisher.

B. **Width**
   1. Narrow
      a. For adaptation to the variety of tooth surfaces and contours.
      b. To prevent damage to the gingival margins as the point is adapted to the curved tooth surfaces.
   2. Wide enough for efficiency in polishing.
   3. Recommended average width: equal to the diameter of the circular wood point holder of the porte polisher.

C. **Shape**
   1. Wedge: for facial, lingual, and proximal surfaces, and inclined planes of cusps.
   2. Cone (pointed): for occlusal pits and grooves.

D. **Sterilization Procedure**
   Autoclave

IV. Techniques for Use of Porte Polisher

The principles of technique described in Chapter 31 are applied during hand polishing. A systematic order of procedure from one tooth surface to the next surface is prerequisite to thoroughness. Applications of the general principles are included here.

A. **Instrument Grasps** (page 463)
   1. Modified pen
      a. Recommended for all surfaces except maxillary anterior facial.

    b. Hold middle finger as near work-
       ing end of instrument as possible
       as a guide and support.
  2. Palm
    a. Recommended for maxillary an-
       terior labial surfaces.
    b. Adapt to posterior maxillary fa-
       cial surfaces when indicated by
       existing stains.

B. **Finger Rest**
   Securely maintained on firm tooth.

C. **Strokes**
  1. Circular: $1/16$ to $1/8$ inch diameter;
    apply at cervical third and when
    adjacent to gingival margin.
  2. Linear
    a. Horizontal: back and forth on
       buccal and lingual of posterior
       teeth and to proximal surfaces as
       applicable.
    b. Vertical: up and down over labial
       and lingual surfaces of anterior
       teeth.
  3. Selection of type and size
    a. Provide greatest protection for
       gingiva.
    b. Provide greatest efficiency in
       technique in accord with the
       anatomy of the tooth and the
       nature and location of the
       plaques and stains.

D. **Manner of Operation**
  1. Apply appropriate grasp and finger
    rest, then position wood point on
    the tooth surface.
  2. Hand, wrist, and arm rotate to
    propel the porte polisher.
    a. Fulcrum remains positioned as
       hand pivots around it.
    b. Fingers remain immobile, ex-
       cept for turning the instrument
       for adaptation.

E. **Pressure Applied**
  1. Apply a directed, firm, moderate
    pressure with the use of slow
    deliberate strokes.
  2. Apply increased pressure when

circular stroke is directed awa
from free gingiva; decrease pres
sure when directed toward fre
gingiva.
  3. Vary pressure with the tenacity o
    the deposit or stain to be removed
  4. Balance pressure applied to woo
    point with finger rest pressure.
  5. Effect of excess pressure
    a. Increases hazard of injury to th
       margin of the free gingiva.
    b. Decreases stability and contro
       during stroke.

TECHNICAL HINTS

   I. Edges of wood points should b
     trimmed and the wood grai
     smoothed to minimize splinter
     which may harm the gingival tis
     sues.
  II. Place wood point flush with port
     polisher attachment to prevent pos
     sible irritation to cheek, lip, o
     tongue.
 III. Change wood point frequently dur
     ing polishing procedure as it be
     comes saturated with moisture an
     splintered.
    A. To prevent wood slivers fron
       damaging free gingiva.
    B. To increase efficiency by havin
       well-shaped wedge for polish
       ing.
  IV. When more than one polishin
     agent is to be applied, use fresl
     wood points to prevent mixing th
     abrasives.
   V. Use cotton roll or patient's partia
     removable denture in place fo
     finger rest where teeth are missing
  VI. Avoid undue pressure on pontic
     and mobile teeth.
 VII. Thorough flossing and irrigation o
     sulci following polishing is impo
     tant as retained particles of polish
     ing agent can be a source of irrita
     tion to the gingiva and increas
     postoperative discomfort.

VIII. An iodine disclosing solution applied to green stain prior to polishing tends to facilitate its removal.

FACTORS TO TEACH THE PATIENT

I. The nature, occurrence, etiology, and detrimental effects of plaques and stains.
II. Reasons for polishing the teeth.
III. Benefits of hand polishing.
IV. Relationship of plaque and stain accumulation to the frequency and thoroughness of patient's personal oral care habits.

Reference

1. Fones, A. C.: *Mouth Hygiene*, 4th ed. Philadelphia, Lea & Febiger, 1934, p. 277.

Suggested Readings

Alper, M. N.: An Evaluation of Tooth Polishing Techniques, *J. Am. Dent. Hyg. Assoc., 43,* 137, 3rd Quarter, 1969.
Beube, F. E.: *Periodontology.* New York, Macmillan, 1953, pp. 87–91.
Fones, A. C.: *Mouth Hygiene,* 4th ed. Philadelphia, Lea & Febiger, 1934, pp. 277–289.
Glickman, I.: *Clinical Periodontology,* 4th ed. Philadelphia, Saunders, 1972, p. 568.
Goldman, H. M. and Cohen, D. W.: *Periodontal Therapy,* 5th ed. St. Louis, Mosby, 1973, pp. 387, 397–398.
Grant, D. A., Stern, I. B., and Everett, F. G.: *Orban's Periodontics,* 4th ed. St. Louis, Mosby, 1972, p. 379.
Hard, D.: Oral Prophylaxis, in Bunting, R. W.: *Oral Hygiene,* 3rd ed. Philadelphia, Lea & Febiger, 1957, pp. 255–258.
Miller, S. C.: *Textbook of Periodontia,* 3rd ed. Philadelphia, Blakiston, 1950, pp. 278–280.
Sorrin, S., ed.: *The Practice of Periodontia.* New York, Blakiston Division, McGraw-Hill, 1960, pp. 182–183.

Chapter 39

Care of Hypersensitive Teeth

Sensitivity in the cervical area of a tooth can produce considerable discomfort. Care must be taken during instrumentation and application of air to prevent a hypersensitive reaction. Since tooth sensitivity is frequently related to the accumulation of plaque in the exposed cervical area, instruction in exacting plaque removal techniques is indicated.

Patients are appreciative of clinical procedures directed at desensitizing the area involved. A number of chemical and mechanical means have been used successfully to reduce or eliminate pain. No known method is universally effective for desensitization.

Factors Contributing to Hypersensitivity

I. **Exposure of Cementum and Dentin**
1. Gingival recession[1,2]
   a. Pathologic (localized or generalized): inflammation which may stimulate proliferation of the junctional epithelium along the root surface.
   b. Traumatic: toothbrush with abrasive dentifrice.
2. Periodontal surgery: for pocket elimination.

B. **Anatomy of the Cementoenamel Junction**
   Zone of dentin occurs between the enamel and the cementum in approximately 10 percent of teeth[3,4] (page 181).

C. **Loss of Cementum Denudes the Dentin**
   Cementum is lost through abrasion, erosion, dental caries, scaling, and root planing.

D. **Sensitivity of Dentin**
   In most teeth the dentin is more sensitive on its outer surface.[5]

II. Types of Pain Stimuli[6]

A. **Mechanical**
   Toothbrush bristles, eating utensils, periodontal and dental hygiene instruments, friction from denture clasps or other appliances.

B. **Chemical**
   Acids formed from fermentable carbohydrates in debris and plaque, citrus fruit acids, or condiments.

C. **Thermal**
   Hot or cold foods or beverages; air entering the oral cavity.

III. Mode of Action of Desensitizing Agents[6]

The exact mechanism of pain transmission is not known. It is probable that basically sensitivity is due to irritation of the organic matter or "nerve elements" in the dentinal tubules.

Agents used for desensitization may be classified as those acting (1) by precipitation of the peripheral ends of the odontoblastic processes (Tomes' fibers), (2) by an attempt to deposit an insoluble salt in the exposed dentin, or (3) by stimulation of the formation of secondary dentin. The specific mode of action of most agents is not known.

IV. Useful Characteristics of a Desensitizing Agent

When selecting a method for desensitization practical aspects are important. When possible, the patient's daily personal care can be used to incorporate treatment on a self-care basis. When an agent is applied professionally, the following considerations are suggested. An agent needs

A. Rapidity of action.

B. Ease of application.

C. Biologic acceptance by the body tissues.

D. Long-lasting, or permanent effects.

E. No side effects such as discoloration of the teeth.

METHODS FOR DESENSITIZATION

Few patients respond to a single form of treatment. For all, keeping the teeth as free of plaque, particularly at the gingival third where sensitivity areas occur, and the use of a form of self-applied topical fluoride are basic procedures. When that program is established, specific agents can be selected for professional application to persistent areas of sensitivity.

I. Self-care by the Patient
A. Plaque Control

Root surfaces subjected to vigorous plaque control measures by brushing, flossing, and using other aids such as a Perio-aid, develop a smooth hard surface with increased luster and lack of hypersensitivity. The dentinal tubules are blocked off by increased mineralization.[7]

When plaque is retained at the cervical third, the root surfaces are soft to touch when explored, may develop root caries, and usually are hypersensitive. A concentrated program of instruction and supervision would be indicated. A sulcular technique (page 315) with a soft nylon brush, flossing, use of the Perio-aid, and other appropriate measures must be instituted.

B. Dentifrice

Dentifrices containing strontium chloride 10 percent[8,9*] and sodium monofluorophosphate 0.76 percent[10] [12†] have been shown to reduce sensitivity when used routinely. Research has compared the two dentifrices.[13,1]

The advantage which the dentifrice with sodium monofluorophosphate has over that with strontium chloride is the caries preventive action. In the prevention of cemental caries, the use of a fluoride dentifrice can be an important part of the total program.

C. Self-Applied Fluoride

In addition to fluoride dentifrice, the patient's treatment plan should include daily, or at least frequent applications of fluoride by mouth-rinsing, custom tray with gel,[15] chewable tablet, brushing with a gel,[16] or other mode for regular use. The various procedures are described on pages 431–441. With an increase in surface fluoride, hypersensitivity usually decreases.

*Sensodyne
†Colgate with MFP

D. Diet

A food diary kept for five to seven days from which a dietary analysis is made with the patient, can be valuable. Foods which aggravate the hypersensitivity can be identified, and substitutes can be selected with the patient. Excessive fermentable carbohydrates, citrus fruits, or condiments of pronounced flavors may initiate a reaction.

II. Professional Applications

Dentists have used albumin precipitants such as 40 percent formalin, 40 percent zinc chloride, or 40 percent silver nitrate to seal the dentinal tubules and hence reduce sensitivity. Cavity varnishes, thin mixes of crown and bridge cement, zinc oxide and eugenol packs, or Gottlieb's solution have been used to protect the tooth surface against thermal shock.

A. Preparation for Desensitization
1. Complete scaling and planing.
2. Anesthesia. When teeth are too sensitive for scaling and planing, a local anesthetic is indicated. Note areas where a desensitizing agent is to be applied before the anesthetic is given.

B. Fluoride Preparations
1. *Sodium Fluoride Aqueous Solution* (two or four percent). Apply as in the topical application for the prevention of dental caries (pages 434–437).
2. *Sodium Fluoride Densensitizing Paste.* 33 percent sodium fluoride, 33 percent kaolin, and 33 percent glycerin.[17]
   a. Clean and isolate the sensitive tooth using cotton rolls, cotton roll holder for mandibular, and saliva ejector.
   b. Wipe exposed area with cotton pellet moistened in two percent sodium fluoride solution.
   c. Dry area thoroughly using cotton pellets or cotton roll.
   d. Place small amount of desensitizing paste on area with tip of wood point in porte polisher. A narrow wood point may fit the cervical area more effectively than a wide one.
   e. Massage paste on area gently but firmly with wood point, using small circular strokes. If patient suffers acute pain response at beginning of application, wipe off paste, have patient rinse with warm water, and begin again immediately.
   f. Continue massage for three minutes: use timer.
   g. Wipe off excess paste with cotton pellet.
   h. Remove cotton rolls and saliva ejector, and request patient to rinse with warm water.
   i. Repeat at future appointment if desensitization has not been accomplished.
3. *Sodium Silicofluoride Solution* (0.7 to 0.9 percent).[18]
   a. Clean and isolate the sensitive tooth using cotton rolls, cotton roll holder for mandibular, and saliva ejector.
   b. Dry the area thoroughly using cotton pellets or cotton roll.
   c. Apply solution from dappen dish with cotton pellet or applicator.
   d. Keep area glistening (but not dripping) wet for five minutes.
   e. Remove excess solution with cotton pellets.
   f. Repeat weekly for maximum of three applications as needed: if desensitization is to occur, it will have occurred after three applications.

C. Iontophoresis[19–21]
Iontophoresis is the impregnation of tissue with ions from dissolved salts

with the aid of an electric current. Iontophoresis utilizes a direct current to promote ionic transport of fluoride, a negatively charged ion, onto a tooth surface. The actual mechanism of action may be deposition of fluoride ions deeper into the dentin to obtain more extensive protoplasmic precipitation, or formation of secondary dentin. It has also been suggested that there may be a short-lived paresthesia of the odontoblastic processes produced.[20] Manufacturer's instructions should be followed for use of the equipment.

1. Low-voltage batteries (1½ to 9 volts) supply positive current to patient's tooth.
2. Circuit completed by contact of brush applicator for negatively charged aqueous fluoride solution (one to two percent sodium fluoride used in dental office).
3. Check patient's medical history before use of a current. A patient wearing a pacemaker should not receive treatment by such means as pulp tester, ultrasonic, or other current-producing instrument.[22]

TECHNICAL HINTS

I. Do not use compressed air on sensitive teeth. Dry only with cotton pellets or cotton roll.
II. Sodium silicofluoride solution and sodium fluoride desensitizing paste contain enough fluoride to cause nausea if swallowed in excess. Prevent by using only small amounts, wiping excess off with cotton pellets before removing cotton rolls, requesting the patient to rinse thoroughly, and using the saliva ejector to prevent the need for swallowing before the mouth can be rinsed.
III. Prepare solution of sodium silicofluoride weekly and store in

polyethylene container. A chemical reaction results when a plain glass bottle is used.[18]
IV. Keep jar containing sodium fluoride desensitizing paste tightly closed. Its shelf-life can be indefinite because of its glycerin base.

FACTORS TO TEACH THE PATIENT

I.   Possible general causes of gingival recession.
II. Possible causes of hypersensitivity of teeth.
III. Importance of toothbrushing for plaque removal in the cervical area as a method of desensitization.
IV. Possibility that the hypersensitivity will subside in time whether a desensitizer is applied or not.
V.   Specific foods which should and should not be used in the diet if relief from sensitivity is to be obtained.

References

1. Grant, D. A., Stern, I. B., and Everett, F. G.: *Orban's Periodontics*, 4th ed. St. Louis, Mosby, 1972, pp. 253–255.
2. Glickman, I.: *Clinical Periodontology*, 4th ed. Philadelphia, Saunders, 1972, pp. 118–122.
3. Permar, D.: *Oral Embryology and Microscopic Anatomy*, 5th ed. Philadelphia, Lea & Febiger, 1972, pp. 74, 124, 129–130.
4. Sicher, H. and Bhaskar, S. N., eds.: *Orban's Oral Histology and Embryology*, 7th ed. St. Louis, Mosby, 1972, pp. 170–171.
5. Ibid., pp. 113–115, 128.
6. Grant, Stern, and Everett: op. cit., pp. 414–416.
7. Hiatt, W. H. and Johansen, E.: Root Preparation I. Obturation of Dentinal Tubules in Treatment of Root Hypersensitivity, *J. Periodont.*, 43, 373, June, 1972.
8. Blitzer, B.: A Consideration of the Possible Causes of Dental Hypersensitivity: Treatment by a Strontium-ion Dentifrice, *Periodontics*, 5, 318, November-December, 1967.
9. Shapiro, W. B., Kaslick, R. S., and Chasens, A. I.: The Effect of a Strontium Chloride Toothpaste on Root Hypersensitivity in a Controlled Clinical Study, *J. Periodont.*, 41, 702, December, 1970.
10. Bolden, T. E., Volpe, A. R., and King, W. J.: The Desensitizing Effect of a Sodium Monofluorophosphate Dentifrice, *Periodontics*, 6, 112, June, 1968.

11. Hazen, S. P., Volpe, A. R., and King, W. J.: Comparative Desensitizing Effect of Dentifrices Containing Sodium Monofluorophosphate, Stannous Fluoride, and Formalin, *Periodontics,* 6, 230, October, 1968.
12. Kanouse, M. C. and Ash, M. M.: The Effectiveness of a Sodium Monofluorophosphate Dentifrice on Dental Hypersensitivity, *J. Periodont.,* 40, 38, January, 1969.
13. Hernandez, F., Mohammed, C., Shannon, I., Volpe, A., and King, W.: Clinical Study Evaluating the Desensitizing Effect and Duration of Two Commercially Available Dentifrices, *J. Periodont.,* 43, 367, June, 1972.
14. Shapiro, W. B., Kaslick, R. S., Chasens, A. I., and Weinstein, D.: Controlled Clinical Comparison Between a Strontium Chloride and a Sodium Monofluorophosphate Toothpaste in Diminishing Root Hypersensitivity, *J. Periodont.,* 41, 523, September, 1970.
15. Sall, H. D.: Technic for Treating Cervical Sensitivity, *Dent. Surv.,* 50, 60, November, 1974.
16. Miller, J. T., Shannon, I. L., Kilgore, W. G., and Bookman, J. E.: Use of a Water-free Stannous Fluoride-containing Gel in the Control of Dental Hypersensitivity, *J. Periodont.,* 40, 490, August, 1969.
17. Hoyt, W. H. and Bibby, B. G.: Use of Sodium Fluoride for Desensitizing Dentin, *J. Am. Dent. Assoc.,* 30, 1372, September 1, 1943.
18. Stout, W. C.: Sodium Silicofluoride as a Desensitizing Agent, *J. Periodont.,* 26, 208, July, 1955.
19. Schaeffer, M. L., Bixler, D., and Yu, P.-L.: The Effectiveness of Iontophoresis in Reducing Cervical Hypersensitivity, *J. Periodont.,* 42, 695, November, 1971.
20. Murthy K. S., Talim, S. T., and Singh, I.: A Comparative Evaluation of Topical Application and Iontophoresis of Sodium Fluoride for Desensitization of Hypersensitive Dentin, *Oral Surg.,* 36, 448, September, 1973.
21. Eshleman, J. R. and Leonard, E. C.: Desensitization of Dentin by Iontophoresis; A Review and Case Reports: Clinical Impressions, *J. Oral Thera. and Pharm.,* 1, 526, March, 1965.
22. Woolley, L. H., Woodworth, J., and Dobbs, J. L: A Preliminary Evaluation of the Effects of Electrical Pulp Testers on Dogs with Artificial Pacemakers, *J. Am. Dent. Assoc.,* 89, 1099, November, 1974.

Suggested Readings

Anderson, D. J.: Human and Animal Studies on Sensory Mechanisms in Teeth, *Int. Dent. J.,* 22, 33, March, 1972.
Chasens, A. I. and Kaslick, R. S., eds.: *Mechanisms of Pain and Sensitivity in the Teeth and Supporting Tissues.* Fairleigh Dickinson University School of Dentistry and the American Academy of Oral Medicine, Workshop sponsored by the Block Drug Company, 1973, 53 pp.
Dayton, R. E., DeMarco, T. J., and Swedlow, D.: Treatment of Hypersensitive Root Surfaces with Dental Adhesive Materials, *J. Periodont.,* 45, 873, December, 1974.
Everett, F. G., Hall, W. B., and Phatak, N. M.: Treatment of Hypersensitive Dentin, *J. Oral Thera. and Pharm.,* 2, 300, January, 1966.
Hodosh, M.: A Superior Desensitizer—Potassium Nitrate, *J. Am. Dent. Assoc.,* 88, 831, April, 1974.
Minkov, B., Marmari, I., Gedalia, I., and Garfunkel, A.: The Effectiveness of Sodium Fluoride Treatment with and without Iontophoresis on the Reduction of Hypersensitive Dentin, *J. Periodont.,* 46, 246, April, 1975.
Seltzer, S.: Hypothetic Mechanisms for Dentine Sensitivity, *Oral Surg.,* 31, 388, March, 1971.

Chapter 40

Evaluation and Recall

The objective of treatment is oral health for the patient, and individually performed services are steps toward total health. To evaluate the health of the gingival tissues a period of time must be allowed for healing to take place and for the benefits of the professional treatment and the patient's self-care on a daily basis to become apparent. After health has been attained, it must be maintained. Dental hygiene care is an integral part of total care and cannot be thought of as isolated appointment procedures.

There are three basic phases for evaluation. The *first* is the immediate observation at the completion of each appointment; the *second* is short-term follow-up one week to ten days after completion of a treatment or series of treatments; and the *third* is long-term recall to evaluate maintenance.

IMMEDIATE EVALUATION

I. Objectives

A. Teeth

Observation and exploration will reveal the immediate effects of instrumentation on the teeth. An objec-

tive has been to produce a smooth glassy tooth surface, free from deposits and stains. The effect of specific instrumentation is to facilitate the patient's self-care by removing signs of disease and local factors, particularly calculus and overhanging fillings which encourage plaque retention.

B. Gingiva

The gingival changes are not apparent immediately after instrumentation. Tissue regeneration and healing takes approximately one week to ten days for initial healing, and even longer for maturation of connective tissue and keratinization of epithelium.

The objective at the treatment appointment is to *create an environment in which the gingival tissue can heal and be maintained in health by the patient.*

II. Inspection

When scaling is accomplished over a series of appointments, each previously scaled quadrant or area is examined and rescaled as needed at each appointment. For the final evaluation, visual and tactile

569

methods are applied carefully to each tooth surface. Instruments, methods and procedures were described on pages 183–201.

A. **Visual**
1. Use compressed air with mouth mirror and adequate lighting for supramarginal examination and just below the gingival margin (page 185).
2. Transillumination methods are applied.
3. A disclosing agent can reveal small areas of remaining deposits.

B. **Tactile**
Use submarginal explorer Number 17 to assure smoothness of tooth surfaces to the bottom of each sulcus/pocket (pages 199–201).

III. Appearance of the Teeth after Instrumentation

The experienced eye will recognize the bright luster of thoroughly clean teeth. Polished enamel has a high gloss which reflects light. All deposits have been removed and the surfaces are smooth to tactile examination.

To evaluate completion of instrumentation, the following observations are made:

A. **Supramarginal Nondecalcified Tooth Surfaces**
1. Surfaces are visually clean and lustrous.
2. No calculus or extrinsic stains are evident after drying the surfaces with compressed air.
3. Metallic restorations are free from tarnish.
4. Enamel surfaces are smooth to tactile examination; root surfaces in areas of gingival recession feel smooth and hard.
5. Gingival surfaces of pontics are free of deposits.

B. **Submarginal Nondecalcified Tooth Surfaces**
1. Surfaces feel free of calculus and diseased cementum.

2. Surfaces are smooth and hard to tactile examination with a submarginal explorer.

C. **Overhanging Fillings**
1. Excess amalgam has been removed.
2. Junctions between restorations and tooth surfaces are smooth and uninterrupted when an explorer tip is passed over.
3. Normal tooth contour has been restored.

D. **Removable Appliance**
1. Outer polished surfaces have no visible calculus, soft deposits, or stains, and are smooth and unscratched.
2. Impression surfaces are free of deposits and unmarred.
3. Attachments or metal parts are smooth and shiny.

POSTOPERATIVE PROCEDURES

Postoperative care immediately following instrumentation includes flossing to remove particles of polishing agents from all proximal surfaces and gingival sulci, as well as the gingival surfaces of pontics, careful irrigation, and postoperative instructions for the patient to carry out after leaving the office or clinic. Depending on the service performed, postoperative care may also include the placing of a periodontal dressing, application of a topical antiseptic, and gingival massage. Postoperative care may also include a postappointment telephone contact concerning patient comfort, adherence to instructions, or other purpose.

Long-range postoperative care may include suture and dressing removal and dressing replacement. These have been described on pages 528–534.

Postoperative care and instruction can have a direct bearing on the progress of healing and hence the follow-up evaluation which is planned for a week or ten days after treatment is completed. Healing may be influenced by rinsing, brushing, and other self-care by the patient.

I. Gingival Massage

A firm but gentle massage of the gingival tissue may be performed after completion of scaling and planing. It would not be wise to massage the tissue over partially completed scaling because of mechanical injury to the pocket lining by the rough calculus. Massage can be soothing to the patient and temporarily stimulating to the circulation of the gingiva. It is performed prior to application of an antiseptic solution.

A. Effects of Massage

Massage is the systematic mechanical application and removal of pressure. The application of pressure forces stagnant blood from the tissues and produces a temporary ischemia; the removal of pressure allows arterial blood to enter the capillaries and produce a temporary hyperemia.

B. Technique for Massage

A flavored toothpaste may be applied to the gingiva as a lubricating agent, or the massage may be performed with the fingers moistened with water.

1. Follow the routine order of technique used for other procedures or start from the midline to massage each quadrant.
2. Place the thumb and index finger over the teeth onto the attached gingiva.
3. Apply moderate, firm pressure, moving the fingers in the direction of the gingival papilla, toward the incisal or occlusal surfaces.
4. Release pressure at the tip of the papilla and return fingers to the attached gingiva above the adjacent tooth. Repeat rhythmically around the mouth.

II. Application of an Antiseptic

When an antiseptic is applied, the limitations should be realized. Although some temporary reduction in bacterial count may be expected, sterilization would be impossible.

The antiseptics usually employed for postoperative applications are iodine or mercury preparations in the proper dilutions for application to the oral mucous membrane. Merthiolate (1:1000), Metaphen (1:200), or Merbromin (2 percent) (Mercurochrome) are commonly used for this purpose.

A. Purposes

1. Reduces the possibility of infection.
2. Reduces postoperative discomfort.

B. Technique for Application

1. Hold small cotton pellet with cotton pliers and saturate it in the antiseptic to be used. Express excess solution.
2. Provide adequate retraction of lip, cheek, and tongue, and apply solution to the crest of each interdental papilla on both facial and lingual surfaces. Solution will flow into sulcus/pocket.
3. Do not allow the patient to rinse.

III. Postoperative Instruction

Instruction pertaining to periodontal dressings is outlined in table 35–1 on page 528. Many of the same principles can be applied for postoperative instruction when a dressing has not been applied.

Postoperative instruction is essential following scaling, particularly when the patient's gingiva have been hypersensitive or have hemorrhaged excessively, or when there has been extensive submarginal instrumentation. Directions for postoperative care include suggestions for rinsing, toothbrushing, and what discomfort may be expected.

Dietary and nutritional factors may be discussed. The temporary use of bland foods lacking in strong, spicy seasonings, as well as continuing use of nutritional foods to promote healing can be helpful.

It is best to prepare directions for

postoperative care in printed or mimeographed form. This can prevent incomplete or inaccurate interpretation of orally delivered directions.

A. **Rinsing**

A warm solution will be soothing to the tissue and improve the circulation for healing. A suggested solution would be one which provides the appropriate concentration for osmotic balance of the salts of the solution with the salts of the oral tissue fluids.

1. Solutions suggested for use:
   a. Hypertonic salt solution: level ½ teaspoonful table salt in four-ounce glass of warm water.
   b. Sodium bicarbonate solution: level ½ teaspoonful baking soda in ¾ glass (eight-ounce) warm water.
2. Directions for rinsing
   a. Every two hours; after eating; after toothbrushing; before retiring.
   b. Use the rinse mouthful by mouthful, forcing the solution between the teeth.

B. **Toothbrushing**

The use of a soft brush is advisable after scaling and root planing, but the patient must clearly understand the need for complete plaque removal.

FOLLOW-UP EVALUATION

In order that the response of the gingival tissues to treatment and the patient's personal daily care can be observed, an appointment is planned for approximately one week after instrumentation is completed. Such reevaluation after an interval in which the tissues can heal provides the opportunity to locate areas where additional treatment and instruction may be indicated.

It should not be assumed that, because the teeth were apparently free from deposits and were smooth and glassy at the immediate evaluation following instrumentation, gingival healing, pocket wall shrinkage, resolution of inflammation, and other favorable treatment effects will inevitably result. Follow-up examination may reveal a variety of complications which may point to a need for additional root planing, curettage, self-care instruction, or referral for periodontal therapy.

A six-step evaluation plan is described here.

I. Evaluate the Gingival Tissue

A. Inspect with the patient to observe
   1. Color, size, shape, consistency, surface texture. By one week to 10 days the tissues should assume normal characteristics. Use table 11–1 on page 172 for guidelines.
   2. Areas of damage to the gingiva resulting from incorrect brushing or flossing.

B. Compare findings and indices with previous examination and notes from treatment appointments when these characteristics were observed before.

II. Evaluate Pocket Depths

A. Use probe, and measure around each tooth, with particular attention to areas showing increased depth at the previous charting.

B. Record and compare with initial measurements recorded.

C. Shrinkage of pockets when tissue is spongy and soft can be expected as healing progresses.

III. Evaluate Gingival Bleeding

A. Run the probe along the inside of the pocket wall. The technique is illustrated in figure 19–1 on page 279. If bleeding was apparent during probing for pocket depth in Step II (above), evaluation can be made without additional probing for bleeding.

B. Ask the patient whether bleeding has occurred during toothbrushing.

C. Healthy tissue does not bleed. As healing progresses, bleeding should be eliminated.

IV. Evaluate Plaque

A. Apply disclosing agent and inspect with the patient for areas where plaque has not been removed by the patient's personal care.

B. Relate areas of plaque on the teeth to the areas of gingival redness, enlargement, and other signs of disease.

V. Evaluate Plaque Control Methods and Techniques

A. Request patient to demonstrate techniques with emphasis on areas where the disclosing agent revealed plaque, and where the gingiva has not responded.

B. Help the patient to evaluate and make corrections.

C. Introduce or substitute new methods when applicable.

D. Learning is a slow process and repeated review and encouragement is usually needed.

VI. Examine for Residual Calculus

A. Use a submarginal explorer to examine areas where gingival redness and enlargement have persisted, whether marginal plaque was observed or not.

B. Remaining particles of calculus or areas of root surface roughness, however small, may be sufficient to encourage plaque collection and prevent complete healing.

C. Because the detection and removal of calculus in a pocket requires intricate and exacting instrumentation, even the most skilled operator must expect to recheck and complete the scaling and planing as indicated. The most frequent areas for residual calculus are proximal surfaces of molars, premolars, and crowded anteriors.

VII. Continuation of Evaluation

In practice a patient should not be placed in the recall category until there is complete healing and the dentist and dental hygienist are satisfied that optimum tissue health has been obtained. Sometimes a series of short appointments can be arranged in conjunction with dental appointments for restorative procedures by the dentist. At each appointment the patient may meet with the dental hygienist for continuing supervision of self-care procedures and observation of tissue response.

Notes concerning the status of gingival health and the instruction for the patient should be made in the patient's permanent record at each appointment. The observations are important to long-range planning for patient care and can provide a basis for determining the frequency of recall.

RECALL: THE MAINTENANCE PHASE

Through common usage, the term "recall" is applied to the system of appointments for the long-term maintenance phase of patient care which has as its primary objective the *prevention of the recurrence of disease* through supervised control. This program requires the cooperative efforts of the patient, the dentist, and the dental hygienist.

Initially the success of the program depends on the understanding of the patient relative to the recall procedure. The patient must realize that oral diseases do recur, but control is possible by combined personal and professional care.

I. Recall Interval

There can be no fixed schedule by which all patients are recalled because the frequency depends on the needs of each patient. Appointments may vary from two to six months, and an occasional patient needs only an annual recall. The time interval needs to be reevaluated periodically and changed in accord with changing needs.

A. **The First Recall**

The gingival or periodontal treatment is generally completed or nearly completed by the time appointments for restorative phases of treatment are under way. The first recall appointment should be dated from the completion of the gingival and periodontal treatment. When there is extensive restorative, prosthetic, or other treatment to follow, tissue maintenance during long-term therapy is essential (pages 295–296).

B. **Frequent Recall Requirements**

Two- and three-month intervals are required by many patients. Examples of patients in this category are those with the following conditions:

1. *Rampant Dental Caries.* Recall for continuation of a caries control effort which includes topical fluoride applications, dietary supervision, and personal care factors for dental plaque control (pages 412–414).

2. *Periodontal Disease.* Following periodontal surgery or deep scaling and curettage, many patients need a long period of supervision before it is certain that the etiological factors are under control.

3. *Orthodontic Therapy.* Appliances make cleaning and plaque control difficult; frequent topical fluoride applications may be indicated; gingival tissue response to irritants can be marked.

4. *Mentally or Physically Handicapped.* There may be difficulty in managing the toothbrush; when the handicap involves the mouth area, there may be problems of opening the mouth.

5. *Diabetes* or other disease which predisposes to a lowered resistance to infection; tissues must not be allowed to develop advanced disease.

6. *Cardiovascular Diseases or Other Conditions.* Brushing is a difficult procedure to carry out and only short appointments at the dental office can be tolerated because of the fatigue factor.

II. Recall Procedures

Preparation of data for the recall follows the same plan as for a new patient. The dental hygienist can prepare a diagnostic work-up with as many of the steps included as designated by the dentist. At least annually, every patient needs a medical history review, an intraoral and extraoral examination for soft tissue lesions particularly for cancer, and a blood pressure determination. At every appointment for recall, whether three, six, or other number of months, a patient of any age who has had periodontal therapy needs special evaluations for the particular problems of previous treatments. The patient with complete oral rehabilitation needs a detailed examination every few months (page 379).

Basic to all recall examination are the periodontal examination (page 288) and the dental examination (page 289) with charting.

Steps in preparation of a recall diagnostic work-up include the following:

A. **Review Patient History**

Supplementary questions are asked to determine the present state of health, recent illnesses, present medications, and other pertinent data (page 70).

B. **Blood Pressure Determination** (pages 85–88).

C. **Extraoral and Intraoral Inspection** for oral pathology particularly cancer (pages 92–93 and table 8–1, page 96).

D. **Radiographs,** frequency in accord with dentist's policy.

E. **Periodontal Examination**
Details are outlined on pages 170 and 186–205. Minimum examination includes clinical tissue examination of color, size, shape, consistency, surface texture, pocket charting, determination of tooth mobility, examination of mucogingival line, furcations, occlusion, and tooth deposits. Bleeding on probing should be correlated with a bleeding index.

F. **Examination of the Teeth** (page 207)
A new charting with restorations and caries, examination for pulp vitality when indicated, and a record of tooth sensitivity if reported by the patient or detected during examination.

G. **Evaluation of Oral Cleanliness and Adequacy of Self-care Measures**
Relate plaque on teeth as observed after applying a disclosing agent, with areas of gingival redness, enlargement, and other signs of disease.

H. **Inspection and Specific Examinations by the Dentist**
Areas of special problems including endodontically treated teeth, post-surgery, occlusal factors, prosthetic appliances.

III. Recall Treatment Plan

The dentist reviews the data collected and a treatment plan is outlined, based on the new diagnosis and evaluation of the patient's oral condition. For the dental hygienist's treatment plan, scaling, planing, topical fluoride or other preventive application, and patient instruction provide the basis for the continuing preventive program.

TECHNICAL HINTS

Methods for maintenance of a recall plan vary. Two systems in current use are:

I. Make each patient's appointment before the patient leaves the office. An appointment card is given the patient who is asked to enter it on his calendar ahead of time, and an envelope is prepared for mailing a duplicate card a week before the appointment is to be held.

II. Individual file cards ($3'' \times 5''$ or $4'' \times 6''$) are maintained for each patient to show name, address, telephone number, and instructions concerning the recall frequency as well as the available appointment time. Cards are filed by the month in which the patient is due for recall. Each month the cards are pulled, and appointments are mailed or telephoned well in advance.

FACTORS TO TEACH THE PATIENT

I. Appearance and feeling of a clean mouth.

II. Relationship of personal oral care habits to maintenance of cleanliness provided through professional scaling and planing.

III. Purposes of postoperative care by the dental hygienist and the patient.

IV. How to prepare solutions for postoperative rinsing.

V. Directions for postoperative care.

VI. Purposes of follow-up and recall appointments.

Suggested Readings
Boggs, D. G. and Schork, M. A.: Determination of Optimal Time Lapse for Recall of Patients in an Incremental Dental Care Program, *J. Am. Dent. Assoc.*, 90, 644, March, 1975.

Ehrlich, A. B. and Ehrlich, S. F.: *Dental Practice Management.* Philadelphia, Saunders, 1969, pp. 126–130.

Goldman, H. M. and Cohen, D. W.: *Periodontal Therapy,* 5th ed. St. Louis, Mosby, 1973, pp. 1014–1033.

Grant, D. A., Stern, I. B., and Everett, F. G.: *Orban's Periodontics,* 4th ed. St. Louis, Mosby, 1972, pp. 683–694.

Ogilvie, A. L.: Recall and Maintenance of the Periodontal Patient, *Periodontics*, 5, 198, July-August, 1967.

Parr, R. W.: *Periodontal Maintenance Therapy.* Berkeley, California, Praxis Publishing Co., 1974, 86 pp.

Powell, R. N. and Alexander, A. G.: The Treatment of Periodontal Disease. II. The Maintenance Phase of Periodontal Treatment, *Br. Dent. J.*, 120, 306, April 5, 1966.

Ward, M. A.: An Effective Recall System, *J. Am. Dent. Hyg. Assoc.*, 40, 24, 1st Quarter, 1966.

VI

Applied Techniques for Patients with Special Needs

INTRODUCTION

To understand each patient's general and/or oral health problems requires particular study. Actually each patient is a "special" patient and must be considered according to his individual needs. However, certain patients have problems peculiar to their age group and/or unusual health factors which may complicate the routine of care generally provided. These special patients require more skillful application of dental hygiene knowledge and ability to accomplish a comparably favorable result than for what might be called the "normal" patient.

Optimum oral health is frequently an important contributing factor in maintaining or restoring the patient's physical, emotional, vocational, economic, and social usefulness to the extent of his capabilities. *The dental hygienist's obligation is to see that no patient needs special rehabilitative dental services because of any condition which could have been prevented by dental hygiene care.*

To consider the patient as a whole requires attention to general physical and emotional problems as well as oral problems. Basic psychological needs for

affection, belonging, independence, achievement, recognition, and self-esteem frequently influence the outcome of treatment as well as the patient's whole attitude toward dental and dental hygiene care. With certain physical conditions, oral health has assumed less importance in the mind of the patient because other health problems have demanded so much attention. For some of these patients neglect has intensified the need for oral care.

The patients with special needs who will be considered in the chapters following include patients with oral and general systemic conditions. Variations with respect to age are considered.

SPECIAL ORAL PROBLEMS

In each specialty of dentistry, patients present problems which can be helped by the services performed by the dental hygienist. For example, patients with removable dentures require particular attention. The care of the denture has been described on page 548 and the instruction for the patient is on page 361. Patients with dentofacial handicaps who have missing teeth or congenital malfor-

577

mations, patients requiring surgery, and patients afflicted with habits conducive to the initiation of dental caries need special adaptations of the preventive care and instruction which the dental hygienist can afford.

SYSTEMIC DISEASES

Oral manifestations may be evident in association with certain acute and chronic systemic diseases, particularly nutritional deficiencies, endocrine disturbances, blood diseases and a number of chronic degenerative diseases. The presence of dental diseases may complicate and delay the rehabilitation of the patient with systemic illness. When an oral manifestation suggests the possibility of an undiagnosed systemic disease, dental personnel have a responsibility in the referral of the patient for medical examination.

As defined by the Commission on Chronic Illness,[1] chronic disease comprises all impairments or deviations from normal which have one or more of the following characteristics: are permanent, are caused by nonreversible pathological alterations, require special training of the patient for rehabilitation, or may be expected to require a long period of supervision, observation, or care. According to the National Health Survey, an estimated 49 percent of the civilian, noninstitutionalized population of the United States had one or more chronic diseases or impairments in 1965–1966. About 11 percent of the total population had some degree of limitation of activity, and 2½ percent were unable to carry on the major activity (school, work, etc.) of their age-sex group.[2]

The percentage of people with chronic conditions increases from approximately 20 percent of persons under 17 years to nearly 85 percent of those 65 years and over. More females have chronic conditions, but a higher percent of males have limited activity in the group unable to carry on major activity.[2] Heart conditions and arthritis and rheumatism are the leading causes of limitation of activity and mobility.

Patients with chronic diseases may or may not be able to go to a dental office for appointments. Certain conditions, particularly during the advanced stages of a disease, require the patient to remain confined and, in some instances, bedridden. Dental hygienists need to understand the special procedures for care in these instances.

The basic approach to oral problems of the chronic disease patient is prevention, and individual initiative is vital in prevention. The public, including dental personnel, must incorporate into their daily living fundamental health practices which contribute to optimum health and hence to the prevention of chronic disease. Dental hygiene care improves the general health and influences the resistance to infection of the oral cavity. Through patient instruction, an important role in the prevention of chronic disease can be performed.

INTEGRATION OF APPLICATIONS TO SPECIAL NEEDS

It should be realized that a patient may have more than one special need. For example, the patient who requires dental hygiene care prior to oral surgery may have a blood disease. The pregnant patient may be diabetic. Here the use of the patient's medical history plays an important role when the total needs of the patient are outlined.

In Part VI there is an attempt to integrate learning in other areas of concentrated study in the dental, dental hygiene, medical, and social sciences. The dental hygienist is encouraged to supplement knowledge and appreciation of the special needs of patients through the use of additional readings such as those suggested at the end of each chapter. By application of understanding of the patient's needs, clinical techniques and patient instruction may be directed more skillfully to provide *complete dental hygiene care.*

References

1. Commission on Chronic Illness: *Chronic Illness in the United States.* I. *Prevention of Chronic Illness.* Cambridge, Harvard University Press, 1957, p. 320.
2. United States Department of Health, Education, and Welfare: Vital and Health Statistics, Data from the National Health Survey, *Limitation of Activity and Mobility Due to Chronic Conditions, United States, July 1965-June 1966.* Washington, D.C., Public Health Service, Publication No. 1000, Series 10, No. 45, May, 1968.

Suggested Readings

American Dental Association, Council on Dental Therapeutics: *Accepted Dental Therapeutics,* 36th ed. Chicago, American Dental Association, 1975, pp. 3–17.

Colbert, M. H.: The Role of the Dental Hygienist in a Chronic Disease Hospital, *J. Am. Dent. Hyg. Assoc., 41,* 139, 3rd Quarter, 1967.

Morris, A. L. and Little, J. W.: Oral Medicine in General Practice, in Morris, A. L. and Bohannan, H. M., eds.: *The Dental Specialties in General Practice.* Philadelphia, Saunders, 1969, pp. 42–80.

Chapter 41

The Patient Who is Homebound, Bedridden, or Helpless

HOMEBOUND PATIENTS

Within recent years, efforts have been made through research and organized programming, to attend to the oral health needs of the chronically ill and handicapped. These patients represent all age groups. Many are confined to hospitals, institutions, nursing homes, or private homes, which means that special adaptations for dental and dental hygiene care are required. Portable equipment is being developed and special training for dental personnel promoted.

Dental care for the chronically ill must be completed in a variety of surroundings. For the hospitalized, dental clinics frequently are available to provide care for inpatients. Those who are not hospitalized may be confined to their homes or may be able to be transported to the dental office in a wheel chair depending on the severity of the case and the extent of disability.

Dentists and dental hygienists in private practice have occasion to attend patients confined to their homes. Dental hygiene techniques lend themselves to care for the bedridden since the entire instrumentation can be completed with manual instruments. Topical fluoride applications can be made by skillful adaptations for keeping the teeth dry. Instruction in personal oral care procedures has particular significance for the comfort as well as the health of the patient. Suggestions relative to planning and conducting a home visit are included in this chapter.

I. Objectives

A. Aid in preventing periodontal diseases which would require extensive treatment.

B. Assist in preventing further complication of the patient's state of health by lessening dental care problems.

C. Contribute to the patient's comfort, mental ease, and general well-being.

D. Encourage adequate personal care procedures, whether performed by the patient or an attendant.

E. Contribute to general rehabilitation or habilitation of the patient.

581

II. Preparation for the Home Visit

A. **Understanding the Patient**
1. Consider the characteristics associated with the particular chronic illness or disease.
2. Consider special problems related to age. (For example, for the gerodontic patient see page 587.)
3. Review patient's medical history (by telephone if preliminary inspection visit is not practical) to determine unusual precautions which must be taken. Arrange with physician and dentist when premedication is indicated (page 71).

B. **Instruments and Equipment**
1. Sterile instruments and other items are transported in the packages in which they were autoclaved.
2. Gauze sponges, cotton rolls and pellets, wood points, and dappen dishes are prepared in packages which will be convenient to open and use at the bedside.
3. Substances such as the disclosing agent, postoperative antiseptic, polishing agent, and topical fluoride preparation are carried in small, tightly closed bottles.
4. Coverall: a large plastic drape is of particular importance since in certain types of illness the patient's coordination during rinsing may be limited. Thoughtfulness in the care of bed linen is appreciated by the patient's attendant.
5. Emesis basin: for patient rinsing. Although a small basin undoubtedly would be available at the home, the kidney-shaped basin facilitates the rinsing process.
6. Lighting: adaptation of available possibilities.
   a. Headlight or reflector: dentist may have as part of his office equipment; with practice the dental hygienist can learn to use with ease.
   b. Photography spot light: might be available either from the dentist or from the patient's home; need a type with a narrow, concentrated beam.
   c. Gooseneck lamp: might be available in patient's home; need bulb of adequate wattage.
7. Miscellaneous facilities usually available at the home: arrangements must be planned (by telephone) in advance of appointment.
   a. Large towels: for covering pillows.
   b. Types of pillows available which may be firm enough to assist in maintaining patient's head in reasonably stationary position.
   c. Hospital bed: can be adjusted most effectively for patient's position.
   d. Mouthwash: inquire as to whether the patient has a favorite kind and whether this would be available for use.

C. **Appointment Time**
Arrange during the patient's usual waking hours at as convenient a time as possible in relation to nursing care and mealtime schedule.

III. Approach to Patient

Since a majority of patients who come to the dental office are active people with good general health, it is sometimes difficult to adjust to the relatively helpless, chronically ill person. There may be a tendency to be oversolicitous which does not contribute to the development of a cooperative patient.

Usually a direct approach with gentle firmness is most successful. Establishment of rapport with the patient depends in part on whether the patient has requested and anticipated the appointment, or whether those caring for the patient have insisted on and arranged for the visit.

A. **Psychological Characteristics of Patient**

Frequently the well-adjusted chronically ill person may be more appreciative of the care provided than the patient who comes to the dental office, and may be well aware of the difficulties under which the dental hygienist is working. The cooperation obtained frequently depends on the patient's attitude toward his illness or disability.

A prolonged illness which may have been accompanied by suffering is not conducive to a healthy outlook on life. Monotonous confinement contributes to the development of characteristics such as those listed below.

1. Difficulty in maintaining a cheerful attitude.
2. Bored or dissatisfied with sameness of daily routine.
3. Easily depressed.
4. Discouragement about recovery leads to mental state which retards recovery.
5. Sensitive and easily offended.
6. Demanding; enjoys being waited on if used to having prompt attention to each request.
7. Indifferent to personal appearance and general rules of personal hygiene.
8. Preoccupied with details of medical examinations, tests, treatment, medicaments, and symptoms.

B. **Suggestions for General Procedure**

1. Request that visitors be asked to remain out of the room during the appointment to prevent distraction of patient.
2. Introduce each step slowly to be sure patient knows what is being done.
3. Do not make the patient feel rushed. Listen attentively; socializing is one of the best ways to establish rapport.

4. Regardless of inconvenience of arrangements, two or more appointments should be planned when extensive scaling is required.
   a. Patient may fatigue.
   b. Need for observing tissue response.
   c. Need to give encouragement in plaque control procedures.

IV. Dental Hygiene Care

A. **The Working Situation**

Since many patients can be up in a chair or wheel chair at least an hour or two each day, only rarely is it necessary to perform procedures with the patient in bed. For the patient in the chair, a kitchen or large bathroom may be most satisfactory for working. In either situation, ingenuity is needed to arrange patient position, head stabilization, and proper lighting to maintain patient comfort and yet provide access for the operator.

1. *Patient in Bed*
   a. Hospital bed: adjust to lift patient's head to desirable height.
   b. Ordinary bed: use firm pillows to support patient.
2. *Patient in Wheel Chair*
   a. Tall back: may provide excellent headrest; back lowered to proper height.
   b. Short back: although it is possible to back the chair against a wall and insert a pillow for the head, it may be better to have patient moved to a davenport or chair where a more stable headrest would be provided.
   c. Portable headrest may be attached to back of plain chair or wheel chair.
3. *Suggestions for Lighting*
   a. Turn off overhead lighting to reduce shadows in the mouth.
   b. Headlight: usually the most convenient and efficient form of

lighting because of concentrated beam.

c. Head reflector: reflect light from bed lamp attached to bed behind patient's head.

d. Gooseneck or photographer's light: care must be taken not to direct light into patient's eyes.

4. *Instrument Arrangement.* On towel on table beside bed or chair.

B. **Instrumentation**

Scaling and porte polishing are complicated by instability of head. A mouth prop may be needed when patient has difficulty in opening.

C. **Fluoride Application**

Selection of method for fluoride application will vary with the patient and the home situation. The use of self-care techniques will depend on the patient's handicap and the cooperation of the parent or other attendant. The most benefit would be obtained from a daily mouthrinse, chewable tablet, or gel application in a mouthguard tray (pages 429, 439–440).

V. Patient Instruction

A. **Personal Oral Care**

Provide specific instruction for attendant of helpless or uncoordinated patient. Demonstrate in patient's mouth. An automatic toothbrush may prove valuable for certain cases (pages 319–322).

B. **Dietary Suggestions**

1. Need for consultation with physician concerning prescribed diet. When important relationships of diet to oral health are suspected they should be reported to the dentist. The patient's problem can then be discussed with the physician.

2. Diet for dental caries prevention can be very important since the patient cannot go to dental office.

Cariogenic foods should be avoided as snacks.

3. Factors influencing suggestions for diet

a. Patient's appetite may be poor, particularly if there is discouragement about the state of health.

b. Patient may be finicky in food selection which may have affected the general nutritional state or have resulted in excessive use of carbohydrate foods.

c. Monotony of meals may have lessened the desire to eat.

THE HOSPITALIZED HELPLESS OR UNCONSCIOUS PATIENT

Personal oral care procedures for the hospitalized patient are accomplished by the attendant member of the nursing staff when self-care by the patient is impossible. Understanding the possible procedures is important to all dental hygienists whether or not they are employed in a hospital if they are to appreciate ramifications of dental hygiene care for the many types of patients with special needs.

Skill is required to carry out routine methods of toothbrushing, rinsing, and cleaning of removable dentures for the conscious patient who is able to cooperate. Methods must be adapted when the patient's head cannot be elevated. When the patient's illness or injury involves the oral cavity, the advice and recommendations of the attending oral surgeon are followed.

Maintenance of oral cleanliness for the acutely ill or unconscious patient requires special procedures because of the complete helplessness of the patient. Objectives and methods described below have application for patients with other special needs as, for example, the patient with a fractured jaw (pages 609–613) or severe mental retardation (pages 641–650).

I. Objectives of Care

A. Prevent debris in the mouth from being aspirated and clogging air passages.

B. Minimize the possibility of oral infection.

C. Clean the mouth and provide comfort for the patient.

II. Removable Denture Care

A. Remove dentures from the patient's mouth. It is usual hospital policy to remove dentures while a patient is unconscious.

B. Procedure for removal is described on page 549.

C. Clean the dentures (pages 549–550) and store in water in a covered container by the patient's bedside.

III. General Mouth Cleansing

A. **Edentulous and Dentulous**
1. Cleanse the mouth at least three times each day to prevent dryness and sordes.
2. Apply a lubricant such as equal parts pure glycerin and lemon juice to the oral mucosa and the lips. Prepared disposable swabs are available for this purpose.

B. **Brushing and Flossing**
1. Patient who can rinse. When helpless for manipulation of brush or floss but can rinse and expectorate, a patient can be propped upright and an emesis basin used.
2. Patient who cannot participate: suction is a necessity. When suction is used, an assistant is needed except for the suction toothbrush described below (IV).
3. Brush. Generally an automatic brush is more efficiently and thoroughly used than a manual brush when an attendant must brush a helpless patient's teeth. A mouth prop can be placed in one side while the other side is retracted.

IV. Toothbrush with Suction Attachment

The toothbrush with attached suction provides an efficient and safe method for patient care.

A. **Description of the Brush[1,2]**
1. Soft-textured nylon brush with hole drilled between the bristles in the middle of the head of the brush.
2. Small plastic tubing inserted into hole; end adjusted slightly below level of brushing plane.
3. Other end of tubing passed across back of brush handle and attached to handle by small rubber bands (figure 41–1).
4. Tubing is connected by an adapter to aspirator or suction outlet.

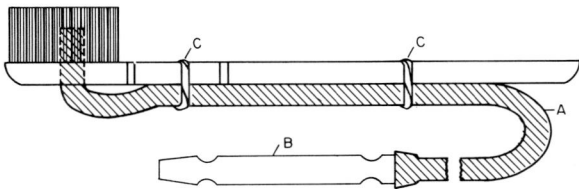

Figure 41–1. Soft toothbrush with suction attachment for care of helpless patient. **A.** Plastic tubing. **B.** Adapter for attachment of tubing to aspirator or suction outlet. **C.** Rubber bands to attach tubing to toothbrush handle.

Plastic tube is inserted through a hole in the head of the brush and extended to a level slightly below the brushing plane.

B. **Procedure for Use of Brush**

The detailed procedure would be outlined for hospital personnel and included in the nursing procedures manual. An abbreviated outline of the basic steps is include here.

1. Preparation of the patient.
   a. The patient may be aware of what is going on although not respond in a usual manner.
   b. Tell patient that the teeth are going to be brushed.
   c. Turn patient on a side and place a pillow at the back for support.
   d. Place a face towel under patient's chin and over bedding.
2. Attach toothbrush to suction outlet and lay brush on towel near patient's mouth.
3. Place a rubber bite block on one side of the patient's mouth between the teeth. String tied to bite block is fastened to patient's gown with a safety pin.
4. Dip brush in fluoride mouthwash; turn on suction.
5. Gently retract lip and carefully apply the appropriate toothbrushing procedures; apply suction over each tooth surface with particular care at each interproximal area. Moisten brush frequently.
6. Move bite block to opposite side of mouth and continue brushing procedure.
7. Place brush in cup of clear water to allow water to be sucked through and clear the tubing both during the procedure if there is clogging and after brushing to clean the tube.
8. Remove bite block; wipe patient's lips with paper wipe and apply petrolatum.
9. Wash brush and bite block; prepare materials for next use.
10. One toothbrush usually is sufficient for the patient's stay in the hospital.

References

1. Capps, J. S.: New Device for Oral Hygiene, *Am. J. Nursing*, 58, 1532, November, 1958.
2. Tronquet, A. A.: Oral Hygiene for Hospital Patients, *J. Am. Dent. Assoc.*, 63, 215, August, 1961.

Suggested Readings

American Dental Association, Council on Dental Health: Dental Care: Views from the Nursing Homes, *J. Am. Dent. Assoc.*, 77, 117, July, 1968.

Bell, C. E., Lasater, T. M., Sawyer, J. F., and Ramirez, A.: Communicating Dental Hygiene Practices to Chronically, Emotionally Ill, Hospitalized Patients, *Am. J. Public Health*, 63, 778, September, 1973.

Carsen, R. A.: Stable Head Support for the Wheelchair Patient, *J. Hosp. Dent. Pract.*, 4, 112, October, 1970.

Cross, W. G.: Oral Hygiene for Patients in Hospital, *Dental Health*, 5, 30, April-June, 1966.

Dunkley, R. P. and Wilson, M.: Oral Hygiene and Mental Hospitals: A Preventive Treatment Program, *J. Am. Dent. Hyg. Assoc.*, 42, 75, 2nd Quarter, 1968.

Kerson, J.: Treatment Planning for Patients in Nursing Homes, *J. Am. Dent. Assoc.*, 89, 640, September, 1974.

Lotzkar, S.: Dental Care for the Homebound, in Davidoff, A., Winkler, S., and Lee, M. H. M.: *Dentistry for the Special Patient.* Philadelphia, Saunders, 1972, pp. 131–155.

Niebel, H. H. and Keough, G.: Oral Hygiene Program for Totally Dependent Patients, *Military Medicine*, 137, 71, February, 1972.

Pickles, T. H.: A Review of the Status of Portable Dental Equipment, *J. Public Health Dent.*, 29, 19, Winter, 1969.

Roddy, P.: Dentistry for an Iron Lung Patient, *Dent. Surv.*, 45, 26, October, 1969.

Terry, J. M. and Shannon, I. L.: Clinical Evaluation of an Ingestible Dentifrice, *J. Oral Thera. and Pharm.*, 4, 426, May, 1968.

Waldman, H. B.: Home Dental Care and the Dental Hygienist, *J. Am. Dent. Hyg. Assoc.*, 40, 27, 1st Quarter, 1966.

Waldman, H. B. and Stein, M.: Dental Care for the Shut-in Patient: A Workable Solution, *Am. J. Public Health*, 56, 1921, November, 1966.

Chapter 42

The Gerodontic Patient

Preventive measures for the aged through care and instruction assume greater importance as the number of people involved in this group increases steadily. Currently the population over age 65 represents nearly 10 percent of the total population of the United States, or approximately 20,000,000 people.

Only between four and five percent of persons 65 or over are in institutions such as mental hospitals, chronic disease hospitals, nursing homes, and homes for the aged. In mental hospitals nearly one-third of the patients are from the older age group. Of the 95 percent that live in the community, almost 70 percent are in urban areas.[1]

Dentists and dental hygienists are challenged by the need to help the aging population to learn about personal care and seek professional care which will provide continuing oral comfort and function. Tooth loss increases with age. While approximately 20 percent of the people in the 45 to 54 age group were edentulous, 50 percent had no teeth by age 65 and over, according to the National Health Survey.[2] With application of current knowledge of preventive methods in younger age groups, hopefully future generations of older people will not be subjected to the severe effects of neglect of oral disease.

The biologic age is not synonymous with the chronologic age and hence signs of aging appear at different chronologic ages in different individuals. In other words, some people are old at 45 years while others are not old at 75 years.

In reality aging begins at birth. Senescence, the process or condition of growing old, has sociocultural implications as well as physiologic and chronologic. Normal aging should not be confused with the effects of pathologic influences which accelerate the aging process.

Each age period brings changes in body metabolism, activity of the cells, endocrine balance, and mental processes. Knowledge and understanding of normal physical and emotional characteristics for each age level provide a guide for planning patient care and instruction.

I. General Physical Characteristics

People between 65 and 75 years of age are usually considered to be "young old" and those over 75, the "old old." The physical changes of aging listed below are more typical of the "old old." Changes with aging vary between individuals and between organs and tissues of the same individual.

A. **General Tissue Changes**
1. Dehydration.
2. Atrophy.
3. Diminished elasticity.
4. Decreased function including diminished reparative capacity.
5. Fibrosis.

B. **Skeletal System**
Skeletal integrity is significantly influenced by an insufficient fluoride intake (page 426). Senile osteoporosis is common in individuals over age 60, and the incidence increases with age. It is also most predominant in postmenopausal women.

C. **Basal Metabolism**
Lowered.

D. **Skin**
Thin, wrinkled, dry, loss of tone, pigmented spots, atrophy of sweat glands.

E. **Special Senses**
1. Sight: reduced visual acuity, increased farsightedness, sensitivity to light, and night blindness.
2. Hearing: loss of sensitivity to high tones, gradual loss of hearing acuity.

F. **Muscular System**
Loss of muscle tone, development of unsteadiness and tremor, lack of muscular strength, decreased speed of response.

G. **Cardiovascular System**
1. Increase in blood pressure.
2. Decreased circulation to tissues.

H. **Blood**
Lowered red blood cell count and hemoglobin.

I. **Respiratory System**
Shortness of breath.

J. **Digestive System**
1. Gradual decrease in production of hydrochloric acid and other secretions necessary for digestion.
2. Peristalsis slowed.

K. **Glandular Secretions**
Diminished.

L. **Stress Reactions**
1. Cannot tolerate extremes of heat and cold.
2. Cannot tolerate muscular strain.
3. Decreased pain threshold.

M. **Healing**
1. Slowed.
2. Resistance to infection decreased.

II. Oral Findings

The same general tissue changes apply alike to oral tissues. Many older people may have lost some or all of their teeth as a result of dental caries or periodontal diseases. Some of the changes listed here may be due to aging, but many are related to the cumulative effects of disease.

A. **Lips**
Dry, purse-string (related to dehydration within tissue).

B. **Mucous Membranes**
1. Loss of elasticity.
2. Diminished keratinization.
3. Dryness.

C. **Tongue**
1. Atrophy of papillae resulting in a smooth appearance; related to nutritional deficiencies and impaired circulation.
2. Taste bud degeneration: reduced or abnormal taste sensations.
3. Loss of muscle tone: tongue may become flabby and less effective for cleansing the teeth.

D. **Salivary and Mucous Glands**
1. Atrophy resulting in diminished secretion.
2. Decrease in amount of saliva (xerostomia).

E. Teeth
1. Color: may be darker (yellow or brown).
2. Attrition: influenced by use, habits, dietary choices, and occupational factors.
3. Tooth loss: Although unnecessary when preventive measures have been continued throughout life, teeth are missing frequently in older people. The teeth most frequently remaining are the canines and the mandibular anteriors.
4. Dental caries: Root (cemental) caries may develop as roots are exposed, salivary flow diminishes, and diet changes to include softer foods which contain more sucrose.
5. Pulp
   a. Narrowing of pulp chamber; formation of secondary dentin.
   b. Fibrotic changes.
   c. Formation of pulp calcifications (pulp stones or denticles).

F. Periodontium
Changes frequently reflect cumulative effects of long standing chronic disease.
1. *Gingiva*
   a. Loss of stippling: shiny appearance.
   b. Diminished keratinization; lowered resistance to irritation and infection.
2. *Junctional Epithelium*
   Migrates apically with continued eruption of tooth related to attrition.
3. *Periodontal Ligament*
   a. Decreased vascularity.
   b. Arteriosclerosis frequently seen.
4. *Alveolar Bone*
   a. Reduction in height.
   b. Increased porousness or rarefaction when there is osteoporosis (I.B. page 588).
   c. Decreased vascularity.
   d. Reduction in metabolism and healing capacity.

III. Psychological Characteristics
The list below should not be considered typical of all elderly patients since many are well-adjusted. These characteristics are suggested to help the dental hygienist understand possible patient attitudes and actions.

A. Insecurity
1. Related to reduced economic status, self-respect, and feeling of being needed due to inability to work.
2. Reduced activity
   a. Physical limitations.
   b. Overprotection by family.
3. Others may be rejected by family and have desire for attention.
4. Anxiety over health.

B. Depression
1. Limited physical power; sensitivity about shortcomings of impaired vision, hearing, and lack of motor control.
2. Changes in physical appearance.
3. Loneliness: desire for attention.

C. Inability to Adjust to Changes in Mode of Life
Tendency to develop fixed habits and ideas.

D. Slowing of Voluntary Responses
As well as slowing of speed of association of thought.

E. Difficulty in Perception and Timing Sequential Events

F. Tendency to Introspection
Narrowing of interests; living in the past.

G. Slowing of Speed of Vocalization

IV. Appointment Procedures
In planning and conducting the appointment for the gerodontic patient, knowledge of the general physical, oral, and psychological characteristics of aging is applied. Suggested factors for consideration are listed in table 42–1.

Table 42–1.   Adaptations in Clinical Techniques for the Gerodontic Patient

Appointment Factors	Characteristic of the Gerodontic Patient	Suggested Relation to Appointment Procedure
Appointment Time	Tires more easily than younger patient Shortness of breath	Plan shorter appointments Need more frequent recall to provide for a high level of preventive care Appreciation of fact that patient has made a real effort to get to the office
	Cannot tolerate extremes of muscular strain; recovery from activity slow	Prevent need for long appointments
	Slower voluntary responses Sensitivity about shortcomings of lack of motor control	Do not rush. Do not make the patient feel old by obviously assisting him into the dental chair
	Lowered tolerance to extremes of heat and cold; less body cooling through perspiration	Adjust room temperature
	Impaired hearing	Speak clearly and slowly; provide written memorandum of date and time of each appointment
Instrumentation	Loss of elasticity of lips and oral mucosa	Difficulty in retraction may provide patient discomfort
	Slowing of voluntary responses Cannot adjust to sudden muscular demands	Do not demand quick response to request for change of position of head, rinsing
	Increased susceptibility to irritations of the tissues Friable tissues; epithelium tears easily Tendency to develop canker sores, traumatic ulcers, or angular cheilosis following mild stress to tissues	Need for unusual care during instrumentation or radiographic film placement to prevent irritation to soft tissues
	Reduction in growth and repair processes Decreased resistance to infection	Provide as little trauma to gingiva as possible during instrumentation Suggest postoperative care procedures to promote healing
	Inability to recover readily from stresses and strains Unsteadiness; tendency to dizziness	At completion of appointment straighten chair and let patient sit up for short time before dismissing; assist out of chair
Radiography	Increased fibrosis of tissues and rarefaction of bone	Adjustment of exposure or processing time

Attention to dental office arrangement which may provide physical barriers is important. The aged person's impaired vision, feebleness, or lack of motor control must be considered. There is need for elimination of hazards such as small rugs which can slide on polished floors, corners of rugs which can be tripped over, and irregularities in floor levels.

A. Patient History

Preparation of a careful and detailed medical and dental history takes on particular significance. Since 85 percent of people 65 years and older have one or more chronic conditions (page 578), knowledge of present and past health, medications, and other treatment is essential to planning dental and dental hygiene care. For example, approximately 65 per 1000 civilian noninstitutionalized persons ages 65 to 74 have diagnosed diabetes, and an estimated 25 per 1000 have undiagnosed diabetes.[3] Principles of dental hygiene care for diabetics (pages 689–700) have special application for the gerodontic patient.

Generally the patient's physician should be contacted since all details of the patient's condition may not have been revealed to the patient. Procedure for the patient history has been described in Chapter 6, pages 63–79. Blood pressure determination is recommended for each visit (pages 85–88).

B. Oral Inspection

The need for careful, periodic inspection of the oral mucosa from lips to throat cannot be overstressed at any age, but especially for the elderly since oral cancer occurs with increasing frequency with advancing years. Many, in fact most, oral lesions exist without the patient being aware of them. In a survey of 785 healthy people most of whom were between ages 60 and 90, 81 percent showed some form of notable, grossly visible pathology in the soft tissues.[4] Two patients were found to have squamous cell carcinoma.

For some early surface lesions, biopsy is definitely indicated. For others, the dental hygienist may prepare the cytologic smear as directed by the dentist (pages 101–103).

V. Patient Instruction

Older individuals need to be as interested in their health and appearance as people of any age. Esthetic deterioration may create emotional unhappiness and when the aged feel insecure or unwanted they may lose their interest in personal oral care and diet. Motivation through expression of sincere interest on the part of dental personnel can be an influencing factor in helping the patient to better health.

In the younger age groups there are still many who believe it inevitable and normal to lose the teeth eventually. With older people who still have their teeth, there is a tendency to be very resistant about the loss of them. Certain people fear dentures because they associate them with "old" people. Patients with partial dentures may already have been impressed with the need for preservation of the remaining teeth. Here, in the desire to save the teeth, lies the appeal for preventive measures for both the teeth and their supporting structures, and good use should be made of this very real motivating force.

In patient instruction it is important not to try to change all life-long habits since this may create frustration and unhappiness. Self-confidence, which has diminished because of lowering of physical capabilities and emotional satisfaction, must be built up. Major changes required because previous habits are detrimental must be brought about gradually if cooperation is to be expected. There is need for a more optimistic attitude about the degree of oral health which the elderly patient can be expected to achieve.

A. **Plaque Control Procedures**
  1. *Needs*
      Periodontal disease incidence and severity increase with age. According to the National Health Survey[5] oral cleanliness decreases with age, primarily related to calculus accumulation. The actual amount of superficial debris, materia alba, and plaque was not found to be different from younger age groups. Periodontal disease was more frequent and severe for older people than for younger people with the same level of oral cleanliness.
  2. *Objectives*
      Basic objectives do not differ from those for younger people: infection must be eliminated, the masticatory apparatus must be maintained for general health related to diet utilization, and esthetic factors are very important for the patient's sense of well-being and importance.
  3. *Specific Recommendations*
      Toothbrushing and other plaque control procedures as well as methods for care of fixed and removable prostheses are selected as for other adult patients (pages 310, 376, 386). Impaired motor functions or chronic conditions, such as arthritis of the hands, alter brush selection and method to some degree. An automatic toothbrush helps certain patients. Addition of acrylic material to enlarge the handle of a manual brush may be effective (pages 656–657).
      Because of increased exposure of root surfaces, attention to the abrasiveness of a dentifrice as well as to the occasional need for a desensitizing dentifrice is necessary (page 564). Delicate, friable gingival tissue may be sensitive to the sharp flavoring of certain dentifrices which may create a burning sensation.
      With the elderly, instruction and motivation techniques may best be applied gently, gradually, yet regularly. Suggestions for adaptation of instruction to physical and psychological characteristics which may be evident are listed in table 42–2.
      Recommendations follow the same pattern as for other adult patients. Each procedure is related to the individual need. With the elderly patient the difference lies in the method of motivation and instruction.

B. **Fluoride**
    To counteract tendencies toward cemental caries related to dry mouth and excess sucrose in the diet, daily exposure to fluoride is advised. Self-applied fluoride by means of a mouthwash, chewable tablet, gel in custom tray, or other form, in addition to using a fluoride dentifrice more than once each day, can contribute to dental caries prevention (pages 429, 439). Desensitization of the teeth can be accomplished by the same technique (page 564).

C. **Dietary Habits**
    Dietary and resulting nutritional deficiencies are common in older people. For example, characteristic changes such as burning tongue, angular cheilosis, and atrophic glossitis may be related to vitamin B deficiencies. Unfortunately, many people believe that a diet rich in nutritive

Table 42–2.   Characteristics Affecting Instruction for the Gerodontic Patient

Characteristic of the Gerodontic Patient	Suggested Relation to Appointment Procedure
Tendency for introspection; desire for attention	Patience needed in taking time to listen to complaints and accounts of past experiences
Feelings of insecurity Deprivation of physical capabilities Mental weakness shown through touchy sensitiveness, exaggerated imaginary or real pains, or attitudes of suspicion	Sympathetic understanding needed Build up self-confidence
Resistance to change; tendency to maintain fixed habits	Should not attempt to change all life-long habits, only detrimental ones
Vision impaired	Provide eyeglasses while giving instruction. Recommend that eyeglasses be worn at home while performing plaque control procedures
Hearing impaired; loss of sensitivity to higher tones	Speak distinctly in normal voice. Look at patient while speaking; many are lip readers (page 672)
Slowing of voluntary responses Slowing of speed of thought associations Difficulty in timing sequential events; skills become separate movements as by a child Least comfortable when must respond quickly to demanding sequential stimuli Rate of learning changed, ability to learn not changed Changes in speed of vocalization	Make suggestions gradually, over a series of appointments Do not demand learning a completely new procedure; adapt procedure already used Guide patient's demonstration of toothbrushing to prevent embarrassment Do not expect perfection; go slow, anticipate difficulties, give cues, clues Distinguish between slowness of learning and inability
Memory shortened due mainly to lack of attention, lack of interest, or more selection of what patient wants to remember	Use motivating factors carefully. Provide written instructions; spoken instructions may be forgotten or misunderstood
Need for personal achievement	Help patient gain sense of accomplishment; commend for any success, however minor

elements is important only for children.

1. *Factors Contributing to Dietary and Nutritional Deficiencies*
   a. Limited budget.
   b. Lives alone or eats alone.
   c. Does not eat regular meals; frequently uses nonnutritious snacks and foods for entertaining.
   d. Lacks interest in shopping for food or preparing it.
   e. Acuteness of senses lowered; may seek highly seasoned or sweetened foods.
   f. Childish likes and dislikes; unusual cravings.
   g. Tendency to follow food habits of lifetime; ignores newer knowledge of food preparation methods and dietary needs.
   h. Inadequate masticatory efficiency through tooth loss or inadequate dentures.

i. Adverse food selection may result from social embarrassment over inability to chew.

j. Adaptations in eating habits made to compensate for deficiency may interfere with adequate digestion and absorption of nutrients.

k. May follow dietary fads which provide only a very limited and unbalanced diet.

l. Loss of appetite: may have physiologic, social, or economic causes.

m. Lack of self-discipline; feeling that aging brings privilege to eat only preferred foods.

2. *Dietary Needs of the Aged*

Adequate nutritional balance is one of the best safeguards for promoting health and efficiency at any age. Because of the factors mentioned above, elderly people frequently use a high carbohydrate diet and neglect other nutritional needs.

The first consideration in making recommendations for aging patients is that a well-balanced diet be used with limited fermentable carbohydrate for dental caries prevention. Food for an adequate diet is listed in table 28–1 on page 403.

Caloric intake must be decreased because of lowered metabolic rate and activity. Protein, vitamins, and minerals are particularly important for body function, repair, and resistance to disease. Reviews of dietary and nutritional needs of older people are available for study.[6,7,8] Recent research shows that fluoride in the diet of the elderly is beneficial in the prevention of osteoporosis and fractures of the bones (page 426).

3. *Instruction in Dietary Habits*

A dietary analysis for evaluation of the patient's problems (pages 402–405) could prove very helpful if handled tactfully. The dietary review would aid in calling deficiencies to the patient's attention.

Appeal to the patient is made through his own personal concern for the relationships of dietary deficiencies to appearance, lowered resistance to disease, and premature aging, which may inspire the patient to improve his daily habits. Educational materials are available to study with and to give to the patient.[9]

References

1. Stotsky, B. A.: *The Elderly Patient.* New York, Grune & Stratton, 1968, p. 2.
2. United States Department of Health, Education, and Welfare: Vital and Health Statistics, Data from the National Health Survey, *Total Loss of Teeth in Adults, United States—1960–1962.* Washington, D.C., Public Health Service, Publication No. 1000, Series 11, No. 27, October, 1967.
3. U.S. Department of Health, Education, and Welfare, Public Health Service: *Diabetes Source Book.* Washington, D.C., Public Health Service Publication No. 1168, Revised 1968, pp. 7–11.
4. Bhaskar, S. N.: Oral Lesions in the Aged Population, a Survey of 785 Cases, *Geriatrics, 23,* 137, October, 1968.
5. United States Department of Health, Education, and Welfare: Vital and Health Statistics, Data from the National Health Survey, *Oral Hygiene in Adults, United States—1960–1962.* Washington, D.C., Public Health Service, Publication No. 1000, Series 11, No. 16, June, 1966.
6. Nizel, A. E.: *Nutrition in Preventive Dentistry: Science and Practice.* Philadelphia, Saunders, 1972, pp. 285–286, 443–460.
7. Schroeder, H. A.: Nutrition, in Cowdry, E. V. and Steinberg, F. U., eds.: *The Care of the Geriatric Patient,* 4th ed. St. Louis, Mosby, 1971, pp. 137–161.
8. Esposito, S. J., Vinton, P. W., and Rapuano, J. A.: Nutrition in the Aged: Review of the Literature, *J. Am. Geriatrics Soc., 17,* 790, August, 1969.
9. *Food Guide for Older Folks.* Washington, D.C., U.S. Department of Agriculture, Home and Garden Bulletin No. 17, Revised July 1969.

Suggested Readings

Burket, L. W.: *Oral Medicine*, 6th ed. Philadelphia, Lippincott, 1971, pp. 523–537, 545–549.

Donahue, W.: Psychologic Aspects, in Cowdry, E. V. and Steinberg, F. U., eds.: *The Care of the Geriatric Patient*, 4th ed. St. Louis, Mosby, 1971, pp. 267–280.

Elfenbaum, A.: Newer Problems of Older Patients: An Introduction to Geriatric Dentistry, *Dent. Clin. North Am.*, p. 217, March, 1968.

Feller, R. P. and Shannon, I. L.: Effect of Fluoride Intake on Osteoporosis and Other Rarefying Bone Disease: A Review, *J. Am. Soc. Prev. Dent.*, 3, 68, January-February, 1973.

Glickman, I.: *Clinical Periodontology*, 4th ed. Philadelphia, Saunders, 1972, pp. 69–73.

Gordon, R. H.: Meeting Dental Health Needs of the Aged, *Am. J. Public Health*, 62, 385, March, 1972.

Grant, D. and Bernick, S.: Arteriosclerosis in Periodontal Vessels of Ageing Humans, *J. Periodont.*, 41, 170, March, 1970.

Grant, D. and Bernick, S.: The Periodontium of Ageing Humans, *J. Periodont.*, 43, 660, November, 1972.

Grant, D. A., Stern, I. B., and Everett, F. G.: *Orban's Periodontics*, 4th ed. St. Louis, Mosby, 1972, pp. 77–96.

Hall, G.: The Dental Hygienist in a Nursing Home, *J. Am. Soc. for Geriatric Dent.*, 3, 1, July, 1968.

Hansen, G. C.: An Epidemiologic Investigation of the Effect of Biologic Aging on the Breakdown of Periodontal Tissue, *J. Periodont.*, 44, 269, May, 1973.

Hartsook, E. I.: Food Selection, Dietary Adequacy, and Related Dental Problems of Patients with Dental Prostheses, *J. Prosthet. Dent.*, 32, 32, July, 1974.

Heath, M. R.: Dietary Selection by Elderly Persons, Related to Dental State, *Br. Dent. J.*, 132, 145, February 15, 1972.

Lutwak, L.: Continuing Need for Dietary Calcium Throughout Life, *Geriatrics*, 29, 171, May, 1974.

Pickett, H. G., Appleby, R. G., and Osborn, M. O.: Changes in the Denture Supporting Tissues Associated with the Aging Process, *J. Prosthet. Dent.*, 27, 257, March, 1972.

Roper, R. E., Knerr, G. W., Gocka, E. F., and Stahl, S. S.: Periodontal Disease in Aged Individuals, *J. Periodont.*, 43, 304, May, 1972.

Vinton, P. W.: The Geriatric Complete Denture Patient, *Dent. Clin. North Am.*, p. 759, November, 1964.

Chapter 43

The Patient With Acute Necrotizing Ulcerative Gingivitis

Acute necrotizing ulcerative gingivitis (ANUG) is, as its name suggests, an inflammatory, destructive condition of the gingiva. Although it may occur at any age, the majority of cases are seen among young people between ages 15 and 30. Other names which are commonly used for the disease include trench mouth, Vincent's infection, Vincent's disease, and ulceromembranous gingivitis.

Dental hygienists frequently participate in the patient care necessary in all phases of treatment. Patient instruction and motivation for self-care are needed along with skillful submarginal instrumentation. After the initial acute symptoms have subsided, complete therapy must be carried out. The tissue destruction usually has left the gingiva deformed, with interdental flattening or cratering. Surgical treatment may be needed to restore a physiologic form which can be maintained by the patient in the plan to prevent recurrence of the disease.

I. Clinical Recognition

A. Initial Signs and Symptoms
The patient reports:
1. Sudden onset.
2. Pain and soreness: caused by slight pressure such as by foods during chewing and toothbrushing; intensified by hot or highly seasoned foods.
3. Bleeding: spontaneous or on slight pressure.
4. Poor appetite.
5. Metallic or other unpleasant taste.

B. Characteristic Clinical Findings
1. Interdental necrosis with ulceration of the papillae. In early disease only the tips of papillae are involved, followed by progressive destruction of the entire papillae and extension to the marginal gingiva facially and lingually.
2. Pseudomembrane. A gray, loose, necrotic slough forms over the necrotic area. When it is wiped off,

597

red and shiny hemorrhagic gingiva is exposed.

3. The membranous ulceration may be seen locally, that is between two or three teeth, or it may be generalized throughout both maxillary and mandibular arches.

C. **Other Clinical Findings**

The following usually accompany the characteristic signs and symptoms:

1. Debris, materia alba, and plaque collect profusely because the patient avoids brushing the sensitive teeth and gingiva.
2. Fetor oris (bad breath) is often severe. It is caused by necrotic tissue, stagnant saliva, and breakdown products of blood and debris.
3. Increased salivation.

D. **Systemic Signs**

An occasional patient will have apparent systemic involvement. Examination should always be made to detect the presence of the following:

1. Fever.
2. Malaise.
3. Lymphadenopathy of submaxillary and cervical nodes.

II. Predisposing Factors

A specific cause has not been determined, but certain predisposing factors are usually associated. When the condition occurs, local factors, stress factors, and factors related to general health and resistance to disease are involved.

A. **Local Factors**

ANUG is rarely, if ever, seen in a clean, healthy, cared-for and professionally supervised mouth. Many of the factors which can be considered predisposing are the same as those which predispose to chronic marginal gingivitis.

Predisposing factors include

1. Preexisting gingivitis.

2. Inadequate personal oral care with general neglect.
3. Smoking.
4. Factors related to retention of microorganisms and deposits (pages 268–271).
   a. Calculus as a retainer for plaque and debris.
   b. Open contacts encourage food impaction and stagnation.
   c. Oral habits, for example, mouth breathing.
   d. Periodontal pockets retain microorganisms and debris.
   e. Malposition of teeth; overcrowding.
   f. Iatrogenic causes: overhanging fillings.
   g. Tissue flap, for example, over a partially erupted third mandibular molar.
   h. Open carious lesions.

B. **Stress Factors**

1. Acute anxiety related to life situations is a common characteristic of patients with ANUG. In susceptible people, the condition has been found to occur or recur during periods of stress. Examples include students during examination periods, military men in combat, and some people at times of important decision-making.
2. Emotional stress is frequently accompanied by poor oral care, improper diet, excessive smoking, overexertion with interrupted sleep, and other deviations in health habits.

C. **Systemic: Disease-resistance Factors**

1. Dietary and nutritional inadequacies; vitamin deficiencies.
2. Recent illnesses; frequent colds, debilitating diseases such as infectious mononucleosis, pernicious anemia.
3. Fatigue; insufficient sleep.

III. Etiology

Bacteriologic and immunologic factors are implicated. For many years, bacteriologic smears were made from the ANUG lesion and examined by microscope for the presence of fusiform bacilli and spirochetes. Because the bacterial findings are not specific, it is now realized that the smear test is not necessary for making a diagnosis.

ANUG is not a communicable disease. Research has shown that a transfer of organisms from an infected patient does not produce the typical disease.

Recent studies suggest strongly that an endotoxin, produced by gram-negative bacteria, is involved in the initiation and progression of ANUG.[1]

IV. Course of Development

A. **Description of the Lesion**
   1. ANUG is superimposed over gingivitis or periodontitis.
   2. Ulceration and necrosis begin in the col area.
   3. Both epithelial tissue and connective tissue are involved.
   4. The disease process progresses to involve the entire papilla and eventually to the marginal gingiva on the facial and lingual.
   5. The pseudomembrane covering the lesion is a necrotic slough of the surface epithelium. It contains leukocytes, bacteria, epithelial cells, and fibrin.
   6. Connective tissue shows the signs of acute inflammation. It is hyperemic and filled with leukocytes, and its capillaries are engorged. When the pseudomembrane is lifted, the red inflamed connective tissue can be seen.

B. **Microscopic Examination**
   There are four layers in the lesion which have been described from observations made by electron microscopy.[2] All layers contain spirochetes.
   1. *Bacterial Zone.* The most superficial zone consists primarily of a mass of varied bacteria, including a few spirochetes.
   2. *Neutrophil-rich Zone.* Under the bacterial zone is a layer of leukocytes, predominantly neutrophils. Microorganisms including many spirochetes are found among the leukocytes.
   3. *Necrotic Zone.* This zone contains disintegrating tissue cells, many spirochetes, and other bacteria.
   4. *Spirochetal Infiltration Zone.* In this non-necrotized layer where tissue components are still preserved, spirochetes have invaded, but other microorganisms have not. In other forms of gingival diseases it is unusual for bacteria to be found within tissues. The action of toxins and other bacterial products was described in pocket formation on pages 177–178.

TREATMENT

I. Preparation for Diagnosis

Initially certain data must be collected for use by the dentist in making the diagnosis and treatment plan. To prepare a complete diagnostic work-up may be impractical considering the emergency nature of the patient's condition. Basic information needed is suggested by the steps described here.

A. **History**
   1. Description of chief complaint. The history of the current disease is recorded by date of onset, duration, symptoms as described, and what self-treatment the patient had already performed. Record whether this is a recurrence and, if so, details of previous episodes with the treatment given.

2. Basic medical history
   a. Obtain information needed for preliminary treatment.
      (1) Conditions needing medical consultation.
      (2) Identify need for premedication for prevention of bacteremia (see the list on page 71).
      (3) Allergies. Inquire in particular concerning drugs which may be used in the current therapy, such as antibiotics or hydrogen peroxide.
   b. Use knowledge of predisposing factors in ANUG to gather pertinent information.
      (1) Smoking habits.
      (2) Recent illnesses.
      (3) Dietary habits: record immediately previous 24-hour food intake. When the mouth has been sore and it has been painful to eat, this recording will not necessarily be typical of the patient's usual intake. Later a five-day or week-long diet diary will be requested as part of the continuing preventive program.
      (4) Sleeping hours: variations of normal routine.

B. **Examination**
   1. Record the patient's temperature.
   2. Extraoral inspections.
      a. Palpate submandibular and cervical nodes (figure 8–6, page 99).
      b. Observe face and skin: flushed, damp, malaise.
   3. Oral inspection. Without instrumentation, the dental hygienist can make a preliminary inspection and record the overall appearance of the gingival tissue. The dentist usually will prefer to see the gingiva as it appeared initially, before instrumentation or rinsing, in order to make the diagnosis and prepare the treatment plan. Instrumentation may be contraindicated for patients requiring premedication.

II. Treatment Plan

The dental hygiene treatment plan is formulated within the total treatment plan. Only a partial treatment plan is made until after the acute phase of the disease has passed. After the initial treatment, the diagnostic work-up can be completed and full evaluation made.

A. **Systemic Treatment**
   1. Antibiotics. After the diagnosis is made, the dentist will designate whether systemic therapy is required. Except for those requiring antibiotic coverage for instrumentation to prevent bacteremia, antibiotics are prescribed conservatively. Generally they are used only when the patient has definite systemic involvement as shown by significant temperature increase, malaise, and lymphadenopathy.
   2. Directions concerning diet, rest, and other systemic influences.
   3. Multivitamin supplements are sometimes prescribed.

B. **Relief of Acute Symptoms**
   1. Debridement of teeth and gingiva.
   2. Scaling and gingival curettage.
   3. Personal care instruction for rinsing, brushing, smoking limitation.

C. **Basic Therapy**
   1. Complete diagnostic work-up.
   2. Reevaluation and preparation of total treatment plan.
   3. Preventive program.
      a. Instruction for prevention of recurrence of ANUG.
      b. Dietary analysis and counseling.
      c. Self-care fluoride; professional application when indicated.
   4. Complete scaling, planing, curettage.

5. Reduction or elimination of predisposing factors to ANUG.
   a. Removal of overhanging margins and other retention factors.
   b. Restoration of teeth and contact areas.
6. Evaluation for periodontal surgery: need for restoration of tissue contour and elimination of craters.
7. Restoration of occlusion; prosthetic replacements and all other dental needs.

DENTAL HYGIENE CARE

A series of appointments for a typical ANUG patient is outlined here. The number of appointments and the exact procedure at each appointment will depend on the severity of the disease and the response of the gingiva as treatment progresses. Usually four or five appointments will be needed during the acute stage, and at least the first three should be at 24-hour intervals. After that, when the acute stage has subsided, a regular appointment is established for continued supervision and for proceeding with basic therapy.

I. Acute Phase: First Appointment

The first part of this appointment has been described under *History* on page 599. After the dentist has examined the patient and made the diagnosis, the dental hygienist will be directed to follow a procedure such as the following:

A. **Check the history for patient requiring prophylactic premedication** for prevention of bacteremia, and arrange accordingly. Parenteral administration may be indicated which should be discussed with the patient's physician.

B. **General Debridement**
   1. Spray the mouth with warm water or mouthwash.
   2. Apply hydrogen peroxide (three percent solution with equal parts of water) with cotton pellets at proximal areas; spray with water, and patient can rinse.
   3. Apply topical anesthetic (one quadrant or one-half mouth to be treated at a time).
   4. Supramarginal instrumentation. Use ultrasonic or manual scaling instruments or both for scaling. Use warm water for frequent irrigation while scaling. When time is limited, more time should be spent on calculus which is at the gingival margin and in the submarginal areas. Supramarginal calculus which does not contact the gingival margin can be left for future appointments since it does not immediately influence gingival healing.[3]

C. **Submarginal Instrumentation**
   The gingiva will respond sooner if submarginal scaling and curettage can be started at the first visit. When necessary, local anesthesia should be given in order that as complete treatment as possible can be done for the area selected.
   1. Perform instrumentation carefully to prevent tissue damage.
   2. Irrigate and evacuate frequently to clear all debris and diseased tissue removed by curettage.

D. **Patient Instruction**
   1. Instructions for home procedures must be carefully explained. Written directions are needed.
   2. Inform the patient that treatment will not be complete when the pain is eliminated. Explain the underlying gingival or periodontal disease and how ANUG recurs if the periodontal condition is not treated and followed.
   3. Rinsing directions. Vigorous rinsing with hot weak salt water (page 342) or hydrogen peroxide (three

percent with equal parts water) is necessary every hour for five minutes during the period of acute symptoms.

4. Toothbrushing. Use a soft nylon brush (.006" filament) gently, but clean the teeth as much as possible after each meal and before going to bed. When a brush is not given the patient at the clinic or office, write down the names of specific brushes for the patient to purchase.

5. Avoid smoking. The heavy smoker can be asked to limit the number.

6. Diet.[4]
   a. Recommend frequent small nutritious meals which incorporate daily requirements from the Basic 4 (table 28–1, page 403).
   b. A liquid diet is advised for the first day, particularly for the patient with systemic symptoms or who has pronounced sensitivity when chewing. A semi-liquid or soft solids diet can be used on the second day. Examples of foods to include in a liquid and a soft solid diet are listed on page 611.
   c. Increased nutrients should be used from the milk and meat food groups, and fruits and juices containing vitamin C.
   d. Avoid highly seasoned foods and alcoholic beverages.

II. Acute Phase: Second Appointment

A. Patient Inspection
In 24 hours it is usual to see a remarkable improvement. It would be expected that the pain and discomfort would have subsided, the pseudomembrane would have disappeared, and the tissue swelling be reduced.

B. Complete the Patient History

C. Scaling and Curettage
Continue from previous appointment after checking areas previously treated. The objective is to be as thorough as possible, since plaque retained over residual calculus can keep the tissues from complete healing.

D. Instruction
1. Rinsing. When healing is progressing favorably, change rinsing schedule to every two hours.
2. Toothbrushing. Emphasize thorough coverage of the entire teeth. Sulcular brushing must be demonstrated for use as soon as the sensitivity of the gingiva has gone.
3. Proximal surfaces. The use of floss is advised and demonstrated at this or the third appointment, depending on the readiness of the patient and the tissues. Other proximal cleaning devices may be useful. The importance of complete plaque removal must be explained.
4. Diet. A liquid diet is not usually indicated after the first day and the patient can use the soft solids diet or a regular diet adapted with bland foods that will not irritate the healing tissues.
5. Provide specific written instructions.

III. Acute Phase: Third Appointment

A. Observe and Evaluate the Gingival Tissues
Continued improvement normally will be noted each day. Note areas where healing has not progressed, as these areas will need additional scaling, planing, and curettage.

B. Instruction in Self-care Procedures
Initial instructions may have been started previously, but as soon as possible, plaque should be explained and disclosed and sulcular brushing instruction presented in detail. Follow Lesson I or Lesson II (pages 388–391), depending on the extent of previous instruction.

C. Scaling, Planing, and Curettage

Treatment is continued, with particular attention to areas where healing has not been complete.

D. Home Care Instruction

1. Rinsing. Discontinue peroxide if that was the selected rinse. Request the patient to use warm mild saline solution vigorously after brushing and flossing.
2. Review and emphasize previous instruction.

IV. Successive Appointments

After daily supervision during the acute stage, regular appointments for basic treatment are planned. The gingiva is evaluated, and repeated scaling, planing, and curettage performed as needed.

A. Preparation of a Diagnostic Work-up

The complete diagnostic work-up is prepared as directed by the dentist, and the patient instructed for continued treatment.

B. Recurrence of ANUG

When the gingival and bony craters which remain after the acute stages disappear are not treated, they are vulnerable to continuing disease and recurrence of ANUG. Plaque and debris can collect readily in the misshapen proximal areas, and the areas are difficult to clean with plaque control techniques. Gingival craters invite further tissue breakdown leading to periodontal pocket formation.

Surgical treatment may involve gingivoplasty when the bone is not involved. When bony craters exist, treatment may involve flap surgery with osseous reshaping.

TECHNICAL HINTS

I. Provide explicit directions concerning rinsing with hydrogen peroxide. Extended use of oxygenating drugs can cause tissue changes such as surface necrosis or "burn," and black hairy tongue.

II. Instructions for patients can be printed or written. Since each day during the acute phase the instructions change, individual slips should be prepared using paper of different colors. Printed instructions can be personalized with added written notations.

FACTORS TO TEACH THE PATIENT

I. Premature discontinuance of therapy because acute signs have subsided can lead to recurrence of the disease.

II. The role of diet, rest, and plaque control in the prevention of ANUG.

References

1. Shapiro, L. and Ruben, M. P.: Acute Necrotizing Ulcerative Gingivitis, in Goldman, H. M., Gilmore, H. W., Irby, W. B., and Olsen, N. H., eds.: *Current Therapy in Dentistry*, Vol. V. St. Louis, Mosby, 1974, pp. 40–45.
2. Listgarten, M. A.: Electron Microscopic Observations on the Bacterial Flora of Acute Necrotizing Ulcerative Gingivitis, *J. Periodont.*, 36, 328, July-August, 1965.
3. Goldhaber, P.: Acute Necrotizing Ulcerative Gingivitis, in Goldman, H. M. and Cohen, D. W.: *Periodontal Therapy*, 5th ed. St. Louis, Mosby, 1973, pp. 167–177.
4. Nizel, A. E.: *Nutrition in Preventive Dentistry: Science and Practice.* Philadelphia, Saunders, 1972, pp. 407–411.

Suggested Readings

American Dental Association, Council On Dental Therapeutics: *Accepted Dental Therapeutics*, 36th ed. Chicago, American Dental Association, 1975, p. 269.

Barnes, G. P., Bowles, W. F., and Carter, H. G.: Acute Necrotizing Ulcerative Gingivitis: A Survey of 218 Cases, *J. Periodont.*, 44, 35, January, 1973.

Brown, R. H.: Necrotizing Ulcerative Gingivitis in Mongoloid and Non-mongoloid Retarded Individuals, *J. Periodont. Res.*, 8, 290, No. 5, 1973.

Davis, R. K. and Baer, P. N.: Necrotizing Ulcerative Gingivitis in Drug Addict Patients Being Withdrawn from Drugs, *Oral Surg.*, 31, 200, February, 1971.

Formicola, A. J., Witte, E. T., and Curran, P. M.: A Study of Personality Traits and Acute Necrotizing Ulcerative Gingivitis, *J. Periodont.*, 41, 36, January, 1970.

Giddon, D. B., Zackin, S. J., and Goldhaber, P.: Acute Necrotizing Ulcerative Gingivitis in College Students, *J. Am. Dent. Assoc., 68,* 381, March, 1964.

Glickman, I.: *Clinical Periodontology,* 4th ed. Philadelphia, Saunders, 1972, pp. 126–138, 799–809.

Goldhaber, P. and Giddon, D. B.: Present Concepts Concerning the Etiology and Treatment of Necrotizing Ulcerative Gingivitis, *Int. Dent. J., 14,* 468, December, 1964.

Grant, D. A., Stern, I. B., and Everett, F. G.: *Orban's Periodontics,* 4th ed. St. Louis, Mosby, 1972, pp. 335–348.

Graykowski, E. A. and Holroyd, S. V.: Therapeutic Management of Primary Herpes, Recurrent Labial Herpes, Aphthous Stomatitis, and Vincent's Infection, *Dent. Clin. North Am., 14,* 721, October, 1970.

Klingsberg, J.: Patient Education about Necrotizing Gingivitis, *N.Y. Dent. J., 37,* 413, August-September, 1971.

Shafer, W. G., Hine, M. K., and Levy, B. M.: *Textbook of Oral Pathology,* 3rd ed. Philadelphia, Saunders, 1974, pp. 724–729.

Shannon, I. L., Kilgore, W. G., and O'Leary, T. J.: Stress as a Predisposing Factor in Necrotizing Ulcerative Gingivitis, *J. Periodont., 40,* 240, April, 1969.

Chapter 44

The Oral Surgery Patient and the Patient with a Fractured Jaw

ORAL SURGERY PATIENT

A mouth is not considered a good surgical risk when the teeth are covered with debris and calculus, and the gingiva show signs of inflammation and possible nutritional deficiency. It is recommended that unless emergency surgery is required, the appointment be postponed until the mouth is in a better state of cleanliness and health.

The patient's medical history will reveal essential information to guide procedures. Presurgery patients may have extensive oral infection and calculus deposits particularly in a neglected mouth. The extent and position of a pathological lesion and the ability of the patient to maintain his mouth in an open position will influence techniques used.

I. Objectives

Dental hygiene care and instruction prior to oral surgery may contribute to the patient's health and well-being by one or more of the following:

A. **Remove Debris and Reduce Oral Bacterial Count**
   1. Aid in the preparation of an aseptic field of operation.
   2. Make postextraction infection less likely.

B. **Reduce Inflammation of the Gingiva and Improve Tissue Tone**
   1. Lessen local hemorrhage at the time of the operation.
   2. Promote postoperative healing.

C. **Remove Calculus Deposits**
   1. Remove a source of irritation to the gingiva and thus improve tissue tone.
   2. Prevent interference with placement of surgical instruments.
   3. Prevent pieces of calculus from breaking away during tooth removal.
      a. Danger of inhalation particularly when a general anesthetic is used.
      b. Possibility of calculus falling into socket or other surgical area

and acting as a foreign body to inhibit healing.

D. **Instruct in Presurgery Personal Oral Care Procedures**

This will contribute to reducing inflammation and thus improve tissue tone.

E. **Instruct in the Use of Foods**

The patient should be instructed about those foods which provide the elements essential to tissue building and repair during pre- and postsurgery periods.

F. **Interpret the Dentist's Directions**

This should be done for the immediate preoperative preparation with respect to rest and dietary limitations, particularly when a general anesthetic is to be administered.

G. **Motivate the Patient Who Will Have Teeth Remaining**

The patient who will have teeth remaining after surgery should be motivated to prevent further tooth loss through routine dental and dental hygiene professional care and personal oral care procedures.

H. **Emphasize the Importance of Diet**

For the patient who will have all teeth removed and dentures inserted, the importance of a diet containing all essential food groups should be emphasized.

II. Psychological Considerations

The extent of the surgery to be performed and previous experiences will affect the patient's psychological attitude. A majority of the patients who are in greatest need for presurgery dental hygiene care and instruction may be people who have neglected their mouths for many years. They have been indifferent toward or unaware of the importance of obtaining adequate care. Their only visits to a dentist may have been to have a toothache relieved by extraction. Their knowledge of preventive measures may be limited. A few of the characteristics which may confront the dental hygienist are suggested below.

A. **Apprehensive and Fearful**
1. Apprehensive and indifferent toward need for cleaning teeth which are to be removed.
2. Fearful of all dental procedures, particularly oral surgery and anesthesia.
3. Fearful of personal appearance after surgery.

B. **Impatient**

When teeth have caused discomfort and pain it is difficult to understand need for delay while dental hygiene procedures are accomplished.

C. **Ashamed**

Of appearance or of having neglected teeth.

D. **Resigned**

Feeling of inevitableness of the situation; lack of appreciation for natural teeth.

E. **Discouraged**

Over tooth loss or development of soft tissue lesions.

F. **Resentful**
1. Toward time lost from work.
2. Toward the financial aspects of dental care.
3. Toward inconvenience and discomfort.

DENTAL HYGIENE CARE

I. Presurgery

At least two appointments frequently are needed, but the pending date for the surgery and the patient's attitude may limit the time to be spent.

A. **First Appointment**

Develop patient rapport, demonstrate toothbrushing procedures, remove calculus deposits, and make suggestions for diet.

B. **Second Appointment**
Observe response of gingival tissue, review toothbrushing and dietary procedures and continue the scaling.

II. Patient Instruction: Plaque Control

A. **Toothbrushing**
1. Brush: soft, nylon type is usually preferable depending on the condition of the tissue.
2. Technique: since many presurgery patients may not have practiced careful brushing on a regular plan, a simple technique is preferred as time for establishing habits may be limited until postoperative healing is complete. Use of disclosing agent for the patient's own evaluation is important.

B. **Auxiliary Procedures**
Interdental plaque removal and care of fixed and removable appliances are included in instruction (pages 331, 335). The patient who will have multiple extractions for an immediate denture or other appliance, or an obturator or other replacement following cleft palate, tumor, or other surgery, will need postsurgical instruction for the specific care of the appliance.

III. Instrumentation

Scaling techniques are of primary importance. Frequently, polishing procedures are contraindicated because of the condition of the gingival tissues.

A. **Scaling**
1. Problems
   a. Teeth with large carious lesions.
   b. Mobile teeth.
   c. Edentulous areas.
   d. Sensitive, enlarged gingival tissue which bleeds readily.
2. Suggestions for technique
   a. Use topical anesthetic when tis-

sue is sensitive and patient is apprehensive (pages 511–513).
   b. Maintain as clear a field as possible preferably using evacuation techniques.
   c. Use alternate finger rests to adapt to mobile teeth or edentulous areas; stabilize mobile teeth during scaling stroke.
   d. Ultrasonic scaling techniques may be particularly appropriate (pages 509–511).
   e. Irrigation: following scaling and root planing, thorough irrigation of the sulcus is advised to prevent debris and calculus from becoming imbedded in the underlying tissues where they can promote inflammation and delay healing.

B. **Polishing**
1. Contraindications
   a. Enlarged, inflamed, sensitive gingiva.
   b. Deep pockets.
   c. Profuse hemorrhage.
2. Effects
   a. Irritation to tissue by polishing abrasive and action of rubber polishing cup.
   b. Movement of rubber cup forces abrasive particles into the gingival tissues.
3. Recommended procedure
For patients whose anterior teeth will not be removed, improvement of appearance by polishing labial surfaces may provide encouragement and motivation for attention to future personal and professional care.
Follow-up evaluation, scaling, and planing should be planned for a few weeks after surgery to complete the procedures. Such an appointment should not be scheduled until healing has progressed favorably.

C. **Rinsing Instruction**
1. Objectives: to promote tissue healing following scaling and to remove
debris; to initiate the habit of
rinsing for postsurgical care later.
2. Rinsing solution: warm mild hypertonic salt solution (page 348) for
healing; mouthwash with flavor for
alleviation of mouth odors following surgery.
3. Frequency: recommended for several times each day; after surgery as
instructed by oral surgeon.

IV. Patient Instruction: Diet Selection[1]

The patient's nutritional state can
influence his resistance to infection and
wound healing, as well as his general
recovery powers. Specific recommendations of what to include and not to include
in the diet should be given to the patient.
Postoperative suggestions may differ from
preoperative; for example, when
difficulty in chewing is a postoperative
problem, a liquid or soft diet may be
necessary. Diets outlined are designed to
include the essential foods from the Four
Food Groups (table 28–1, page 403).

A. **Nutritional and Dietary Needs**
1. Essentials for promotion of healing:
protein and vitamins, particularly
vitamin A, vitamin C, and riboflavin.
2. Essential for building gingival tissue resistance: a varied diet which
includes adequate portions of all
essential food groups.
3. Essential for providing gingival
stimulation: detergent foods which
require mastication, especially
fresh fruits and vegetables. Possibilities for making recommendations in this area are limited by the
patient's masticatory deficiencies.
4. Essential for dental caries prevention: foods without fermentable
carbohydrate. When a patient has
not been able to masticate properly,

the diet employed frequently may
have included many soft carbohydrate foods.

B. **Suggestions for Instruction**
1. Provide instruction sheets which
show specific meal plans for pre-
and postsurgery. Foods for liquid
and soft diets are listed on pages
611–612.
2. Express nutritional needs in terms
of quantity or servings of foods so
that the patient clearly understands.
3. For the patient who will receive
dentures, extensive and careful instruction must be provided over a
period of time. At the presurgery
appointment only an introduction
can be given, particularly because
the patient is probably more concerned about the operation than
about the after effects.

When the patient will lose the
teeth because of dental caries, the
diet has likely been high in fermentable carbohydrates. Emphasis
should be placed on helping the
patient include nutritious foods for
the general health of the body and
more specifically the health of the
alveolar processes which will support the dentures.

V. Postsurgery Care

A. **Immediate**
Examples of items usually included
in printed instructions for postoperative care by the outpatient are listed in
Technical Hints, pages 613–614.

B. **Follow-up Care**
The dental hygienist may participate in suture removal, irrigation of
sockets, and other postoperative procedures when the patient returns to
the dental office or surgery. Appropriately, instruction concerning
plaque control, rinsing, oral irrigation,

and other personal care as well as diet supervision can be continued.

FRACTURED JAW PATIENT

The limited access to the gingiva for personal oral care procedures and the effect of the liquid diet required for most cases define the need for special dental hygiene care for the patient with a fractured jaw. Attention to rehabilitation of the oral tissues during the period following the removal of appliances takes on particular significance lest permanent tissue damage result or inadequate oral care habits be continued indefinitely.

Many fractured jaw cases are hospitalized. A dental hygienist employed in a hospital would be called upon to assume a part of the responsibility for patient care and instruction. After dismissal from the hospital, the patient may require special attention in the private dental office for a long period of time.

Fractured jaw cases may be very complex and the patient may suffer considerably, both physically and mentally. Some basic knowledge of the nature of fractures and their treatment is helpful in understanding the patient's needs.

I. Causes

1. Trauma: from automobile injuries, industrial accidents, and physical violence (blows, fistfights).
2. Predisposing: pathologic conditions such as tumors, cysts, or osteomyelitis weaken the bone, thus permitting slight trauma to cause fracture.

II. Types

The fracture or fractures are classified by using any combination of those listed below under mandibular and maxillary, and described by their nature and severity. Fractures may be single or multiple.

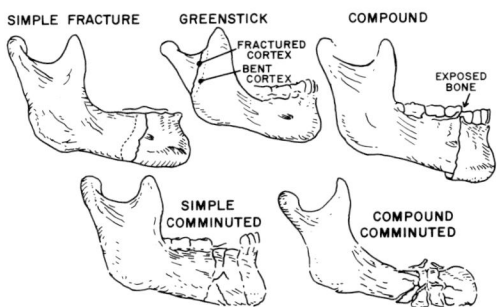

Figure 44–1. Types of fractures. (From Kruger, G.O.: Textbook of Oral Surgery, 4th ed. St. Louis, Mosby, 1974.)

A. **Mandibular** (described by location)
   1. Condyle
   2. Angle
   3. Body
   4. Symphysis
B. **Maxillary**
   1. Horizontal
   2. Pyramidal
   3. Transverse Facial
C. **Classification by Nature of the Fracture** (figure 44–1).
   1. Simple: has no communication with outside.
   2. Compound: has communication with outside.
   3. Comminuted: shattered.
   4. Incomplete: "greenstick" fracture has one side of a bone broken and the other side bent. It occurs in incompletely calcified bones (young children usually). The fibers tend to bend rather than break.

III. First Aid

Immediate attention must be paid to first aid measures for care of the patient's general condition. *First aid care is given for impaired airway, hemorrhage, shock, and skull or internal head injuries, in that order.*

Almost any category of first aid may be required (pages 724–733). Although treatment for the fractured jaw must not be postponed for any great length of time, its immediate care takes second place in the light of the vital aspects of patient care.

IV. Treatment

A. Objectives

To permit healing through *reduction* of the fracture, *fixation* of the fragments, and *immobilization* of the parts in correct anatomic relationship with the teeth in occlusion.

B. Types of Treatment

Each fracture differs from the next, and the methods used in treatment vary with the individual case. Many factors are involved when the oral surgeon selects the methods to be used, particularly the location of the fracture or fractures, the presence or absence of teeth, existing injuries to the teeth, other head injuries, and the general health and condition of the patient.

Maxillary fractures are more difficult to handle because of the number of bones, the associated anatomy, and the complications of basal skull fractures. Undisplaced maxillary or mandibular fractures occasionally require no fixation but the patient must avoid all masticatory stresses.

Treatment is generally composed of *reduction* and *fixation*. These consist of the following two categories:

1. *Closed reduction.* Immobilization is accomplished by applying arch bars to the teeth and tying the teeth (or dentures) in occlusion by wires or elastic bands. Other types of fixation involve the use of head-caps, circumferential wiring, and metal or acrylic splints.
2. *Open reduction.* An incision is made and the broken segments are positioned by direct manipulation. Fixation is usually by bone wiring. The surgery is performed with the patient under general anesthesia in an operating room. One of the most common sites for this type of surgery is the angle of the mandible.

V. Healing

Union is affected by the location and character of the fracture. Much depends on the patient's general health and resistance and cooperation. Six weeks is considered the average for the uncomplicated mandibular case and four to six weeks for the maxillary. The major cause of complication is infection.

DENTAL HYGIENE CARE

I. Problems

Fixation apparatus, however carefully placed to prevent tissue irritation, interferes with normal function. The length of time the appliances must be in place is sufficient for considerable disturbance of tissue metabolism. Identification of possible effects of treatment provides the basis for planning dental hygiene care.

A. **Development of Gingivitis or Periodontal Complications**
   1. Rapid calculus formation in susceptible patients, and debris accumulation resulting from a nondetergent diet and saliva stagnation, provide sources of irritation to the gingiva.
   2. Lack of normal stimulation to the circulation of the periodontium usually provided by the excursion of food may lower tissue resistance.
   3. Tender, sensitive gingiva makes plaque control more difficult even on available surfaces.

B. **Dental Caries Initiation**
   It is difficult to plan an interesting diet using limited fermentable carbohydrates for dental caries prevention.

C. **Loss of Appetite**

Loss of appetite related to monotonous liquid or soft diet leads to weight loss and lowered physical resistance. Secondary infections, including those of the oral tissues, may result.

D. **Difficulty in Opening the Mouth**
1. When there has been injury to the temporomandibular joint, the patient wearing fixation appliances which involve only the mandible has difficulty in applying a toothbrush to the lingual surfaces of teeth.
2. After removal of appliances, all patients have a degree of muscular trismus which hinders toothbrushing and mastication.

II. Instrumentation

A. **Presurgery**

Gross calculus is removed insofar as possible before wiring or the placement of metal or acrylic splints.

B. **During Treatment**

Periodic scaling in conjunction with plaque control.

C. **After Removal of Appliances**

A few weeks after removal of appliances, when the patient can open the mouth normally and plaque control procedures have been initiated, complete scaling and planing can be performed.

III. Diet

Many fractured jaw patients tend to lose weight which is generally related to an inadequate nutrient and caloric intake. Objectives in planning the diet are to help the patient maintain an adequate nutritional state, to promote healing, and to increase resistance to infection.

Attention must be given to the patient's willingness and ability to follow the recommendations made. The patient may be in the hospital for a few days to a week, depending on the severity of other injuries, so a greater length of time is spent as an outpatient when the diet is much more difficult to supervise. It has been suggested that the patient's understanding of dietary instructions and what is expected appears to be much more significant than the actual type of diet recommended.

A. **Nutritional Needs**

After any surgery the diet must be planned to promote tissue building and repair.[1,2]
1. All essential food elements.
2. Emphasis on protein, vitamins, particularly A and C, and minerals, particularly calcium and phosphorus.
3. Usual caloric requirements for patient's age, taking into consideration lack of physical exercise and loss of appetite while ill.

B. **Liquid Diet**
1. Indications
   a. All patients with jaws wired together.
   b. All patients with no appliance or single jaw appliance who have difficulty in opening mouth due to condition such as temporomandibular joint involvement, or tongue or lip injury which will hinder insertion of food or manipulation of food in the mouth.
2. Examples of foods: fruit juices; milk; eggnog; meat juices and soups; cooked thin cereals; canned baby foods. Strained vegetables and meats (baby foods) may be added to meat juices and soups.

C. **Soft Solids Diet**
1. Indications
   a. Patients with no appliance or with single jaw appliance without complications in opening

mouth or in movement of lips and tongue.

b. Patient who has been maintained on liquid diet throughout treatment period: after appliances are removed the soft diet is recommended for several days to a week to provide the stomach with foods which are readily digestible rather than making drastic change to regular diet. A soft solids diet can also aid by protecting tender oral tissues from rough textures of regular diet until tissues have a chance to respond to softer foods and regular plaque control routine.

    2. Examples of foods: soft poached, scrambled, or boiled eggs; cooked cereals; mashed soft cooked vegetables including potato; mashed fresh or canned fruits; soft, finely divided meats; custards, plain ice cream.

D. **Methods of Feeding**
    1. Glass drinking tube: liquid is sucked from the tube through the teeth, or the tube can be inserted through an edentulous area.
    2. Cup or bowl, small pitcher or teapot.
    3. Spoon-feeding: when patient's arms are not functional.
    4. Oropharyngeal, nasopharyngeal, or rectal feeding for severely injured or unconscious patients.

E. **Hints for Diet Planning With the Nonhospitalized Patient**
    1. Provide instruction sheets which show specific meal plans.
    2. Express nutritional needs in quantities or servings of foods.
    3. Show methods of varying the diet. A liquid or soft diet is at best monotonous because of sameness of texture.
    4. Suggest limitation of foods containing high content of fermentable

carbohydrate as an aid to prevention of dental caries.

IV. **Personal Oral Care Procedures**

Every attempt to keep the patient's mouth as clean as possible and to provide some degree of tissue stimulation should be made for both health and comfort. The extent of possible care depends on the appliances, the condition of the lips, tongue, and other oral tissues, and the cooperation of the patient. Encouragement must be given to the patient to begin toothbrushing as soon as possible after the surgery, but until the patient is able, a plan for care is outlined for an attendant.

A. **While Appliances Are in Place**
    1. Irrigation by attendant
        a. Indications: during first few days after surgery while mouth may be too tender for brushing, frequent irrigations are required; irrigation also serves as an adjunct to toothbrushing.
        b. Method: spray bottle and suction tube. Power spray at least once each day aids in removing microorganisms which have accumulated interproximally.
        c. Mouthwash used
            (1) Physiologic saline solution to aid healing.
            (2) Sodium bicarbonate as a detergent.
            (3) Fluoride mouthwash may increase resistance to dental caries.
            (4) Oral surgeon may recommend an astringent or oxidizing mouthwash for special cases.
    2. Cleansing before a toothbrush can be used: a cotton roll can be wiped over gingiva, exposed tooth surfaces, and appliances.
    3. Use of toothbrush with suction
        This method can be effective particularly during the early days

after the appliances are placed. For method of use see page 585.

4. Toothbrushing by the patient

As soon as possible the patient is instructed in personal care. A toothbrushing method and other aids such as are used for orthodontic appliances are recommended and demonstrated (page 357). The patient must be shown why care must be taken not to entangle the toothbrush bristles with the wires. When the patient's tongue is not injured he can be instructed to use his tongue as an aid in cleaning the lingual surfaces of the teeth and massaging the gingiva.

5. Massage: in addition to the massage provided by the cotton roll and toothbrush, the patient may be instructed in digital massage for the gingival tissue.

6. Oral irrigation (page 342): Specific instruction with the irrigator should be provided. The spray should be carefully directed to prevent tissue injury (figure 23–15, page 343).

B. **After Appliances Are Removed**

A thorough review of toothbrushing procedures should be provided. A step-by-step series of lessons is usually necessary before the patient can carry out adequate plaque control.

A method for daily self-applied fluoride, such as a mouth rinse or gel tray, should be introduced along with the use of a fluoride dentifrice. Decalcification and dental caries can result from plaque retention about the appliances as well as the nature of the sticky liquid diet used.

DENTAL HYGIENE CARE PRIOR TO GENERAL SURGERY

Complete scaling prior to general surgery has significance particularly when a general inhalation anesthetic is to be administered, and when a long recovery period and convalescence are anticipated. Providing a clean mouth with gingival irritants removed is one means of treating the patient as a whole: it contributes to comfort and protection against complications.

Plaque control and professional instrumentation aid in reducing the oral bacterial count. Since the mouth is the entrance to the respiratory chamber, there is always the possibility of the inhalation of debris and fluids from the mouth. This could occur during the administration of an anesthetic, or when the patient coughs.

When the patient has a clean mouth initially, the problems of postoperative oral care are lessened. If a patient is very ill he will not be attending to his own personal oral care for some time. Certain types of surgery require that the patient convalesce for a long period. In these cases oral care must be provided by an attendant, and at best the results are limited.

When emergency surgery is performed, procedures of dental hygiene care are obviously impossible. However, when surgery is planned in advance, the patient should be informed of the importance of a clean mouth, and be encouraged to have an appointment. The dental hygienist in private practice has an important role to play in this phase of dental hygiene care.

TECHNICAL HINTS

I. Surgery is not provided to minors without consent of parent or guardian. Written consent is mandatory.

II. Basic instructions following tooth extraction and other dental operations: printed or mimeographed postsurgical instructions should be given to each patient after the prepared material is reviewed with the patient after surgery. Specific details will vary with the individual dentist but basic information for postoperative instruction sheets includes the following:

A. Keep the sponge in the mouth over the surgical area for one-half hour, then discard it. When bleeding persists at home, place a gauze pad or cold wet teabag over the area and bite firmly for 30 minutes.

B. Rinsing: do not rinse for 24 hours after the surgery. Then use warm salt water (about one-half teaspoonful salt in an eight-ounce glass of warm water), after toothbrushing and every two hours.

C. Brush the teeth as usual; use dental floss.

D. Rest: get plenty of rest: at least eight to ten hours sleep each night. Avoid strenuous exercise during the first 24 hours and keep the mouth from excessive movement.

E. Diet: use a liquid or soft solid diet high in protein. Drink water and fruit juices freely. Avoid foods that require excessive chewing.

F. Pain: take aspirin or other pain-relieving preparation prescribed by the dentist.

G. Icepack: following a flap operation or when there is swelling, apply icepack (ice cubes in a plastic bag) for 30 minutes followed by 30 minutes off, or apply for 15 minutes after 30 minutes off, as directed by the dentist. Heat is not used for swelling.

H. Instructions should include the telephone number to call after office hours, should complications arise; complications may include uncontrollable pain, marked bleeding, temperature rise, difficulty in opening the mouth, or unusual swelling a few days after the surgery.

III. Booklet: *What to Do After Extraction of a Tooth* is available from the American Dental Association, Order Department, 211 E. Chicago Avenue, Chicago, Illinois, 60611 (Catalog Number G20).

IV. Accident prevention: encourage patients to use the seat belts in their cars. Professional people should set the example by using their own seat belts.

References

1. Nizel, A. E.: *Nutrition in Preventive Dentistry: Science and Practice.* Philadelphia, Saunders, 1972, pp. 427–442.
2. Byrne, J. E. and Byrne, L. R.: The Dietary Management of the Patient with a Fractured Jaw, *Oral Surg.*, 29, 666, May, 1970.

Suggested Readings

Archer, W. H.: *Oral Surgery*, 4th ed. Philadelphia, Saunders, 1966, pp. 758–905.
Boyer, H. E. and DeJean, E. K.: Principles of Management of Oral Surgery Patients, *Dent. Clin. North Am.*, p. 349, July, 1964.
Goracy, E. and Stratigos, G. T.: Successive Mandibular Fractures in the Alcoholic-epileptic Patient, *Oral Surg.*, 32, 701, November, 1971.
Huelke, D. F. and Harger, J. H.: Maxillofacial Injuries: Their Nature and Mechanisms of Production, *J. Oral Surg.*, 27, 451, July, 1969.
Jones, N. B.: Dietary Needs of the Oral Surgery Patient with Comparison of Dietary Supplements, *J. Oral Surg.*, 28, 892, December, 1970.
Kruger, G. O., ed.: *Textbook of Oral Surgery*, 4th ed. St. Louis, Mosby, 1974, pp. 314–329.
Mitchell, D. F., Standish, S. M., and Fast, T. B.: *Oral Diagnosis/Oral Medicine*, 2nd ed. Philadelphia, Lea & Febiger, 1971, pp. 404–406.
Rowe, N. L.: Fractures of the Jaws in Children, *J. Oral Surg.*, 27, 497, July, 1969.
Shapiro, D. N.: Reactions of Children to Oral Surgery Experience, *J. Dent. Child.*, 34, 97, March, 1967.
Shira, R. B.: Emergency Treatment of Patients with Facial Trauma, in Douglas, B. L., ed.: *Introduction to Hospital Dentistry*, 2nd ed. St. Louis, Mosby, 1970, pp. 129–144.
Simpson, P. M.: Work in an Oral Surgery Unit, *Dental Health*, 6, 47, July-September, 1967.
Smith, J. F.: Nutritional Maintenance of the Oral Fracture Patient, *Oral Surg.*, 19, 705, June, 1965.
Stanton, G.: Applied Nutrition in Hospital Dentistry, in Douglas, B. L., ed.: *Introduction to Hospital Dentistry*, 2nd ed. St. Louis, Mosby, 1970, pp. 154–158.
Thoma, K. H.: *Oral Surgery*, 5th ed. St. Louis, Mosby, 1969, pp. 178, 524–571.
Williamson, R. and Davis, C. L.: Drug-dependent, Alcohol-dependent, and Mental Patients: Clinical Study of Oral Surgery Procedures, *J. Am. Dent. Assoc.*, 86, 416, February, 1973.

Chapter 45

The Patient With Oral Cancer

Care of the cancer patient before, during, and after therapy has as its main purposes attaining and maintaining oral health at the highest possible level and contributing to the patient's general and mental health. The patient may be under the care of a team of medical and dental specialists including the dentist, oral surgeon, dental hygienist, physician, radiation oncologist, registered nurse, and other paramedical auxiliaries. Special rehabilitation personnel, such as a plastic surgeon, speech therapist, psychiatrist, and a maxillofacial prosthodontist, are frequently involved after the treatment phase.

DESCRIPTION

A *neoplasm* is an abnormal, uncontrolled new growth generally classified as benign or malignant. A *benign tumor* is slow-growing, does not invade, does not metastasize to other organs, and is not a threat to life. A *malignant tumor*, in contrast, is faster-growing, invades surrounding tissues, may metastasize to other parts of the body, and is life-threatening. The principal locations of oral tumors are shown in the diagram in figure 8–7 on page 100.

I. Incidence

The prevention of oral cancer through early recognition of suspicious lesions was described on pages 95 and 100. Since the patient suffers no pain or other symptoms from early cancer, detection is dependent on oral inspection by a dentist and a dental hygienist during routine examinations. When discovered early, removal or other treatment can increase the cure rate at the local site, before invasion to adjacent tissues and lymph nodes of the neck.

A. **Number of Oral Cancers**

Including the lips and salivary glands, there are approximately 17,000 new cancers of the oral cavity proper, and another 6400 of the oropharynx annually in the United States. Of those in the oral cavity, about 50 percent occur on the lip and tongue.[1] Males between ages 40 and 65 have the highest numbers of lip and tongue cancers.

B. **Deaths**

Cancer is the second ranking cause of death in the United States. Only diseases of the heart rank higher in adults, and accidents in children under 15 years of age. Approximately 8200 deaths result from cancers of the oral cavity proper and the oropharynx. Of the 4600 in the oral cavity, nearly 2000 are from cancers of the tongue. Estimated annual deaths from lip cancer total 225, of which 200 are males and 25 females.[1] The fewer deaths from lip cancer can be attributed to the accessibility and visibility for early treatment.

II. Etiology and Predisposing Factors

Although the specific etiology of cancer is not known, extensive research is being conducted. There are a number of factors which are considered predisposing to oral cancers. These are very important in the prevention, control, and particularly in early recognition by dentists and dental hygienists. Factors which are believed to contribute to the initiation and development of oral cancer in susceptible people are listed here.[2]

A. **Long-term Exposure to the Sun's Rays**
 1. Squamous cell carcinoma of the lower lip has been related to overexposure. Occupations which require outdoor activity and work have been found in a high percentage of those with lip cancer.
 2. Pigmentation appears to intervene, so that carcinoma of the lower lip is relatively rare in black people.

B. **Heavy Smoking**
 1. Smoking increases the chances of developing oral cancer. Long term exposure to the chemical carcinogens of tobacco as well as trauma from the heat on the tissues are significant.
 2. Holding chewing tobacco or snuff on an area of the oral mucosa will lead to tissue changes and premalignant lesions.
 3. The risk of developing a second

primary oral cancer is greatly increased by continued smoking.[3]

C. **Chronic Alcoholism**
 Chronic alcoholism increases the tendency to develop cancer. Chronic alcoholics have more lesions of the tongue and floor of the mouth than other locations in the oral cavity.

D. **Chronic Inflammation**
 Irritation brought about by ill-fitting dentures, jagged edges of restorations or broken down teeth may lead to a chronic inflammatory response of the mucosa or tongue in the specific area. Such an area has been shown to have a predilection for malignancy.

III. Types of Treatment

A. **Surgical Incision**
 1. Biopsy. Small lesions are removed completely when a biopsy is made.
 2. Radical neck dissection. When the oropharynx and neck are involved, and/or to prevent the spread of cancer to the lymph nodes, there is a wide removal of parts on the affected side, which is called radical neck dissection.

B. **Radiation**
 Therapeutic radiation may be given as the only treatment or it may be used in conjunction with surgery.
 1. Given as a total treatment. Exposures are usually made in fractions, as daily doses.
 2. Given in conjunction with surgery
  a. Preoperative: to reduce the size of the tumor as an aid to surgery by limiting the surgical area.
  b. Postoperatively: to control residual disease.
 3. Types
  a. External
   (1) Orthovoltage. Low-yield radiation may be used for superficial lesions. It has high skin and bone absorp

tion factors, and is not used currently as much as it was in the past before megavoltage radiation was developed.

   (2) Supervoltage or megavoltage. High-yield radiation, which includes cobalt-60, has a sparing effect on skin and bone, but is more penetrating.

  b. Internal: radium implant.

C. **Chemotherapy**

Chemotherapy may be used in conjunction with other types of treatment.

IV. Psychological Considerations

Patient attitudes and feelings are similar to those of any patient with a major chronic disease or disability.[4] As with other diseases with limited hope for cure, strong feelings of hopelessness and despair predominate.

The course of the illness of cancer patients and their survival rates are well known. The very word *cancer* brings fear and anxiety to the patient who knows the diagnosis and of what the treatment will consist. The concerns of a patient may differ at different stages of treatment.

A. **Patient Problems**
1. Early fears and anxieties
   a. Imminent surgery, radiation, or other treatment.
   b. Disfigurement, changes in appearance, and pain.
   c. Extended hospitalization.
   d. Financial stress for family and medical care.
   e. Outcome of the treatment.
2. During and following therapy
   a. Preoccupation with details of examinations, treatments, symptoms, or medications.
   b. Depression and grief which may lead to withdrawal and isolation.
   c. Major concerns include obvious facial deformity, speech difficulty, swallowing difficulty, drooling, and odors from debris collection and tissue changes.

B. **Suggestions for Patient Approach**
1. Provide explanations before and after therapy to prevent misconceptions and apprehensions, and attempt to allay fears.
2. Provide paper and pencil for patient with a speech difficulty to write questions and requests.
3. Show acceptance. Acknowledge the appropriateness of the patient's concerns.
4. Express empathy, but avoid oversolicitousness.
5. Focus on what the patient has, and help to direct thoughts and efforts to restoration of activity.
6. Instill trust and security by demonstrating genuine interest.
7. Assist the patient who was an alcoholic, smoked heavily, or had other habits which have to be eliminated. The patient may need the help of psychiatry, Alcoholics Anonymous, or other type of organization.

V. Preparation for Treatment

Time may be a factor for the patient with advanced malignancy. The aim is to restore the mouth to optimal health in the time provided. The extent and severity of the after effects of radiation are directly related to the condition of the teeth and soft tissues before therapy.

Basic preparation of a patient for whom immediate radiation is not planned follows the same general outline as described on page 606 for a patient with oral surgery. Objectives and treatment include steps to reduce the oral microbial count and provide a better environment for surgical procedures, as well as improving the conditions for healing.

A. **Oral Findings**

Many patients with an oral cancer have not sought dental treatment for many years and have neglected personal care which could maintain oral cleanliness. Therefore it is not unusual to find some or all of the following:

1. Broken-down teeth, some with exposed pulps.
2. Severe periodontal involvement.
3. Ill-fitting dentures.
4. Very poor oral hygiene.

B. **Dental Treatment Plan**

When the patient is to have therapy by radiation, particular attention must be paid to eliminating sources of infection in the oral cavity. Radiation has a detrimental effect on bone and teeth, and bone necrosis and postirradiation dental caries can result. It has been shown, however, that when consideration is given to proper preparation for treatment and supervision of preventive measures during and after treatment, the incidence of harmful effects can be reduced.

Because of the effect of radiation on the bone and other tissues, dental procedures, such as tooth removal, periodontal surgery, and endodontic treatment which could open a channel for infection to reach the bone, are contraindicated after therapy. Therefore the objectives in dental and dental hygiene care prior to radiation are to reduce the incidence of complications of radiation, particularly osteoradionecrosis and postirradiation caries.

The patient's total treatment plan should include at least the following:[5]

1. Removal of nonrestorable teeth. Extensively involved teeth may need extraction due to severity of bone loss, mobility, and other signs of advanced periodontal disease, large carious lesions with pulpal exposures not conducive to endodontic therapy, or periapical pathology.

In the past, treatment frequently called for complete extraction of all teeth that would be in the pathway of radiation whether or not they were broken down or diseased. Now, only teeth that are definitely beyond salvaging are removed. There are patients with such badly broken-down teeth that all will have to be removed. When extractions are needed, trimming of the bone and careful surgical removal of all spicules is necessary. As long a healing period as possible should be allowed before starting radiation because, when bone is irradiated, healing and remodeling will stop.

2. Removal of residual root tips and other subsurface pathology in edentulous areas.
3. Endodontic therapy for essential abutment teeth. Treatment planning for prosthetic replacements must be made in advance so that abutment teeth can receive proper treatment before radiation.
4. Periodontal therapy
   a. Complete scaling and planing with curettage as indicated.
   b. Surgical procedures when time permits follow-up for healing.
   c. Occlusal adjustment.
5. Restoration of carious lesions.
6. Complete preventive program for plaque control and fluoride therapy started at the first appointment.

VI. Effects of Radiation Therapy

Irradiation is the exposure of tissues to x rays or other forms of radiation. The purpose is to destroy cancerous cells. Damage to surrounding normal tissue cannot be avoided, but the severity of damage can be minimized.

Ionizing radiation induces tissue changes, some of which are apparent during the treatment period and may continue for a few weeks or months after cessation of irradiation. Other changes may not be evident until after treatment and may have long-term significance.

Principal effects are on the mucosa, salivary glands, bone, teeth, and taste sensations.[6,7]

A. **Mucosa**
1. Mucositis. Inflammation of the mucosa may appear as early as one week after radiation therapy is started. An unpleasant odor usually results.
   a. Cellular changes. Initially there is an inflammatory response with edema. The tissues may become ulcerated and necrotic with sloughing. Later there is fibrosis.
   b. Clinical signs. Sensitivity to temperature extremes and pressure with an unpleasant odor from the necrotic tissue and plaque collection are commonly found. The patient with dentures may not be able to tolerate wearing them.
   c. Recovery. The severe signs will heal and disappear within a few weeks after radiation is stopped, but the epithelium never completely recovers and tends to be thin and more fragile than normal.
2. Effects on Patient. Toothbrushing and other personal care may be neglected because of the sensitivity of the tissues. A flavored dentifrice may not be tolerated. A soft diet may be required.

B. **Salivary Glands**
Radiation to the salivary glands may be unavoidable depending on the location of the cancerous lesion. The radiation primarily affects the serous gland cells with a lessening of secretion.

1. Xerostomia. A reduced quantity of saliva may be noticed as early as the third or fourth day after the beginning of radiation.
2. Saliva is thickened and sticky, which makes swallowing difficult.
3. Increased acidity with lowered pH.
4. Effects on patient
   a. Difficulty in wearing dentures
   b. Increased dental caries.

C. **Bone**
Radiation damages bone cells and blood vessels within the bone. Changes in the endothelial cells lead to sclerosis of the vessels. The result is change in the growth potential of the bone and lowered resistance to infection.
1. Osteoradionecrosis predisposes the bone to an infection called osteomyelitis. This occurs when microorganisms reach the bone through an ulcer in the mucosa, deep periodontal pocket, periapical lesion, open socket from tooth extraction, or other potential channel for microorganisms. Such infection may develop many years after radiation. It occurs more frequently in the mandible because of the limitation of the blood supply.
2. Symptoms. The early infection may have no symptoms, which complicates control of the disease. Advanced lesions create pain, will be suppurative, and cause halitosis. Treatment is difficult.
3. Prevention. Correct pre- and postradiation procedures have a definite effect on the incidence of osteoradionecrosis. Maintenance of oral cleanliness and health are contributing preventive factors.

D. **Teeth**
1. Dental caries
   a. Description. A distinct form of postirradiation caries can de-

velop in all teeth, not just those in the path of radiation. The lesions develop in the cervical thirds and gradually encircle the necks of the teeth. They appear black or dark brown.

b. Etiologic factors. Xerostomia, neglect of plaque control measures, soft diet related to sore mouth, and changes in oral flora are responsible, not radiation directly.

c. Prevention. Intensified preventive measures for fluoride application and plaque control are needed.

2. Tooth development. Radiation in children can affect the odontogenic cells. A tooth bud may be completely destroyed if irradiated before calcification has started.

3. Sensitivity of teeth. The teeth with marked dental caries are particularly sensitive, but all teeth may react to temperature extremes.

E. **Taste**

Taste can be influenced by direct effects which destroy taste buds, or by changes in the saliva quantity. The loss of taste which occurs soon after the initiation of radiation therapy can be expected to return about six months after therapy ends.

F. **Loss of Appetite**

Because of sore mouth, loss of taste sensation, diminished saliva, and related symptoms, interest in eating fades, and there is a loss of appetite followed by weight loss. Denture wearers who cannot wear their dentures have an added eating problem.

G. **Trismus**

Trismus is spasm of the muscles of mastication. It can result from fibrosis in the muscle fibers which were irradiated. It may occur three to six months after therapy has stopped, and

it makes opening of the mouth very difficult. Exercises and stretching appliances have been used for treatment.[8]

DENTAL HYGIENE CARE

In the not too distant past, the oral cancer patient was doomed to complete tooth removal or at least removal of all teeth in the line of radiation. When the teeth were left in the mouth, inevitable severe radiation caries developed. A high percentage of patients had osteoradionecrosis. Now many teeth are saved, restored, and preserved by an intensive daily preventive program of plaque control and self-applied gel trays.

The dental hygienist's contribution to the preparation of the patient for surgery and radiation, and the continued supervision of oral health and preventive techniques, has special significance. Plaque control, irrigation, rinsing, fluoride application, dietary factors for general health and dental caries prevention, along with specific instrumentation for the health of the periodontal tissues, are major areas of attention for the dental hygienist.

I. Patient Instruction

A. **Plaque Control**

A complete instruction series (pages 388–393) should be started prior to cancer treatment with daily supervision. The patients must understand the reasons for intensive oral health care. Scaling and planing can be accomplished within the same series of appointments as those for the series of lessons for plaque control. Time is usually an important factor when a malignant tumor is involved.

1. Toothbrushing. Sulcular brushing with a soft nylon brush is recommended for the following reasons:

a. Radiation caries occurs primarily at the cervical third, about the necks of the teeth. Emphasis must be placed on keeping the cervical areas plaque-free.

b. Control of gingival health with prevention of gingivitis is necessary. When surgery for oral cancer must be performed before periodontal therapy can be completed, maintenance of the tissues following complete scaling, planing, and curettage is especially needed.

c. Sensitivity of teeth is most frequently associated with the cervical third. Brushing with monofluorophosphate dentifrice can help alleviate sensitivity and prevent dental caries (page 564).

2. Tongue brushing. Bacteria and debris collect on the dry tongue.

3. Dental floss. Proximal surface plaque must be removed. Other interdental devices may be helpful.

B. **Irrigation**

Warm water lavage can be soothing to the oral tissues during radiation therapy. It also provides moisture to counteract the xerostomia. By training the patient prior to therapy in the correct method for use of an irrigator, a habit can be developed.

C. **Rinsing**

Commercial mouthwashes with strong flavoring agents and other ingredients which may irritate the gingiva will not be tolerated by the patient during therapy or for several months following. Warm water rinses with salt or soda in weak solution can be recommended. Hydrogen peroxide, diluted, may prove helpful in debris removal. To minimize oral odors, weak solutions of commercial bleaching agents have been used.[9]

D. **Nutrition and Diet**

Every possible attempt to improve the general health must be made. If the patient is malnourished and debilitated, a high protein diet is needed. Reduction of dietary sucrose is essential to the dental caries prevention program.

A hospitalized patient will be under the supervision of a physician who gives diet prescription orders to the hospital dietitian. The private or clinic physician may make specific recommendations to the patient. Within the framework of the physician's orders, the dental hygienist may also help the patient and the person who will prepare the patient's food at home. Instructions in the preparation of food in a blender may be needed.

Because the mouth is sore and tender, a topical anesthetic in the form of a troche may be needed before eating. During the treatment phase and immediately following radiation therapy, there will be difficulty in swallowing and, because of xerostomia, liquids with a meal will be needed to moisten the food for swallowing. Since the patient suffers from a loss of appetite and difficulty in eating, weight loss is common. Diet selection can be very important so that proper nutrients will be included within the limited diet.

E. **Other Instruction**

1. Reduction of sources of irritation to the mucosa: there must be no smoking or use of alcohol.

2. Care of dental appliances: meticulous plaque removal from new and previous appliances may aid in preventing mouth sores and ulcers.

II. Instrumentation

A. **Mouth Preparation for Radiation and Surgery**

Although complete periodontal treatment prior to treatment of oral cancer would be ideal, time frequently contraindicates prolonged procedures. Minimum preparation, therefore, would include complete calculus removal with root planing.[10] Excessive manipulation of tissues and instrumentation within the few days preceding oral surgery should be avoided.

Whenever possible the following should be completed:

1. Complete scaling, planing, and curettage. These may be accomplished in conjunction with plaque control instruction in a series of quadrant treatments.
2. Removal of all rough and overhanging margins and polishing of all restorations.

B. **Continuing Treatment**

Repeated scaling and planing is needed at each appointment to supplement plaque control efforts by the patient.

III. Fluoride

A. **Dentifrice**

Basic to fluoride therapy is the use of a fluoride dentifrice. When the dentifrice is highly flavored, the tissues may not tolerate it during the period when the mucosa is inflamed.

B. **Gel Tray Applications**

The patient must receive daily fluoride applications while receiving radiation therapy. The incidence of postirradiation caries has been shown to be reduced by use of a custom tray with a fluoride gel or by brushing with the gel after regular brushing.[5,12]

1. Application by patient. The patient can be trained to make the application. During radiation therapy the patient may be preoccupied or too uncomfortable to have interest in carrying out the procedure since it may appear to have no immediate benefit. When it seems apparent that the patient may neglect the fluoride, the dental hygienist or other dental or medical auxiliary must plan to make the daily application. If that is not feasible, a family member can be trained in the procedure.
2. Procedure. Prepare custom trays before the radiation therapy starts, one for each dental arch. Fluoride gel is placed in the tray and fitted over the teeth for five minutes.[5] The patient does not rinse after removal.
3. Effect on sensitivity of the teeth. Topical fluoride on a daily basis benefits the patient by lessening tooth sensitivity.

IV. Recall and Maintenance

A. **Preventive Self-care**

The importance of prevention and control throughout the patient's life cannot be overemphasized. All the steps for care of the gingiva and teeth should be continued daily.

B. **Frequency of Recall**

Examination of the oral mucosa and supervision of gingival and dental health are carried out weekly following the completion of therapy and then monthly as indicated by the condition of the oral tissues.

The dental hygiene recall will include at least the following:

1. Extraoral and intraoral soft tissue inspection (pages 93–95).
2. Gingival examination with pocket measurements and evaluation of bleeding, tooth mobility, and other checks of periodontal disease.
3. Evaluate plaque and plaque removal procedures. Review techniques to motivate and encourage the patient.
4. Instrumentation. Scaling and planing must be completed at each recall.

5. Review of fluoride procedures with a check to be certain the patient has refilled the fluoride prescription.

TECHNICAL HINTS

I. Source of material for professional and patient education:
    American Cancer Society, 219 East 42nd Street, New York, New York 10017.
    State cancer society addresses can be obtained from the New York office.

II. Preparation of a medical and dental history should include questions relative to radiation therapy received by all patients. The effects of radiation on the bone, particularly the mandible, last indefinitely, and osteomyelitis has been known to develop many years after radiation therapy.

III. Patient Referral. When a patient is referred to a specialist or specialty clinic, a check must be made to ascertain that the patient arrives for the appointment. Frightened patients may become confused or may postpone the visit if they do not realize the urgency of the condition.

FACTORS TO TEACH THE PATIENT

I. Plaque control methods, use of irrigation, gel-tray application, and all other details of personal care.

II. Why smoking and use of alcohol must be stopped.

III. Instruction for family members in oral health care for the sick and helpless patient.

References

1. Cancer Statistics, 1975. *CA—A Cancer Journal for Clinicians*, 25, 8, January-February, 1975.
2. Osterkamp, R. W. and Whitten, J. B.: The Etiology and Pathogenesis of Oral Cancer, in *Oral Cancer, Diagnosis, Treatment and Rehabilitation*. American Cancer Society, Professional Education Publication, 1972, 1973, pp. 48–52.
3. Silverman, S. and Griffith, M.: Smoking Characteristics of Patients with Oral Carcinoma and the Risk for Second Oral Primary Carcinoma, *J. Am. Dent. Assoc.*, 85, 637, September, 1972.
4. Rosillo, R. H., Welty, M. J., and Graham, W. P.: The Patient with Maxillo-facial Cancer. II. Psychologic Aspects, *Nurs. Clin. North Am.*, 8, 153, March, 1973.
5. Hayward, J. R., Kerr, D. A., Jesse, R. H., Castigliano, S. G., Lampe, I., and Ingle, J. I.: The Management of Teeth Related to the Treatment of Oral Cancer, in *Maintenance of Oral and General Health in the Management of the Oral Cancer Patient*. American Cancer Society, 1968, 1969, pp. 29–37.
6. Masella, R. P., Cupps, R. E., and Laney, W. R.: Dental Management of the Irradiated Patient, *Northwest Dent.*, 51, 269, September-October, 1972.
7. Sapp, J. P.: The Role of the Dentist in the Management of Patients Irradiated for Oral Cancer, *J. Can. Dent. Assoc.*, 38, 104, March, 1972.
8. Rahn, A. O. and Drone, J. B.: Dental Aspects of the Problems, Care, and Treatment of the Irradiated Oral Cancer Patient, *J. Am. Dent. Assoc.*, 74, 957, April, 1967.
9. Jesse, R. H.: The Treatment of Oral Cancer, in *Oral Cancer, Diagnosis, Treatment and Rehabilitation*. American Cancer Society, Professional Education Publication, 1972, 1973, pp. 36–42.
10. Zegarelli, E. V., Kutscher, A. H., Cohen, D. W., Ketcham, A. S., Ochoa, M., and Stanton, G.: Maintaining the Oral and General Health of the Oral Cancer Patient, in *Maintenance of Oral and General Health in the Management of the Oral Cancer Patient*. American Cancer Society, 1968, 1969, pp. 1–28.
11. Edgerton, M. T., Hoopes, J. E., Marchetta, F. C., Powers, W. E., Gaisford, J. C., Frazell, E. L., and McKee, D.: The Management of Soft Tissue Before, During and After Treatment for Oral Cancer, in *Maintenance of Oral and General Health in the Management of the Oral Cancer Patient*. American Cancer Society, 1968, 1969, pp. 48–61.
12. Miller, J. T. and Shannon, I. L.: A Clinical Report. Water-free Stannous Fluoride Gel and Post-irradiation Caries, *J. Public Health Dent.*, 32, 127, Spring, 1972.

Suggested Readings

Bass, E. B.: Management of Teeth in Jaws To Be Irradiated for Malignancy, in Goldman, H. M., Gilmore, H. W., Irby, W. B., and Olsen, N. H., eds.: *Current Therapy in Dentistry*, Vol. 5. St. Louis, Mosby, 1974, pp. 396–400.
Beumer, J., Silverman, S., and Benak, S. B.: Hard and Soft Tissue Necroses Following Radiation Therapy for Oral Cancer, *J. Prosthet. Dent.*, 27, 640, June, 1972.

Billingsley, L.: Effects from Radiation Therapy of Oral Carcinoma, *J. Am. Dent. Hyg. Assoc.*, 45, 305, September-October, 1971.

Bottomly, W. K. and Ebersole, J. H.: Guidelines for Dental Care When Patients Receive Radiation Therapy to the Head and Neck, *Oral Surg.*, 22, 252, August, 1966.

Carl, W., Schaaf, N. G., and Chen, T. Y.: Oral Care of Patients Irradiated for Cancer of the Head and Neck, *Cancer*, 30, 448, August, 1972.

Elzay, R. P., King, E. R., and Dettman, P.: Dental Prostheses and Radiation to the Jaws: A Survey of Prosthodontists and Radiotherapists, *J. Am. Dent. Assoc.*, 77, 856, October, 1968.

Goode, R. L.: Head and Neck Operations after Radiation Therapy, *Oral Surg.*, 36, 170, August, 1973.

Marciani, R. D. and Piezia, R. A.: Management of Teeth in the Irradiated Patient, *J. Am. Dent. Assoc.*, 88, 1021, May, 1974.

Miller, R. N.: Psychological Problems of Patients with Head and Neck Cancer, in *Rehabilitation of the Cancer Patient*, Chicago, Year Book, 1972, pp. 19–24.

Poyton, H. G.: The Effects of Radiation on Teeth, *Oral Surg.*, 26, 639, November, 1968.

Rahn, A. O. and Boucher, L. J.: *Maxillofacial Prosthetics*. Philadelphia, Saunders, 1970, pp. 31–82.

Shafer, K. N., Sawyer, J. R., McCluskey, A. M., Beck, E. L., and Phipps, W. J.: *Medical-Surgical Nursing*, 5th ed. St. Louis, Mosby, 1971, pp. 571–575.

Stark, R. B.: Oral Cancer: Reconstruction and Rehabilitation, in *Oral Cancer, Diagnosis, Treatment and Rehabilitation*. American Cancer Society, Professional Education Publication, 1972, 1973, pp. 43–47.

Stern, D.: The Influence of Systemic Cancer on the Oral Tissues, *Oral Surg.*, 29, 229, February, 1970.

Strauss, S. I. and Spatz, S. S.: Irradiated Dentitions: The Dentist's Responsibilities, *J. Prosthet. Dent.*, 27, 209, February, 1972.

Welty, M. J.: The Patient with Maxillofacial Cancer. I. Surgical Treatment and Nursing Care, *Nurs. Clin. North Am.*, 8, 137, March, 1973.

Types and Pathology of Tumors

Bhaskar, S. N.: *Synopsis of Oral Pathology*, 4th ed. St. Louis, Mosby, 1973, pp. 461–488.

Castigliano, S. G.: Oral Cancer, in Burket L. W.: *Oral Medicine*, 6th ed. Philadelphia, Lippincott, 1971, pp. 581–640.

Giunta, J.: Oral Pathology, in Dunn, M. J., ed.: *Dental Auxiliary Practice*, Module 3. Baltimore, Williams and Wilkins, 1975, pp. 98–115.

Kerr, D. A. and Ash, M. M.: *Oral Pathology*, 3rd ed. Philadelphia, Lea & Febiger, 1971, pp. 111–131.

Scopp, I. W.: *Oral Medicine*, 2nd ed. St. Louis, Mosby, 1973, pp. 325–368.

Shafer, W. G., Hine, M. K., and Levy, B. M.: *A Textbook of Oral Pathology*, 3rd ed. Philadelphia, Saunders, 1974, pp. 81–211.

Chapter 46

The Patient with a Cleft Lip or Palate

The patient with a cleft lip or palate or both may be a dental cripple without prolonged rehabilitative supervision. Treatment and care require the united efforts of nearly all of the dental specialists as well as the plastic surgeon, speech therapist, psychiatrist, otolaryngologist, social worker, and vocational counselor. The dental hygienist is an important member of the team responsible for preventive oral care measures.

Cleft lip, cleft palate, or both are found in one out of approximately 750 live births. Speaking ability and appearance are necessarily the first factors considered when the long-range treatment program is planned since the objective is to help the patient lead a normal life. Dental personnel need to maintain a current list of the health agencies, clinics, and other community resources where the patient and his family may obtain assistance for the various phases of treatment and habilitation.

DESCRIPTION

Classification of Cleft Lip and Palate

The classification is based on the interference with embryologic formation of the palate as it develops from the premaxillary region toward the uvula in a definite pattern. There may be an interference with normal development of the palate at one age level of the embryo and the normal pattern may be reestablished at a later age. Such interferences would modify the classification suggested below.

All degrees are found from an insignificant notch in the mucous membrane of the lip or uvula which produces no functional disability, to the complete cleft defined by Class 6 of this classification. The first six classes are illustrated in figure 46–1.

Class 1. Cleft of the tip of the uvula.
Class 2. Cleft of the uvula (bifid uvula).
Class 3. Cleft of the soft palate.
Class 4. Cleft of the soft and hard palates.
Class 5. Cleft of the soft and hard palates which continues through the alveolar ridge on one side of the premaxilla; usually associated with cleft lip of the same side.
Class 6. Cleft of the soft and hard palates which continues through the alveolar ridge on both sides, leaving a free premaxilla; usually associated with bilateral cleft lip.
Class 7. Submucous cleft in which there is imperfect muscle union across

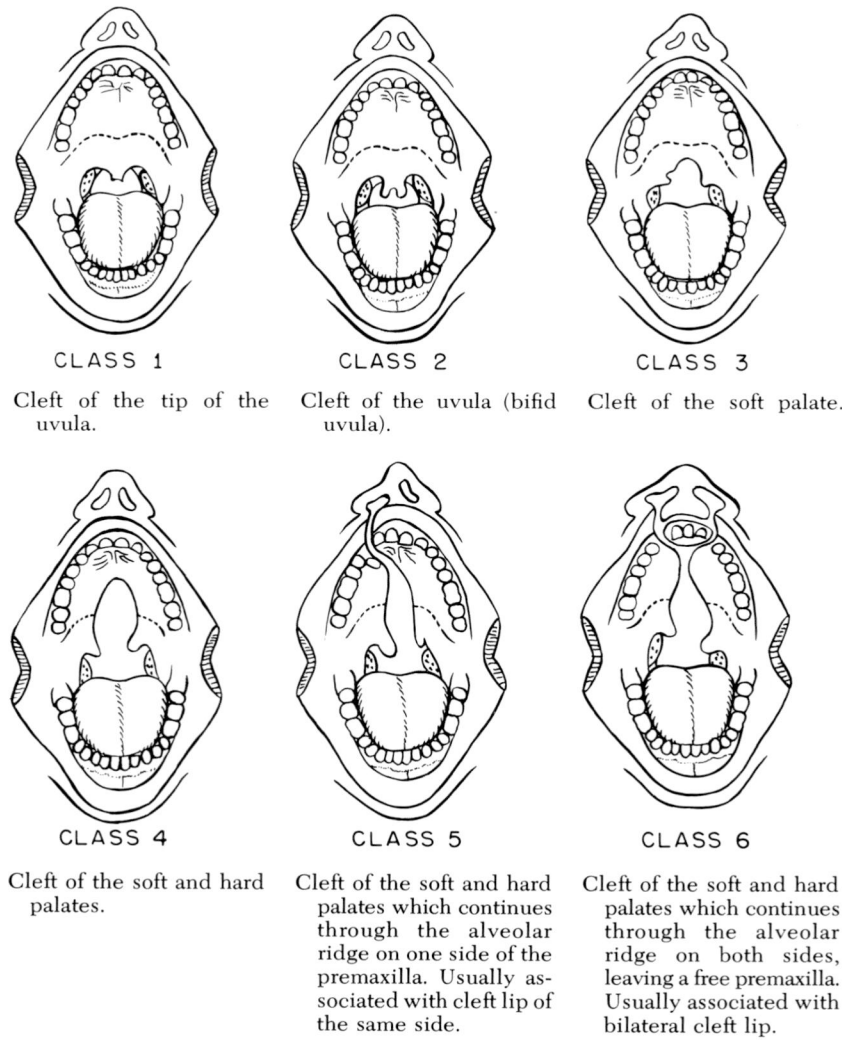

CLASS 1 — Cleft of the tip of the uvula.

CLASS 2 — Cleft of the uvula (bifid uvula).

CLASS 3 — Cleft of the soft palate.

CLASS 4 — Cleft of the soft and hard palates.

CLASS 5 — Cleft of the soft and hard palates which continues through the alveolar ridge on one side of the premaxilla. Usually associated with cleft lip of the same side.

CLASS 6 — Cleft of the soft and hard palates which continues through the alveolar ridge on both sides, leaving a free premaxilla. Usually associated with bilateral cleft lip.

Figure 46–1. Classification of cleft lip and palate. (Courtesy of O. E. Beder.)

the soft palate. The palate is short, the uvula often bifid, a groove is situated at the midline of the soft palate, and the closure to the pharynx is incompetent.

II. Etiology

A. Embryology[1,2]

Cleft lip and palate represent a failure of normal fusion of embryonic processes during development. For-mation of the lip occurs between the fourth and seventh weeks in utero. The development of the palate takes place during the eighth to twelfth weeks. Fusion begins in the premaxillary region and continues backward toward the uvula.

B. Predisposing Factors

Heredity is believed to exert a major influence. A number of other factors have been considered and some of these have been shown effective in animal experimentation. Examples are infectious diseases in the mother, nutritional deficiencies, or mechanical interferences in the fetus. It is generally believed that both genetic and environmental forces are involved.

III. Oral Characteristics

A. Tooth Development

Disturbances in the normal development of the tooth buds are more marked in patients with clefts, and there is a higher incidence of missing and supernumerary teeth, as well as other abnormalities of tooth form.[3,4]

B. Malocclusion

A high percentage of cleft lip and palate patients require orthodontic care.

C. Open Palate

Provides direct communication with the nasal cavity.

D. Muscle Coordination

A lack of coordinate movements of lips, tongue, cheeks, floor of mouth, and throat may exist and lead to compensatory habits formed in the attempt to produce normal sounds while speaking.

E. Gingival Disturbances

These are created by effects of local irritants as they are influenced by malocclusion, displaced teeth, possible inability to keep lips closed, as well as difficulties in accomplishing adequate personal oral care.

F. Dental Caries

The incidence of dental caries should be no different from noncleft patients, except that predisposing factors such as malocclusion, problems of mastication, and dietary selection factors may be intensified.

G. Treated Case

1. Suture lines from surgery may be evident.

2. Removable prosthodontic appliance (page 628).

IV. General Physical Characteristics

A. Other Congenital Anomalies

Incidence is higher than in noncleft people.

B. Facial Deformity

Depression of nostril on the side with the cleft lip; deficiency of upper lip in which it may be short or retroposed, lower lip may be overprominent.

C. Infections

Predisposition to upper respiratory and middle ear infections.

D. Hearing Loss

This may result from improper ventilation and drainage of the Eustachian canals which can lead to infection. The cleft exposes the nasopharynx region to oral debris and microorganisms which can enter the Eustachian canals. Adenoid tissue sometimes grows over the openings of the canals and prevents drainage.

E. Speech

Difficulty in making certain sounds; nasal tones produced. Anatomical structure is not considered the only contributing factor to the speech problem. It may be related to the hearing loss or psychological factors related to inferior feelings or parental attitude.

F. Undernourishment

Undernourishment may result when feeding problems continue for a long period.

V. Psychological Characteristics

Most cleft lip and palate patients do not have personality problems but realization of the social effects of speech and appearance makes it easy to understand why some of them exhibit evidences of maladjustment. The ridicule of contemporaries soon teaches even the small child that he is "different." Parental acceptance or rejection no doubt can be a strong influence in adjustment. A few possible characteristics are suggested here.

A. **Self-consciousness**

Hypersensitivity to taunts or obvious pity.

B. **Feelings of Inferiority**

The result may be a person who is quiet, unresponsive, and withdrawn or one who is openly brash or rebellious until rapport is established.

C. **Interference with Educational Adjustment**

Some drop out of school when they reach high school age because of personality difficulties.

VI. Treatment

A. **Cleft Lip**

Surgical union of the cleft lip is made early, usually between two and twelve weeks of age. The infant's general health is a determining factor, and some surgeons wait until the birth weight is regained or the weight has reached twelve pounds.

The closure aids in feeding, helps development of the premaxilla and growth of the lip, and may also help to close partially the palatal cleft. The psychological effect on parents and family members can be more favorable when the lip operation is performed before the infant is taken home from the hospital although this is not always indicated.

B. **Cleft Palate**

It is generally agreed that treatment should be undertaken as soon as technically possible during the preschool years after the eruption of the primary teeth, which is usually between 30 and 36 months. Occlusion has a strong influence on the development of palatal dimensions and

growth is rapid during this period. If surgery were to be performed too early there would be interference with normal growth. The combined efforts of many specialists are required.

1. Purposes for early treatment
   a. Improve child's well-being.
   b. Aid child's mental development.
   c. Prevent malnourishment by improving the feeding apparatus.
   d. Aid in development of the speech pattern.
   e. Reduce possibilities of repeated infections of the nasopharyngeal region.
2. Maxillofacial surgery: closure of the palate is accomplished by surgery or prosthodontics or both. Surgery provides direct union of the existing tissue that has been moved to a more desirable position for function.

C. **Prosthodontics**

A removable appliance is designed to provide closure of the palatal opening and/or to complete the palatopharyngeal valving required for speech.

1. Types of appliances
   a. *Prosthesis.* Artificial replacement for a missing part.
   b. *Obturator.* Removable appliance designed to close an opening such as a cleft of the hard palate.
   c. *Speech Aid.* A removable appliance related to the soft palate which provides a means for palatopharyngeal valving for speech.
2. Purposes of the appliance (it may be designed to accomplish one or all of the following factors)
   a. Closure of the palate.
   b. Replacement of missing teeth.
   c. Scaffolding, to fill out the upper lip.
   d. Masticatory function.

e. Restoration of vertical dimension.

f. Postorthodontic retainer.

D. **Orthodontics**

Treatment may be initiated as early as three years of age depending on the problems of dentofacial development.

E. **Speech Therapy**

Training may be started with very young children and is particularly emphasized after the surgical or prosthodontic treatment has been accomplished.

F. **Operative Dentistry (Pedodontist or General Dental Practitioner)**

A major problem can be dental caries leading to tooth loss. With missing teeth, major difficulties arise related to all phases of treatment particularly the retention of the prosthesis. Preservation of the primary teeth is very important.

DENTAL HYGIENE CARE

Preventive measures for preservation of the teeth and their supporting structures are essential to the success of the special care needed for the habilitation of the cleft palate patient. Each phase of dental hygiene care and instruction which is important for all patients takes on even greater significance in the light of the magnified problems of the dental cripple.

Every attempt should be made to avoid the need for removal of teeth since this patient has enough oral problems without also being edentulous. Primary and permanent teeth are needed for the stabilization of a speech aid or obturator and success of all treatment procedures. Understanding by the patient and the parents of the value of preventive procedures is accomplished through explanation and instruction.

When the patient has not had specialized care, the dental hygienist has a responsibility in working with the dentist to arrange referral to an available agency, clinic, or private practice specialist.

I. Objectives for Appointment Planning

Frequent recall appointments, scheduled every three or four months, are usually needed during the maintenance phase of the patient's care.

A. To review plaque control measures and provide encouragement for the patient in maintaining the health of the supporting structures and the cleanliness of the obturator or speech aid.

B. To remove all calculus and smooth the surfaces as a supplement to the patient's personal daily care procedures.

C. To make topical fluoride applications at proper intervals for both primary and permanent dentitions, and supervise self-applied daily fluoride.

II. Appointment Psychology

A. Speech may be almost indiscernible, although with repeated contact, understanding is developed.

1. Avoid embarrassment produced by constantly asking the patient to repeat what has been said.

2. Provide pencil and paper for the older child to write his requests or comments.

3. Let parent or other person accompanying small child interpret.

B. Hearing loss: depending on severity, approach is similar to that for speech difficulties listed above. Suggestions for care of patients with hearing problems are described on page 672.

C. Avoid solicitousness or obvious pity. Approach as a normal patient.

D. Provide motivations for quiet unresponsive or bold rebellious types which will help them gain an objective approach to the care of their mouths.

III. Sterile Techniques

Although procedures should be the same for all patients, it should be remembered that the open fissure lines make the cleft palate patient particularly susceptible to infections.

IV. Instrumentation

Techniques are adapted to the oral characteristics. All objectives of scaling and other instrumentation have particular implications for the cleft palate patient.

A. Malaligned teeth: adjust scaling and polishing procedures.

B. Free premaxilla related to bilateral cleft of alveolar ridge: avoid undue pressure with finger rests or instrument to prevent movement of the part.

C. Area of recent surgery: avoid pressure.

D. Sensitive, enlarged gingival tissue which bleeds readily.
   1. Begin plaque control instruction first before any instrumentation.
   2. Continue plaque control instruction as small sections of scaling are done over several appointments.
   3. Arrange follow-up appointments to check response of tissue.

E. Open fissures: prevent debris, pieces of calculus, or polishing abrasive particles from passing into or being retained in the clefts.

F. Lack of coordinated movements: small children especially may need instruction in how to rinse when this is a new procedure for them.

G. Prosthesis or speech aid: use same procedures and precautions as for cleaning a removable denture (pages 548–550).

V. Topical Application of Fluoride Agent

Free premaxilla or short upper lip may complicate cotton roll placement.

VI. Patient Instruction

A. **Personal Oral Care Procedures**

The self-conscious patient with an inferiority complex may actually fear or exhibit rejection toward his oral cavity. With a small child the parents may be afraid of damaging the deformed areas or hurting the child if cleansing methods are employed. The dental hygienist must have an empathetic and sympathetic approach and plan for continued instruction over a long period of time.

1. Teeth and gingiva
   a. Select toothbrush, brushing method, and auxiliary aids according to the individual needs.
   b. Adapt techniques for patient with free premaxilla to prevent its movement. A soft nylon brush is usually indicated.
   c. Suggest rinsing procedures (page 342).
      (1) Mild hypertonic salt solution for tissue healing.
      (2) Solution of bicarbonate of soda when there is a tendency for heavy mucinous plaques to form.
   d. Instigate daily self-applied fluoride: oral rinse and fluoride dentifrice (pages 439–441).

2. Prosthesis or speech aid
   Halitosis may be a real problem when the prosthesis forms the soft palate and the floor of the nasal cavity because of the accumulation of mucus secreted by the nasal cavity surfaces.
   a. Instruct patient in the need for frequent removal of appliance for cleansing, particularly following eating.
   b. Method for cleaning prosthesis: same as for removable partial denture (pages 368–370).

B. Diet

1. Need for a varied diet which includes adequate proportions of all essential food groups (table 28–1, page 403).
2. Need for providing gingival stimulation: fibrous foods, particularly fresh fruits and vegetables. Patient's malocclusion and cleft may present difficulties, but usually the patient can adapt.
3. Need for prevention of dental caries: limitation of foods containing sucrose, particularly for between-meal snacks. Procedures of the dental caries control study are recommended (pages 410–414).

VII. Dental Hygiene Care Related to Oral Surgery

A. Presurgery (pages 605–608).

Objectives have particular significance because the cleft palate patient is unusually susceptible to infections of the upper respiratory area and middle ear. Every precaution should be taken to prevent complications.

B. Postsurgery Personal Oral Care

In certain of the palate operations, arm restraints are applied to prevent accidental damage to the repaired region. After each feeding (liquid diet for several days, soft diet for the next week), the mouth must be rinsed carefully. Brushing must be accomplished with great care, usually by the parent or hospital attendant, to avoid damage to the healing suture lines. In certain cases the toothbrush with suction attachment may be useful (page 585).

References

1. Sicher, H. and Bhaskar, S. N., eds.: *Orban's Oral Histology and Embryology*, 7th ed. St. Louis, Mosby, 1972, pp. 14–15.
2. Permar, D.: *Oral Embryology and Microscopic Anatomy*, 5th ed. Philadelphia, Lea & Febiger, 1972, pp. 2–14.
3. Olin, W. H.: Dental Anomalies in Cleft Lip and Palate Patients, *Angle Orthodont.*, *34*, 119, April, 1964.
4. Jordan, R. E., Kraus, B. S., and Neptune, C. M.: Dental Abnormalities Associated with Cleft Lip and/or Palate, *Cleft Palate J.*, *3*, 22, January, 1966.

Suggested Readings

Dennis, C. G.: Preventive Therapy in the Prosthetic Treatment of Congenital and Developmental Anomalies, *Austral. Dent. J.*, *10*, 292, August, 1965.

Fishman, L. S.: Factors Related to Tooth Number, Eruption Time, and Tooth Position in Cleft Palate Individuals, *J. Dent. Child.*, *37*, 303, July-August, 1970.

Greene, J. C., Vermillion, J. R., Hay, S., Gibbens, S. F., and Kerschbaum, S.: Epidemiologic Study of Cleft Lip and Cleft Palate in Four States, *J. Am. Dent. Assoc.*, *68*, 387, March, 1964.

Honke, A.: Total Rehabilitation of the Cleft Lip—Cleft Palate Child, *J. Am. Dent. Hyg. Assoc.*, *47*, 155, May-June, 1973.

Jacobson, B. N. and Rosenstein, S. W.: The Cleft Palate Patient: Dental Help Needed, *J. Dent. Child.*, *37*, 105, March-April, 1970.

Kay, B. S.: Anomalies of Speech in Cases of Cleft Lip and Palate, *Br. Dent. J.*, *120*, 20, January 4, 1966.

Marshall, D.: Cleft Lip and Palate Deformities, *Dent. Radiogr. Photogr.*, *46*, 3, No. 1, 1973.

Moller, P.: Treatment of the Handicapped Child, in Finn, S. B.: *Clinical Pedodontics*, 4th ed. Philadelphia, Saunders, 1973, pp. 562–578.

Nizel, A. E.: *Nutrition in Preventive Dentistry: Science and Practice.* Philadelphia, Saunders, 1972, pp. 440–441.

Olin, W. H.: Cleft Lip and Palate Rehabilitation, *Am. J. Orthodont.*, *52*, 126, February, 1966.

Poole, A. E.: Genetics of Cleft Lip and Cleft Palate, *Dent. Clin. North Am.*, *19*, 171, January, 1975.

Pruzansky S.: Cleft Lip and Palate: Therapy and Prevention, *J. Am. Dent. Assoc.*, *87*, 1048, October, 1973 (Special Issue).

Rosen, M. S.: The Function of Maxillofacial Prosthetics for Congenital Oral Facial Defects, *J. Prosthet. Dent.*, *30*, 632, October, 1973 (Part 2).

Scott, J. H.: The Embryology of Cleft Palate and Hare Lip, *Br. Dent. J.*, *120*, 17, January 4, 1966.

Stark, R. B., ed.: *Cleft Palate; a Multidiscipline Approach.* New York, Harper & Row, 1968, 339 pp.

Williams, A. C., Rothman, B. N., and Seidman, I. H.: Management of a Feeding Problem in an Infant with Cleft Palate, *J. Am. Dent. Assoc.*, *77*, 81, July, 1968.

Wong, L. P. and Weiss, C. E.: A Clinical Assessment of Obturator-wearing Cleft Palate Patients, *J. Prosthet. Dent.*, *27*, 632, June, 1972.

Wylie, H. L. and McWilliams, B. J.: Guidance Materials for Parents of Children with Clefts, *Cleft Palate J.*, *2*, 123, April, 1965.

Chapter 47

The Patient with Epilepsy

Epilepsy is not a disease entity but is rather a term used to describe a symptom or group of symptoms of disordered function of the central nervous system. A person with epilepsy is susceptible to recurrent involuntary loss of consciousness or awareness with or without convulsive movements or spasms.

It has been estimated that two million people over the age of six in the United States have some form of epilepsy. A small percentage are hospitalized.

The patient's medical history should reveal a susceptibility to seizures and the physician must be contacted when additional information other than that provided by the patient is required. The well-controlled patient who is under anticonvulsant therapy usually presents no specific problems. An uncontrolled patient may require special treatment such as extra sedation or an increase of the anticonvulsant. A knowledge of symptoms is important in all cases and dental personnel should know and be able to apply first aid measures in or out of the dental office.

Except for effects left by accidents occurring during a seizure, oral manifestations are limited to epileptics being treated with sodium diphenylhydantoin

(Dilantin) which may induce a gingival hyperplasia. All patients are advised by their physicians to live a moderate life and pay strict attention to general health rules. Care of the oral cavity becomes important both for its relationship to general health and to oral accidents which may occur during a severe convulsion.

DESCRIPTION[1,2]

I. Precipitating Factors Which May Occur in Those Not Medicated

A. Arousal of anxiety through some immediate interpersonal conflict or through fantasy of such a conflict.

B. Emotional disturbances from excitement, fear, frustration, or tensions, particularly in teenage patients.

C. Fatigue secondary to sleep deprivation.

D. Sleep, or arousal from sleep.

E. Flickering lights, sudden sounds, or other physical or sensory stimuli.

II. Types of Seizures

The three major types of seizures are *grand mal*, *petit mal*, and psychomotor.

Loss of awareness or a change in level of consciousness is characteristic. The frequency of attacks varies from several a day to one every few years in those that are not completely controlled.

A. **Grand Mal (Major Epilepsy)**
 1. *The Aura or Warning.* Lasts from a moment to several seconds and may consist of one of a number of sensations suggested below. Not all of the patients experience an aura.
   a. Numbness or tingling.
   b. Strange feeling over stomach.
   c. Hallucination of a special sense: flashes of light, noises, peculiar taste or smell.
   d. Twitching or stiffness of certain muscles.
 2. *The Seizure*
   a. Loss of consciousness: sudden and complete; patient falls. If patient is in dental chair he may slide out.
   b. Entire voluntary musculature experiences continuous contraction: lasts from one to three minutes, occasionally longer; bladder, and rarely rectum, may be emptied.
   c. Muscles of chest and pharynx may contract at same time thus forcing air out which results in a peculiar sound known as the "epileptic cry."
   d. Color: pale at first, then superficial veins become gorged; chest becomes fixed and aeration of blood ceases, leading to cyanosis of face.
   e. Pupils dilate.
   f. Intermittent muscular contractions follow, rapidly at first, then less frequently. If tongue is between the teeth it may be bitten.
   g. Respiration begins to return. Saliva which could not previously have been swallowed may become mixed with air and appear as foam.
   h. Postconvulsive coma: rigid pupils, noisy respiration, profuse perspiration, cyanosed lips, and complete relaxation of body muscles.
   i. Patient emerges in a cloudy state.
 3. *Postconvulsive Phase.* Headache, muscle aches, and drowsiness; usually falls into a deep sleep.
 4. *Occurrence.* Some patients have seizures only during sleep or an hour or so after waking. Others have a random distribution day and night.
 5. *Status Epilepticus.* Series of seizures without regaining total awareness between; danger to life.

B. **Petit Mal (Minor Epilepsy)**
 1. *The Seizure*
   a. Loss of consciousness for five to thirty seconds.
   b. Patient does not fall; posture becomes fixed; may drop whatever he has in his hand.
   c. May become pale.
   d. May have rhythmic twitching of eyelids, eyebrows, or head.
   e. Resumes activities: may or may not be aware of attack.
 2. *Occurrence.* Most common in children 3 to 15 years. Seizures may occur up to as many as 100 times each day. Individual *petit mal* seizures occur more frequently than *grand mal.*

C. **Psychomotor**
 1. *The Seizure*
   a. Trance-like state with confusion: usually for few minutes, sometimes for hours.
   b. No loss of consciousness.
   c. May manifest purposeless move-

ments or actions followed by confusion, incoherent speech, ill humor, bad temper; frequently does not remember what happened during the attack.

2. *Occurrence.* Primarily a disorder of adults and older children.

III. Etiology[1,2]

Epilepsy is a symptom of a disorder of the central nervous system, the explanation for which has not been clearly defined. During infancy seizures can be related to congenital maldevelopment or a birth injury, while in older children and adolescents trauma, infections, or idiopathic causes also are possible. In middle age and older, tumors, vascular disease, and the other symptomatic factors listed below are predominant.

A. **Idiopathic or Cryptogenic Epilepsy**
1. May have innate flaw in brain which causes nerve cells to effect the seizure.
2. Includes approximately 77 percent of all epilepsies.
3. Tends to manifest early in life; majority of cases between ages 2 and 14.
4. Heredity.

B. **Symptomatic or Acquired Epilepsy**
1. Known cerebral lesion brings about dysfunction leading to seizures.
   a. Tumor.
   b. Trauma.
   c. Infection.
   d. Degenerative brain disease.
   e. Alcoholism and drug addiction may bring related symptoms.
2. Occurrence: not related to age, but generally a symptomatic cause is suspected in epilepsy which manifests after age 20.

V. Oral Manifestations[3,4,5,6,]

Epilepsy in itself has no oral manifestations. Patients being treated with the

anticonvulsant, sodium diphenylhydantoin (Dilantin), are subject to gingival enlargement. The enlarged tissue results from hyperplasia and inflammation. The condition is known as diphenylhydantoin-induced hyperplasia or Dilantin-induced hyperplasia.

When inflammation is kept to a minimum through strict plaque control and oral physical therapy measures, the hyperplasia is not as great or may be completely prevented.[6] Other oral structures may show the effects of accidents during severe seizures.

A. **Gingiva: Diphenylhydantoin-induced Hyperplasia**
1. *Occurrence*
   a. From 25 to 50 percent of patients treated with the drug develop hyperplasia. The greatest frequency is in younger persons after initiation of the drug.
   b. Manifests from a few weeks to a few years.
   c. Size of lesion: affected by duration of treatment and dosage.
   d. Does not occur in edentulous areas.
2. *Primary Lesion*
   a. Hyperplasia of isolated interdental papillae.
   b. Granular, highly stippled.
   c. Firm, pale coral pink, resilient.
   d. Size: gradual increase to form an elevated mass (bulb-like); clefts may form within individual papillae.
   e. No tendency to hemorrhage.
   f. No pain.
3. *Advanced*
   a. Massive tissue fold partially obstructs tooth from view.
   b. Level of gingival attachment not disturbed.
4. *Most Severe*
   a. Attached gingiva becomes involved.

b. Hyperplasia appears continuous from tooth to tooth.

c. Interference during mastication: pain.

5. *Secondary Inflammation*

a. Causes: local irritants including calculus and soft deposits, and the effects of overhanging restorations or large carious lesions in retaining debris and dental plaque.

b. Appearance: edema and other signs of inflammation with increased tissue size greater than that of a primary lesion; increased bleeding tendency and soreness.

c. Orthodontic appliances: marked enlargement with hyperplastic tissue extending over the fixed appliances, continually bleeding gingiva, bad odor, and virtually impossible to keep clean.

6. *Treatment*

a. Rigid plaque control and oral physical therapy measures starting when the drug is first prescribed when possible.

b. Prescription: although diphenylhydantoin is the drug of choice for frequent *grand mal* seizures, other drugs have been used in order to reduce the gingival hyperplasia.

c. Positive pressure appliance: the use of a custom-fitted rubber mouthpiece designed to exert pressure against the gingival margin has been shown effective for certain patients.[7,8] In one study, wearing of the pressure device was a stimulus to improved personal daily care.[9]

d. Surgical removal: gingivectomy-gingivoplasty, followed by plaque control and oral physical therapy measures.[10]

B. **Other Oral Structures: Effects of Accidents During Seizure**

1. Scars of lips and tongue.
2. Fractured teeth.
3. Cuspal wear due to bruxism.

V. Psychological Characteristics[1,11]

There is no characteristic personality of epileptics. A good part of any maladjustment exhibited by the noninstitutionalized patients can be blamed on the attitude of society toward them. They react individually according to their feelings toward themselves and how others look upon their illness.

Occupation is limited as the epileptic cannot be permitted to participate in activities which provide hazards in the event of a seizure. This is particularly depressing to adults who have acquired epilepsy since reaching the working age and who must change their vocation.

In studying the behavior and personality of the epileptic, it should be clear that the symptoms suggested below may appear in part or may not appear at all.

A. **Injury to Central Nervous System**

1. Variability of mood without apparent cause; changes in disposition.
2. Restlessness; overactivity; at times has seeming excess energy; difficulty at times in sitting still.
3. Irritability: related to impatience and ease in becoming aroused to aggressive activity.
4. Short attention span due to medications
   a. Varying difficulty in powers of concentration and remembering what has been learned.
   b. Distractibility; difficulty in continuous application to task at hand.
5. Difficulty in reasoning, problem-solving situations: difficulty in mathematics for school-age child.

B. **Attitude Toward Illness**

1. Dread or anxiety toward having a seizure.
2. Irritation: oversolicitousness of

parents or others hampers activity and provides aggravation.

3. Despair and resentment: over being excluded from school and community activities; may create antisocial tendencies.

4. Aggressiveness: reaction to parental rejection.

5. Shyness: related to state of insecurity.

6. Depression over appearance of enlarged gingiva.[12]

DENTAL HYGIENE CARE

I. Objectives

A. Maintain oral health as a part of general health. One fundamental in the treatment of epileptics is the maintenance of optimum physical health.

B. Prevent tooth loss leading to need for dentures.
1. Severe bruxism can cause wear and fracture of a denture.
2. Denture is a hazard during seizures.

C. For epileptics with diphenylhydantoin-induced hyperplasia: strict oral care.
1. To prevent complications of inflammation and hemorrhage resulting from deposits on the teeth which cause irritation to the gingival tissue.
2. To prevent halitosis resulting from debris accumulation in clefts and crevices of the hyperplastic gingiva.

II. Appointment Planning

A. **Recall Intervals**
1. Sufficient to maintain tissues in optimum health.
2. Patient with diphenylhydantoin-induced hyperplasia may require frequent appointments.

B. **Length of Appointment**
1. Adjust time to degree of illness.
2. Patients are advised by physician to avoid fatigue.
3. Recognize restlessness, particularly in children.

C. **Time of Day**
Avoid stressful times when fatigue or other possible precipitating factors may become involved. Advice of patient's physician may be helpful.

D. **Appointment Keeping**
Drugs used in treatment, if hypnotic, tend to make patient drowsy; may sleep more than an average person.
1. Be understanding when patient is late or misses an appointment.
2. Plan telephone reminder at opportune time if patient is chronically late.

III. Patient Approach

Each of the physical and possible psychological characteristics should be given consideration during the appointment.

A. Treat as an ordinary individual with patience and sympathy, but avoid oversolicitousness.

B. Impress the patient with his importance and responsibility; express confidence in him.

C. Avoid discussions or actions which may create anxiety; explain procedures to be used.

D. Encourage self-expression particularly if the patient tends to be quiet and withdrawn and has narrowed interests.

E. Do not mistake drowsiness (effect of drugs) for inattentiveness.

F. Recognize possible impairment of memory when reviewing personal oral care procedures.

G. Plan instruction for short periods, in accord with patient's shortened attention span.

H. Appeal to patient's lagging interest in personal appearance: develop interest in caring for his mouth; commend his successes.

IV. Clinical Techniques

A. Submarginal Examination

In patients without periodontal involvement, pockets which result from gingival hyperplasia will be relative (page 176), and instrumentation will be applied to enamel.

B. Instrumentation

Tissue evaluation: the gingival pocket wall is firm and hard. The effect of the diphenylhydantoin is to produce a fibrotic connective tissue hyperplasia.

C. Irrigation

Following scaling and polishing, thorough irrigation to remove particles and polishing agent is important to tissue response.

V. Patient Instruction

A. Plaque Control and Oral Physical Therapy

1. Rigid toothbrushing routine to aid in prevention of accumulation of deposits. An automatic brush is recommended particularly when the patient requires assistance in brushing.
2. Interdental cleaning methods as well as oral physical therapy are helpful. Use of an interdental stimulator for gingival massage, pressure, and reshaping may help. Instruction with each device used should be meticulous, exacting, and repeated frequently.

B. Diet

1. Physician's recommendations frequently include the following:

   a. Normal diet: same as for other members of the family.
   b. Moderate amount of food; no alcohol.
   c. Avoid long periods without food: low blood sugar may precipitate a seizure.
2. Dental caries control: since patient may eat frequently, need for suggestions for foods which do not contain sucrose.
3. Gingival health: need for helping patient understand nutritive foods of basic groups and detergent foods.

C. Instruction Related to Seizure

1. Preservation of natural teeth: to prevent need for removable dentures which may provide a hazard during a *grand mal* seizure.
2. Removable dentures should be removed at night as seizures frequently occur shortly after patient retires.

VI. First Aid[13]

No attempt should be made to stop the convulsion or to restrain the patient. An outline for procedure appears in table 54–1 on page 732. Some additional suggestions for application to the dental office are included here. First aid is generally required only for *grand mal* seizures.

A. Objectives

1. To prevent body injury.
2. To prevent accidents related to the oral structures, such as:

   a. Tongue bite.
   b. Broken or dislocated teeth.
   c. Dislocated or fractured jaw.
   d. Broken fixed or removable dentures.

B. Preparation for Appointment

When patient's medical history indicates epilepsy, precautions may prevent complications should a seizure occur.

1. First aid materials should be readied in a convenient place.

2. Have patient remove dentures for duration of appointment.

3. Provide a calm and reassuring atmosphere.

C. **First Signs of Seizure**
   1. Lower the dental chair and tilt back.
   2. Do not restrain the patient in any way.
   3. Clear aside movable dental equipment and sharp, potentially injurious instruments.
   4. Turn patient's head on side to prevent aspiration of saliva.
   5. Check for breathing obstruction.
   6. Loosen tight belt, collar, necktie.
   7. *Do not* force anything between the teeth. If an instrument becomes clamped between the teeth during a sudden attack, do not attempt to remove it.
   8. Observe patient's actions and be prepared to submit report for the patient's dental record as well as for the physician if one is called.

D. **Postconvulsive Phase**
   1. Allow patient to rest
   2. When there are repeated convulsions, promptly obtain medical help.
   3. Check oral cavity for trauma to teeth or tissues. Palliative care can be administered. Should a tooth be broken, it is urgent that the piece be located so that aspiration is prevented.

TECHNICAL HINTS

I. Never use a glass syringe or other breakable instrument when a seizure could occur.

II. If an impression tray or instrument becomes clamped between the patient's teeth because of a sudden seizure, do not try to remove it by force. Wait until the spasm subsides.

III. When a patient vomits during a seizure, use high power evacuator with wide tip to remove material from the mouth as a first aid measure against inhalation.

References

1. Kolb, L. C.: *Modern Clinical Psychiatry*, 8th ed. Philadelphia, Saunders, 1973, pp. 242–257.

2. Blum, H. L. and Keranen, G. M.: *Control of Chronic Diseases in Man.* American Public Health Association, 1966, pp. 116–119.

3. Burket, L. W.: *Oral Medicine*, 6th ed. Philadelphia, Lippincott, 1971, pp. 382–385.

4. Glickman, I.: *Clinical Periodontology*, 4th ed. Philadelphia, Saunders, 1972, pp. 93–96.

5. Grant, D. A., Stern, I. B., and Everett, F. G.: *Orban's Periodontics*, 4th ed. St. Louis, Mosby, 1972, pp. 269–272.

6. Hall, W. B.: Dilantin Hyperplasia: A Preventable Lesion, (Abstr.), *J. Periodont. Res.*, p. 36, Supplement 4, 1969.

7. Sheridan, P. J. and Reeve, C. M.: Effective Treatment of Dilantin Gingival Hyperplasia, *Oral Surg.*, 35, 42, January, 1973.

8. Davis, R. K., Baer, P. N., and Palmer, J. H.: A Preliminary Report on a New Therapy for Dilantin Gingival Hyperplasia, *J. Periodont.*, 34, 17, January, 1963.

9. Babcock, J. R.: The Successful Use of a New Therapy for Dilantin Gingival Hyperplasia, *Periodontics*, 3, 196, July-August, 1965.

10. Glickman: op. cit., pp. 795–796, and Figure 49–2, p. 793.

11. Adelson, J. J.: The Dental Management of Epileptic Children, *J. Dent. Child.*, 28, 52, 1st Quarter, 1961.

12. Trott, J. R. and Neuman, K.: Improved Gingival and Mental Condition Following Reduction of Diphenylhydantoin Medication for Epilepsy, *J. Can. Dent. Assoc.*, 30, 518, August, 1964.

13. American National Red Cross: *Standard First Aid and Personal Safety.* Garden City, N.Y., Doubleday, 1973, pp. 175–176.

Suggested Readings

Angelopoulos, A. P.: Diphenylhydantoin Gingival Hyperplasia, A Clinicopathological Review. I. Incidence, Clinical Features and Histopathology, *J. Can. Dent. Assoc.*, 41, 103, February, 1975.

Ciancio, S. G., Yaffe, S. J., and Catz, C. C.: Gingival Hyperplasia and Diphenylhydantoin, *J. Periodont.*, 43, 411, July, 1972.

Donnenfeld, O. W., Stanley, H. R., and Bagdonoff, L.: A Nine-month Clinical and Histological Study of Patients on Diphenylhydantoin Following Gingivectomy, *J. Periodont.*, 45, 547, August, 1974.

Epilepsy Foundation of America: *You, Your Child and Epilepsy* and *Current Information, Epilepsy.* Suite 1116, 733 15th St., N.W., Washington, D.C. 20005.

Klar, L. A.: Gingival Hyperplasia During Dilantin Therapy; A Survey of 312 Patients, *J. Public Health Dent.*, 33, 180, Summer, 1973.

Livingston, S. and Livingston, H. L.: Hypertrophic Gingival Lesions from Use of Epilepsy Drug, *Dent. Surv.*, 46, 38, March, 1970.

Livingston, S. and Livingston, H. L.: Diphenylhydantoin Gingival Hyperplasia, *Am. J. Dis. Child.*, 117, 265, March, 1969.

Chapter 48

The Patient with Mental Retardation

Mental retardation refers to subaverage intellectual functioning which originates during the developmental period and is associated with impairment in adaptive behavior.[1] Sometimes the terms mental retardation and mental deficiency are used interchangeably but more generally *mental deficiency* is used to designate those children whose potential is below normal, and even though everything possible is done to help them, the deficiency remains evident. In contrast, the term *mental retardation* refers to the child who has the possibility, with optimal training and treatment, to approximate a normal range of intelligence.

Mental retardation must not be confused with mental illness. The term mentally ill refers to the person with normal ability who has severe emotional disturbances. Symptoms and treatment for mental illness are very different from those of mental retardation. It is possible for a mentally retarded person to become disturbed or mentally ill, at which time special treatment would be needed.

The background for understanding the problems and needs of the mentally retarded is a clear knowledge of what constitutes normal growth and development and the behavioral manifestations of normal children at each age level. The approach to any dental patient depends on his physical, mental, and emotional capabilities for cooperation and comprehension.

Dental hygiene care for the mentally retarded requires patience and ingenuity for a skillful application of clinical and educational techniques. The dental hygienist's efforts contribute to the overall habilitation of the patient along with other health service personnel.

DESCRIPTION

I. Types and Etiology[2,3]

Mental retardation represents a more or less important symptom in well over 200 different conditions. Many of these are rare. A variety of means of classification is found in the literature, and it has been convenient to divide the causes into factors operating before birth, at birth, and after birth before mental development has been completed.

A majority results from prenatal influences, whereas only a small number are effected as injuries at birth. It should be appreciated that diagnosis may be very complicated and difficult and many cases can only be classified as of unknown etiology. The classification given below provides general etiological categories and is not all-inclusive.

A. **Prenatal**
1. *Familial.* Physiological heredity; factors inherent in genes which transmit intelligence in everyone.
2. *Metabolic.* Effected by genes responsible for absence of or interference with enzymatic activity related to metabolism of specific carbohydrates, proteins, or lipids.
   a. *Phenylketonuria.* An inborn error of metabolism in which one of the enzymes (phenylalanine hydroxylase) essential for digesting protein is defective or missing. Excessive amounts of phenylalanine accumulate in the blood and are excreted in the urine. With early diagnosis and treatment of phenylketonuria (PKU), retardation is not as severe.[4,5,6]
   b. *Galactosemia.* A defect of carbohydrate metabolism in which galactose and lactose cannot be utilized. The condition can be diagnosed by blood test at birth, and with the use of substitutes for foods containing galactose, permanent cerebral damage can be prevented.
3. *Prenatal Infections.* Toxoplasmosis, congenital syphilis, or viral infections including rubella (German measles), mumps, and pertussis.
   a. *Congenital Rubella.* Associated with illness of the mother during the first trimester. Mental retardation and other congenital anomalies including congenital heart disease, deafness, cataracts, or glaucoma can result.[7] More abnormalities occur when the mother is infected during the first month of pregnancy.
   b. *Congenital Syphilis.* Retardation varies with the severity of neurological damage, which occurs primarily with late syphilis and is associated with other manifestations including Hutchinson's teeth and interstitial keratitis.[8]
4. *Kernicterus.* High level of bilirubin in infant's blood, one cause of which is erythroblastosis fetalis due to Rh factor (when fetus is Rh positive and mother Rh negative).
5. *Endocrine Deficiency.* Particularly thyroid: cretinism.
6. *Mongolism* (Down's syndrome, trisomy 21, trisomy G). There is a deviation from the normal chromosomal pattern, usually related to chromosome 21. Characteristics are described on page 645.

B. **Natal**
1. Cerebral birth injury: it should be realized that approximately one-half the children with evidence of brain injury are mentally retarded.
2. Asphyxia with resulting anoxia.

C. **Postnatal**
1. Inflammations of central nervous system: meningitis, encephalitis.
2. Cerebral trauma: accidents of infancy (rare).
3. Prolonged toxemia, malnutrition, or vitamin deficiency (rare).
4. Accidental poisoning: lead, carbon monoxide, or coal-tar derivatives (rare).

D. **Pseudoretardation**
   Heredity, physical environment and social environment are all influential in the development of the child. I

is evident that the rate of intellectual growth can be changed by altering the child's life circumstances. Causes for slow development which are not related or not related directly to central nervous system involvement lead to pseudoretardation.[9,10] Some of the causes are:

1. Prematurity with slow development.
2. Nutritional disturbances: may be related to poverty, deprivation, or ignorance.
3. Prolonged systemic illness.
4. Prolonged hospitalization such as for plastic or reconstructive surgery.
5. Slow motor development such as in muscular dystrophy.
6. Certain types of speech defects which limit communication.
7. Congenitally blind and deaf: because of lack of stimulation from the environment, a degree of retardation can result unless special training is introduced.

E. **Psychological Retardation**
1. Psychiatric illness such as autism or severe neuroses.
2. Sensory, cultural, emotional, or educational deprivation.

F. **Dementia**
   Impairment of intellect which occurs as a result of brain damage after adolescence.

II. Capabilities and Limitations[2,3,11]

The degree of subnormal intelligence or mental deficiency ranges from borderline deficiency down to an intellectual level too low to measure.

Various criteria have been used to classify the mentally retarded including the following: scholastic educability, mental ability test scores, social capacity (that is, to what degree self-support is possible), and legal definitions. Probably the most descriptive and useful classification is based on educability, trainability, and dependency as described below.

A. **Educable**
   Mildly retarded (50 percent of all mentally retarded)
1. Make slow progress in elementary grades in school; may complete fourth grade or continue in special classes.
2. Usually learn to read and write.
3. Do not have mental capacity for successful independent social adjustment.
4. Not capable of consistent planning.
5. Low capacity for sustained effort under pressure.
6. With supervision can perform simple routine work to contribute towards own support, provided competition is kept at a minimum.

B. **Trainable**
   Moderately retarded (40 percent of all mentally retarded).
1. Capable of learning to walk and talk.
2. Poor motor control: awkwardness increases with severity of mental defect.
3. Many show constant overactivity.
4. May develop special motor tics with age: performed deliberately when not interested in surroundings.
   a. Frowning or knitting of the eyebrows.
   b. Blinking.
   c. Grimacing.
   d. Head nodding, shaking, rolling, or bumping.
   e. Shoulder shrugging.
   f. Rocking and swaying of the body.
   g. Oral habits: tongue thrusting and sucking, thumb sucking, nail biting.

5. Can learn to recognize and avoid ordinary physical dangers such as fire and traffic.
6. May be trained to follow simple instructions and assist in simple tasks but cannot contribute to own support.
7. Will always need a protective, supportive environment.

C. **Dependent**

Severely retarded (approximately 10 percent of all mentally retarded)

1. Cannot guard against common physical dangers; need continuous care.
2. Do not learn to form sentences; rarely form articulate words; many cannot speak at all.
3. Many remain inert and placid throughout early years; later movements are slow and clumsy; many never learn to sit up.
4. Usually have to be fed.

III. Physical Characteristics

Certain physical variations appear more frequently in the mentally retarded than among individuals of normal intelligence. Visual diagnosis by physicians is possible in many conditions or syndromes because of a facial or other specific physical characteristic.

Skull anomalies include microcephaly (smaller), hydrocephalus (larger, contains fluid), spherical (occurs in mongolism), conical, or otherwise asymmetrical shapes. Other features such as asymmetries of the face, malformations of the outer ear, anomalies of the eyes, or unusual shape of the nose, may be present. Growth and physiological development are generally delayed.

IV. Oral Characteristics

In the retarded, a higher incidence of oral developmental malformations has been observed, some specifically associated with particular syndromes or conditions.[12] Oral findings which have been observed to occur more frequently in mentally retarded than in people with normal intelligence include the following:

A. Underdeveloped maxilla.
B. Thickness of the lips.
C. Tooth anomalies: imperfectly formed or irregularly erupted.
D. Malocclusion: increased incidence.
E. Periodontal conditions: common, with increased incidence of local irritants related to inability or lack of training in carrying out personal plaque control procedures.
F. Dental caries: mongoloids have shown consistently less dental caries than other retardates, and generally less than the normally intelligent. Surveys which were conducted for nonresident retarded patients tend to show higher dental caries rates than for those in institutions or resident schools.
G. Summary: generalizations from the above items should not be made. Some of the surveys reported in the literature are listed with *Suggested Readings* at the end of the chapter.

V. Psychological Factors

Many factors affect the patient's approach to the dental appointment including environment, training, and parental attitude. Mentally retarded children present no constant personality pattern since some are quiet, subdued, and easily managed whereas others are restless, unstable, and aggressive.[13] Problems of the patient, parents, and the dental personnel need identification when dental hygiene care is planned. The generalities suggested below require thought and adaptation.

A. **The Mentally Retarded Patient**
1. Fears and anxieties: intensified because of slow development, limited

comprehension, and previous medical care experiences.

2. Emotional immaturity
   a. No capacity for setting long-range goals and exercising self-discipline in achieving them; lives in immediate present.
   b. Desires are simple and pass quickly.
   c. Lacks control of emotions if desires are thwarted.
   d. Instability: upset by trivial difficulties.
   e. Lack of self-confidence.
3. Lack of feeling of security: apprehensive; needs attention and praise.
4. Feeling of dependence and helplessness: a reaction to parental overprotection.
5. Easily discouraged: particularly when goals are set too high for the capabilities.
6. Irritability with tenseness and aggression: if attempt is made to push beyond the capabilities.
7. Older patient
   a. Needs feeling of adequacy and usefulness as do other adolescents but frequently lives in atmosphere of frustration and rejection.
   b. May become increasingly lonely.
   c. Discouragement and lowered morale may result when not employed regularly.

B. **The Parents**

Everything that applies to normal parent-child relationships applies alike to parents and their subnormal children. Parents of the mentally retarded have additional emotional problems since the child is so completely dependent on parental care. Some of the difficulties mentioned below are more characteristic while the child is very young.

1. Sense of shame or guilt: disappointment over having retarded child: in part at least, this characteristic is socially determined. Found more in intelligent parents; less intelligent ones tend to accept the child more readily.
2. Overprotectiveness and overindulgence; failure to realize that although the mentally retarded child needs attention and love as does any child, an excess can seriously affect the child's future.
3. Failure to accept the child for what he is; need to limit goals set for the child to those which can be accomplished.

C. **The Dental Personnel**

With an understanding of mental retardation and the particular problems of this group of people, and motivated by a realization of their neglected oral needs, experience can be gained and apprehensions overcome. At first one or more of the psychological reactions listed below may be experienced.[13] Dental personnel must guard against manifesting their own anxieties and will need to analyze their own feelings as they attempt to overcome any reactions which may interfere with the progress and success of dental and dental hygiene care.

1. Curiosity: diminishes with added experience.
2. Pity: need for understanding the problems and needs of the patient.
3. Oversolicitousness.
4. Mild dislike; feeling of discomfort or uneasiness.
5. Rejection.
6. Fear: of doing or saying something offensive.
7. Sympathetic understanding.

VI. The Mongoloid[14,15]

Approximately ten percent of institutionalized mentally retarded patients are mongoloids. It is rare for more than one mongoloid to be born within a family. Other names for this condition are Down's syndrome, trisomy 21, and trisomy G.

Mongoloids represent a distinctive group with a combination of characteristic abnormalities which are relatively constant. They tend to resemble one another.

A. **Mental Characteristics**

Greatest percentage is moderately retarded, in the trainable group.

B. **General Characteristics**
1. Infants
   a. Quiet and placid.
   b. Development: retarded.
   c. Speech: frequently delayed.
2. Head
   a. Skull: small, round, flattened on facial and occipital sides.
   b. Eyes: slanting, Asiatic appearance; widely spaced; opening between eyelids narrow; fold of skin continues from upper eyelid over inner angle of eye.
   c. Nose: short, broad with depressed bridge.
   d. Hair: at first soft, later coarse and scanty.
3. Hands: broad, flat, clumsy-looking; fingers spread, short incurved little finger.
4. Abdomen: large.
5. Joints: unusual range of movement.
6. Circulation: poor.
7. Respiration: shallow, irregular: frequent mouthbreathing.
8. Vitality and resistance: low, subject to infections.
9. Disease incidence: high incidence of congenital heart disease and leukemia.

C. **Oral Characteristics**[15,16]
1. Lips: often thickened, cracked.
2. Jaws: prognathic profile.
3. Palate: high and narrow.
4. Tongue
   a. Protruded: may appear large, but when the nasal and maxillary bones are underdeveloped there may not be sufficient room for the tongue, hence it may protrude.[16]
   b. Fissured.
   c. Papillae hypertrophied.
5. Teeth
   a. Eruption: delayed, partial anodontia.
   b. Microdontia; peg-shaped teeth.
   c. Poor alignment.
   d. Enamel hypoplasia.
6. Periodontal disturbances: high incidence, even in very young.[17–19]
7. Dental caries: low incidence.

D. **Psychological Characteristics: Personality**
1. Lovable; affectionate.
2. Like attention; require affection for feeling of security.
3. Cheerful disposition: rarely irritable.
4. Sociable: social development is ahead of physical; easily amused.
5. Tendency to imitate; mischievous.
6. Full of initiative; observant.
7. Fondness for music: have sense of rhythm (not usually observed in other mentally retarded).
8. Stubbornness: related to their inability to shift quickly from one object to another.

DENTAL HYGIENE CARE

The mentally retarded patient may be afflicted with a physical handicap or a systemic disease which requires additional special adaptations. In conjunction with the appointment suggestions described briefly below, it is recommended that the information in the chapter concerning physical and sensory handicaps also be utilized (pages 653–672) as well as other chapters which describe systemic conditions or diseases.

Basic objectives for care of the mentally retarded patient are related to prevention of tooth loss and maintenance of the teeth in function. Preventive dental hygiene care on a continuing plan is very important. Mental retardation is handicap enough without added oral problems which can even further reduce the already limited potential.

I. The Severely Retarded Patient

A. **Patient Preparation**
   1. Premedication: on prescription of the dentist, a premedicating drug may provide sufficient patient relaxation for dental hygiene procedures.
   2. General anesthesia: some severely retarded children need general anesthesia if any dental or dental hygiene treatment is to be performed. The dental hygienist can join the dentist, anesthetist, and other members of the hospital team for the completion of necessary procedures.

B. **Radiographs**
   Use of a film holder and the assistance of the parent or attendant to support the patient's head may be necessary. Exposures may also be accomplished while the patient is under general anesthesia. Extraoral, panoramic, and occlusal views can be used to supplement intraoral.

C. **Instrumentation**
   With assistance for evacuation, necessary scaling and polishing can be accomplished in less time. Because of the high incidence of periodontal disease in mentally retarded patients, thorough scaling is important to the preventive program.

D. **Fluoride Application**
   Applications should be made routinely. They can be performed while the patient is under general anesthesia.

E. **Restorative Dentistry**
   Restoration of teeth including endodontic treatment can be accomplished under general anesthesia. Several carious lesions or an entire quadrant may be restored at an appointment.

II. The Less Severely Retarded

Procedures used depend upon the cooperation which the patient is able to give. Time should be devoted to training the child to become a good dental patient. Experience helps to develop necessary adaptations for procedures and techniques.

A. **Objectives**
   All of the principles for care of the normal patient apply with greater intensity.
   1. Oral cleanliness contributes not only to oral health through prevention of periodontal diseases, but to appearance; the mentally retarded have difficulty in being accepted by society. An untidy, slovenly person with debris-covered teeth and halitosis is much less socially acceptable.
   2. Improvement of oral appearance helps to minimize the patient's self-consciousness.
   3. All objectives related to prevention of tooth loss leading to malocclusion and/or the need for dentures have particular importance. Dentures are difficult even for the normal person to wear, and with limited patient cooperation, problems are increased for the mentally retarded.

B. **Appointment Planning**
   1. Recall intervals: ideally, three or four times each year.
      a. To prevent development of acute conditions.
      b. To help the patient adjust to

dental and dental hygiene procedures.

c. To provide repetition and encouragement for patient's personal care.

2. Time of appointment: selected on the basis of individual characteristics of each patient and the severity of his retardation.

a. Morning: when the patient, parent, and dental hygienist are in their most responsive state.

b. Early afternoon: some of the patient's morning energy may have worn off and premedication may be more effective; the child may be relaxed when it may be customary to have an afternoon nap.

c. The patient should not be kept waiting for an appointment.

3. Length of appointment

a. Patient's lowered vitality and increased fatigability indicate need for shorter appointments. However, with premedication, appointment time may be extended.

b. Allow time for proceeding slowly as patient may become confused when hurried.

C. **Preparation for the Appointment**

1. Parental preparation of child: prior to appointment instruct parent to talk about the anticipated visit; repetition of statements concerning the dentist and dental hygienist as friends who are kind and helpful, description of the chair that goes up and down, and practice by the parent of putting fingers in the patient's mouth may help to prepare both parent and child. The parent's own attitude toward going to the dental office reflects in the mentally retarded as in the normal child.

2. Patient history

a. Determine other health problems: many will have multiple complications; for example, heart disease is not uncommon and indicates possible need for premedication.

b. Determine drugs used in treatment: some patients may be heavily medicated.

c. Need for close integration of services with physician.

d. Be a good listener: parent may be reluctant to talk at first but, after rapport is established, may offer background information of importance to the various phases of care, management, and instruction.

3. Premedication to produce sedation and relaxation: used upon prescription by dentist for highly active or inadequately trained patients of any degree of deficiency.

D. **General Suggestions for the Appointment**

1. Never hurry but be direct. Patient should not be rushed.

2. Be cheerful and hopeful; work to develop child's confidence; exhibit confidence in child's ability to cooperate.

3. May assist in child's general training.

a. Questioning at time of taking patient's medical history may bring out possibilities: learn the type of school situation the child is in and whether considered educable or trainable.

b. Example: child being trained to speak; effort may be being made to have child state what is wanted instead of pointing.

4. Observe interaction of child and parent: may get clues to ways of obtaining cooperation.

5. Presence of parent in operatory:

overprotected, completely dependent child may be impossible to handle without parent's presence and assistance.

6. Training of patient to open his mouth: may accomplish by mimicry.

7. Child may hold something in his hands to keep him busy.

8. Praise the patient at the end of the appointment.

E. **Instrumentation**

1. Use of instruments at first may be contraindicated. Retract lips with fingers and inspect oral tissues until patient becomes accustomed to the idea.

2. Introduce each instrument slowly: avoid surprise or "sneak" procedures.

3. Motor-driven handpiece may be particularly terrifying to the patient: if so, use of a porte polisher is indicated.

4. When necessary to postpone completion of dental hygiene treatment, parent may be given a plastic mouth mirror to practice placing in patient's mouth daily until the next appointment.

5. Use of compressed air or water syringe can be very frightening to the unsuspecting patient or even to the forewarned one.

F. **Caries Preventive Measures**

1. Topical application of fluoride
   a. Use of cotton roll holder is frequently contraindicated because of lack of understanding leading to resistance by patient.
   b. May be advisable to make separate applications for each quadrant, using the fingers to hold the cotton rolls. This also aids in stabilizing the head. Parent may assist in holding the cotton rolls.

2. Fluoride mouth rinse or other self-applied procedure for daily use may be possible for a trainable patient.

3. Institutionalized patients: when the water supply to the school or institution is not fluoridated, a school fluoridation procedure such as described on page 427 may be recommended.

4. Pit and fissure sealants have been used for mentally retarded children.[20]

III. Patient Instruction

A. **Toothbrushing: Suggestions for Instruction**

Personal daily oral care ordinarily may be limited to toothbrushing, and a simple method is advised. Instruction for the person who cares for the patient is often more important than instruction given to the patient. The mentally retarded learn by constant drilling on a day-to-day basis, as a part of their regular schedule. Some parents may have an organized plan of instruction, working from goal to goal.

For the severely retarded, manipulation of the toothbrush may be beyond the capability so that the cleansing of the oral cavity must be accomplished by the parent or, when the child is in an institution, by an attendant. The toothbrush with suction attachment may be used effectively for institutional care (page 585). An automatic toothbrush has been shown to be particularly adaptable for this group of patients.[21,22]

1. For the patient
   a. Short attention span: present only a little instruction at a time.
   b. Coordination is acquired with difficulty.
   c. Repetition important: teaching of a procedure may take five or six visits; need for continuous supervised practice.

d. Plastic toothbrush handles may be bent if a better grasp can be provided; when the patient uses a curved handled spoon for eating, the toothbrush handle curved in the same manner may be helpful.

e. Teaching must be specific: mentally retarded patients cannot grasp generalities; give directions in simple parts and demonstrate slowly, letting the patient participate.

2. For the parent

a. Help the parent integrate toothbrushing into the child's daily routine: immediately after eating, particularly after eating foods containing fermentable carbohydrates.

b. Show recommended toothbrushing position. A rolling stroke or scrub technique may be the best most of these patients can manage. A soft brush should be used.

c. Parent may have developed special methods of teaching for the individual child: teach principles to the parent for working with the child.

d. Repetition for the mentally subnormal parent: repeated visits with review and redemonstration.

3. Training for the child who will not tolerate toothbrush.

a. Take cotton-tipped applicator dipped in a small amount of dentifrice containing fluoride and touch child's tongue: do this at the usual times for toothbrushing throughout the day for several days, gradually increasing from a touch to moving the swab over the tongue.

b. Run applicator over tongue and over anterior teeth.

c. Add more and more areas until all of the teeth are covered, several times each day, particularly after meals and before going to bed.

d. Continue after a week with soft toothbrush with a small head: go over each area, gradually working up to using a systematic brushing technique.

B. **Diet**

1. For dental caries control

a. Help parent and the older, mildly retarded child to understand role of fermentable carbohydrates in caries initiation.

b. Make specific suggestions for the use of foods which do not contain concentrated sweets, particularly for between meals (pages 410–411).

2. For gingival health and cleansing effect on teeth

a. Dietary suggestions should be checked with the physician to determine any specially prescribed diet and to insure consistency in teaching.

b. Fibrous foods are recommended within the child's capability for mastication.

References

1. United States Department of Health, Education, and Welfare: *The Problem of Mental Retardation.* Washington, D.C., Office of the Secretary, Secretary's Committee on Mental Retardation, 1969. Available from Superintendent of Documents, United States Government Printing Office.
2. Kolb, L. C.: *Modern Clinical Psychiatry,* 8th ed. Philadelphia, Saunders, 1973, pp. 564–582.
3. Bakwin, H. and Bakwin, R. M.: *Behavior Disorders in Children,* 4th ed. Philadelphia, Saunders, 1972, pp. 323–342.
4. Gellis, S. S. and Feingold, M.: *Atlas of Mental Retardation Syndromes.* Washington, United States Department of Health, Education, and Welfare, Division of Mental Retardation, 1968, pp. 118–119.
5. Myers, H. M., Dumas, M., and Ballhorn, H. B.: Dental Manifestations of Phenylketonuria, *J. Am. Dent. Assoc.,* 77, 586, September, 1968.

6. King, W. C.: Oral Characteristics of Phenyl-ketonuric Children, *J. Dent. Child.*, 36, 61, January, 1969.
7. Gellis and Feingold: op. cit., p. 135.
8. Ibid: p. 149.
9. Poser, C. M.: Mental Retardation: The Need for Changing Concepts, *Mod. Treatm.*, 4, 741, July, 1967.
10. Huntley, C. J.: Treatment of Pseudoretardation from Non-neurologic Causes, *Mod. Treatm.*, 4, 747, July, 1967.
11. Bensberg, G. J., ed.: *Teaching the Mentally Retarded*. Atlanta, Southern Regional Education Board, 1965, pp. 19–29.
12. Gellis and Feingold: op. cit., pp. 2–167.
13. Kleiser, J. R.: Psychological Approach to Mental Retardation in Dental Practice, *J. Dent. Child.*, 28, 199, 3rd Quarter, 1961.
14. Kolb: op. cit., pp. 580–581.
15. Tannenbaum, K. A.: The Oral Aspects of Mongolism, *J. Public Health Dent.*, 35, 95, Spring, 1975.
16. Cohen, M. M. and Winer, R. A.: Dental and Facial Characteristics in Down's Syndrome (Mongolism), *J. Dent. Res.*, 44, Supplement, 197, January-February, 1965.
17. Baer, P. N. and Benjamin, S. D.: *Periodontal Disease in Children and Adolescents*. Philadelphia, Lippincott, 1974, pp. 194–200.
18. Goyings, E. D. and Riekse, D. M.: The Periodontal Condition of Institutionalized Children; Improvement Through Oral Hygiene, *J. Public Health Dent.*, 28, 5, Winter, 1968.
19. Sznajder, N., Carraro, J. J., Otero, E., and Carranza F. A.: Clinical Periodontal Findings in Trisomy 21 (Mongolism), *J. Periodont. Res.*, 3, 1, No. 1, 1968.
20. Ripa, L. W. and Cole, W. W.: Occlusal Sealing and Caries Prevention: Results 12 Months After a Single Application of Adhesive Resin, *J. Dent. Res.*, 49, 171, January, 1970.
21. Kelner, M.: Comparative Analysis of the Effects of Automatic and Conventional Toothbrushing in Mental Retardates, *Penn. Dent. J.*, 30, 102, April, 1963.
22. Lucente, J.: Use of an Electric Toothbrush in Severely Retarded Children, *J. Dent. Child.*, 33, 25, January, 1966.

Suggested Readings

Brown, R. H.: Necrotizing Ulcerative Gingivitis in Mongoloid and Nonmongoloid Retarded Individuals, *J. Periodont. Res.*, 8, 290, No. 5, 1973.
Cohen, M. M.: Chromosomal Disorders, *Dent. Clin. North Am.*, 19, 87, January, 1975.
Corcoran, J. W. and Bender, P. A.: Stabilization of the Retarded Child for Dental Procedures, *Ment. Retard.*, 9, 26, December, 1971.
Dicks, J. L.: Effects of Different Communication Techniques on the Cooperation of the Mentally Retarded Child During Dental Procedures, *J. Dent. Child.*, 41, 283, July-August, 1974.

Ford, A. O.: A Training Experience with Mentally Retarded Children, *J. Am. Dent. Hyg. Assoc.*, 39, 156, 3rd Quarter, 1965.
French, E. L. and Scott, J. C.: *How You Can Help Your Retarded Child*. Philadelphia, Lippincott, 1967, 190 pp.
Garn, S. M., Stimson, C. W., and Lewis, A. B.: Magnitude of Dental Delay in Trisomy G, *J. Dent. Res.*, 49, 640, May-June, 1970.
Gertenrich, R. L. and Lewis, M. J.: A Study of Automatic and Hand Tooth Brushing as Used on Retarded or Handicapped Patients, *J. Dent. Child.*, 34, 145, May, 1967.
Greene, N. M. and Falcetti, J. P.: A Program of General Anesthesia for Dental Care of Mentally Retarded Patients, *Oral Surg.*, 37, 329, March, 1974.
Gullikson, J. S.: Oral Findings of Mentally Retarded Children, *J. Dent. Child.*, 36, 59, March-April, 1969.
Gullikson, J. S.: Oral Findings in Children with Down's Syndrome, *J. Dent. Child.*, 40, 293, July-August, 1973.
Harrison, C. C.: Desirable Characteristics of an Electric Toothbrush for Institutional Use, *J. Periodont.*, 39, 270, September, 1968.
Jackson, E. F.: Orthodontics and the Retarded Child, *Am. J. Orthodont.*, 53, 596, August, 1967.
Keyes, P. H., Bellack, S., and Jordan, H. V.: Studies on the Pathogenesis of Destructive Lesions of the Gums and Teeth in Mentally Retarded Children. I. Dentobacterial Plaque Infection in Children with Down's Syndrome, *Clin. Pediatr.*, 10, 711, December, 1971.
Miller, S. L.: Dental Care for the Mentally Retarded: A Challenge to the Profession, *J. Public Health Dent.*, 25, 111, Summer, 1965.
Poole, A. E.: Variation in Protein Structure and Inborn Errors in Metabolism, *Dent. Clin. North Am.*, 19, 47, January, 1975.
Powell, D.: Dental Health Care for the Special Child, *Dent. Hyg.*, 47, 215, July-August, 1973.
Powell, E. A.: A Quantitative Assessment of the Oral Hygiene of Mentally Retarded Residents in a State Institution, *J. Public Health Dent.*, 33, 27, Winter, 1973.
Reynolds, W. E. and Block, R. M.: Evaluating the Effectiveness of Instruction in Oral Hygiene for Mentally Retarded Boys, *J. Public Health Dent.*, 34, 8, Winter, 1974.
Rich, M. H.: Treatment of the Mentally Handicapped, *Br. Dent. J.*, 133, 27, July 4, 1972.
Sandler, E. S., Roberts, M. W., and Wojcicki, A. M.: Oral Manifestations in a Group of Mentally Retarded Patients, *J. Dent. Child.*, 41, 207, May-June, 1974.
Swallow, J. N., Davies, D. E., and Hawkins, H. D.: Gingival Disease Prevalence in Mentally Handicapped Adults, *Br. Dent. J.*, 127, 376, October 21, 1969.
Usher, P. J.: Oral Hygiene in Mentally Handicapped Children, *Br. Dent. J.*, 138, 217, March 18, 1975.
Wells, A.: The Forgotten Three Per Cent, *J. Am. Dent. Hyg. Assoc.*, 41, 19, 1st Quarter, 1967.

Chapter 49

The Patient with a Physical or Sensory Handicap

It is not possible to describe in detail the many diseases of the locomotor system, nervous system, and organs of special senses which have as a symptom or leave as a chronic after effect, loss of sensory or motor function in the form of a handicap. The purposes of this chapter are to outline a few of the types of problems of handicapped patients, to provide brief descriptions of selected diseases to illustrate the types of conditions which may occur, and to suggest adaptations which may be required in dental hygiene care and instruction for an afflicted patient. References and suggested readings are included for additional information.

Oral health for the handicapped takes on more than usual significance and presents a challenge to dental personnel. The handicap provides enough of a burden without additional oral problems which can reduce an already lowered potential for normal living. Preventive measures, particularly fluoridation and other means for supplying the teeth with fluoride (pages 424–442), must be encouraged and promoted through community effort and personal instruction.

It is expected that imagination and ingenuity will help to develop applications for procedures for handicapped patients in addition to those included in this chapter. Calmness, patience, and kindness are keys to patient approach.

I. Objectives

A. To make dental hygiene appointments pleasant and comfortable experiences for each patient.

B. To motivate the patient and others who help care for him, to develop personal oral care practices conducive to health within his range of ability.

C. To contribute to the patient's general health, of which oral health is an integral part. Prevention of tooth loss increases the ability to masticate food, which in turn, is essential to prevent malnutrition and to increase resistance to infection.

D. To prevent the need for extensive dental and periodontal treatment which the patient may not be able to undergo because of his lowered physical stamina or ability to cooperate.

Dentures or other removable appliances can be hazardous for certain handicapped patients or impossible for others.

E. To aid in the improvement of appearance which contributes to social acceptance. An untidy person with unclean teeth and halitosis (from local causes) is much less acceptable socially than one with a clean mouth.

II. Types of Conditions

No specific list can be designated which would describe the symptoms of all physically handicapped patients. The list below is suggestive of types of characteristics which may be observed in certain patients.

A. **Lowered Physical Stamina**
They fatigue easily.

B. **Lowered Resistance to Infection**

C. **Signs and Symptoms Associated with Neurological Diseases**
1. Speech disturbances (aphasia).
2. Convulsive states: example, epilepsy (pages 633–637).
3. Narcolepsy: uncontrollable desire for sleep or sudden attack of sleep.
4. Headaches.
5. Paralysis
   a. Hemiplegia: paralysis of one side of the body; most frequent cause is cerebrovascular accident.
   b. Paraplegia: paralysis of lower extremities or lower part of body; caused by trauma or diseases including poliomyelitis and multiple sclerosis.
   c. Quadriplegia or triplegia: four or three extremities involved.

D. **Symptoms Associated with Muscular Involvements**
1. Weakness and atrophy of muscles.
2. Limitation of motion including functional problems of the muscles

of facial expression and muscles of mastication.
3. Pain: spontaneous or evoked by movement or pressure.

III. Psychological Factors

Psychological and emotional factors enter into the picture with greater intensity than with nonhandicapped patients. Knowledge of the characteristics of the variety of handicapping conditions can prevent personal emotional reactions by professional people to a patient's distorted appearance, postural deformity, or inability to cooperate with the usual procedures.

Handicapped people show the same wide range of individual differences found in others of the same ages. Patients with handicaps may have intellectual and emotional disabilities because of the attitudes of other people toward them or the degree of acceptance by their families.

Loss or lack of ability to function independently or predict one's movements is psychologically traumatizing. Lack of esthetic appearance may have a tremendous influence on a person's life. The general factors suggested below may apply to a child, an adult, or in most instances, either.[1]

A. **Emotional Problems of Patients**
1. Overprotection by family
   a. Decreases incentive to make full use of own abilities.
   b. Prevents acceptance of new situations such as would confront a patient in a dental office; may react aggressively or may be retiring.
   c. May be apprehensive or undisciplined.
   d. May have resistance against assuming responsibility.
2. Rejection by family and others: may feel inadequate and inferior.
3. Parents may deny existence of

disability; patient may be pushed beyond his capabilities which can lead to frustration.

4. Inability to act independently and control movements may lead to irritability, defensiveness, or fear.
   a. Most difficult time to adjust is frequently when symptoms are relatively slight.
   b. Anxiety from increasing help-lessness; fear of helplessness.
   c. Frustration from limitation and restriction of activities.
   d. Increased desire for attention, affection, and protection.

B. **Suggestions for Patient Approach**
   1. Avoid oversolicitousness.
   2. Respect personal pride of patient: encourage patient's interest in personal appearance.
   3. Avoid mention of patient's symptoms.
      a. Help patient from becoming self-centered.
      b. Prevent embarrassment or self-consciousness.
   4. Encourage patient in all achievements, however small.
   5. Maintain cheerful atmosphere: contribute to patient's happiness and peace of mind.

IV. General Appointment Suggestions

Most handicapped patients can be treated in a private dental office. Pre-medication is indicated for certain patients for dental hygiene as well as dental procedures. Others will need hospitalization either because of their inability to cooperate without general anesthesia, or because of a systemic condition which requires special supervision, particularly should an emergency arise.

A. **Patient History**

In addition to the history items covered routinely (tables 6–1, 6–2, and 6–3, pages 69–78), information con-cerning the handicapping condition in more detail can be both helpful and necessary. Consultations with the physician, the social worker, and other specialists who may have treated the patient provide data to guide patient management and treatment. Suggested pertinent information to include is as follows:

1. Specific handicapping condition: when diagnosed; history of treatment; hospitalizations; current medication or other therapy.
2. Muscular coordination: walking, sitting, balance, grasping.
3. Seizures: frequency, treatment.
4. Speech, vision, hearing, mentality.
5. Abilities: dresses self, feeds self, toilet trained, attends school, special training classes.
6. Dependency on parent; relationships with parents and siblings.
7. Previous dental experiences.

B. **Appointment Planning**
   1. Time of appointment
      a. Morning: less fatiguing while patient is rested. When medication is to be administered, early afternoon may be preferable since some of the patient's early morning alertness has worn off. A child may be more relaxed prior to nap time.
      b. Hour: convenient to patient's daily care schedule.
   2. Allow sufficient time so that patient does not feel rushed; many handicapped people cannot hurry.
   3. Recall: frequent
      a. To decrease length of single appointment.
      b. To assist patient whose handicap limits ability in personal oral care procedures.

C. **Reception and Seating**
   1. Assist patient only as needed: let patient feel independent.

2. Learn the way to help patient as he walks which will contribute most to his support.
3. Position chair to give patient feeling of security.
4. Wheel chair patient
   a. Lower or detach arm of dental chair to permit transfer of patient.
   b. Obtain portable headrest which can be attached to back of wheel chair; more effective stabilization may be obtained when patient remains in his own chair.

D. **Techniques**
1. Skillful adaptations are required for all techniques when the patient is unable to cooperate because of muscular involvement of the face or tongue or disturbance of temporomandibular joint function.
2. Radiographs[2,3]
   a. Complete survey should be made. Extraoral, panoramic or occlusal film may be used to supplement intraoral radiographs.
   b. Film holder is indicated (page 122); when the patient cannot hold a film holder, the parent or other attendant can be instructed to hold it. Dental personnel never hold films in a patient's mouth.
   c. Radiographs for severely handicapped patient unable to cooperate may be made under general anesthesia.
3. Rinsing
   a. Assistant applies evacuator during scaling and for rinsing.
   b. Emesis basin: when unassisted and when patient can cooperate except for reaching cuspidor, an emesis basin can be helpful.

E. **Procedures for Bedridden Patient**
   See pages 581–586.

V. Patient Instruction

A. **Plaque Control**
1. Periodontal and gingival conditions are generally more severe in people with handicaps. Causes of inadequate self-care are related to the following:
   a. Lack of professional care and instruction and therefore a lack of knowledge about proper care may result. The need for increased emphasis on general health problems may have limited the effort for oral health maintenance.
   b. Restrictions of movements of hands and arms, ability to grasp, or lack of coordination make mouth cleaning difficult or impossible.
2. *Procedure for Instruction*
   a. Begin instruction for the patient and the parent or attendant first, before instrumentation.
   b. Explain and demonstrate each step carefully. A disclosing tablet may be used when the patient is able to chew and rinse, otherwise a spray or topical application of disclosing solution is indicated.
   c. Review, practice, and continue instruction in short sessions to prevent frustration, fatigue, and discouragement.
   d. Instruction for parent in standing position with child's head supported can be applied for the child who can stand (page 394).
3. *Adaptations of Manual Toothbrush*
   Although a parent or attendant may be willing to brush the patient's teeth, as much as possible should be carried out by the patient. Psychological benefits to the patient result in feelings of self-esteem and accomplishment when

able to manage the important and worthwhile task of brushing. Aids to brushing have been devised.

a. Enlarged handle for manual toothbrush: patient with difficulty grasping the small-handled brush and controlling its motions may benefit from the use of an enlarged handle.[4] Obtain an impression of the patient's hand grasp by having him grasp a cylinder of base plate wax; then fill the wax cylinder with quick-cure acrylic. Insert the toothbrush handle before the acrylic sets. The angle may be adjusted to set the brush head for the patient's convenient use. Polish the acrylic.

b. Attach the toothbrush to the patient's hand by means of an elastic cuff, small strap, or other means. This may facilitate brushing for the patient whose main problem is grasping and holding.

c. Provide a long-handled holder with a socket for insertion of toothbrush for the patient who cannot raise his arms or is otherwise limited in range of motion. These devices are available commercially and are used by the handicapped for other tasks such as hair combing.

4. *Automatic Brush*

An automatic brush has been shown to be particularly effective in improving oral cleanliness and reducing gingivitis in the handicapped. Reports are listed in the *Suggested Readings* at the end of this chapter.

a. The automatic brush handle is thick and easier for grasping.

b. An elastic cuff around the hand and the brush is effective for brush control.[5]

c. For use without hands: attach brush by means of a clamp in a stationary upright position lower than the patient's mouth when he is bent over. Patient can insert the brush into the mouth and apply to the teeth.[6]

5. *Dental Floss:* Use of a floss holder can make flossing possible for certain patients. It may also be useful for attendants, nurses, or family members who perform plaque control for the patient (page 335).

6. *Stationary Denture Brush*[4,7]: a hand brush with attached suction cups can be held to the inside of a sink. The denture may then be cleaned with one hand by the hemiplegic.

B. **Fluoride Therapy**

In addition to the use of a fluoride dentifrice, another form of daily fluoride application should be planned. Depending on the patient's abilities, a chewable tablet, mouth rinse, or gel tray can be used. If none of these is applicable, a fluoride solution can be applied with a cotton applicator after brushing and flossing. The patient should not eat or drink for at least 30 minutes for the full benefit.

C. **Diet**

A varied diet with all essential food elements is important to the general health of the patient; prevention of dental caries has particular significance since performance of techniques required for dental care can be very difficult.

DISEASES OF MUSCLES

Muscular Dystrophy

Muscular dystrophy is a hereditary disease characterized by progressive loss of use and atrophy of symmetrical groups of muscles with eventual involvement of practically the entire voluntary musculature. Pain is rarely evident until the late stages of the disease when there is muscular contracture. Muscular dystrophy is one of the many diseases of the muscles for which the etiology is unknown and therefore specific treatment has not been possible.

I. Characteristics

Several different types of muscular dystrophy have been identified, but classification does not imply any differences in the underlying pathologic processes. Classification is based on the distribution of muscles affected most in the early stages, the presence or absence of pseudohypertrophy of muscles, and the age of onset. The two types described below illustrate characteristics and classification.[8,9] Most of the afflicted are males.

A. **Pseudohypertrophic Muscular Dystrophy**
  1. Most severe type.
  2. Age of onset: childhood, usually from two to five years.
  3. Effects of muscular involvement
      a. Enlargement (pseudohypertrophy) of certain muscles, particularly the calves, is present in early years.
      b. Weakness of hips: child falls frequently, has increasing difficulty in standing erect.
      c. Lordosis; abdominal protuberance.
      d. Progressive muscular wasting: eventual involvement of thighs, shoulders, trunk; inactivity is detrimental and increases helplessness.
  4. Prognosis: disablement severe by age 15; patients rarely live to reach third decade.

B. **Facioscapulohumeral Muscular Dystrophy**
  1. Age of onset: from early childhood to 30 or 40 years, most commonly after adolescence.
  2. Effects of muscular involvement
      a. Facial muscles weak: expression impaired.
      b. Lips: prominent, gaping; patient cannot whistle or purse lips.
      c. Eyes: cannot be closed completely.
      d. Shoulder muscles weakened; shoulders slope.
      e. Upper arms: difficulty in raising arms above shoulders.
  3. Prognosis: progresses more slowly than pseudohypertrophic form of the disease; occasional case may go into remission after six to twelve years leaving permanent disability in proportion to the severity of disease in its active stage.

C. **General Physical Characteristics**
  1. Appearance: two types
      a. Thin, emaciated: typical of majority of ambulatory patients.
      b. Heavy, obese, flabby: typical of nonambulatory.
  2. Gait
      a. Waddling: either walk on toes or flatfoot; results from muscle contracture.
      b. Balance: precarious; patient arches back in attempt to find center of gravity; gait is slow as balance must be attained with each step.
  3. Fatigue readily and do not recover promptly.

II. Dental Hygiene Care

Adaptations will depend on the patient's disability. Patients may have slight muscular involvement, be ambulatory but have balancing difficulties, be in a wheel chair, or bedridden. All factors listed for general consideration of handicapped patients (page 655) have application. Suggestions listed below will be useful for certain patients.

A. **Patient Reception and Seating**
  1. Assistance while patient is walking
    a. Certain patients are better without assistance as they have developed their own method of balancing and the merest touch may upset them.
    b. Many gain balance by holding both hands on partially flexed forearm of person walking beside them.
  2. Seating preparation
    a. Raise chair: when patient does not have strength to lower himself into chair.
    b. Remove conventional chair arm: allow patient to sit directly.
  3. After seating patient: tilt chair back; balance is precarious while sitting as well as standing; patient may fall forward.
  4. Assistance for patient while rising from chair
    a. Stand directly in front of him: lock arms around lower back and pull forward near hips.
    b. Allow patient to sway upper trunk back as he rises to standing position.
    c. Provide support until he obtains balance for walking.

B. **Patient Instruction**
  1. Problems of oral cleanliness
    a. Facial muscle weakness may interfere with self-cleansing mechanisms and prevent adequate rinsing.
    b. Gaping lips: effect on oral tissues similar to that of mouthbreathing.
    c. Weakness of arm and shoulder: difficulty in applying toothbrush. An automatic brush may have advantages.
  2. Patient response to instruction
    a. Tendency to sluggishness in mental response.
    b. Speech is slow; word-forming difficult.
    c. Lack of facial expression: not necessarily an indication of lack of attention or understanding.
  3. Toothbrushing instruction
    a. Instruct parent or other person who cares for patient.
    b. When patient is receiving physical therapy treatments, solicit assistance and advice from the physical therapist.

Myasthenia Gravis[8,10]

Myasthenia gravis is a neuromuscular disease characterized by varying weakness of the voluntary muscles. It is caused by a defect in nerve impulse transmission at the neuromuscular junction, possibly with a decrease in output of acetylcholine from the nerve endings. Anticholinesterase drugs are used in the treatment to relieve symptoms.

I. Characteristics

A. **Early Signs**
  Weakness of eye movements, drooping eyelids, and lack of facial expression; weakness in arms and legs.

B. **Progressive Involvement**
  Voluntary muscles about the head and neck become weak, and gradually other muscles of the body are involved.

C. **Oral and Facial Problems**
  Difficulty in mastication and swallowing; dropping of the jaw.

D. **Speech**
  May be slow and slurred.

II. Occurrence

Chiefly in middle-age group; more frequent in women under 50 and men over 50 years.

III. Dental Hygiene Care

A. Appointment Planning

Short appointments are necessary since the patient fatigues easily. The time of day should be selected when the patient will be most rested.

B. Patient Position

When neck muscles are weak, difficulty in holding the head up may complicate rinsing, therefore the use of the evacuation system is necessary.

C. Plaque Control

1. Mastication difficulties may encourage the use of a soft diet, which in turn encourages the formation of tooth deposits.
2. Toothbrushing: weakness and fatigability may discourage sufficient routine brushing. An automatic brush may be indicated. Instruction must be provided the nurse or attendant who cares for the severely ill bedridden patient who is unable to brush or care for a removable appliance.

DISEASES OF CONNECTIVE TISSUE

Scleroderma[11–13]

Scleroderma is a collagen disease of connective tissue in which there is immobility and rigidity of the skin. It may be localized or generalized and develop as an external manifestation of a progressive systemic sclerosis. Etiology is not known, therefore there is no specific treatment.

I. Occurrence

It usually begins between ages 30 and 50; may develop over months or years; is more common in females.

II. Characteristics

A. Skin

Hard and fixed; ivory-white, yellow, or gray, sometimes with brown pigmentation in the late stages.

B. Face

Masklike and expressionless.

C. Oral Characteristics

1. Lips: thin, rigid, with difficulty in opening and closing.
2. Mucosa: thin, pale, tender, rigid with poor healing capacity.
3. Gingiva: pale, and unusually firm.
4. Teeth: mobility which relates to radiographic findings.
5. Radiographic findings: marked widening of the periodontal ligament space. This finding is sometimes considered pathognomonic for scleroderma.
6. Mastication: difficult; temporomandibular joint movement is limited.
7. Tongue: may be immobile; speech difficult.

III. Dental Hygiene Care

The tightening of the skin and lip limits opening of the mouth and complicates all dental and dental hygiene procedures as well as daily self-care by the patient. Every effort for preservation of the teeth and gingiva in health should be made to prevent the need for extensive treatment.

Patients with scleroderma are sensitive to cold and dampness, stress, undue emotional tension, and fatigue. All of these factors can be considered for the dental hygiene appointment.

DISEASES OF THE JOINTS

Arthritis

Diseases of the joints, including arthritis, are among the most common causes of chronic illness in the United States. They are second only to heart conditions in the list of most frequent causes of activity limitation.[14] In addition to arthritis as a disease entity, arthritic manifestations are produced as part of various other chronic diseases. Cases involve temporary or permanent, partial or complete disability.

Arthritis means inflammation in a joint. It may occur in the acute or chronic form. The etiology varies and is not completely defined, which makes classification difficult. A patient may suffer from more than one type at the same time.

Causes relate to a variety of conditions including specific infectious diseases such as tuberculosis, syphilis, gonorrhea, or rheumatic fever; disturbances of metabolism such as gout; direct trauma; or neoplasms of the joints. In addition there are rheumatoid arthritis of unknown etiology and osteoarthritis, a degenerative joint disease associated with the aging process. The latter two are the most prevalent types of arthritis and a few of the symptoms and characteristics of these are listed in this chapter. For detailed information concerning these and other forms of arthritis, references are listed as *Suggested Readings* at the end of the chapter.

I. Rheumatoid Arthritis

A. Occurrence
More common in females; onset in early adulthood more frequent although it may occur at any age; tendency to recurrence.

B. Early Symptoms
1. Migratory swelling and stiffness of the joints particularly fingers, hands, and knees; varying degree of pain when exercised.
2. Weakness, fatigue, loss of weight, anemia.

C. Subsequent Symptoms
1. Joint symptoms tend to be symmetrical; painful.
2. Subcutaneous nodules in elbows, wrists, or fingers in approximately 15 percent of the patients.
3. Temporomandibular joint in-

volvement occurs in some patients; may have pain with movement of the jaw; ankylosis may develop.[15,16]
4. Progressive anterior open bite related to remodeling of the condyle.[17]
5. Atrophy of muscles leads to deformities; progressive disability: eventually may be bedridden.

II. Osteoarthritis (Degenerative Arthritis)

A. Occurrence
Onset in middle-aged or elderly; associated with aging process.

B. Early Symptoms
Insidious, with slight stiffness in a single joint.

C. General Physical Characteristics
Obesity, poor posture, limping.

D. Joint Symptoms
1. Hips, knees, fingers, vertebrae affected most frequently.
2. Swelling is rare; ankylosis does not occur.
3. Stiffness after rest, diminishes with exercise.
4. Pain aggravated by temperature changes and bearing body weight.
5. Temporomandibular joint may become involved without pain or other clinical symptoms.[15,16] Crepitation, clicking, or snapping may occur when the joints are exercised.

III. Psychological Factors

With long-range illnesses patients are frequently discouraged or apprehensive. Certain patients may be worried, pessimistic, or resigned. Some may be impatient and tend to harm themselves by overexercise. A few are irritable, a characteristic related to the pain which has been suffered.

Psychological causes for temporomandibular joint dysfunction have been demonstrated. In certain instances, treatment of the psychological factors can result in relief of physical symptoms.[18] Facial abnormalities and occlusal discrepancies have also been implicated in temporomandibular joint problems. Any of these other conditions may occur with arthritis of the joint.

IV. Dental Hygiene Care

There is no other specific oral manifestation in arthritis except when the temporomandibular joint is affected. Such involvement presents difficulty in performing techniques for the patient who has limited ability and comfort in opening his mouth.

A high standard of general health contributes to the well-being of the arthritic. Maintenance of oral health contributes to general health. Although the characteristics and requirements of the various types of arthritis differ, the general suggestions below can be applied.

A. **Room Temperature**
Adjust, prevent drafts; patients are susceptible to cold and dampness.

B. **Patient Positioning**
Make adaptations for limited and painful movement.
1. Lower arm of chair to permit patient to sit directly rather than having to step up to a foot rest of a conventional chair.
2. Arrange chair seat so that flexion of knees and hips is at a minimum.
3. Adjust foot rest so that feet may be placed squarely to avoid strain on knee joints.
4. Suggest that patient flex and extend knees a few times before rising from chair: joints become stiff after being seated for a while.
5. Offer hand as patient rises from chair: provides secure hold and usually is more helpful than assistance under the arms since many patients are used to devices for pulling themselves up.

C. **Instrumentation**
1. Adapt instrumentation to minimal opening of jaws: do not expect patient to strain, particularly since pain may result.
2. Avoid traumatizing joint by prolonged pressure on mandible.
3. Use of evacuator is indicated, particularly for the patient whose body motion is limited by generalized arthritic symptoms.

D. **Plaque Control**
Because of hand and arm involvement, a patient may have difficulty grasping a toothbrush or lifting the arm for sufficient periods to clean the mouth completely. Adapted brushing procedures may be applied (pages 656–657).

E. **Diet and Nutrition**
1. No special nutritional factors are known to be associated with the course or treatment of arthritis. Physicians generally recommend a normal, well-balanced diet with a controlled caloric intake for weight control. Encouragement of restriction of sweets and selection of noncariogenic between-meal snacks can help to improve oral health.
2. Dietary analysis: obtaining a food diary for several days to a week can be very important for counseling, especially for the gerodontic arthritic patient (pages 402–405).

DISEASES OF THE NERVOUS SYSTEM
Multiple Sclerosis

Multiple sclerosis is an acute or chronic, remittent or progressive disease of unknown origin. It is characterized by nervous dysfunction. Pathologically the white matter of the central nervous system degenerates in patches and is replaced by sclerotic tissue. There is interference with the transmission of nerve impulses.

The marked variability in onset, course, and degree of dysfunction implies that the illness is not a disease entity but a syndrome. There are no specific oral manifestations but the muscles of the tongue and face are involved in some cases.

I. Occurrence[19]

A. Onset
Usually between late teens and middle thirties; affects males and females alike.

B. Geographic
More prevalent in cold and temperate climates.

II. Characteristics[19,20]

A. Initial Symptoms: Vary
1. May be minor visual impairment, difficulty in coordination, tremor, fatigue, weakness, or numbness of a part of the body; tend to disappear without treatment.
2. May have a sudden onset of severe illness with paralysis or marked weakness.

B. Course of Disease
Characterized by attacks and remissions; patient may live for 20 years or much longer after first attack; bronchopneumonia is the most common immediate cause of death.

C. Physical Symptoms
There is a wide distribution of areas affected which results in a variety of symptoms. Symptoms fluctuate and there may be several years between attacks. They may be brought on by fatigue, psychological or emotional disturbances, malnutrition, chilling or infections, particularly with fever. With extended rest, symptoms usually subside.
1. Involuntary motion of eyes (nystagmus); may later become partially or completely blind.
2. Speech disorders: possble loss of speech in advanced stages.
3. Changes in muscular coordination and gait: one side of body usually affected more than the other; loss of balance.
4. Paralysis of one or more extremities; occasionally facial paralysis.
5. Autonomic derangements such as urinary frequency and urgency; later urinary incontinence.
6. Susceptibility to infection, particularly upper respiratory.

D. Personality Factors
1. Optimism and cheerfulness out of proportion to the degree of disability and seriousness of the illness; euphoria.
2. Subject to sharp deviations of mood: emotional outbursts with spells of laughing and crying.
3. Poor memory; poor judgment.
4. Passive dependency; lack of responsibility.

III. Treatment

A. No specific treatment since the cause of the disease is unknown.

B. General hygienic care: adequate nutrition, rest, avoidance of strain, prevention of infections.

C. Physical therapy; exercise is very important.

D. Psychotherapy for personality problems and morale building: frequently necessary.

E. Drugs: primarily prescribed for alleviation of symptoms.

F. Patient should continue in a usual occupation as long as possible; activity should be encouraged.

IV. Dental Hygiene Care

Knowledge of physical, personality, and treatment factors listed above can be applied during appointment procedures. Since attacks may be initiated by infection, dental hygiene care for the prevention of oral infection assumes particular significance.

A. **Psychological Considerations**
   1. Provide a quiet, comfortable atmosphere: the patient needs to remain relaxed mentally and physically, therefore people around cannot be tense and restless.
   2. Prepare for emotional outbursts of laughing or crying by the patient.
      a. May be initiated by something as simple as the sudden introduction of hot or cold into the mouth, or being startled by a sudden air blast from the compressed air syringe.
      b. When an outburst occurs, change the subject of conversation to something impersonal: suggest something serious if the patient is laughing or something humorous if the patient is crying.

B. **Patient Instruction**
   1. Problems of personal oral care
      a. Involvements of the tongue and facial muscles interfere with the self-cleansing mechanisms.
      b. Involvements of hands or arms make grasping and manipulating a toothbrush difficult or impossible.
   2. Factors affecting teaching
      a. Slow response of patient; give instruction slowly and simply.
      b. Poor memory: instruction should be reviewed frequently.
      c. Visual disturbances: (pages 669–671).

Cerebral Palsy

Palsy means paralysis, and cerebral palsy means a condition in which injury to parts of the brain has resulted in paralysis or disruption of motor parts. Such a condition can occur at any age as a result of brain injury from a variety of causes, and therefore cerebral palsy is not really a disease entity. Through common usage the term is frequently applied to cases of congenital spastic paralysis.

Causes relate to cerebral birth injuries, diseases *in utero*, or, less frequently, a developmental anomaly. Symptoms usually can be observed during the first year but may not appear for a number of years. Deafness, visual disturbances, speech problems, or lowered mentality may accompany the paralysis, weakness, and incoordination of the motor system.

I. General Characteristics[21,22]

The three main types of cerebral palsy are described briefly below. Two other types, rigidity and tremor, may have mixed symptoms and frequently are associated with the major classifications. In each type different parts of the brain are affected and the symptoms vary respectively.

Approximately 60 percent are categorized as spastic and 30 percent athetoid. The remaining 10 percent includes those with ataxia, rigidity, tremor, or mixed involvements.[21]

A. **Spastic Paralysis**
   1. Condition characterized by spasms which are sudden, involuntary contractions of single muscles or groups of muscles.
   2. Muscles have excess tone, tension, and activity.
   3. Patient has complete or partial loss of ability to control muscular movement, therefore movements are awkward; mental effort toward control can result in less control.
   4. Activity: lack of control causes patient to fall easily; tends to avoid activity; may gain weight, particularly during teen years; caloric requirement is therefore low.[23]

B. **Athetosis**
1. Condition characterized by constant involuntary unorganized muscular movement.
2. Patient lacks ability to direct muscles in the motions desired; probably the most difficult dental patient.
3. Factors influencing movements
   a. May be initiated and aggravated by stimuli outside body.
   b. Made worse by attempts of patient to control them.
   c. Intensity influenced by emotional factors: patient is least in control in an emotionally charged environment such as the dental office.
4. Activity: constantly in motion; burns up energy; usually very thin; caloric requirement of diet is therefore high.[23]

C. **Ataxia**
1. Loss of equilibrium: balance and orientation difficult; walk uncertain; has difficulty in sitting straight.
2. Difficulty in control of eye muscles; some dizziness and nausea.
3. Activity: inactive because of balance disturbance; tends to put on weight; caloric requirement in diet is therefore low.[23]

II. Oral Characteristics

A. **Disturbance of Facial, Masticatory, and Tongue Musculature**
1. Prevents normal chewing pattern and swallowing process.
2. Intraoral forces produce varying degrees of orthodontic involvement.
   a. Tongue thrusting may result from faulty swallowing reflex: may tend to push maxillary anterior teeth forward.
   b. Mouth breathing and tissue biting may occur.

3. Interferes with voluntary opening of mouth.
4. Drooling may result from inability to swallow and control facial muscles.
5. Hyperactive reflexes cause patient to clamp jaws together suddenly.

B. **Dental Caries**
   High incidence in children with cerebral palsy.[24,25]

C. **Attrition**
   Severe; constant, involuntary grinding of teeth wears down tooth structure and restorations. Bruxism is most extensive in athetoid group.[26]

D. **Fractured Teeth**
   Patients fall frequently; accidents to anterior teeth result.

E. **Problems in Oral Cleanliness**
1. Soft diet used to compensate for difficulty during mastication.
2. Lack of effects of natural self-cleansing mechanisms in cleansing the teeth; increased food retention.
3. Increased calculus deposits may be observed as an effect of mouth breathing, lack of self-cleansing processes, and inability to carry out personal care.
4. Inability to manipulate toothbrush: abnormal movements of arms, lack of control of hands, disturbance of facial and tongue musculature prevent success in personal care procedures; difficult for others to accomplish for patient because of involuntary movements.

III. Dental Hygiene Care

Dental hygiene care is complicated by the difficulties which the patient has in cooperating and by the oral manifestations listed above. Psychological factors have been listed on page 654. Understanding the physical characteristics is particularly necessary to the success of the appointment. Athetoid movements should not be interpreted as lack of cooperation and a patient's inability to communicate does not mean lack of comprehension. Dentists use general anesthesia in a hospital situation for the unmanageable patient.[25,27]

There are dangers for both the patient and dental personnel which may result from the uncontrolled movement of the patient. The sudden forceful closure of the mouth on the finger of the operator or on a glass mouth mirror, or movement of the patient which diverts a sharp instrument into the patient's tissues, are examples.

Skill, alertness, patience, and application of principles from the experience of others as listed below are needed. Assistance usually is required and it may be advisable to solicit the aid of the parent or other person who accompanies the patient and who would be familiar with the characteristics of the patient. Overprotective parents, particularly if they are not cooperative dental patients themselves, may be of limited help.

A. **Preparation for the Appointment**

Premedication to obtain a degree of relaxation would be given on recommendation of the dentist and advice of the patient's physician.

B. **Patient Positioning**

To help patient overcome feeling of insecurity.

1. Tilt chair back so patient cannot slide forward.
2. Use canvas or leather bands or belts.
   a. Place around patient under arms, around abdomen and attach to back of the chair.
   b. When patient wears leg braces, tie them to the chair.
3. Arm restraint: restraint can serve as an irritant which could result in increased involuntary movement.
   a. Have parent or assistant hold arms.

   b. Arm splint made of cloth: not a straight jacket, but a simple enclosure for the arms; must be fully understood and approved by the patient.
4. Wheel chair patient: it may be best to keep patient in his own chair and attach portable headrest.

C. **Techniques**

1. Position of operator: may be effective to operate standing with arm around patient's head; use crotch of elbow for stabilization.
2. Mouth mirror: use metal-surfaced mirrors.
3. Avoid placing fingers between patient's teeth: use facial surfaces for fulcrum rests. Improvised finger protectors may be used such as a metal thimble covered with a rubber finger cot.
4. Mouth prop: may be helpful with a few patients, but lateral uncontrolled movements of jaw may dislodge it; long wooden wedge wrapped in gauze and placed between the patient's teeth may be held by assistant.
5. Avoid sudden movements, noises, blasts of compressed air, bright light in patient's eyes, or other effects which may startle the patient and cause muscle reaction.

D. **Instruction**

1. Give instruction in simple toothbrushing method to parent or other person who cares for the patient; training the patient is a long-range process.
2. Parents can be shown how to use a mouth prop placed on one side of the mouth while brushing teeth on opposite side.
3. Patient with some coordination may be able to use a toothbrush with a built-up or large handle, or an automatic brush (pages 319–322).

Bell's Palsy[28,29]

Bell's palsy is a paralysis of the facial muscles innervated by the facial or seventh cranial nerve. Although the cause is unknown, various possible agents have been implicated including inflammation, trauma, exposure to cold, surgery of the parotid gland or the removal of a mandibular third molar with damage to the facial nerve.

I. Characteristics

A. Initial Signs

Abrupt paralysis of facial muscles usually without preceding pain, and usually on one side of the face only.
1. Mouth: corner droops and uncontrollable salivation with drooling may occur; speech and eating become difficult.
2. Eye: inability to close lids; watering and drooping of lower lid may invite infection.

B. Progress

Patient with a mild case may return to normal within a month; others may have lasting residual effects or permanent paralysis.

C. Occurrence

Women tend to be affected more frequently than men.

II. Dental Hygiene Care

A. Appointment

Complications may relate to difficulty of patient rinsing or other problems related to facial movements.

B. Plaque Control

Painstaking efforts by the patient are needed since self-cleansing is difficult or impossible. Because of loss of cheek action food frequently collects in the vestibule and about the teeth of the affected side.

Paralysis Agitans[30,31]

Paralysis agitans, also known as *parkinsonism* or *parkinsonian syndrome*, is a progressive disorder of the central nervous system characterized by muscular rigidity and tremor. There may be no apparent precipitating cause or it may be associated with cerebral arteriosclerosis, head trauma, or other conditions.

I. Characteristics

A. General

1. Body posture bent, with bent head.
2. Motion and responses slowed.
3. Speech: monotonous.
4. Tremor of hands and feet when at rest; frequently one extremity or one side is affected more than the other.
5. Intellect is seldom influenced.

B. Face and Oral Cavity

1. Expression: fixed, mask-like.
2. Tremor in muscles of mastication and tongue.
3. Salivation excessive.

II. Occurrence

Affects middle-aged and elderly persons primarily; higher incidence in men than women.

III. Dental Hygiene Care

Various adaptations can be anticipated from knowledge of the characteristics noted above. General suggestions for working with gerodontic patients can be helpful (table 42–1, page 590, and table 42–2, page 593).

Since medical treatment for paralysis agitans sometimes includes atropine-like drugs, problems associated with excess salivation may be lessened.

CEREBROVASCULAR DISEASES

Stroke[7,32]

Cerebrovascular accident or stroke is a process which causes brain damage and leads to disturbances of body functions. It may follow a thrombosis, hemorrhage, embolism, or shortage of blood supply to the brain. These conditions may be caused by arteriosclerosis, hypertension, or an aneurysm, and may be associated with vascular disease of the heart and other systemic diseases. Cardiovascular diseases are described on pages 675–677.

I. Characteristics

The effects of a stroke depend on the location of the damage to the brain as well as the degree or extent of involvement. Acute symptoms and first aid procedures are included in table 54–1, page 730. Some of the effects which may result include the following:

A. **Paralysis**
   Hemiplegia (one side of the body) or portions such as an arm, leg, or the face.

B. **Articulation**
   Difficulty of speech which may be due to involvement of the tongue, mouth, or throat as well as brain damage related to the speech centers.

C. **Salivation**
   Difficulty in control of saliva complicated by difficulty in swallowing.

D. **Sensory**
   Loss in affected parts with superficial anesthesia; or the opposite may occur with increased sensitivity to pain and touch.

E. **Visual Impairment**
   Blurred vision, or diminished visual acuity.

F. **Mental Function**
   May be unaffected, but slowness with poor memory and loss of initiative are common. Brain deterioration may occur over a period of time.

G. **Personality**
   Changes related to emotional trauma, fear, discouragement, and dependency are common.

II. Occurrence

A. Cerebral thrombosis is the most common cause of stroke: it accounts for 50 to 90 percent in people over 45. Cerebral hemorrhage causes up to 20 percent in the 30 to 60 age group, and aneurysms occur more in younger people between 20 and 30.

B. Stroke is the third leading cause of death in the United States.

III. Dental Hygiene Care

Patients may be homebound (pages 581–584) or may be brought to the dental office or clinic in a wheel chair, so that a wide variety of adaptations apply to the care of the patient. Every attempt should be made to provide thorough treatment rather than emergency or superficial only.

Because of the problems of self-care by the hemiplegic, the threat of advanced periodontal disease development has serious implications. As with most handicapped patients, it is not possible to cope with the rigors of complicated dental treatment.

Suggestions for the appointment described on page 655 can be applied for the stroke victim. Assistance during instrumentation particularly for evacuation is important since the patient has difficulty in rinsing because of facial paralysis, as well as to shorten the operating time and accomplish more in the time available.

Techniques for plaque control may need special adaptations. When the right-handed patient is paralyzed on the right side (or vice versa), development of dexterity for the manipulation of the toothbrush with the left hand may take time and patience. The patient needs to be as self-sufficient as possible.

DISORDERS OF PERCEPTION AND COMMUNICATION

Visual Impairment

Limitations of sight cover a broad spectrum from the slightly affected to the completely blind with no perception of light. Adaptations during the appointment vary then from a procedure as simple as providing a patient's eyeglasses before demonstrating a toothbrushing procedure to those required for the nearly or completely sightless as described in this section.

Loss of sight is a major physical deprivation. In many people blindness is secondary only to a primary condition which may have been the cause of the blindness and in itself may be disabling.

I. Causes of Blindness[33]

Senile cataract, glaucoma, diabetes, vascular disease, and infectious diseases, in that order, are the leading causes of blindness.[34] At least one-half of the blindness in children is of prenatal origin. Other causes are injuries, neoplasms, and retrolental fibroplasia. Retrolental fibroplasia was a major cause of blindness in premature infants but now is rare since it has been shown that it can be prevented by proper control of the oxygen exposure of an infant.

Approximately two-thirds of those who are blind lose their vision after age 20. According to the National Health Survey, 68 percent of the blind population is 65 years of age or older.

II. Psychological Considerations

Each blind person must be considered in relation to his aptitudes, interests, abilities, and potentialities, with blindness only one factor involved and frequently not the most important. No pattern of patient attitudes and personality characteristics can be described. The only thing this group of patients has in common is difficulty in seeing. A few suggestions of factors involved are mentioned below.

A. **Child**
   1. *Learning Ability*
      a. Sensory defects often mask the child's intellectual capacity since he cannot respond as other children.
      b. Blind children learn to speak later than sighted children and frequently start school when they are a year or two older.
      c. It takes a blind child longer to cover the same amount of material, therefore there may be a different educational level than for the sighted child of the same chronologic age.
      d. Blind children are deprived of the opportunity to learn by imitation.
   2. *Personality Factors*
      Environment influences the child's adjustment, and parental attitude affects the blind child as it does the sighted child. When the parent is overindulgent and protective, the child may be self-centered, dependent, and emotionally less stable.[35]

B. **Adult**
   The adult who has always been blind or since childhood has made adjustments and may be employed in a limited but useful occupation. The greater number who become blind after adulthood experience an immediate natural reaction of depression and feeling of helplessness. When there is incipient loss of vision there usually is less shock and upheaval, but there may be many years of dread, worry, and anxiety in anticipation. When the patient begins to accept the handicap, efforts for rehabilitation are made easier. Independence and self-confidence need to be developed and

the patient must be helped not to be-come helpless.

III. Dental Hygiene Care

A. **Totally Blind**

1. *Factors in Patient Care*

   a. A blind person can perceive a new experience readily if told about it in detail.

   b. Because of the visual handicap, the patient must rely more on other senses and cultivate them.

   c. A blind person has to be neat and orderly: if something is put down it must be readily located again.

   d. A blind person does things de-liberately and slowly to gain perception and prevent acci-dents.

   e. Effective conversation with a blind person can best be ac-complished by speaking as on a telephone.

   f. A blind person learns to interpret tone of voice and put more reliance on this than people with sight who can watch facial ex-pressions.

2. *Patient Reception and Seating*

   a. Lower dental chair prior to re-ceiving patient; move other den-tal equipment such as bracket table, motor arm, operating stool from pathway.

   b. Guide to dental chair: patient holds arm and is led without being held.

   c. Provide forewarnings of poten-tial hazards in the pathway.

   d. Instruct patient of step up to conventional dental chair.

   e. For recall patient: when patient has become familiar with office arrangement from previous ap-pointments, changes should be mentioned to prevent embar-rassment.

   f. When leaving operatory during the appointment explain ab-sence; prevent embarrassment of patient speaking to someone who is not there; speak when reentering the room.

3. *Techniques*

   a. Describe each step in detail before proceeding: instruments, materials, and how each will be applied; mention flavors.

   b. Permit patient to handle instru-ments before they are used while describing how each will be used; this applies particularly to child patient who is not familiar with dental procedures.

   c. Use second set of instruments in order to maintain sterile proce-dures.

   d. Use other instruments of a simi-lar size and shape when describ-ing scalers or explorers since handling sharp instruments would be dangerous for the pa-tient.

   e. Moving rubber cup may be applied to child's finger: if motor-driven instruments dis-turb the patient, use porte polisher for entire procedure.

   f. Avoid surprise applications of compressed air, water from syringe, or motor-driven instru-ments.

   g. Speak before touching the pa-tient: by maintaining contact of a finger on a tooth or through retraction while changing in-struments, repeated orientation is avoided.

   h. Rinsing: use evacuator when possible; without evacuation, explain the water syringe or place rinsing cup in the hand each time rather than expect the patient to pick it up from unit; help avoid patient's embarrass-ment if water is spilled.

4. *Patient Instruction*
   a. Give instructions clearly and concisely.
   b. Visual aids such as models may be used if described in detail and given to the patient to handle.
   c. Toothbrushing: demonstration in patient's mouth.
   d. Educational materials have been prepared in braille or on tapes.[36,37]

B. **Partially Blind**

People with sight often underestimate degree and fail to realize how useful a little vision can be. Patience in helping a patient make full use of available vision, without oversolicitousness, is important. Although many of the procedures described for the totally blind can be applied to the partially blind, a few additional hints are suggested below.

Elderly patients with failing sight will rarely admit such a handicap. Sight failure in the aged or lowered vision at any age may be suspected from the patient's unusual squinting, blinking, or lack of continuing attention. Techniques can be adapted without mention of sight to the patient.

1. Avoid glare of operating light in patient's eyes: this is true of all patients in helping to preserve sight.
2. Do not expect patient to see fine detail as in a radiograph or on a small model.
3. Work patiently and give instruction slowly: patient may have slow accommodation.
4. Present the patient's eyeglasses before beginning instruction.

Hearing Impairment

When there is impairment of hearing to the extent that it has no practical value for the purpose of communication, a person is considered deaf. When hearing is defective but functional with or without a hearing aid, the terms "hard of hearing" or "partially deaf" are used.

I. Causes of Hearing Impairment[38]

Inability to hear may be temporary or permanent. There is a wide variety of factors which contribute to deafness. In young children, heredity, prenatal influences particularly rubella, perinatal conditions notably kernicterus, and postnatal influences particularly infectious diseases (meningitis) are important causes.

Deafness beginning during school-age years can result from complications of upper respiratory infections. Older people may develop deafness following chronic infection of the middle ear, toxicity from various chemotherapeutic drugs, and trauma. Deterioration of hearing range may occur with aging.

II. Characteristics

A. **Major Types**
   1. *Conduction or Bone Deafness*
      a. Part involved: middle ear, external canal, or drum membrane.
      b. Hearing aid: plate behind ear; sound is conducted by bone.
      c. Speech: soft and low; person hears own voice louder than others.
   2. *Perception or Nerve Deafness*
      a. Part involved: inner ear; injury to nerves.
      b. Hearing aid: button in ear; sound conducted by air.
      c. Speech: loud; person cannot hear own voice.

B. **Characteristics Suggesting Hearing Impairment**

Partial deafness may not have been diagnosed or certain patients, particularly the elderly, may not admit hearing limitation. Clues to the identification of a hearing problem are listed below.

1. Lack of attention; fails to respond to conversational tone.
2. Intentness; strained facial expression; stares at others.
3. Turns head to one side; hearing may be good on one side only.
4. Gives unexpected answer unrelated to question; does one thing when told to do another.
5. Frequently asks others to repeat what was said.
6. Unusual speech tone.
7. Inaccurate pronunciation: characteristic in child who repeats what is heard; with defective hearing certain sounds are missing in the hearing range.

C. **Psychological Factors**

People with hearing loss tend to have more emotional difficulties than those with sight loss. Hard of hearing people are inclined to withdraw. They are bothered when they do not know what others are saying. This is mostly true of older people who develop paranoid tendencies and believe that when they cannot hear, other people are talking about them. Children do not have this problem but live in their own little world and watch others.

III. The Dental Hygiene Appointment

A. **Patient With Hearing Aid**

Allow time for adjustment.

B. **Patient With Partial Hearing Ability**

1. Speak clearly and distinctly; direct speaking to side of "good" ear if hearing is impaired on one side only.
2. Eliminate interfering noises: from street outside or saliva ejector suction.

C. **Lip Reader**

1. Be sure patient is looking; do not turn to side; speak directly.
2. Speaker's faces must be lighted so patient can read lips easily; difficult because dental light is directed to patient's face; operator may have back to window.

3. Speak in normal tone; do not accentuate words.
4. Do not raise voice; raising voice aggravates the situation; patient may be inclined to withdraw.
5. When patient cannot understand: use alternate words to express the same thought; many letters and combinations of letters look the same on the lips; others are not visible at all.
6. Keep calm; display of irritation or annoyance over difficulties in conversing will discourage or upset the patient.
7. Write proper names or unusual words which the patient fails to understand.

D. **Patient Without Hearing Aid Who Does Not Lip Read**

Use gestures and written notes.

E. **General Instructions**

1. Do not startle the patient by tapping to gain attention.
2. Watch for patient's motions and facial expressions to determine reaction or discomfort.
3. Teach by demonstration.
   a. Open mouth wide each time patient is to open.
   b. Small child may be taught to rinse by watching and imitating.
4. Appointment making: hard of hearing person should always have written appointment card to assure complete understanding; appointments made by telephone should be confirmed by mail.
5. Use judgment in prolonging conversation with deaf person: certain patients are under tension and tire easily whereas others enjoy the opportunity to be the center of attention.

References

1. Bakwin, H. and Bakwin, R. M.: *Behavior Disorders in Children*, 4th ed. Philadelphia, Saunders, 1972, pp. 131–132.
2. Adelson, J. J.: Handicapped and Problem Patient—Radiodontic Examination and Treatment, *Dent. Radiogr. Photogr.*, 34, 27, No. 2, 1961.
3. Groper, J. N., Nishimine, K., and O'Grady, C.: A Simplified Radiographic Technique for the Difficult Patient, *J. Dent. Child.*, 32, 269, 4th Quarter, 1965.
4. Hall, G.: A. Holly Patterson Home for Nassau County Aged and Infirm, Uniondale, Long Island, New York 11553, personal communication.
5. Fuller, L. and Dunn, M. J.: An Occupational Therapist's Role in Oral Hygiene for the Handicapped, *Am. J. Occup. Ther.*, 20, 35, January-February, 1966.
6. Birch, R. H. and Mumford, J. M.: Electric Toothbrushing, *Dent. Pract.*, 13, 182, January, 1963.
7. Zafran, J. N. and Zayon, G. M.: Prosthodontics and the Stroke Patient, *J. Am. Dent. Assoc.*, 74, 1250, May, 1967.
8. Blum, H. L. and Keranen, G. M.: *Control of Chronic Diseases in Man*. American Public Health Association, 1966, pp. 97–101.
9. Shafer, W. G., Hine, M. K., and Levy, B. M.: *A Textbook of Oral Pathology*, 3rd ed. Philadelphia, Saunders, 1974, pp. 807–808.
10. Ibid., p. 811.
11. Burket, L. W.: *Oral Medicine*, 6th ed. Philadelphia, Lippincott, 1971, pp. 113–114.
12. Shafer, Hine, and Levy: op. cit., pp. 788–790.
13. McCarthy, P. L. and Shklar, G.: *Diseases of the Oral Mucosa*. New York, Blakiston Division, McGraw-Hill, 1964, pp. 138–140.
14. United States Department of Health, Education, and Welfare: Vital and Health Statistics, Data from the National Health Survey, *Chronic Conditions Causing Activity Limitation*, United States, July 1963-June 1965. Washington, D.C., Public Health Service Publication No. 1000, Series 10, No. 51, February, 1969.
15. Blackwood, H. J. J.: Pathology of the Temporomandibular Joint, *J. Am. Dent. Assoc.*, 79, 118, July, 1969.
16. Mayne, J. G. and Hatch, G. S.: Arthritis of the Temporomandibular Joint, *J. Am. Dent. Assoc.*, 79, 125, July, 1969.
17. Marbach, J. J.: Arthritis of the Temporomandibular Joints, *Dent. Radiogr. Photogr.*, 42, 51, No. 3, 1969.
18. Lupton, D. E.: Psychological Aspects of Temporomandibular Joint Dysfunction, *J. Am. Dent. Assoc.*, 79, 131, July, 1969.
19. Blum and Keranen: op. cit., pp. 125–127.
20. Scheinberg, L. C.: The Demyelinating Diseases, in Beeson, P. B. and McDermott, W., eds.: *Textbook of Medicine*, 14th ed. Philadelphia, Saunders, 1975, pp. 718–720.
21. Blum and Keranen: op. cit., pp. 112–116.
22. Bakwin and Bakwin: op. cit., pp. 143–153.
23. Krause, M. V. and Hunscher, M. A.: *Food, Nutrition and Diet Therapy*, 5th ed. Philadelphia, Saunders, 1972, p. 548.
24. Album, M. M., Krogman, W. M., Baker, D., and Colwell, F. H.: Evaluation of the Dental Profile of Neuromuscular Deficit Patients: A Pilot Study, *J. Dent. Child.*, 31, 204, 3rd Quarter, 1964.
25. Horowitz, H. S., Greek, W. J., and Hoag, O. S.: Study of the Provision of Dental Care for Handicapped Children, *J. Am. Dent. Assoc.*, 71, 1398, December, 1965.
26. Rosenbaum, C. H., McDonald, R. E., and Levitt, E. E.: Occlusion of Cerebral-Palsied Children, *J. Dent. Res.*, 45, 1696, November-December, 1966.
27. Young, W. O. and Shannon, J. H.: Providing Dental Treatment for Handicapped Children, *J. Dent. Child.*, 35, 225, May, 1968.
28. Shafer, Hine, and Levy: op. cit., pp. 800–801.
29. Burket: op. cit., pp. 371–373.
30. Blum and Keranen: op. cit., pp. 129–131.
31. Burket: op. cit., p. 385.
32. Blum and Keranen: op. cit., pp. 64–68.
33. Ibid., pp. 18–30.
34. National Society for the Prevention of Blindness: *Estimated Statistics on Blindness and Vision Problems*. NSPB Fact Book, 1966.
35. Bakwin and Bakwin: op. cit., pp. 164–174.
36. State of Iowa Commission for the Blind, 4th and Keosauqua Way, Des Moines, Iowa 50309.
37. Braille Volunteers of Huntington, 152 Green Oak Drive, Huntington, West Virginia 25703.
38. Blum and Keranen: op. cit., pp. 30–33.

Suggested Readings

Adelson, J. J.: The Effects of Dental Treatment on Behavior of Handicapped Patients, *J. Am. Dent. Assoc.*, 71, 1411, December, 1965.

Anderson, C. F.: Modified Dental Chair for Patients in Wheelchairs, *J. Am. Dent. Assoc.*, 74, 1255, May, 1967.

Baer, P. N. and Benjamin, S. D.: *Periodontal Disease in Children and Adolescents*. Philadelphia, Lippincott, 1974, pp. 255–270.

Barber, T. K.: The Handicapped Adolescent, *Dent. Clin. North Am.*, 13, 313, April, 1969.

Cloran, A. J.: Telescopic Mouth Instruments for Severely Handicapped Patients, *J. Prosthet. Dent.*, 32, 435, October, 1974.

Coffee, L. and Anderson, J. L.: Preventive Dental Care for the Handicapped, *J. Am. Soc. Prev. Dent.*, 3, 55, November-December, 1973.

Cramer, J. J. and Wright, S. A.: The Bean Bag Chair and the Pedodontic Patient with Cerebral Palsy, *Dent. Hyg.*, 49, 167, April, 1975.

Durnan, J. R. and Thaler, R.: Dental Care for the Patient with a Spinal Cord Injury, *J. Am. Dent. Assoc.*, 86, 1318, June, 1973.

Fox, L. A.: The Handicapped Child, *Dent. Clin. North Am.*, 18, 535, July, 1974.

Hall, R. K.: Management of the Sick and Handicapped Child in General Dental Practice, *Austr. Dent. J.*, 12, 323, August, 1967.

King, W. C.: Mouthstick Habilitation, *J. Am. Dent. Assoc.*, 87, 839, October, 1973.

Kroll, R. G.: The Effect of Premedication on Handicapped Children, *J. Dent. Child.*, 36, 29, March-April, 1969.

Law, D. B., Lewis, T. M., and Davis, J. M.: *An Atlas of Pedodontics.* Philadelphia, Saunders, 1969, pp. 307–317.

Miller, J. B. and Taylor, P. P.: A Survey of the Oral Health of a Group of Orthopedically Handicapped Children, *J. Dent. Child.*, 37, 331, July-August, 1970.

Moore, M. J., Behan, P. O., and Lisak, R. P.: Multiple Sclerosis, *Postgrad Med.*, 53, 75, April, 1973.

Myasthenia Gravis Foundation: *Myasthenia Gravis. A Handbook for Patients.* National Headquarters, 2 East 103rd St., New York, New York 10029.

Schweiger, J. W., Netsell, R., and Sommerfeld, R. M.: Prosthetic Management and Speech Improvement in Individuals with Dysarthria of the Palate, *J. Am. Dent. Assoc.*, 80, 1348, June, 1970.

Swallow, J. N.: The Dental Management of the Physically Handicapped Child, *Br. Dent. J.*, 120, 35, January 4, 1966.

United States Department of Health, Education, and Welfare: *Feeding the Child with a Handicap.* Social and Rehabilitation Service, Children's Bureau, Publication No. 450–1967. Superintendent of Documents, U.S. Government Printing Office, Washington, D.C. 20402.

Walter, D. C.: Parkinson's Disease: The Effect of Levodopa Therapy on the Dentition: Report of Case, *J. Am. Dent. Assoc.*, 85, 133, July, 1972.

Wiesjahn, V.: Scoliosis: The Dentist's Role in the Team Approach, *J. Hosp. Dent. Pract.*, 4, 7, January, 1970.

Plaque Control

Albertson, D. and Johnson, R.: Plaque Control for the Institutionalized Child, *J. Am. Dent. Assoc.*, 87, 1389, December, 1973.

Aronovitz, R. and Conroy, C. W.: Effectiveness of the Automatic Toothbrush for Handicapped Persons, *Am. J. Phys. Med.*, 48, 193, August, 1969.

Doykos, J. D., Sweeney, E. A., and Glass, R. L.: Oral Hygiene Maintenance in Handicapped Children, *J. Dent. Child.*, 34, 511, November, 1967.

Holcomb, F. H., Taylor, P. P., and Saunders, W. A.: Comparison of Two Oral Hygiene Devices for the Physically Handicapped, *J. Dent. Child.*, 37, 325, July-August, 1970.

Johnson, R. and Albertson, D.: Plaque Control for Handicapped Children, *J. Am. Dent. Assoc.*, 84, 824, April, 1972.

Levenson, M. F.: Oral Hygiene and Self-care. A Method of Oral Hygiene and Self-care for the Teeth or Gingiva, *Am. J. Occup. Ther.*, 22, 209, May-June, 1968.

Arthritis

American Rheumatism Association: *Primer on the Rheumatic Diseases.* New York, The Arthritis Foundation, 1212 Avenue of the Americas, New York, New York 10036.

Blum, H. L. and Keranen, G. M.: *Control of Chronic Diseases in Man.* Committee on Chronic Disease and Rehabilitation, American Public Health Association, 1966, pp. 104–112.

Burket, L. W.: *Oral Medicine*, 6th ed. Philadelphia, Lippincott, 1971, pp. 346–351.

Collins, L. H. and Crane, M. P.: *Internal Medicine in Dental Practice*, 6th ed. Philadelphia, Lea & Febiger, 1965, pp. 379–422.

Crum, R. J. and Loiselle, R. J.: Incidence of Temporomandibular Joint Symptoms in Male Patients with Rheumatoid Arthritis, *J. Am. Dent. Assoc.*, 81, 129, July, 1970.

Lamont-Havers, R. W.: Arthritis of the Temporomandibular Joint, *Dent. Clin. North Am.*, p. 621, November, 1966.

Shafer, W. G., Hine, M. K., and Levy, B. M.: *A Textbook of Oral Pathology*, 3rd ed. Philadelphia, Saunders, 1974, pp. 657–661.

Zampelli, M., Salkin, L. M., Vandersall, D. C., and Denbo, J. A.: Rheumatoid Arthritis of the Temporomandibular Joint: Case Report, *J. Periodont.*, 45, 26, January, 1974.

Cerebral Palsy

Fishman, S. R., Young, W. O., Haley, J. B., and Sword, C.: The Status of Oral Health in Cerebral Palsy Children and Their Siblings, *J. Dent. Child.*, 34, 219, July, 1967.

Gelbier, S.: Dentistry and the Handicapped Child, *Dent. Health*, 5, 1, January-March, 1966.

Rosenstein, S. N. and King, M. B.: *Dental Care for Adult Patients with Cerebral Palsy.* United Cerebral Palsy of New York City, Inc., 339 E. 44th Street, New York, New York 10017.

Sullivan, S.: Dental Hygiene Patients with Special Needs, The Cerebral Palsy Patient, *J. Am. Dent. Hyg. Assoc.*, 40, 77, 2nd Quarter, 1966.

Scleroderma

Cummings, N. A.: Oral Manifestations of Connective Tissue Disease, *Postgrad. Med.*, 49, 134, January, 1971.

DePalma, R. A.: Case Report: Dental Treatment of Scleroderma, *Dent. Surv.*, 48, 26, August, 1972.

Hoggins, G. S. and Hamilton, M. C.: Dentofacial Defects Associated with Scleroderma, *Oral Surg.*, 27, 734, June, 1969.

Parel, S. M.: Scleroderma: A Prosthetic Problem, *J. Prosthet. Dent.*, 27, 560, May, 1972.

Perception and Communication

Davis, R. L.: The Blind Dental Patient, *Ill. Dent. J.*, 34, 783, December, 1965.

Rapp, R., Kanar, H. L., and Nagler, B.: Pedodontic Care for the Deaf and Blind, *Dent. Clin. North Am.*, p. 21, March, 1966.

Chapter 50

The Patient with a Disorder of the Circulatory System

The circulatory system includes the heart, blood vessels, blood, and the lymphatics. A wide variety of complicated diseases may affect these vital parts. Since many of the conditions are prolonged or even incurable, maintenance of oral health and preventive care assumes particular significance. There should not be further complications of the already existing general health problems by the addition of oral diseases, particularly dental caries or periodontal involvements.

In certain instances the physical condition of the patient is not such that the complicated and time-consuming oral or dental operations which might be required if the health of the mouth were neglected could be endured. The oral comfort of the patient is also important, particularly when there may be a long period of disability involving confinement.

The patient's medical history may reveal the existence of a circulatory disease although frequently the patient may not know the specific nature or seriousness of the disorder. Undiagnosed cases may be suspected by information from the patient history or the general physical condition observed, and the dental hygienist may have the opportunity to assist in the recognition of conditions which should be referred to a physician.

In either the diagnosed or suspected case, consultation with the patient's physician must precede dental and dental hygiene procedures. When the physician is called it is necessary to explain the details of the techniques to be performed and to inquire concerning medication which the patient may be receiving. The physician will suggest precautions which should be observed and the extent of treatment which the patient can be expected to withstand.

Application of knowledge of the characteristics of the particular disease can aid in the prevention of complications which may arise from, for example, excessive hemorrhage, the patient's lowered resistance to infection, or emergencies requiring first aid. Premedication may be mandatory, as in the case of the patient with a damaged heart valve.

CARDIOVASCULAR DISEASES

Cardiovascular, as the name implies, includes diseases of the heart and blood vessels. Diseases of the heart are the leading causes of death in the United States and, of these, coronary heart disease is responsible for at least 80 percent.

Patients with cardiovascular conditions are encountered frequently in the dental office and may be from any age group although the highest incidence is among older people. A heart disease may be present for many years prior to the time symptoms are recognized. The patients seen in the dental office, therefore, range from those with no obvious symptoms to the nearly disabled. In severe cases, the nonambulatory patient may require care in the home.

Classification of the diseases is made either on an anatomic or etiologic basis. In the anatomic system diseases of the pericardium, myocardium, endocardium, heart valves, and blood vessels are defined. In the etiologic system the diseases are named by the cause, as for example, congenital, rheumatic, arteriosclerotic, or hypertensive. Characteristics and symptoms are complex and overlapping.

The five major types of cardiovascular diseases are congenital heart disease, rheumatic heart disease, coronary heart disease, hypertensive heart disease, and bacterial endocarditis. These are defined below and their major symptoms listed. Additional reading is recommended for greater detail.[1-4]

Bacterial endocarditis is considered in a separate section because of its marked relationship to dental and dental hygiene treatment. The necessity for specific preventive procedures has been clearly defined.

I. General Complications of Heart Diseases

Since cardiac arrhythmias and cardiac insufficiency (leading to congestive heart failure) are the causes of many symptoms associated with various heart diseases, these conditions will be described briefly before the specific diseases.

A. **Arrhythmias**
1. Variations in the normal rhythm of the heartbeat may be a normal physiological response or may be a complication of heart disease.
2. Abnormal rates and rhythm in a patient with heart disease may mean that the ventricle is not pumping an adequate amount of blood into the systemic circulation to take care of body needs. Congestive heart failure may then occur.
3. Symptoms: patient reports palpitations or flutterings; may feel weak or faint.

B. **Congestive Heart Failure**
The heart is no longer able to circulate the amount of blood required by the body.
1. Causes
   a. Degenerative changes in the muscles of the heart.
   b. Increased demand on a damaged heart.
   c. Insufficient return of blood to the heart because of failure in the peripheral vessels.
2. Symptoms
   a. Shortness of breath following moderate exertion.
   b. Swelling of ankles.
   c. Cough.
   d. Oral: cyanosis of the lips, tongue, oral mucosa; marked distention of veins on undersurface of tongue.
   e. General fatigue.

II. Major Types of Cardiovascular Diseases

A. **Congenital Heart Disease**
Abnormalities in the anatomic structure of the heart or major blood vessels due to faulty or arrested development during fetal life.

1. Major symptom: cyanosis involving lips and tissues of the oral cavity.
2. Susceptibility of damaged heart to infection may predispose to subacute bacterial endocarditis (page 680).

B. **Rheumatic Heart Disease**

A complication of rheumatic fever which frequently results in heart valve damage. As with the damaged heart valve of congenital heart disease, there is susceptibility to infection predisposing to subacute bacterial endocarditis.

C. **Coronary Heart Disease**

Insufficient blood supply to the heart muscles; also called ischemic heart disease or coronary artery disease. It is usually caused by atherosclerosis with narrowing of the coronary vessels.

1. *Atherosclerosis and Arteriosclerotic Heart Disease.* Hardening and thickening of the arteries which diminish their capacity to supply blood, thus requiring additional work by the heart. In the heart muscle this condition can cause a temporary shortage of oxygen such as occurs in angina pectoris, or there may be a complete obstruction of the blood supply to a portion of the myocardium such as occurs in myocardial infarction.
2. *Angina Pectoris*
   a. Transient sharp pain in the chest over the region of the heart accompanied by sense of suffocation; pain may radiate to left arm and to neck and mandible in certain cases.
   b. Induced by exertion, emotions, excess food.
3. *Acute Myocardial Infarction* (coronary thrombosis, coronary occlusion).
   a. Prolonged severe pain in the cardiac region accompanied by fall in blood pressure and other symptoms of shock; sometimes pain in abdominal region.
   b. Cause: inadequate coronary blood supply resulting from occlusion of coronary arteries by embolism or thrombosis.

D. **Hypertensive Heart Disease**

Result of increased load on the heart because of elevated arterial blood pressure.

1. Primary hypertension: no underlying pathologic abnormality can be found to explain the cause. Frequently it can be related to emotional stress reactions to problems of daily living.
2. Secondary hypertension: pathologic elevation of the blood pressure secondary to an underlying disturbance such as a nephritis.
3. Effects of hypertension. Elevation of blood pressure accompanies and is a symptom in other cardiovascular diseases, particularly hypertension-aggravated coronary heart disease.
   a. Contributes to the acceleration of atherosclerosis.
   b. Contributes to cardiac failure, cerebral hemorrhage, and coronary thrombosis.
4. Symptoms which suggest secondary hypertensive disease[5]
   a. Headache in occipital area.
   b. Failing vision.
   c. Ringing in ears.
   d. Weakness and tingling of hands and feet.
   e. Angina pectoris.
   f. Symptoms of congestive heart failure (I,B, above).
   g. Symptoms of renal failure, including vomiting, general muscle weakness, pruritus, anorexia.

III. Dental Hygiene Care

A. Medical History

A carefully prepared history for each patient should reveal necessary information relative to a history of rheumatic fever, rheumatic heart disease, a heart murmur, or a congenital heart lesion. Other routine questions can lead to a suspicion of a condition as yet undiagnosed (figure 6–1, page 66 and table 6–2, page 73). When the patient or family member is unable to be specific a consultation with the patient's physician is indicated.

For the patient who knows and names the heart condition, details relative to past and present treatment must be obtained. Knowledge of medications, previous or anticipated heart surgery, presence of a valvular prosthesis, and other details or restrictions is essential for planning safe dental and dental hygiene care.

B. Determination of Vital Signs

Blood pressure determination should be a routine part of a diagnostic work-up. For a patient with a disorder of the circulatory system blood pressure should be determined and recorded at the beginning of each appointment. The procedure is described on page 87.

C. Preliminary Procedures

1. *Consultation with Physician.* Generally the dentist will discuss the patient with the physician. The dental hygienist may assist in obtaining the necessary information.
2. *Premedication.* A sedative is frequently indicated for the patient with angina pectoris, postmyocardial infarction, or secondary hypertension.
3. *Prophylactic Antibiotic Therapy.* For prevention of bacterial endocarditis in patients with rheumatic fever history, damaged heart valve, congenital heart defect, or valvular prosthetic replacement. Others requiring premedication are listed on page 71. Special precautions for these patients are discussed on page 681.

D. Appointment Planning

1. Time: morning, before patient becomes fatigued.
2. Length: short to conserve patient's limited reserve. Instrumentation may be performed by quadrants or other segments depending on the extent required.
3. Recall: frequent, to prevent need for extended appointments for extensive dental or periodontal treatment.

E. Characteristics Affecting Appointment Procedures

1. *Physical Handicaps*
   a. Diminished tolerance for exercise.
   b. Readily fatigued.
   c. Shortness of breath.
2. *Psychological Handicaps*
   a. Fear of sudden death; overconcern about the heart; anxiety.
   b. Depression; feelings of rejection or hostility.
   c. Unwillingness to accept limitations required by the physical condition.
   d. Attitude of family: when cooperative and understanding may make complete difference in patient's attitude; overprotective or fearful family influences patient's attitude.
   e. Fear and anxiety over the dental appointment can result in detrimental cardiovascular reactions.

F. Suggestions for Appointment Procedure

1. Patient position: patient who has difficulty breathing usually requires an upright position.

2. Room temperature: should be adjusted and maintained. Sudden chilling can initiate attack of angina pectoris in the susceptible patient.
3. Avoid anxiety or undue apprehension on part of patient: explain carefully in nontechnical language what is going to be done, how long it will take, the type of discomfort which the patient may expect, and what cooperation is required.
4. All procedures should be carried out efficiently and quickly, consistent with thoroughness and patient comfort, and with a minimum of manipulation of oral tissues.
   a. Work with an assistant so that evacuation can decrease operating time and time required for rinsing. Patient fatigue from rinsing activities can also be lessened.
   b. Use an anesthetic: a topical anesthetic may suffice, but local anesthesia is not usually contraindicated for patients with heart diseases. Vasoconstrictors may be used with concentrations kept to a minimum of 1:100,000 or less.[6]

G. **Special Treatment Situations**
1. *Heart Valve Prosthesis*[7]
   a. Problems
      (1) High susceptibility to bacterial endocarditis.
      (2) Nearly all who have a prosthesis receive anticoagulant therapy.
   b. Preoperative: before the heart surgery, the patient's mouth should be brought to a state of optimum health with all sources of infection removed, all teeth restored, and a preventive program under way.
      (1) Complete plaque control: patient must understand the need for daily plaque removal using toothbrush, floss, and other aids as needed; and must learn to evaluate the mouth, using a disclosing agent.
      (2) Removal of all overhanging fillings and other sources of sharp edges and areas for plaque retention.
   c. Postoperative
      (1) Frequent recall for supervision and maintenance of health.
      (2) Antibiotic coverage for *all* procedures, especially scaling, root planing, and other procedures which touch gingival tissues.
   d. Prevention of dental caries: a specific plan for daily application of fluoride using a mouth rinse, gel tray, chewable tablet, or other method (pages 429, 439–442).
2. *Pacemaker*
   a. Definition and types: a pacemaker is an electrically operated mechanical device which stimulates ventricular heart action. There are portable and implantable types. The implantable one is a tiny self-contained transistorized unit that is implanted subcutaneously.
   b. Contraindication: electrosurgical and ultrasonic equipment (pages 218, 510).
3. *Anticoagulant Drug Therapy*
   Continuous anticoagulant therapy is commonly prescribed by the physician to prevent blood coagulation in patients susceptible to thrombosis or embolism. Current evidence indicates that generally it is safer to continue the patient's medication and take precautions to control bleeding.[8,9] The dentist and the physician determine the best procedure for the individual pa-

tient. When extensive surgical procedures are required, they may be performed in a hospital.

Instrumentation can be performed for most patients without complication provided precautions are taken to minimize tissue trauma, to control bleeding, and not to dismiss the patient until bleeding has stopped. Pressure with a gauze sponge or with cotton pellets packed between the teeth aids to hasten control.[10] Placement of a periodontal dressing is sometimes indicated.

Postoperatively, the patient is advised to avoid vigorous toothbrushing for several hours or until the next day. Use of a soft diet, cool rather than hot foods and beverages, and avoiding the area in general should be emphasized.

4. Emergency care: see table 54–1 on pages 729–731.

IV. Patient Instruction

A. Plaque Control

1. Stress the importance of meticulous care.
2. Distribute teaching over several appointments to avoid patient fatigue.
3. Instruct attendant of patient who is not capable of caring for his own mouth.

B. Diet

1. Suggestions may be limited by diet prescribed by physician: this should always be checked.
2. Example: patients with arteriosclerosis are frequently required to omit fats and other foods with high cholesterol content: substitutes frequently may be carbohydrates which are cariogenic; practical suggestions should be made accordingly.

BACTERIAL ENDOCARDITIS

Bacterial endocarditis is a serious disease and the prognosis depends on the degree of cardiac damage, valves involved, duration of the infection, and treatment. Patients are prone to develop heart failure leading to death unless the infection is promptly controlled.

Bacterial endocarditis is characterized by the formation of vegetations composed of masses of bacteria and blood clots on the heart valves. The vegetations may arise on normal valves but are most likely to occur on previously damaged valves. When a bacteremia occurs, the heart valves may become infected and bacterial endocarditis can develop.

Bacteremias frequently follow dental and dental hygiene treatment procedures. The relationship of bacteremias to scaling and curettage was described on page 496 with references.

I. Etiology

A. Microorganisms

Formerly a nonhemolytic streptococcus (particularly *Streptococcus viridans*) caused 70 to 80 percent of all cases, but because of antibiotic therapy there has been a marked change. The streptococci are currently responsible in 30 to 40 percent, while staphylococci now have increased involvement and are found to be the causative agent in about 23 percent of the cases of bacterial endocarditis.[11]

B. Predisposing Factors

1. Previous damage to heart valves by rheumatic fever; congenital malformations of the valves; or defects in the walls of the heart.
2. Site of cardiac surgery and the tissue about a valvular prosthesis are particularly vulnerable.
3. Presence of infection at portals of entrance of microorganisms into the

blood stream, for examples, periodontal disease, infected tonsils, renal infections.

C. **Exciting Factors**
1. Trauma: general or oral surgery, scaling, curettage.
2. Upper respiratory infections.

D. **Disease Process**
1. Trauma from oral surgery, scaling, and curettage ruptures blood vessels in the gingival sulcus.
2. Pressure from trauma forces oral microorganisms into blood stream thereby initiating a bacteremia.
   a. Ease of bacterial entry directly relates to amount of trauma.
   b. The greater the trauma, the greater the ease of bacterial entry.
3. Circulating microorganisms attach to endocardium of defective heart valve.
4. Microorganisms proliferate to form bacterial masses.
5. Heart valve becomes inflamed and cannot function properly.
6. Clumps of bacteria may break off, get into the systemic circulation, and be spread throughout the body.

II. Preventive Measures[12]

Bacteremias have been demonstrated following toothbrushing, chewing hard foods, as well as dental, dental hygiene, and periodontal treatment, and tooth removal. When infection is present, bacteremia has been shown to occur with greater frequency and severity.

The dental hygienist has an important part to perform with the cardiac patient in improving and maintaining the overall health of the oral cavity. Continuing efforts for the prevention of periodontal involvement and dental caries through professional care and motivation and instruction for self-care contribute to the safety and well-being of the patient.

A. **Patient History**
   It cannot be overemphasized that a complete patient history followed by consultation with the susceptible patient's physician is mandatory before any manipulation of oral tissues. This includes the use of the probe and explorer during patient examination prior to treatment planning.

B. **Prophylactic Antibiotic Medication**
1. *Purposes*[13]
   a. Prevent bacteremia or reduce its magnitude and duration should it occur.
   b. Eradicate bacteria that may implant on heart valves before a vegetation is formed.
2. *Indications* (page 71)
   a. Patients with rheumatic or congenital heart disease: treatment is started one to two hours prior to appointment, and continued for two days after. Penicillin is the drug of choice except when a patient is allergic, and then erythromycin is used.[13]
   b. Patients with rheumatic heart disease who receive long-term antibiotic prophylaxis: additional coverage is needed.[14]
   c. Patients who have had heart surgery and wear a valvular prosthesis: increased dose of antibiotic is needed.[7]

C. **Dental Hygiene Care**
1. *Plaque Control*
   a. Initial instruction in brushing and flossing should be provided while the patient is under antibiotic coverage.
   b. Instruction is given prior to instrumentation for calculus removal as for any patient, and the same basic procedures should be followed.
   c. Because of the importance of gingival health and conscien-

tious self-care, it is better not to tell the patient that brushing can create a bacteremia. Patients who fear bacteremia may be afraid to brush and floss thoroughly. Far more harm can result from persistent gingivitis or developing periodontal disease than from routine brushing. Furthermore, routine brushing for plaque control can prevent or control gingivitis and periodontal disease.

2. *Instrumentation.* Use particular care in all instrumentation to prevent unnecessary trauma.

BLOOD DISEASES

Oral tissue changes, lowered resistance to infection, and tendencies to hemorrhage are the major factors to be considered for patients with blood disorders. Oral symptoms of blood diseases are exaggerated as a result of neglect of health of the mouth. Routine professional care and instruction in personal oral care are indicated to aid in the prevention of the need for complicated dental and periodontal treatments.

I. Clinical Findings

The patient's medical history may not reveal the existence of a blood disorder. Oral manifestations which may be indicative of a blood disease should be called to the dentist's attention. The oral findings are not conclusive evidence that a disease exists and reference for medical study and blood tests is necessary. The findings listed below are important indications for recommending further clinical study for the patient.[15]

A. Spontaneous hemorrhage from the gingiva or mucous membranes.

B. Numerous petechiae.

C. History of difficulty in controlling postoperative hemorrhage by usual procedures.

D. Marked pallor of the mucous membranes.

E. Chronic oral infections which do not respond to treatment.

F. Atrophy of the papillae of the tongue without apparent cause.

G. Persistently sore tongue and mouth without evidence of local irritation.

H. History of prolonged bleeding episodes or ready bruising.

I. Severe ulcerations in the mouth associated with signs of severe illness or lack of response to treatment.

J. Acute infections of the oral mucosa which do not respond promptly to treatment.

II. The Red Blood Cells[16,17]

A. **Anemias**

Reduction in number of red blood cells, hemoglobin, or both.

1. Due to blood loss: hemorrhage from trauma or surgery.

2. Due to defective blood production: deficiencies in required nutrients.

   a. Iron-deficiency anemia: caused chiefly by inadequate intake of iron, chronic blood loss, or pregnancy.

   b. Pernicious anemia: caused by deficiency in vitamin B_{12}.

3. Due to depression of bone marrow activity: caused by x ray, radium, toxic chemicals, tumor invasion, or chronic infection.

4. Sickle cell anemia: a hereditary hemolytic form of anemia with sickle-shaped red blood cells resulting from a hemoglobin abnormality.[18,19]

B. **Oral Characteristics**[20,21]

Anemia is most frequently a symptom of a systemic disease remote from the tissues of blood formation or destruction. Because of reduced oxygen-carrying capacity of the blood, the patient exhibits signs of fatigue, weakness, lethargy, and shortness of breath.

1. General characteristics: all anemias
   a. Prolonged healing time.
   b. Lowered resistance to infection.
   c. Pale mucous membranes.
2. *Iron-deficiency anemia*
   a. Interdental papillae and free gingiva: purplish-red when inflammation is present.
   b. Tongue: atrophic, hypersensitive, loss of muscle tone.
   c. Lips: angular cheilosis.
   d. Black stain of teeth and tongue: related to using liquid preparation of iron.
3. *Pernicious anemia*
   a. Glossitis: atrophy of papillae leaves smooth red tongue which is painful and flabby.
   b. Mucosa and lips: pale and atrophic; susceptible to ulceration following minor trauma.
4. *Sickle cell anemia*[18,19]
   a. Radiographic change: generalized osteoporosis of the alveolar bone, with loss of trabeculation and large irregular marrow spaces. No change in the lamina dura or periodontal ligament space is seen.
   b. May be pallor of the gingiva and mucosa, but it may go unnoticed because of melanin pigmentation; the condition is found almost exclusively in negroes.

C. **Polycythemias**

Increase in hemoglobin concentration due to increase in number of red blood cells.

1. Mucous membranes, tongue, and gingiva: deep reddish-blue.
2. Gingiva appears engorged and tends to bleed easily.

D. **Dental Hygiene Care and Instruction**
1. *Appointment Planning*
   a. Short appointments: for patients with physical symptoms of weakness.
   b. Recall: frequent enough to prevent complications of oral diseases which require extensive, traumatic dental or periodontal treatment.
2. *Instrumentation.* Apply unusual care to prevent trauma to delicate tissues; apply petrolatum or cream for protection of angles of lips particularly when there is evidence of cheilosis.
3. *Patient Instruction*
   a. Emphasize personal oral care to promote healthy gingival tissues to mimimize hemorrhage and infection.
   b. Describe need for diet containing a variety of foods representing all of the basic food groups to compensate for nutritional deficiencies.
   c. Recommend that liquid iron preparations be taken through a straw and that the mouth be rinsed with water immediately following to prevent stains.

III. The White Blood Cells[16,17]

Leukopenia is a condition where the white blood cells are markedly reduced due to a depression of bone marrow activity as a result of infections, drugs, or radiation. *Leukemia*, on the other hand, is characterized by an abnormal proliferation of mature and immature white blood cells and is considered a neoplasm. Although the cause of the leukemias is not known, ionizing radiation, genetic predisposition, and viruses are implicated.

A. **Acute Leukemia**
1. Occurs in young people; has a high incidence in children under five.
2. Symptoms include an abrupt onset with fever, extreme fatigue, upper respiratory infection, and, after a few weeks to months, infections

and hemorrhages are present with increasing severity. Bleeding from the gingiva is fairly common.

B. **Chronic Leukemia**
1. Occurs less frequently in children and more in adults.
2. Onset is insidious with weakness, anemia, weight loss, enlargement of spleen and lymph nodes, and recurrent persistent infections. Hemorrhages may be a major manifestation and occur as profuse nosebleeds, bleeding from the gastrointestinal tract, or unusual bleeding from the gingiva.

C. **Oral Manifestations**[20,21]
Gingival signs may be among the earliest evidence, particularly of the chronic type of leukemia. It behooves the dental hygienist to watch for the various changes which may occur in the oral tissues. When patients are seen on a regular plan for recall, the opportunity is available to observe tissue changes and bring the changes to the attention of the dentist.

Oral signs appear generally the same in both acute and chronic leukemia. In acute there tends to be a more severe tissue response.
1. Gingiva
   a. Bluish-red color; enlargement which tends to obscure the teeth as the disease progresses; interferes with mastication.
   b. Bleeding on slight provocation and sometimes spontaneously.
   c. Ulceration, necrosis, and epithelial sloughing; unpleasant odor.
   d. Debris is retained and deposits accumulate in the deepened sulci. The patient may not brush adequately because of soreness and bleeding. Local irritants increase the severity of the tissue reaction.
2. Mucosa: pale, with ulcerations and petechiae.

3. Increased susceptibility to infection.
4. Cervical and submandibular lymph node enlargement.

D. **Dental Hygiene Care**
1. *Referral.* When oral signs are noted that suggest leukemia in the undiagnosed patient, referral for thorough medical examination is mandatory.
2. *Treatment.* In the patient with diagnosed leukemia, preventive care to restore the health of the gingiva and teeth can be accomplished during periods of remission. Such periods are usually relatively short, so that long extensive periodontal therapy or reconstruction may be contraindicated.
3. *Appointment Planning*
   a. Short appointments: techniques limited to a few teeth at a time.
   b. Recall: frequent to attempt to maintain tissues in best possible condition.
4. *Antibiotic Premedication.* Arranged at advice of dentist and physician to minimize possibility of postoperative infection.
5. *Instrumentation*
   Because of the severe tissue reaction from local irritation, dental hygiene care is directed at the removal of deposits for the alleviation of symptoms. Gingivitis in leukemia is a conditioned response: patients may be free of tissue changes when local irritants from dental plaque, materia alba, food impaction, poorly contoured restorations, or ill-fitting prostheses are missing.[20]
   a. First appointment: instruction for personal daily care including brushing with a soft brush and rinsing. Scaling can be started at the first or second appointment and continued at successive appointments.

b. Topical anesthetic may be used to aid patient comfort.

c. Techniques adapted to enlarged tissue with extreme care to prevent unnecessary trauma.

d. Sterile technique: use of antiseptic solution on tissue; unusual care in sterilization of instruments.

e. Polishing is usually contraindicated to avoid gingival irritation by abrasive polishing agent and rubber cup.

6. *Patient Instruction*

a. Toothbrushing with a soft nylon brush (.006″ diameter filaments) is recommended.

b. Mouthwash: to combat unpleasant taste and odor from necrotic tissues.

IV. Hemorrhagic Disorders

Hemorrhagic disorders are characterized by spontaneous bleeding or excessive bleeding following trauma. Hemorrhage from a blood vessel depends on two major factors: the susceptibility of the vessels to injury, and the adequacy of the hemostatic responses. Hemorrhagic disorders may be categorized by two factors, the vessels and the clotting mechanism.[17]

The blood vessels, especially the capillaries, may be damaged or may become susceptible to injury in many disease conditions, for example, bacterial infections, bacterial endocarditis, and scurvy. Disorders of the blood which affect the hemostatic response may be related to a deficiency of platelets (thrombocytopenia), prothrombin deficiency associated with insufficient availability or utilization of vitamin K, and a deficiency of clotting factors of which Classical Hemophilia A is an example.

A. Hemophilia A

Classical hemophilia is a hereditary bleeding disorder resulting from a deficiency of factor VIII, the antihemophilic factor. Hemophilia A can be distinguished from hemophilia B which is a similar but less common disorder resulting from a deficiency of factor IX, the plasma thromboplastin component. Hemophilia B is also known as Christmas disease. In addition to factors VIII and IX there are other factors associated with more rare conditions.[22]

1. Heredity: Hemophilia A is inherited by males through the mother. Nearly 30 percent have no traceable history.

2. Degree of severity: of the hemophilia patients, only about half are severely affected and in these, the presence of a bleeding tendency is generally discovered early in life. Those with less severe conditions may not be aware of them until they are subjected to surgical trauma.

B. Dental Hygiene Care

Preventive education, treatment, and follow-up are all-important to the patient with a bleeding disorder. It is essential that the need for extensive dental and periodontal procedures that may involve excess bleeding be avoided.

1. *Consultation.* The dentist and physician need to consult to provide cooperative patient care and determine the correct procedure for the dental hygienist and dentist to follow relative to the bleeding problem of the individual patient.

2. *Instrumentation*[22,23]

a. Thorough removal of calculus is necessary if gingival health is to be obtained. Meticulous care to minimize tissue trauma is indicated. The standard of service should not be compromised because the patient is a bleeder.[22]

b. Length of appointment: shortened, and fewer teeth involved, when hemorrhage can be expected because of the clinical appearance of the gingiva.

3. *Fluoride Application.* All possible preventive measures should be included in the patient's treatment plan. A combined fluoride therapy program is advised. With fluoridation, topical fluoride and the use of a fluoride dentifrice; without fluoridation, a prescription for tablets should be provided.

4. *Plaque Control.* A strict program of self-care, which is fully understood by the patient, is needed. Instruction is carried out over several appointments and reviewed with each recall (pages 388–393).

References

1. Blum, H. L. and Keranen, G. M.: *Control of Chronic Diseases in Man.* American Public Health Association, 1966, pp. 46–64.
2. Burket, L. W.: *Oral Medicine,* 6th ed. Philadelphia, Lippincott, 1971, pp. 240–258.
3. Robbins, S. L.: *Pathologic Basis of Disease.* Philadelphia, Saunders, 1974, pp. 643–680.
4. Boyd, W.: *A Textbook of Pathology,* 8th ed. Philadelphia, Lea & Febiger, 1970, pp. 519–572.
5. Little, J. W. and Jakobsen, J.: Management of the Hypertensive Patient in Dental Practice, *J. Oral Med.,* 29, 13, January-March, 1974.
6. Bennett, C. R.: *Monheim's Local Anesthesia and Pain Control in Dental Practice,* 5th ed. St. Louis, Mosby, 1974, pp. 214–223.
7. Bottomley, W. K., Willis, P. W., and Fekety, F. R.: The Dental Patient with a Heart Valve Prosthesis: Preoperative and Postoperative Considerations, *J. Mich. Dent. Assoc., 51,* 149, April, 1969.
8. Kutscher, A. H., Zegarelli, E. V., Hyman, G. A., McLean, P., and Kutscher, H. W.: *Pharmacology for the Dental Hygienist.* Philadelphia, Lea & Febiger, 1967, pp. 141–142.
9. Fay, J. T.: Dental Procedures for the Patient with Cardiovascular Disease, *J. Am. Dent. Assoc.,* 78, 105, January, 1969.
10. Glickman, I.: *Clinical Periodontology,* 4th ed. Philadelphia, Saunders, 1972, pp. 974–975.
11. Robbins: op. cit., pp. 673–676.
12. Myall, R. W. T. and Gregory, H. S.: Current Trends in the Prevention of Bacterial Endocarditis in Susceptible Patients Receiving Dental Care, *Oral Surg.,* 28, 813, December, 1969.
13. American Heart Association: Prevention of Bacterial Endocarditis, *J. Am. Dent. Assoc.* 85, 1377, December, 1972.
14. Tarsitano, J. J. and O'Hara, J. W.: Rheumatic Fever: In-Depth Appraisal with a Discussion of Penicillin, *J. Am. Dent. Assoc.,* 77, 1074, November, 1968.
15. Collins, L. H. and Crane, M. P.: *Internal Medicine in Dental Practice,* 6th ed. Philadelphia, Lea & Febiger, 1965, p. 373.
16. Boyd: op. cit., pp. 1109–1155.
17. Robbins: op. cit., pp. 703–726.
18. Shafer, W. G., Hine, M. K., and Levy, B. M.: *A Textbook of Oral Pathology,* 3rd ed. Philadelphia, Saunders, 1974, pp. 672–674.
19. Catena, D. L.: Oral Manifestations of the Hemoglobinopathies, *Dent. Clin. North Am.* 19, 77, January, 1975.
20. Glickman: op. cit., pp. 102–103, 394–406, 971–972.
21. McCarthy, P. L. and Shklar, G.: *Diseases of the Oral Mucosa.* New York, Blakiston Division McGraw-Hill, 1964, pp. 255–264.
22. Webster, W. P., Roberts, H. R., and Penick G. D.: Dental Care of Patients with Hereditary Disorders of Blood Coagulation, *Mod Treatm.,* 5, 93, January, 1968.
23. Chiono, O.: The Role of the Dental Hygienist in the Care of Hemophilic Patients, *J. So. Calif. Dent. Hyg. Assoc.,* 11, 7, Winter, 1968.

Suggested Readings
Cardiovascular

American Dental Association, Council on Dental Therapeutics: *Accepted Dental Therapeutics* 36th ed. Chicago, American Dental Association, 1975, pp. 4–10, 169.

Archard, H. O. and Roberts, W. C.: Bacterial Endocarditis After Dental Procedures in Patients with Aortic Valve Prostheses, *J. Am. Dent. Assoc.* 72, 648, March, 1966.

Baer, P. N. and Benjamin, S. D.: *Periodontal Disease in Children and Adolescents.* Philadelphia, Lippincott, 1974, pp. 233–240, 241–253.

Burch, G. E. and DePasquale, N. P.: Arterial Hypertension and the Dental Patient, *J. Am Dent. Assoc.,* 73, 102, July, 1966.

Prudoff, S. H. and Stratigos, G. T.: Successful Management of Patients with Cardiac Valvular Prosthesis, *N. Y. State Dent. J.,* 38, 207, April 1972.

Scopp, I. W.: *Oral Medicine, A Clinical Approach with Basic Science Correlation,* 2nd ed. St Louis, Mosby, 1973, pp. 267–285.

Sorenson, H. W.: The Pedodontic Patient with Heart Disease, *Dent. Clin. North Am.,* 17, 173, January 1973.

Tocker, J. and Weibert, E.: The Dental Significance of Corticosteroids, Antihypertensive Drugs and Anticoagulants, *Dent. Hyg.,* 49, 11, January, 1975.

Waldrep, A. C. and McKelvey, L. E.: Oral Surgery for Patients on Anticoagulant Therapy, *J. Oral Surg.* 26, 374, June, 1968.

Blood Diseases

Burket, L. W.: *Oral Medicine*, 6th ed. Philadelphia, Lippincott, 1971, pp. 290–319.

Herschfus, L.: Oral Manifestations of Blood Disorders, *J. Oral Med.*, 25, 56, April-June, 1970.

Kerr, D. A. and Ash, M. M.: *Oral Pathology*, 3rd ed. Philadelphia, Lea & Febiger, 1971, pp. 279–294.

Stamps, J. T.: The Role of Oral Hygiene in a Patient with Idiopathic Aplastic Anemia, *J. Am. Dent. Assoc.*, 88, 1025, May, 1974.

Weiss, J. I.: Thrombocytopenic Purpura: The Dentist's Responsibility, *J. Am. Dent. Assoc.*, 87, 165, July, 1973.

Hemophilia

Glogoff, M., Baum, S. M., Sussman, R., Stewart, S., and Stoopack, J. C.: Management of the Hemophilic Oral Surgery Patient, *J. Oral Surg.*, 30, 252, April, 1972.

Leake, D. and Deykin, D.: The Diagnosis and Treatment of Bleeding Tendencies, *Oral Surg.*, 32, 852, December, 1971.

Lewis, B.: Dental Care for the Hemophiliac, *J. Am. Dent. Assoc.*, 87, 1411, December, 1973.

Lucas, O. N. and Prescott, G. H.: Hemophilias and Other Hemorrhagic Disorders, *Dent. Clin. North Am.*, 19, 63, January, 1975.

Powell, D. and Bartle, J.: The Hemophiliac: Prevention Is the Key, *Dent. Hyg.*, 48, 214, July-August, 1974.

Simpson, W. J. and Strelioff, M. G.: Postextraction Complications in Haemophilia: Report of Case and Discussion, *J. Can. Dent. Assoc.*, 34, 636, December, 1968.

Tarsitano, J. J. and Cohen, S. M.: Revelation and Initial Diagnosis of Mild Hemophilia from Dental Findings: Report of a Case, *J. Am. Dent. Assoc.*, 76, 823, April, 1968.

Leukemia

Arthur, A. L. and Salman, S. J.: Leukemia, *Oral Surg.*, 27, 460, April, 1969.

Carey, J. A. and Chilcote, R. R.: Dental Treatment for the Child with Acute Lymphocytic Leukemia 1974, *J. Dent. Child.*, 42, 191, May-June, 1975.

Curtis, A. B.: Childhood Leukemias: Initial Oral Manifestations, *J. Am. Dent. Assoc.*, 83, 159, July, 1971.

Lynch, M. A. and Ship, I. I.: Initial Oral Manifestations of Leukemia, *J. Am. Dent. Assoc.*, 75, 932, October, 1967.

Lynch, M. A. and Ship, I. I.: Oral Manifestations of Leukemia: A Postdiagnostic Study, *J. Am. Dent. Assoc.*, 75, 1139, November, 1967.

Sarnquist, J. L.: Oral Manifestations of Leukemia, *J. Am. Dent. Hyg. Assoc.*, 43, 145, 3rd Quarter, 1969.

White, G. E.: Oral Manifestations of Leukemia in Children, *Oral Surg.*, 29, 420, March, 1970.

Sickle Cell Anemia

Bhaskar, S. N.: *Synopsis of Oral Pathology*, 4th ed. St. Louis, Mosby, 1973, pp. 553–554.

Mourshed, F. and Tuckson, C. R.: A Study of the Radiographic Features of the Jaws in Sickle-cell Anemia, *Oral Surg.*, 37, 812, May, 1974.

Powell, E. A. and Januska, J. R.: Sickle Cell Anemia: Chronology, Natural History, and Implications for Dental Practice, *Quart. Nat. Dent. Assoc.*, 31, 72, July, 1973.

Schabel, R. W.: Diagnosis of Sickle-Cell Anemia in the Prosthetic Patient, *J. Prosthet. Dent.*, 20, 116, August, 1968.

Chapter 51

The Patient with Diabetes Mellitus

A preventive dental hygiene program is vital for the patient with diabetes mellitus. The diabetic patient, particularly one whose condition is unstable or uncontrolled, has a lowered resistance to infection and a delayed healing process. Gingival reactions to local irritants are exaggerated. Periodontal disease tends to develop with increased severity at an earlier age in the diabetic than in the nondiabetic patient.[1-4]

The presence of infection, including infection in the oral cavity, tends to intensify the diabetic symptoms and to contribute to difficulty in insulin regulation. The dental hygienist has a significant responsibility to assist the dentist in providing the patient with oral care and instruction for self-care aimed to maintain health and prevent gingival and periodontal diseases which may be potential sources of infection.

Modifications of dental and dental hygiene procedures for the diabetic patient may be indicated depending on the severity and control of the diabetes. No treatment involving tissue manipulation, including submarginal probing and scaling, should be attempted until the diabetic state has been controlled as confirmed by the patient's physician. Many well-controlled diabetics may be treated as healthy patients.

I. Occurrence[5]

A. Population Involved

It has been estimated that 4.4 million people in the United States are diabetic, but only slightly over one-half of these have been diagnosed and are under medical care. In addition, there are some five million nondiabetics who carry the genetic make-up that can lead eventually to symptomatic diabetes.[6] Together these figures represent approximately five percent of the population.

B. Age

There are ten times more people with diabetes in the over-45 age group than under 45; prevalence rises rapidly with age to the highest rate in the 65 to 74 age group.

C. Increased Incidence

An increased incidence of diabetes in recent years can be related to various factors including the following:

1. Improved methods of diagnosis.
2. Concentrated professional and community efforts to find undiagnosed cases and bring them to treatment.
3. Increased longevity of life
   a. More people live to the older age groups when diabetes is more prevalent.
   b. Diabetics live longer; they may marry and have children who are diabetic.
4. Generalized increased food consumption, more obesity, and tendency for less physical exercise.

II. The Diabetic Syndrome: Definition

Clinical diabetes has been known as a genetic (and less frequently an acquired) disorder of the metabolism of carbohydrate, fat, and protein, in which there is a disturbance in the production and action of insulin, a hormone secreted by the beta cells of the islets of Langerhans in the pancreas. In addition, it is recognized that certain clinical signs and symptoms such as increased blood glucose (hyperglycemia) may represent an advanced stage in the progression of the diabetic state.

There are manifestations, particularly those related to pathology of the small blood vessels (microangiopathy), which occur before detectable hyperglycemia or other clinical symptoms and can be demonstrated in prediabetic people.[6,7] Such findings contribute to a broadened concept of the definition of diabetes. It is now recognized to be a lifelong, complex syndrome with potential for control of marked complications.[8]

III. Classification

The classification outlined here was prepared by the Committee on Professional Education of the American Diabetes Association.[9] It is based on abnormalities of carbohydrate metabolism. No attempt was made to categorize vascula disease (microangiopathy) because it ma occur at any stage, even in prediabetes Changes from one stage to another may be slow or rapid, or may not occur at all.

A. **Overt Diabetes (Clinical or Symptomatic Diabetes)**
   1. Characteristic symptoms are present (symptoms are listed on page 694).
   2. Abnormal glucose tolerance i shown by all tests.
   3. It may be acute or chronic.

B. **Chemical or Latent Diabetes (Asymptomatic)**
   1. No clinical symptoms are apparent
   2. Oral glucose tolerance test* give results in the range for diabetes.

C. **Suspected Diabetes (Latent Chemical, Stress, or Subclinical Diabetes)**
   1. A temporary carbohydrate intolerance is shown in a period o physiologic or pathologic stress particularly when there is a family history of diabetes. Stress situation include pregnancy, severe infection, trauma, burns, impaired nutrition, or severe emotional disturbances.
   2. Abnormal glucose tolerance can be shown by the cortisone–glucose tolerance test.†

D. **Prediabetes ("Before Diabetes")**
   1. This stage represents the interva between fertilization of the ovum to

*Oral glucose tolerance test: a generally used test fo diagnosis of diabetes. Following the ingestion of a specific amount of glucose in solution in a non diabetic, the fasting blood glucose rises promptly then falls to normal within two hours. In a diabetic the blood glucose increase is greater and the return to normal prolonged. (Fasting blood glucose mean the glucose determination on a specimen of bloo drawn after at least nine and one-half hours o fasting.)

†Cortisone-glucose tolerance test: by giving cor tisone prior to the oral glucose tolerance test, the demand for insulin increases and more sensitive results are obtained.

the time when an impaired glucose tolerance can be shown in an individual predisposed to diabetes on genetic grounds.

2. Current tests cannot diagnose this state. The only positive diagnoses are in the nondiabetic identical twin of a diabetic patient and the offspring of two diabetic parents.

V. Categories of Diabetes

A. **Primary Diabetes (Hereditary, Idiopathic)**

1. *Juvenile and Adult Onset*

Juvenile–onset diabetes generally means that which has its onset during the growth period, particularly by age 20. However, the rapid onset and more severe symptoms frequently seen in the young can occur at older ages.

Earlier diagnosis in children than in adults may be related either to the need to treat acute symptoms or the probability that parents seek medical supervision for their children more regularly than for themselves. A comparison of characteristics of juvenile–onset and adult–onset is made in table 51–1.

2. *Susceptible Individuals*[5,8]

Predisposition to diabetes is present at birth. Not all who are genetically predisposed to develop diabetes will, as there appears to be an interaction between genetic susceptibility and environmental factors. Diabetes is most likely to occur in the following situations:

a. The identical nondiabetic twin of a diabetic.

b. Individuals with diabetic close

Table 51-1. Comparison of Characteristics of Juvenile–Onset and Adult–Onset Diabetes

Characteristic	Juvenile-Onset	Adult-Onset
Age of Onset	Under 20 years	Adulthood, particularly over 40 years
Body Weight	Normal or thin	High percent obese at the time of diagnosis
Rate of Onset of Clinical Symptoms	Rapid	Slow
Severity	Severe	Mild
Diabetic Emergency (Ketoacidosis)	Common	Rare
Stability	Unstable	Stable
Insulin Treatment Required	Almost all	Less than 25 percent
Chronic Manifestations	Uncommon before 20 years; prevalent and severe by age 30	Develop slowly with age.
Incidence (percent of all diabetics)	Less than five percent	Increase with age; peak in 65 to 74 years age group.

relatives: when both parents are diabetic, all offspring are liable to develop diabetes.

c. Women with abnormal obstetrical history: tendency to large babies over 10 pounds; perinatal mortalities; repeated miscarriages.

d. Obese individuals.

e. Individuals with diabetes-like vascular manifestations: retina or kidney pathology, coronary artery disease.

B. **Secondary Diabetes (Acquired, Nonhereditary)**

1. Due to malfunction in endocrine glands other than the pancreas, for example, hyperpituitarism, hyperadrenalism, hyperthyroidism.

2. Due to surgical removal or destruction of pancreatic islet tissue as by a destructive neoplasm or an inflammatory disease.

C. **Stable and Unstable Diabetes**

1. *Stable:* when nearly normal blood glucose levels are maintained on relatively convenient regimens of treatment. Most stable diabetics are in the adult-onset group.

2. *Unstable* (labile): about 15 percent of insulin-dependent patients have excessive fluctuations of blood glucose levels despite apparent optimal therapy. Most unstable diabetics are of the juvenile-onset category.

3. *"Brittle"* diabetes: very unstable with marked variations from high to low blood glucose levels; requires extra care to prevent emergencies.

V. Action of Insulin

A. **Functions of Insulin**

As a powerful hormone, insulin directly or indirectly affects every organ in the body.

1. Facilitates conversion of glucose to fat in adipose tissue.

2. Speeds the conversion of glucose to glycogen in the liver and muscles.

3. Facilitates the transmission of glucose into cells.

4. Speeds the oxidation of glucose within the cells for energy.

B. **Effects of Decreased Insulin**

In diabetes insulin is decreased in amount or function.

1. With decreased insulin, less glucose is transmitted through cell walls into the cells.

2. Glucose increases in the circulating blood until a threshold is reached when glucose spills over into the urine.

3. Without glucose in the cells to use for energy, the cells utilize fats.

a. End products of fat metabolism (ketones) accumulate in the blood.

b. Ketones are acid. Usually when they accumulate they are neutralized in the blood stream. When there is such a large quantity, the neutralizing effect is depleted rapidly and an acid condition (acidosis) results.

c. In severe, untreated or inadequately controlled diabetes, acidosis leads to diabetic coma (ketoacidosis).

C. **Insulin Complications**

With earlier diagnosis, improved treatment procedures, and better informed patients and their families, there has been a decrease in emergencies. It now becomes increasingly important to recognize the earliest symptoms in order to arrest the development of a crisis stage.

1. Insulin reaction: too much insulin (hyperinsulinism) with lowered blood glucose.

2. Diabetic coma (ketoacidosis): too little insulin (hypoinsulinism). See table 51–2 for a comparison of the characteristics of insulin reaction

Table 51-2. Comparison of Insulin Reaction and Diabetic Coma

	Insulin Reaction (Hypoglycemia)	Diabetic Coma (Ketoacidosis)
History (Predisposing Factors)	Too much insulin Too little food: delayed or omitted Loss of food by vomiting or diarrhea Excessive exercise	Too little insulin: omitted medication or failed to increase dose when requirements increased Too much food Infection Stress Illness of any sort
Cause	Lowered blood glucose with excess insulin in proportion	Decreased glucose utilization when insufficient insulin leads to prolonged increasing acidosis
Occurrence	In insulin-dependent diabetics particularly the unstable, severe type	Juvenile-onset primarily Adult-onset: poorly controlled, unstable, who omit or reduce insulin for emotional or other reasons
Onset	Sudden Slower when long-acting insulin is used	Gradual, over many hours, even days
Physical Findings	Skin: moist, increased perspiration Hunger Headache Tremor Pallor Dilated pupils Dizziness, staggering gait Weakness	Skin: flushed and dry Nausea, vomiting Lack of appetite Weak, rapid pulse Dry mouth, thirst Soft, sunken eyeballs Increased urination Deep difficult breathing Abdominal pain
Behavior	Drowsiness Restless, anxious, irritable Incoordination Stupor, confusion Eventual coma, with or without convulsions	Progressive drowsiness Confusion Lethargy Weakness Eventual coma
Treatment	Give sugar to raise the blood glucose level (orange juice, candy, sugar cubes) Revival: prompt Unconscious or unresponsive: treated by injection of glucagon* or may require intravenous glucose	Immediate professional care, hospitalization Keep patient warm Fluids for the conscious patient Insulin injection by physician
Prevention	Smooth regulation of diabetes with steady diet, insulin, exercise	Early diagnosis of diabetes Well-indoctrinated, regulated patient

Glucagon is a hormone produced by the alpha cells of the pancreas, which increases blood glucose.

and diabetic coma, and the respective treatment procedures.

VI. Signs, Symptoms, Effects

A. **Signs and Symptoms of Uncontrolled Diabetes**
1. Increased urine (polyuria).
2. Excessive thirst (polydipsia).
3. Dehydration from fluid loss.
   a. Dry, itchy skin.
   b. Dry mouth; decreased saliva.
   c. Burning tongue.
4. Increased appetite (polyphagia).
5. General weakness, drowsiness, fatigue.
6. Weight loss from inability to utilize foods.
7. Elevated blood glucose (hyperglycemia).
8. Glucose in the urine (glycosuria).
9. Slow wound healing; persistent infections such as boils or carbuncles.
10. Pain and/or numbness in the fingers and toes.
11. Changes in vision.

B. **Infection and Diabetes**[10,11]
1. Diabetics, particularly the inadequately controlled, are more susceptible to infections.
2. Failure to treat an infection increases the severity of the diabetic state and intensifies the symptoms; can precipitate diabetic coma.
3. With infection present, insulin requirements may increase; with elimination of the infection, it may be possible to decrease the prescribed insulin.
4. Frequently encountered infections involve the urinary tract, skin, lungs (pneumonia or tuberculosis), and the oral cavity, particularly the periodontium.
5. Factors involved: impaired circulation, alterations in carbohydrate and protein metabolisms, altered

nutritional state, or abnormal immunological response.

C. **Diabetes in Pregnancy**[12,13]
1. Insulin adjustment, carefully supervised prenatal care, and improved obstetrical practices have lessened much of the potential danger for the mother.
2. Effects on offspring
   a. Infants are larger; premature births more frequent; incidence of congenital malformations high.
   b. High perinatal death rate, less with improved prenatal care.

D. **Long-term Complications**
   Patients with controlled diabetes may develop complications later than those less well controlled. The principal involvements are in the nervous system (neuropathy), kidney (nephropathy), retina (retinopathy), and blood vessels (arteriosclerosis and atherosclerosis).
   Kidney disease is most severe in juvenile-onset diabetes, while atherosclerotic coronary heart disease is common in the older diabetics. Retinopathy occurs frequently, and diabetes is the third leading cause of blindness in the United States.[5]

VII. Psychological Factors

A. **Impact of Personality on Diabetes**[14]
1. Problems during treatment may be related to an imbalance between diet and insulin, but often can be influenced by the patient's conscious or subconscious attempt to resist.
2. Periods of emotional distress bring on alterations in the blood glucose.
3. Changes which lead to acidosis and coma may start during periods of depression, hostility, or anxiety, particularly when such symptoms lead to neglect of diet or insulin.

B. **Impact of Diabetes on Personality**[15]

1. Reaction to an initial diagnosis may be extremely traumatic with long-range effects, particularly in a child.
   a. Adult-onset patient may suffer fear, frustration, and confusion. Less mature adults show less acceptance and may reject the diagnosis and try to control their treatment.
   b. Parents of a child diabetic may be acutely disturbed and experience feelings of guilt and rejection of the "imperfect" child.
2. Adult behavior during the course of treatment can vary from reckless neglect of treatment to the opposite extreme where there can be obsession with details to the point of preoccupation with weighing of foods and extreme attention to personal hygiene.
3. Adolescents may find the restrictions nearly intolerable and their hopes for the future seemingly destroyed. Growing independence and rejection of authority figures (parents and physician) makes diabetes control difficult.[16]
4. Younger children may exhibit feelings of oppression, restriction, or suppressed emotions because of subordination and control by the diabetic regimen.
5. Parents' attitudes influence the diabetic child's adjustment.[17]
   a. Overanxious, overprotective parent may precipitate anxiety states or complete dependence of the child.
   b. Overindulgent parent may indirectly lead the child to exploitation or even complete control.
   c. Indifferent or nonchalant parent may give the child feelings of desertion, neglect, or depression.

VIII. Treatment for Diabetes Control

Objectives in patient care are directed to correct metabolic disturbances, attain the best possible state of general health, and prevent or postpone complications or chronic effects of diabetes. Treatment methods depend on the severity of the disease, age, activity, vocation, and psychological needs as well as the nutritional and weight problems of the patient.

A. **Methods Used**
1. Immediate treatment: management of acute symptoms.
2. Elimination of sources of infection present, including oral diseases.
3. Patient education: self-care.
4. Diet and exercise.
5. Medication: insulin or oral hypoglycemic agents.
6. Personal hygiene: physical and mental.

B. **Self-Care**[18]

There is no known cure for diabetes. The success of treatment depends on the knowledge, understanding, and attitude of the patient, and how well he manages his condition on a day-to-day basis throughout life.

1. *Instruction*

Continuing instruction must be provided the patient and his parents by the health team, including the physician, registered nurse, dietitian, and other specialists. The dentist and dental hygienist participate to instruct and supervise the patient's oral health practices for the prevention and control of oral diseases.

2. *Components of Self-Care*
   a. Objectives: to prevent infections and injuries; prevent glycosuria; and maintain the best possible general health.
   b. Specific instruction: the American Diabetes Association has

prepared a check list of nine elements of treatment in a minimum program. These are: diet, urine testing, action of insulin and other hypoglycemic agents, technique of insulin injection and sites for it, care of syringe and of insulin, symptoms of hypoglycemia, symptoms of uncontrolled diabetes, care of the feet, and what to do in case of acute complications.[19]

c. Instruction materials: a number of excellent books and other printed materials have been prepared specifically for the diabetic patient. Review of some of these materials can provide the dental hygienist with greater insight into the background and knowledge of the patient in preparation for oral health instruction.*

C. **Diet Therapy**[20,21]

Diet planning is essential to all diabetics. Approximately one-third of all diabetics can be controlled by diet alone.[22]

1. *Fundamentals of the Diabetic Diet*
   a. Elimination of concentrated carbohydrates (sugar, frostings, pastries, candy, syrup, and others) with limitations on all carbohydrates.
   b. Caloric intake may be identical with normal for the patient's age and stature, with appropriate adjustments for growth in the young patient, degree of activity, occupation and especially the need for weight loss or gain in the obese or debilitated patient respectively.
   c. Nutritional aspects: the diet

*List of educational materials is available from the American Diabetes Association, 18 East 48th Street, New York, New York 10017.

should supply nutrients essential for better than average general health (Basic 4 Food Groups, table 28–1, page 403).

2. *Eating Habits*
   a. Distribution of food: daily regulation of eating a prescribed caloric intake is essential to balance insulin and blood glucose.
   b. Meals: spaced, on time, with or without planned between-meal eating. All food including that used between meals is counted into the day's total intake.
   c. Patient must eat all the food prescribed at the prescribed times. Rejected foods or food lost through vomiting must be reported as these may explain changes in glucose balance.

D. **Insulin Therapy**[20]

1. *Indications.* All diabetics suffering acute complications (ketoacidosis) most juvenile-onset patients; and adult-onset patients with diabetes too severe for control by diet and/or oral hypoglycemic agents. Daily injection is required.

2. *Types of Insulin.* There are several available types. They are classified as short-acting, intermediate-acting or prolonged-acting.

3. *Dosage.* Depends on the severity of the individual case.
   a. Objective: to attain optimum utilization of glucose throughout each 24 hours.
   b. Factors affecting the need for insulin: food intake, emotional disturbances, variations in exercise, or infections.

E. **Oral Hypoglycemic Agents**[20,23]

1. *Indications.* Primarily for mild stable diabetes, newly diagnosed adult-onset patients (over 40 years) who do not require insulin.

2. *Sulfonylureas*
   a. Action: to stimulate insulin production by the pancreas.
   b. Types: tolbutamide (Orinase), chloropropamide (Diabinese), acetohexamide (Dymelor), and tolazamide (Tolinase).
3. *Biguanides*
   a. Action: not clearly understood, they do not stimulate insulin production, but act to make more effective use of the insulin which is available.
   b. Type: phenformin (DBI).

ORAL RELATIONSHIPS

The oral mucosa, tongue, and periodontal tissues of a patient with diabetes mellitus may show unusual susceptibility to and tendency toward more marked reactions to injury, infections, and all local irritants than tissues of nondiabetics. Such a response is related to the diabetic's general lowered resistance and delayed healing processes.

Many different oral signs and symptoms of the teeth, mucosa, tongue, pulp, and periodontium have been described in the literature.[24-27] None of these can be attributed to diabetes, except as they may be more severe or acute or may develop more rapidly than in a nondiabetic patient. Such reactions are most typical in the uncontrolled or irregularly controlled patient.

I. Periodontal Involvement

A. Juvenile-Onset
Marked periodontal disease may be observed at early ages. There may be heavy calculus, alveolar bone resorption, pocket formation, and increased tooth mobility, all of which are relatively rare in young nondiabetics.[28]

B. Adult-Onset
Characteristic findings for periodontal disease are observed in the presence of local irritants, but with more severe symptoms which develop more rapidly at an earlier age than in nondiabetics.[1-4,29,30]

C. Contributing Factors
1. Diabetes acts as a conditioning, modifying, and accelerating factor with local irritants having an important role in the development of periodontal symptoms.[31]
2. Local irritants elicit more severe tissue response because of decreased resistance.
3. Pathology of small blood vessels (microangiopathy) in the periodontium alters the normal tissue metabolism.[7,32-34] The thickening of the vessel walls and narrowing of the lumen lead to diminished blood supply which interferes with the nutrition and respiration of the cells. This can reduce the tissue's ability to resist trauma, infection, and the effects of local irritants.

II. Dental Caries

A. Uncontrolled Diabetes
Dental caries rate is generally consistent with own age group or may be slightly higher related to diminished saliva and dry mouth, or a high carbohydrate diet in the obese.

B. Controlled
With a well-regulated diet, necessarily low in or free of sugar-containing foods, and with a regular eating pattern that excludes permissive and unaccounted-for between-meal snacks, a reduced dental caries experience is frequently observed.

DENTAL HYGIENE CARE

Since infection in the oral cavity can alter the course of diabetes and its treatment, the control of oral diseases has a vital role in the maintenance of the patient's health. Frequent and thorough care with regular supervision of the patient's self-care is required. This in turn requires gaining the patient's utmost cooperation and confidence.

I. Patient History

To supplement the basic history obtained (pages 71–78), additional questioning will provide other essential information such as the type and schedule of medication, dietary requirements, meal schedule, and frequency of medical appointments.

II. Consultation with Physician

Consultation between the dentist and the physician is necessary before any instrumentation involving tissue manipulation is performed.

A. **Information Obtained**
1. Degree of control, stability, and severity of the diabetes; susceptibility of the patient to emergency reactions.
2. Other health problems which may influence oral care.
3. Advice relative to the prescription for antibiotic therapy or sedative in preparation for dental and dental hygiene appointments.
4. Instructions which have been given the patient about diet, personal care, medication adjustment, or other.

B. **Use of Information**
   The dental hygienist should study and apply information from the patient history and the physician-dentist consultation in order that dental hygiene phases of care and instruction be conducted in accord with the health requirements of the patient.

III. Appointment Planning

Except for relief of pain or other emergency performed after initial consultation with the physician, treatment, *including dental hygiene appointment procedures, should not be started until the diabetes is under control.*

A. **Time**
1. Choice: morning, 1½ to 3 hours after the patient's normal breakfast and medication, during the descending portion of the blood glucose level curve.
2. Long-acting medication: adjust time accordingly.

B. **Precautions**
1. Avoid long periods of stressful procedures: dental and dental hygiene care should be divided into units for short appointments appropriate to the individual needs.
2. The patient should not be kept waiting unduly.
3. Do not interfere with the patient's regular meal and between-meal eating schedule.
4. Prepare for diabetic emergency when the patient's history reveals diabetic instability or susceptibility to emergencies. Keep sugar cubes or other sweets as part of the office emergency supplies.

C. **Maintenance Phase: Recall Frequency**
1. Appoint for supervision and examination on a regular two to three months' basis.
2. Calculus and other local irritants cannot be permitted to accumulate, therefore routine scaling and planing may be required.
3. Soft tissue examination for areas of irritation related to fixed and removable prosthesis must be carried out at each recall.

IV. Clinical Procedures

A. **Instrumentation**
1. Prophylactic antibiotic therapy is frequently indicated to prevent postoperative infection.[27,35] The pa-

tient must have the information and prescription prior to the scheduled appointment.

2. Aseptic technique: scrupulous procedures for sterile instrument and tray preparation should be the same for all patients. However, it is important to keep in mind the diabetic's susceptibility to infection and take any necessary precautions.

3. Undue trauma to tissues must be avoided to encourage postoperative healing without complications.

B. Fluoride Application

When the gingival tissue has been inflamed or scaling has been extensive, it is advisable to postpone a topical fluoride application until the gingival tissue shows improvement following healing and personal oral care by the patient.

V. Patient Instruction

A. Influence of Diabetes Instruction

Many patients with diabetes are already education-oriented since instruction relative to diabetes and self-care procedures by the physician, nurse, and dietitian is an integral part of therapy (page 695). Some emphasis on the care of the mouth may have been made. The interrelation of oral tissue infection and the control of diabetes can be reinforced as personal instruction is given.

B. Plaque Control

Self-care measures for plaque control are selected on the basis of individual needs (page 386). Continuing supervision and review of recommended procedures is critical to the patient with diabetes because of increased susceptibility to periodontal tissue involvement.

C. Diet

1. Correlate information about dental caries prevention with the elimination of concentrated sweets. Since the diabetic diet contains no concentrated sweets, cooperation in caries control measures can be expected.

2. Reinforce principles of a nutritious diet in accord with the instruction provided by the physician, as a contribution to general health. Emphasis on the texture of the diet to avoid soft foods which cling to the teeth and gingiva is important to the periodontal disease-prone patient.

PREVENTION OF DIABETES

Primary prevention is not possible because the cause is not known. However, detection can be made before the advanced clinical symptoms appear. When the disease is detected and treated early, most complications can be minimized, postponed, or possibly prevented.[8]

Mass screening has been used for many years to locate those persons who may have diabetes. Both blood and urine tests have been used for screening, but blood tests have been shown to be the most reliable.[5]

In the universal effort of the health professions and community groups to find early diabetes, it is becoming increasingly evident that dental offices and clinics may become important screening centers. The history-taking and oral examination procedures for dental patients can be extremely useful for singling out diabetic suspects. Suspects can then be referred for a blood test, or an initial screening test can be performed in the dental office.

In addition to the objectives related to the health and well-being of individuals and the community health aspects of case finding, the dentist and dental hygienist have a responsibility to seek out diabetic patients in order that safe and successful dental and periodontal treatment, including the phases of care assigned the dental hygienist, may be carried out. Before proceeding with traumatic, stress-creating treatment in an infection-prone patient, every effort should be made to discover the true systemic condition of each patient.

I. Diabetic Suspects Among Dental Patients

A. Patients in a Diabetes-Susceptible Group

From observation and through questions in the patient history the following may be identified:
1. Individuals with close relatives who have diabetes.
2. Women with abnormal obstetrical history, particularly large babies.
3. Obese persons, particularly in the over-40 age group.
4. Those with eye, kidney, or coronary artery disease.

B. Patients with Symptoms Suggestive of Diabetes

Questions in the patient history can be directed to obtain information such as the following:
1. Weight changes: weight loss with increased appetite.
2. Thirst; frequent urination.
3. Slow healing cuts, bruises, or skin infections such as boils or carbuncles.
4. Pain in extremities: fingers and toes.
5. Fatigue and drowsiness.
6. Most recent blood tests: whether test was made for blood glucose.

C. Repeat of Patient History

With long-standing patients it is not unusual for the history to have been completed at an initial visit without follow-up reviews periodically. Illnesses, hospitalizations, or other involvements, including a diagnosis of diabetes, may have occurred subsequent to the original history record. At each recall appointment a review history is indicated (page 70).

II. Screening Tests

A. Test Subjects

It is not necessarily practical to test every patient, therefore attention is directed to people from susceptible groups and others who present with suggestive general or oral symptoms.

B. Test for Urine

Although urine tests have been used for screening in dental offices and clinics, urinalysis is not as reliable as blood testing for early diabetes.

C. Test for Blood Glucose

1. Results of blood tests for screening are most reliable when the blood sample is taken two hours after the intake of 50 to 100 grams of carbohydrate. A commercially available product, Glucola,* is a flavored carbonated liquid containing the measured amount of carbohydrate in individual containers which are convenient for use in a dental clinic or office.
2. Dextrostix* has been used for dental patients.[36-38] In this test a drop of fingertip blood is applied for one clocked minute to a paper strip which is chemically treated with glucose oxidase. After one minute the paper is washed with water and the color compared with a standard chart which indicates milligrams percent of blood glucose. After adequate instruction and experience in comparing the color chart with the test material, the dental hygienist appropriately can conduct the blood testing program as directed by the dentist.
3. Referral for oral glucose tolerance test (footnote, page 690) is made when Dextrostix yields blood glucose values over 140 milligrams percent. The normal fasting blood glucose ranges from 80 to 120 milligrams percent.

*Ames Company, Elkhart, Indiana

References

1. Sandler, H. C. and Stahl, S. S.: Prevalence of Periodontal Disease in a Hospitalized Population, *J. Dent. Res.*, 39, 439, May-June, 1960.
2. Belting, C. M., Hiniker, J. J., and Dummett, C. O.: Influence of Diabetes Mellitus on the Severity of Periodontal Disease, *J. Periodont.*, 35, 476, November-December, 1964.
3. Finestone, A. J. and Boorujy, S. R.: Diabetes Mellitus and Periodontal Disease, *Diabetes*, 16, 336, May, 1967.
4. Glavind, L., Lund, B., and Löe, H.: The Relationship Between Periodontal State and Diabetes Duration, Insulin Dosage and Retinal Changes, *J. Periodont.*, 39, 341, November, 1968.
5. United States Department of Health, Education, and Welfare: *Diabetes Source Book.* Public Health Service Publication No. 1168, Revised 1968.
6. Conn, J. W.: Expanding Concepts of Diabetes Mellitus, *Modern Med.*, 32, 130, April 13, 1964.
7. McMullen, J. A., Legg, M., Gottsegen, R., and Camerini-Davalos, R.: Microangiopathy Within the Gingival Tissues of Diabetic Subjects with Special Reference to the Prediabetic State, *Periodontics*, 5, 61, March-April, 1967.
8. Camerini-Davalos, R. A.: Prevention of Diabetes Mellitus, *Med. Clin. North Am.*, 49, 865, July, 1965.
9. Hamwi, G. J.: Special Report. Classification of Genetic Diabetes Mellitus, *Diabetes*, 16, 540, July, 1967.
10. Warren, S., LeCompte, P. M., and Legg, M. A.: *The Pathology of Diabetes Mellitus*, 4th ed. Philadelphia, Lea & Febiger, 1966, pp. 167–177.
11. Bleicher, S. J.: Infections and Trauma in the Patient with Diabetes Mellitus: General Considerations, in Hamwi, G. J. and Danowski, T. S., eds.: *Diabetes Mellitus; Diagnosis and Treatment*, Volume II. New York, American Diabetes Association, 1967, pp. 155–159.
12. White, P.: Pregnancy and Diabetes, Medical Aspects, *Med. Clin. North Am.*, 49, 1015, July, 1965.
13. Freinkel, N.: Pregnancy and Diabetes Mellitus, in Hamwi, G. J. and Danowski, T. S., eds.: *Diabetes Mellitus: Diagnosis and Treatment*, Vol. II. New York, American Diabetes Association, 1967, pp. 161–165.
14. Kolb, L. C.: *Modern Clinical Psychiatry*, 8th ed. Philadelphia, Saunders, 1973, pp. 473–476.
15. Isenberg, P. I. and Barnett, D. M.: Psychological Problems in Diabetes Mellitus, *Med. Clin. North Am.*, 49, 1125, July, 1965.
16. White, P. and Graham, C. A.: The Child with Diabetes, in Marble, A., White, P., Bradley, R. F., and Krall, L. P., eds.: *Joslin's Diabetes Mellitus*, 11th ed. Philadelphia, Lea & Febiger, 1971, pp. 353–354.
17. Bakwin, H. and Bakwin, R. M.: *Behavior Disorders in Children*, 4th ed. Philadelphia, Saunders, 1972, pp. 136–138.
18. Bradley, R. F.: Importance and Technics of Patient Education, in Hamwi, G. J. and Danowski, T. S., eds.: *Diabetes Mellitus: Diagnosis and Treatment*, Vol. II. New York, American Diabetes Association, 1967, pp. 83–90.
19. Hamwi, G. J.: Treatment of Diabetes, *J. Am. Med. Assoc.*, 181, 1064, September 22, 1962.
20. Krall, L. P.: Diabetes Mellitus in Adults, in Conn, H. F., ed.: *Current Therapy, 1969.* Philadelphia, Saunders, 1969, pp. 365–376.
21. Krause, M. V. and Hunscher, M. A.: *Food, Nutrition and Diet Therapy*, 5th ed. Philadelphia, Saunders, 1972, pp. 399–414.
22. *Facts About Diabetes.* New York, American Diabetes Association, 1966, p. 7.
23. Ferguson, D.: The Oral Hypoglycemic Compounds, *Med. Clin. North Am.*, 49, 929, July, 1965.
24. Sheridan, R. C., Cheraskin, E., Flynn, F. H., and Hutto, A. C.: Epidemiology of Diabetes Mellitus: I. Review of the Dental Literature, *J. Periodont.*, 30, 242, July, 1959.
II. A Study of 100 Dental Patients, *J. Periodont.*, 30, 298, October, 1959.
25. Gottsegen, R.: Dental Considerations in Diabetes Mellitus, *N.Y. State J. Med.*, 62, 389, February, 1962.
26. McCarthy, P. L. and Shklar, G.: *Diseases of the Oral Mucosa.* New York, Blakiston Division, McGraw-Hill, 1964, pp. 249–250.
27. Burket, L. W.: *Oral Medicine*, 6th ed. Philadelphia, Lippincott, 1971, pp. 466–472.
28. Adelson, J. J.: Dental Treatment of the Diabetic Child, *J. Dent. Child.*, 27, 55, 1st Quarter, 1960.
29. Williams, R. C. and Mahan, C. J.: Periodontal Disease and Diabetes in Young Adults, *J. Am. Med. Assoc.*, 172, 776, February 20, 1960.
30. Campbell, M. J. A.: Periodontal Disease in the Diabetic Patient and Its Treatment, *Aust. Dent. J.*, 12, 117, April, 1967.
31. *World Workshop in Periodontics.* Ann Arbor, University of Michigan, 1966, p. 141.
32. Stahl, S. S., Witkin, G. J., and Scopp, I. W.: Degenerative Vascular Changes Observed in Selected Gingival Specimens, *Oral Surg.*, 15, 1495, December, 1962.
33. Schallhorn, R. G.: Diabetes Mellitus and Periodontal Disease, *Periodont. Abstr.*, 14, 9, March, 1966.
34. Russell, B. G.: The Periodontal Membrane in Diabetes Mellitus, *Acta Path. et Microbiol. Scand.*, 70, 318, Fasc. 2, 1967.
35. Glickman, I.: *Clinical Periodontology*, 4th ed. Philadelphia, Saunders, 1972, p. 386–389, 973.
36. Kaplan, H.: The Reagent-strip Method for Estimating Blood Glucose Concentration, *J. Am. Dent. Assoc.*, 74, 1261, May, 1967.

37. Myall, R. W. T.: An Evaluation of the Dextrostix as a Diabetic Screening Tool in the Dental Office, *I.A.D.R. Program and Abstracts* of Papers, No. 16, March, 1969, p. 44.
38. Stein, G. M. and Nebbia, A. A.: A Chairside Method of Diabetic Screening with Gingival Blood, *Oral Surg.*, 27, 607, May, 1969.

Suggested Readings

Bay, I., Ainamo, J., and Gad, T.: The Response of Young Diabetics to Periodontal Treatment, *J. Periodont.*, 45, 806, November, 1974.

Benveniste, R., Bixler, D., and Conneally, P. M.: Periodontal Disease in Diabetics, *J. Periodont.*, 38, 271, July-August, 1967.

Bernick, S. M., Cohen, D. W., Baker, L., and Laster, L.: Dental Disease in Children with Diabetes Mellitus, *J. Periodont.*, 46, 241, April, 1975.

Burns, R. L. and Krebs, K. A.: The Detection of Diabetic Tendencies in Periodontal Practice, *J. Periodont.*, 40, 535, September, 1969.

Campbell, M. J. A.: Epidemiology of Periodontal Disease in the Diabetic and the Non-diabetic, *Austr. Dent. J.*, 17, 274, August, 1972.

Cohen, D. W., Friedman, L. A., Shapiro, J., Kyle, G. C., and Franklin, S.: Diabetes Mellitus and Periodontal Disease: Two-year Longitudinal Observations. Part I, *J. Periodont.*, 41, 709, December, 1970.

Collins, L. H. and Crane, M. P.: *Internal Medicine in Dental Practice*, 6th ed. Philadelphia, Lea & Febiger, 1965, pp. 270–287.

Danowski, T. S.: *Diabetes as a Way of Life*, revised. New York, Coward, 1974.

Harps, N.: Dental Hygiene Patients with Special Needs. The Diabetic Child, *J. Am. Dent. Hyg. Assoc.*, 40, 74, 2nd Quarter, 1966.

Hove, K. A. and Stallard, R. E.: Diabetes and the Periodontal Patient, *J. Periodont.*, 41, 713, December, 1970.

Kaplan, H.: Further Experience in Diabetes Detection Using a Standard Carbohydrate Drink, *J. Oral Med.*, 25, 51, April-June, 1970.

Kutscher, A. H., Zegarelli, E. V., Hyman, G. A., McLean, P., and Kutscher, H. W., eds.: *Pharmacology for the Dental Hygienist*. Philadelphia, Lea & Febiger, 1967, pp. 207–210.

Lavine, M. H.: Diagnosis and Management of the Diabetic Patient, *Oral Surg.*, 24, 16, July, 1967.

O'Driscoll, P. M.: Incidence and Management of Diabetes in Oral Surgery, *Br. J. Oral Surg.*, 4, 38, July, 1966.

Stein, G. M.: Current Thinking on the Relationship of Diabetes Mellitus to Oral Disease, *J. Am. Dent. Hyg. Assoc.*, 45, 100, March-April, 1971.

Stein, G. M. and Shannon, I.: Glucose Tolerance and the State of Periodontal Health, *J. Periodont.*, 41, 520, September, 1970.

Tahl, H. and Colwell, A. R.: The Dental Surgeon and the Diabetic Patient, *Oral Surg.*, 23, 721, June, 1967.

Truelove, E. L., Burden, R., and Goebel, W.: Evaluation of a New Chairside Test for Diabetes Mellitus, *J. Oral Med.*, 26, 139, December, 1971.

Tuckman, M. A., Kaslick, R. S., Shapiro, W. B., and Chasens, A. I.: The Relationship of Glucose Tolerance to Periodontal Status, *J. Periodont.*, 41, 513, September, 1970.

Wegner, H.: Increment of Caries in Young Diabetics, *Caries Res.*, 9, 91, No. 1, 1975.

World Health Organization: *Diabetes Mellitus*. WHO Technical Report Series #310. Geneva, World Health Organization, 1965, 44 pp.

Chapter 52

Patients During Puberty, Adolescence, and Menopause

INTRODUCTION

The endocrine glands are glands of internal secretion. They secrete highly specialized substances—the hormones—which, with the nervous system, maintain body homeostasis.

A hormone is a chemical product of an organ or certain cells within an organ, which has a specific regulatory effect upon cells remote from its origin. Hormones are transported by the blood or lymph. They may act directly on body cells or may act to control the hormones of other glands. Their complex and unified action augments and regulates many vital functions, including growth and development, energy production, food metabolism, reproductive processes, and the responses of the body to stress.

The major endocrine glands are the pituitary, thyroid, parathyroids, pancreas, adrenals, and gonads. The anterior pituitary is called the master gland because it is the regulator of the output of hormones by other glands. In turn, the pituitary itself is regulated by the hormones of the other glands.

Both hyposecretion and hypersecretion of a hormone can cause physical and mental disturbances. Regulation of hormonal secretion is complex, and the mechanisms are not fully known. Normally, hormones are secreted when needed. The external temperature, for example, can influence the production of thyroxin of the thyroid gland, and the calcium level of the blood affects parathyroid activity.

Treatment for endocrine disturbances is accomplished either by decreasing the output of an overactive gland or, when there is a hormone deficiency, by stimulating glandular activity or supplying the deficient hormone. As an example, the use of insulin or a hypoglycemic agent in the treatment of diabetes was described in the previous chapter (page 696).

Hormones of the reproductive system have a marked controlling influence on the development and function of the individual. Some of the relationships to oral health and patient care will be discussed in this chapter.

PUBERTY AND ADOLESCENCE

Puberty is the period during which the gonads mature and commence to function. *Adolescence* is the period extending from the time of puberty to the attainment of complete maturity.

I. Pubertal Changes

Chronological age is an unreliable means for designation because puberty may begin normally in either sex between 9 and 17 years of age. In a majority, the secondary sex characteristics will begin to appear between 10 and 13 in girls, whereas in boys changes are later, starting about 13 or 14 years. The major changes are usually complete in three to four years.

A. **Hormonal Influences**

Pituitary hormones control the hormones produced by the ovaries and testes. The several hormones produced by the ovaries are known collectively as *estrogens,* and those produced by the testes are called *androgens.* They are responsible for the development of the sex organs, the accessory sex organs, and the secondary sex characteristics, and have strong influences throughout the body.

B. **Female Development**
   1. Beginning of menstruation and ovulation. Menstruation precedes ovulation (page 708).
   2. Growth of accessory sex organs: Fallopian tubes, uterus, vagina, and breasts.
   3. Appearance of secondary sex characteristics
      a. Growth of pubic and axillary hair.
      b. Skeletal development: especially enlargement of the pelvis.
      c. Fat deposition on the hips.
      d. Voice drops one or two tones.

C. **Male Development**
   1. Increase in size of testes and beginning of spermatogenesis.
   2. Growth of accessory sex organs: vas deferens, seminal vesicles, prostate, and penis.
   3. Appearance of secondary sex characteristics
      a. Growth of beard and pubic hair.
      b. Voice deepens.

II. Characteristics of Adolescence

A. **Growth Spurt**
   1. Varies in age of occurrence, extent, and duration; with boys generally between 12 and 16, girls 11 to 14.
   2. Marked by rapid, extensive growth in height, weight, and muscle mass.
   3. Obesity: overeating with underexercise along with psychological problems make obesity a difficult and serious problem particularly among those young adolescents where food is not limited by scarcity or cost.[1]
   4. Young adolescents: poor coordination and awkwardness may result from irregular, uneven stages of growth.

B. **Nutritional Requirements**
   1. Highest of any time in life for the boys; will be exceeded only during pregnancy for the girls.[2]
   2. Undernutrition is common; boys because of overactivity and poor food selection; girls because of voluntary diet restrictions with poor food selection, and fad diets in the attempt to keep slim.
   3. Iron-deficiency anemia is not uncommon among teen-age girls, particularly after menstruation starts.

C. **Skin Disorders**
   Acne vulgaris is common; improves with improved diet and skin care.

D. **Fatigue**

Many adolescents require an unusual amount of sleep.

III. Psychological Factors

Adolescents are no longer children, and yet they have not reached adulthood. They may respond and wish to be treated as adults or children at different times. They are learning to adapt to body changes, sexual impulses, and secondary sex characteristics. The most likely causes of anxiety in adolescents are sex, performance in school, family relationships, acceptance by their own age group, confusion over their beliefs, and their futures.[3]

There is no fixed picture which can be described, but characteristics listed here are exhibited to one degree or another by many adolescents.[3,4]

A. **Increased Self-interest**
  1. Adolescents have a great deal of concern for themselves and respond best to those who show concern for them.
  2. They want attention and tend to reject those who do not listen.

B. **Growing Independence**
  1. Adolescence is a period of rapidly growing independence of thought and action.
  2. Childhood dependence on parents is given up: idea of infallibility of parents is lost; teachers and others in authority are questioned.
  3. Personal identity is sought: they are uncertain about their place and role in society.
  4. Independence from parents frequently means increased confidence and respect for other adults.

C. **Concern over Physical Characteristics**
  1. Girls mature earlier than boys, and young female adolescents are usually taller than males, which presents social problems.

  2. Increased interest in personal appearance: want to dress and be like their peers.
  3. Problems such as delayed growth and sexual development, and obesity can be of extreme importance.

IV. Oral Conditions

A. **Dental Caries**

The incidence of dental caries is higher during adolescence than in any other age group. This can be directly related to the dietary and eating habits of most adolescents. Appetite becomes intensified by the demands of rapid growth as well as by the emotional problems confronted, which leads to frequent eating. Many cariogenic foods are utilized, particularly for between-meal use.

B. **Gingivitis**

A large majority of adolescents have gingivitis.[5-7] An exaggerated response to local irritants sometimes occurs during puberty and may be related to hormonal influences which may be conditioning factors.[8,9]

The tissue presents with gingival enlargement, particularly of the papillary gingiva, relative pockets, bluish-red color, and pronounced inflammation. Local aggravating factors include dental plaque, other tooth deposits, mouth breathing, erupting teeth, and orthodontic appliances (pages 268–271).

C. **Acute Necrotizing Ulcerative Gingivitis**

Although found infrequently in children, acute necrotizing ulcerative gingivitis has its highest frequency in older adolescents and young adults. Stress, undernutrition, lack of plaque control, neglect of oral health, as well as psychosomatic factors are implicated as predisposing influences in its development (page 598).

D. **Periodontal Disease**

Bone destruction and other signs of early periodontal involvement may be found in adolescents. Careful radiographic examination is indicated for each patient in order that all precautions can be taken and early treatment initiated.

DENTAL HYGIENE CARE

Dental and dental hygiene care during adolescence can influence oral health throughout the patient's lifetime. Preventive measures are even more critical than in younger age groups because of the increased incidence of dental caries and gingival diseases.

Adolescents will be parents within a few years. Knowledge, attitudes, and practices acquired and developed during adolescence can influence the oral health of their families.

A. **Patient Approach**

Adolescence is a period of transition. Working with adolescents offers a real challenge and each situation requires its own approach. Some of the physical and psychological characteristics have been listed in this chapter to provide framework for what may be expected. A few basic suggestions for approach include the following:

1. Treat adolescents as adults. Physically many of them are mature, although their emotional development may be at various levels.
2. Set the stage to let them know of your interest in them and their problems. Encourage them to talk and then listen.
3. Suggest and advise but do not become impatient or take offense when they try to make their own decisions.
4. They are usually interested in health matters and details about

their physical condition, although they may act indifferently. Cleanliness and attractiveness are important to the teen-age patient.
5. Health, including oral health, may be a real concern of adolescents. They need to be well-informed about their oral conditions, and explanations on a scientific basis are generally appreciated.

B. **Patient History**

Adolescents should provide their own information for the medical and dental histories. It may also be necessary to consult the parents for information, but not in the same interview with the patient and not without the patient's knowledge.[10]

Adolescents need to begin to take increasing responsibility for their own health. Although frequently the initial dental visit may be at the insistence of the parents, every effort of the dentist and dental hygienist should be to focus the evaluation and treatment on the patient, not his parents.

The adolescent patient may present with other health problems. The patient with diabetes, heart disease, a mental, physical, or sensory handicap, or other systemic involvement will require special methods for approach as described in the various chapters of this book. Medical clearance will be necessary for conditions requiring antibiotic coverage or other medication.

C. **Preventive Dental Hygiene Program**

A clear explanation of the causes of dental caries and periodontal conditions with the methods for prevention is important. Adolescents need to understand the effects of accumulation of local irritants, the purposes of calculus removal and the relation of the daily self-care plaque control program to the health status of the gingiva.

For dental caries prevention they must appreciate the effects of fluoride and the need for restriction of dextrose-containing foods which cling to the teeth. The program is outlined and conducted on the basis of these clear-cut preventive measures.

D. **Plaque Control**
1. Instruction in self-care procedures is given in sequential steps (pages 388–393).
2. Continuing review over a series of appointments is necessary to develop daily practices which can be carried on into adult life.
3. Gingival enlargement: when gingival response to local irritants appears unusually pronounced, the treatment plan outlined by the dentist may call for gingival curettage along with root planing, or gingival surgery. The dental hygienist will be responsible for providing postsurgical instruction for a rigid plaque control program to prevent recurrence of the gingival enlargement.

E. **Instrumentation**
1. Schedule: a series of appointments is frequently required for the patient with gingivitis associated with puberty depending on pocket depth and extent of calculus deposits. Careful and complete removal of all local irritants is the basic treatment.[8,9]
2. Relation to gingival surgery: when the gingival enlargement has developed over a long period of time and the tissue is firm (fibrotic) rather than spongy (edematous) which can be treated with gingival curettage, surgery may be necessary. Follow-up root planing with frequent recall is indicated for adequate supervision.

F. **Fluoride Treatment Program**
A combined fluoride program is generally indicated for most adolescent patients. In addition to the topical applications made in conjunction with dental hygiene appointments, self-administered methods may include a fluoride dentifrice, a mouthwash following toothbrushing, or a daily application of a fluoride gel in a custom-made tray. The methods are described in Chapter 29 and the combined fluoride program discussed on pages 441–442.

G. **Diet Control**
1. Dietary analysis (pages 402–405).
   A study of the patient's diet and counseling relative to general nutrition and dental caries control can provide important learning experiences for many adolescents. The parent or other person who is in charge of shopping and food preparation will have to be included in order that appropriate foods will be available for selection. As much responsibility as possible should be placed on the patient himself.
2. Instruction suggestions
   a. Advise foods from the Four Food Groups (page 403) for growth, energy, clear complexion, and prevention of illness.
   b. Emphasize having a good breakfast: teen-agers tend to slight or omit breakfast, particularly if they have to prepare it for themselves.
   c. Snack selection: from the nutritious foods, with recognition of the foods which contain dextrose; suggest including raw fruits and vegetables, nuts, milk, use of sugarless foods when possible, and sugarless chewing gum if used.

MENSTRUATION

The menstrual cycle refers to the cyclic structural changes in the uterus, instigated by hormones, which represent periodic preparation of the lining of the uterus for fertilization of the ovum and pregnancy. When fertilization does not take place, changes in the mucous membrane lining the uterus (the endometrium) lead to the menstrual discharge. The fluid discharged is composed primarily of blood with fragments of the disintegrated endometrium.

I. Characteristics

A. **Occurrence**

The cyclic changes occur from puberty to menopause except during pregnancy. Although the average cycle is complete in about 28 days, there is a range of normal from 22 to 34 days.[11]

B. **Menarche**

Menstruation may commence any time from age 9 to 17. The mean age in the United States is between 12 and 13 years.

Menarche, the beginning of menstruation, frequently occurs before ovulation, that is, before the pituitary and ovarian hormones are synchronized and ovulation becomes a part of the menstrual cycle. There may be irregularity in timing and extent of flow for several months or even a few years after the start of menstruation.

II. Irregularities

Variations in menstruation and the cycle are common. The pattern of the cycle may be upset by such factors as changes in climate, changes in work schedule, emotional trauma, or acute or chronic illnesses.

Menstruation may have strong emotional impact and associated disturbances may have psychological bases. Some girls have intense conflicts with a major problem related to the inability to accept the feminine role and assume the responsibilities of womanhood. Some or all of the symptoms of premenstrual tension and dysmenorrhea described below may continue beyond adolescence and even to menopause.

A. **Premenstrual Tension**

This disorder is associated with fluid retention in the body and psychological depression occurring within ten days prior to menstruation. Symptoms include headache, fatigue, weight gain, heaviness in the lower abdomen and fullness and tenseness of the breasts. Feelings of depression and irritability with mood variations are common. The symptoms disappear when menstrual flow begins.[11]

B. **Dysmenorrhea**

Difficult or painful menstruation may be due to conditions such as tumors or inflammatory diseases in women past adolescence. In adolescents causes are generally related to physiologic and psychologic factors. Dysmenorrhea is frequently an indication of the adolescent's emotional status, which may result from poor preparation for the arrival of puberty and menstruation, or from parental example.

Although a high percentage of girls may have some discomfort, a smaller percentage suffer severe pain with "cramps" sometimes accompanied by nausea and vomiting. They may be bedridden, seek sympathy, and behave in a dependent, childlike manner. A few girls may need psychiatric help, but others are relieved of the severity of their symptoms when a mature relationship with their parents has been acquired, when they obtain security about maturing into womanhood, or with childbirth.[11]

III. Dental Hygiene Care

A. Patient History

Menstruation is a normal process and should not be referred to as a "sick period" or a "monthly illness." When presenting questions for the patient history, use of terms such as the "period" or "monthly period" is preferable.

The menstrual history may provide indicators of a woman's general health. Regular excessive menstrual flow may be related to an anemic state.

B. Oral Findings[12,13]

There are no specific gingival changes related to the menstrual cycle. An exaggerated response to local irritants or unusual gingival bleeding during or following scaling may be noted in an occasional patient. With control of local irritants by plaque control, self-care measures, and removal of calculus at regular recall appointments, bleeding can be controlled.

Recurrent aphthous ulcers have been associated with the menstrual cycle in the susceptible patient. A recurrence of more severe symptoms of acute necrotizing ulcerative gingivitis when treatment has not been completed has been observed.

MENOPAUSE AND CLIMACTERIC

Menopause is the cessation of menstruation. It occurs normally between the ages of 42 and 55, with the average between 47 and 49. It may be induced by surgical removal of the ovaries or by radiation therapy.

The female *climacteric* is that period of change during the gradual decline of ovarian efficiency when ovulation is less regular and finally ends, through the menopause, and including the period after menopause when the body is adjusting to endocrine and other changes. While adolescence is considered the transitional period from childhood into maturity, climacteric has been described as the transitional period from maturity into senescence. The male climacteric occurs at a later age with few if any definite symptoms.

I. Characteristics

Prior to menopause menstruation decreases in frequency, duration, and amount of flow over a period of about 12 to 24 months. Although many women may experience minor symptoms, only about 10 percent have any pronounced effects from menopause.

A. General Symptoms

With diminishing estrogen as ovarian function declines, physiologic changes in body function take place. Vasomotor reactions in the form of hot flashes in which there are sudden periodic surges of heat involving the whole body and accompanied by drenching sweats may occur during the day or night. Although a strict distinction is not always made between flush and flash, the term hot flush may be used to mean a reaction of lesser degree in which there is a wave of warm feeling over the face, neck, and upper thorax. Headaches, heart palpitations, and sleeplessness may occur.

Emotional disturbances are not caused specifically by estrogen deficiencies but are frequently related to personal and family circumstances and a fear of growing old. Reactions generally are most severe in women who had premenopausal neurotic or prepsychotic tendencies. Anxiety, tension, irritability, with depression and feelings of uselessness may appear.

B. Postmenopausal Effects

1. Reproductive organs atrophy.
2. Bone: changes may lead to osteoporosis. This condition is less

frequent among people using drinking water containing fluoride (page 426).

3. Skin and mucous membranes: decreased thickness with decreased keratinization.

4. Predisposition to other conditions including atherosclerosis, diabetes, hypothyroidism, and cancer of the sex organs.

II. Oral Findings

Oral disturbances are relatively uncommon. Findings are nonspecific and may be noted only because they appear when the patient has reached menopause, a time when she may be more sensitive to minor changes.

A. **Gingiva**

Gingival changes associated with menopause usually represent an exaggerated response to local irritation which reflects the conditioning influence of the hormonal changes taking place. When local factors are controlled through preventive dental hygiene recall and personal oral care, unusual gingival changes will rarely be noted.

Desquamative gingivitis has a tendency to occur more in women of the 40 to 55 age group, although it may occur in either sex and in younger and older people. Desquamative gingivitis is a painful condition characterized by inflammation of the gingiva in which the epithelium tends to peel away, leaving red denuded areas interspersed with grayish epithelium.[14] It is a rare condition and its etiology and treatment are still incompletely explained. The condition improves with the removal of local factors such as overhanging restorations and calculus.

B. **Mucous Membranes and Tongue**

1. Dryness, with burning or unusual taste sensations may be present.

2. Epithelium may become thin and atrophic with decreased keratinization; there may be diminished tolerance for removable prostheses.

3. Relation to diet and undernutrition: inadequate diet and eating habits may contribute to the adverse changes of the mucosal tissues. The appearance and symptoms frequently resemble those associated with vitamin deficiencies particularly B vitamins.

III. Dental Hygiene Care

In the approach to the patient a specific relation of oral conditions to menopause should not be made because the patient may tend to overemphasize such a relationship and deemphasize the need for self-care measures. Because of the importance of local factors, attention should be directed to the need for regular and frequent professional care as well as increased efforts for plaque control.

A. **Appointment Suggestions**

The symptoms of physical and emotional changes should be kept in mind when planning and conducting the appointment. The patient's possible tenseness and irritability can be anticipated, and attention to details, such as not keeping the patient waiting unduly, handling materials and instruments with calm assurance, and maintaining conservativeness in conversation to prevent annoyances, may be significant.

B. **Patient Instruction**

Preservation of oral health is of particular importance to the woman who has her natural teeth. Because of the difficulties and discomforts of wearing prostheses, every effort should be made to prevent the need for tooth removal.

Measures for the prevention of periodontal diseases need to be carefully explained, and emphasis placed on reasons for frequent calculus removal supplemented by meticulous daily care. Since good general health practices are very important to this age group, the relationship of general and oral health can be brought out.

C. Diet

A dietary survey may prove to be a helpful teaching–learning experience (pages 402–405). Because of the tendency toward inadequately balanced food selection, the patient can see and analyze her own inadequacies better when illustrated by a daily food diary. When a patient tends to indulge in between-meal eating, caries prevention through selection of nutritious and non-sucrose-containing foods is emphasized.

References

1. Gallagher, J. R.: *Medical Care of the Adolescent*, 2nd ed. New York, Appleton-Century-Crofts (New Century), 1966, p. 178.
2. Nizel, A. E.: *Nutrition in Preventive Dentistry: Science and Practice*. Philadelphia, Saunders, 1972, pp. 283–284.
3. Gallagher: op. cit., pp. 10–14.
4. Hollon, T. H.: Psychology of Adolescence, *Dent. Clin. North Am.*, 13, 289, April, 1969.
5. Marshall-Day, C. D., Stephens, R. G., and Quigley, L. F., Jr.: Periodontal Disease: Prevalence and Incidence, *J. Periodont.*, 26, 185, July, 1955.
6. Parfitt, G. J.: A Five-Year Longitudinal Study of the Gingival Condition of a Group of Children in England, *J. Periodont.*, 28, 26, January, 1957.
7. James, P. M. C.: The Prevalence of Gingivitis in School Children, *Dent. Health*, 5, 71, October-December, 1966.
8. Glickman, I.: *Clinical Periodontology*, 4th ed. Philadelphia, Saunders, 1972, pp. 101–102, 146, 797, 980.
9. Wentz, F. M. and Pollack, R. J.: Periodontics, *Dent. Clin. North Am.*, 13, 495, April, 1969.
10. Gallagher: op. cit., pp. 16–27.
11. Ibid., pp. 266–299.
12. Glickman: op. cit., pp. 146–147, 981–982.
13. Burket, L. W.: *Oral Medicine*, 6th ed. Philadelphia, Lippincott, 1971, pp. 322–323.
14. Glickman: op. cit., pp. 150–154, 977–980.

Suggested Readings

Hugoson, A.: Gingival Inflammation and Female Sex Hormones, *J. Periodont. Res.*, Supplement No. 5, 1970, 18 pp.

Kerr, D. A. and Ash, M. M.: *Oral Pathology*, 3rd ed. Philadelphia, Lea & Febiger, 1971, pp. 263–267.
Kerr, D. A., Ash, M. M., and Millard H. D.: *Oral Diagnosis*, 4th ed. St. Louis, Mosby, 1974, pp. 65–66.
McCarthy, P. L. and Shklar, G.: *Diseases of the Oral Mucosa*. New York, Blakiston Division, McGraw-Hill, 1964, pp. 180–191, 218–219, 246–248.
Nikai, H., Rose, G. G., and Cattoni, M.: Electron Microscopic Study of Chronic Desquamative Gingivitis, *J. Periodont. Res.*, Supplement No. 6, 1971, 30 pp.
Storer, R.: The Effect of the Climacteric and of Ageing on Prosthetic Diagnosis and Treatment Planning, *Br. Dent. J.*, 119, 349, October 19, 1965.
Tuttle, W. W. and Schottelius, B. A.: *Textbook of Physiology*, 16th ed. St. Louis, Mosby, 1969, pp. 448–473, 490–505.

Puberty and Adolescence

Bakwin, H. and Bakwin, R. M.: *Behavior Disorders in Children*, 4th ed. Philadelphia, Saunders, 1972, pp. 84–111.
Cohen, L.: Oral Manifestations of Systemic Diseases in the Adolescent, *Dent. Clin. North Am.*, 13, 329, April, 1969.
Holmes, C. B. and Collier, D.: Periodontal Disease, Dental Caries, Oral Hygiene and Diet in Adventist and Other Teenagers, *J. Periodont.*, 37, 100, March-April, 1966.
Massler, M.: Teen-age Cariology, *Dent. Clin. North Am.*, 13, 405, April, 1969.
Ravinett, S.: Factors Influencing Fixed Partial Dentures for Adolescents, *J. Prosthet. Dent.*, 15, 880, September-October, 1965.
Ritsert, E. F. and Binns, W. H.: Adolescents Brush Better with an Electric Toothbrush, *J. Dent. Child.*, 34, 354, September, 1967.
Schreiber, E. H. and Scales, J. L.: Anxiety and Dental Health in Institutionalized Delinquent Adolescents, *J. Am. Dent. Assoc.*, 82, 600, March, 1971.
Sutcliffe, P.: A Longitudinal Study of Gingivitis and Puberty, *J. Periodont. Res.*, 7, 52, No. 1, 1972.
Taano, J.: Correlation of Frequency of Prophylaxis with Habits and Attitudes of High School Freshmen, *J. Am. Dent. Hyg. Assoc.*, 44, 34, 2nd Quarter, 1970.
Tjossem, T. D.: Psychologic Considerations in the Care of the Adolescent Dental Patient, *Dent. Clin. North Am.*, p. 449, July, 1966.
Tofani, M. I.: Mandibular Growth at Puberty, *Am. J. Orthod.*, 62, 176, August, 1972.
Wheatcroft, M. G. and Arnim, S. S.: An Effective Program of Oral Hygiene the Dentist Can Teach Adolescents, *Dent. Clin. North Am.*, 13, 375, April, 1969.
Workshop on Periodontal Disease in the Circumpubertal and Adolescent Periods, *J. Periodont.*, 42, 452–537, August, 1971.
World Health Organization: *Health Problems of Adolescence*. WHO Technical Report Series No. 308, Geneva, World Health Organization, 1965, 28 pp.

Chapter 53

The Pregnant Patient

During pregnancy, attention is focused on good health practices for the mother. She is anxious and concerned for the health of her baby and for herself. This alertness to total health, of which oral health is an important part, provides an unusual opportunity to help the patient learn principles which may be applied to the future care of the child.

The term *prenatal care* refers to the supervised preparation for childbirth which helps the mother enjoy optimum health during and after her pregnancy and the reward of a healthy baby. Such a program involves the combined efforts of the obstetrician, nurse, dentist, dental hygienist, and the expectant parents. Pregnancy is arbitrarily divided into three periods of three months each, referred to as the first, second, and third trimesters, respectively.

Unfortunately there are still many women who do not seek care until delivery. Oral health is neglected along with general health. Some of these patients will appear for emergency dental service, and may be receptive to a program of care and instruction to prevent further emergencies. The dental hygienist in public health will participate in community educational programs with public health nurses whereby some of the less informed or less motivated women may learn of the need for professional dental care and advice during pregnancy.

Obstetricians routinely recommend dental care early in pregnancy. This brings to the dental office many women who previously would not have had a regular plan for obtaining professional service. Many of these have not known the advantages of personal habits of daily care and diet related to the health of the oral tissues. There are numerous misconceptions or "old wives' tales" to counteract when providing up-to-date information about the relationship of pregnancy and oral health.

I. Gingival Conditions During Pregnancy[1-4]

The condition of the gingiva is related to the presence of local irritants primarily produced by dental plaque. When the mouth is in good health and the patient practices adequate personal oral care procedures, no adverse gingival changes may be expected.

Pregnancy will tend to aggravate an existing gingival condition and is therefore a secondary or conditioning factor. Since the principal gingival reaction in pregnancy is an inflammatory one, the pregnancy itself cannot be the cause.

From 50 to 100 percent of pregnant patients have been shown in surveys to have gingival inflammation.[1,5,6] The severity increases during pregnancy when untreated, and there is a partial remission of symptoms postpartum.[5,6]

Gingivitis may be particularly noticed during the second trimester or late in the first trimester. During that period the patient may become more aware of her mouth than she was during the earlier emotional period.

Exaggerated symptoms abate after the birth of the child, but it should not be expected that a completely healthy condition will result. Patients with a gingival disturbance during pregnancy will continue to have the disturbance somewhat lessened in degree.

A. Generalized Gingival Enlargement

1. *Clinical Appearance*

    Symptoms are generally limited to the free gingiva. The appearance varies as suggested by the possible characteristics of inflamed tissues listed below.

    a. Enlargement: hyperplasia, edema.

    b. Shiny, smooth surface.

    c. Hemorrhages readily with probing and slight trauma.

    d. Color: may be bluish-purple or raspberry red.

    e. Loss of normal resiliency.

2. *Predisposing Factors*

    a. Local irritation due to an unhygienic oral condition and deposits on the teeth related to laxity in personal care procedures.

    b. Hormonal changes during pregnancy may alter the tissue reaction.

B. Isolated Gingival Enlargement

An isolated or discrete gingival enlargement occurs which has been called a "pregnancy tumor." The use of the word tumor is misleading since the lesion is not a tumor but a hyperplasia.[7] In one survey these lesions were shown to occur in about 0.5 percent of pregnant women.[1]

1. *Clinical Appearance*

    a. Location: superficially on the free gingiva, usually associated with an interdental papilla.

    b. Mushroom-like flattened mass.

    c. Smooth glistening surface.

    d. Color: purplish-red, magenta, or deep blue, sometimes dotted with red; color depends on vascularity.

2. *Symptoms*

    a. Hemorrhages readily with slight trauma.

    b. Painless unless it becomes large enough to interfere with occlusion and mastication.

II. Psychological Characteristics

Mental hygiene of the expectant mother is influenced by her attitude toward herself, her husband, her other children, and her unborn child. Normally, in a large majority of cases, when the husband is pleased and there is security in the marriage, there will be genuine happiness and anticipation or at least tranquil acceptance. When there is emotional instability, the mother may exhibit degrees of apprehension or even open rebellion in her rejection of the baby.

The first few months are usually the most difficult, and anxiety may be observed since pregnancy provides an emotional experience with many adjustments to be made. Generally these early problems resolve themselves and, if they continue throughout the pregnancy, may disappear when the baby is born. A few of the possible characteristic emotional manifestations of pregnancy are listed below with suggestions for the dental hygiene appointment.

A. **Changes in Mood from Happiness to Depression**

At times the change may be abrupt. Adapt conversation and instruction to receptiveness of patient.

B. **Hypersensitivity**

Be cautious about joking over personal matters and avoid calling attention to size or appearance.

C. **Irritability**

Minimize disturbances, interruptions, or noises; make operations smooth; adjust room temperature; avoid topics of discussion which might bring patient reaction.

D. **Increased Introversion, Passivity, Dependence on Others**

Help patient to feel the concern for her oral health being taken by the dentist and dental hygienist, yet interest her in the need for her own personal care.

E. **Physical and Mental Indifference**

May explain lack of conscientiousness in the patient's personal oral care habits.

1. Plan sufficient appointments for dental hygiene care to counteract patient's own limited care.
2. Plan for special reminders such as telephone to help a patient who is indifferent to keeping appointments.
3. Be firm with patient instruction in plaque control; take advantage of teachable moments.

F. **Impaired Judgment**

Be specific in outlining the plan for oral care, both professional and personal. Help the patient visualize realistically the possible effects of neglect.

G. **Hidden Fears Not Recognized or Admitted**

Fear of the pregnancy, the child's health, her own health or of adjustments which must be made after the birth of the child. Offer reassurance. Conversation should dwell on positive factors, not morbid.

H. **Changes in Appetite; Craving for Unusual Foods**

Provide specific information concerning the use of foods other than fermentable carbohydrates, particularly as snacks.

III. Aspects of Patient Care

The dental hygienist needs to be well-informed concerning aspects of dental care in order to motivate the patient and dispel fears related to certain services. The patient may consult the dental hygienist for reassurance and interpretation concerning the dentist's recommendations and procedures.

A. **Oral Examination and Treatment Planning**

The patient should be seen as early in pregnancy as possible. Consultation with the patient's physician is of particular importance in order that the total prenatal care may be integrated.

B. **Radiography**

There is no contraindication for routine radiographs being made since the oral cavity is sufficiently removed from the pelvic region. Ordinary precautions of ultra-speed film, extended target-film distance, and the use of an adequate diaphragm and filter should be observed as for any patient. The number of exposures should be restricted to a minimum. A lead apron placed across the patient's lap will reduce hazards of secondary radiation to that region (page 116).

C. Periodontal Treatment

Areas of food impaction should be corrected and all overhanging restorations replaced. All scaling and root planing procedures should be carefully and thoroughly completed.

The patient's general health, the severity of the periodontal disease, and particularly the advice of the obstetrician will determine the plan of action when surgery is indicated. In general the second trimester is considered most favorable when surgery cannot be postponed.[3,8]

D. Restorative Dentistry

All required work should be completed with permanent restorations. One important contraindication for the use of temporary restorations lies in the fact that after the baby is born the mother may be much too busy to attend to appointments and may postpone them.

DENTAL HYGIENE CARE

Severe gingival involvement need not be expected when the teeth are kept free of deposits, all other local irritants are removed, and the patient is motivated to practice conscientious self-care procedures for oral cleanliness and plaque control. This calls for a specific recall appointment plan for scaling and instruction.

A concentrated plan for dental caries control is indicated. A multiple fluoride program and limitation of dietary sucrose are basic to the preventive efforts.

I. Appointment Planning

A. Recall Intervals

Monthly appointments or three times during the nine-month period may be required depending on the individual mouth and the patient's motivation in personal care.

B. Length of Individual Appointments

Short, for patient comfort. A series of appointments is needed when there is heavy calculus.

C. Recall Postpartum

For the patient who has not been on a regular recall plan prior to pregnancy, emphasis must be placed on motivating the patient to continue regular appointments for dental hygiene and dental care.

II. Appointment Procedures

A. Patient History

The history must be reviewed carefully since the prenatal patient may require applied techniques for conditions other than pregnancy. For example, diabetes or cardiovascular diseases can involve serious complications. Special procedures for these and other systemic conditions have been described in other chapters.

When the expectant mother is an adolescent, consideration for her own health takes on a different perspective than for the matured woman. Aspects of adolescent development and psychology were described on pages 704–705.

B. Consultation with Physician

The dentist and the physician benefit mutually through discussion of patient treatment. The need for particular precautions before, during, and after treatment becomes known to the dentist and dental hygienist.

When a patient seeks dental and dental hygiene care and is not under the care of a physician, she should be strongly urged to obtain medical supervision, have examinations, and therefore improve her health as well as that of the baby. She must understand the relationship of general health and oral health.

Table 53-1.   Appointment Adaptations for the Prenatal Patient

Characteristic	*Dental Hygiene Implication*
Fatigues easily, may even fall asleep	Short appointments; several in series, as needed
Discomfort of remaining in one position too long	Interrupt in middle of appointment to change chair position. Assistance with evacuation during scaling and polishing can lessen operating time.
Backache	Adjust chair appropriately for comfort.
Frequent urination	Allow long enough appointment time for interruptions. Suggest at beginning of appointment that patient mention need for interruption.
General awkwardness because of size and shape	Move bracket table out of way when patient is rinsing. Attend to details such as gently lowering chair and straightening it for patient to get out. Make sure rinsing facilities are convenient; or preferably an assistant attends to evacuation.
Faintness and dizziness	Be prepared for first aid (table 54–1, page 730). Place the patient on her *side* and not in supine or Trendelenburg position because pressure from the enlarged uterus and the abdominal organs on the inferior vena cava can interfere with venous return. Placental separation could result.
Nausea and vomiting *a.* Unpleasant taste in mouth *b.* Gagging *c.* Reactions to odors and flavors of medicaments and other office materials *d.* Physician's recommendations for alleviation of symptoms: frequent eating of small amounts of foods	Suggest toothbrushing or rinsing at frequent intervals. Care in instrument and radiographic film placement Attention to cleanliness of cuspidor Determine particularly obnoxious odors for an individual patient and remove them. Encourage use of foods which do not contain dextrose and which are retained on the teeth readily because of the consistency, particularly if the problem continues for several months; relate to dental caries initiation.
Unusual food cravings	If cravings are for sweets, clearly define relationship of frequent nibbling of fermentable carbohydrate to dental caries.

III. Clinical Techniques

It is not within the scope of this book to review all of the physiologic changes which occur during pregnancy. There are common disturbances which should be identified since they can affect appointment procedures. Nearly every pregnant woman is bothered by one or more minor complaints.

Attention to small details will provide the patient with comfort and motivate her to continued oral care. Table 53–1 lists the more common minor physical disturbances of pregnancy and suggests a few appointment considerations.

A. **Instrumentation**

When the patient is seen with gingival enlargement and inflammation, the first appointment should consist entirely of instruction in plaque control measures. At the second appointment evaluation is made and instruction continued (page 390).

As the local irritants are removed, careful instrumentation is indicated. Bleeding may be excessive. If polishing is needed, it is usually advisable to postpone until the tissue has responded to the plaque control measures.

B. **Fluoride Application**

As described in the chapter on fluoride treatment (pages 433, 438), applications are not advised on inflamed, enlarged gingival tissue immediately following scaling. At a second appointment, after the patient has practiced the recommended plaque control procedures and the tissue has healed, the teeth can be polished and the fluoride application made.

PATIENT INSTRUCTION

During pregnancy, the emphasis on general health provides the ideal situation for the dental hygienist to instruct relative to many aspects of oral health for the mother, her expected new child, as well as for other members of the family. New developments in disease prevention and control need to be explained.

Printed materials concerning the prevention of periodontal diseases and dental caries, and the development and care of children's teeth are available from the American Dental Association.* Reading material to supplement personal discussions can contribute to patient understanding and appreciation.

I. **Plaque Control**

A rigid schedule for self-care must be demonstrated and supervised. A series of instructional periods is usually needed (pages 388–392).

Emphasis should not be placed on the hormonal changes of pregnancy as influential in producing gingival changes. The patient may be all too willing to use the systemic factor as an excuse for her lack of attention to adequate self-care.

II. **Diet**

A majority of expectant mothers will base their diets on the recommendation of their physicians. However, instruction must be provided in the relationship of dental caries prevention and the health of the supporting structures of the teeth to the use of a varied diet containing the essential protective foods.

A. **Purposes of Adequate Diet During Pregnancy**
1. To maintain daily strength.
2. To prepare for labor by building up the muscle tone of the body to meet the crisis of labor and delivery.
3. To shorten the period of convalescence after delivery.

---

*An American Dental Association catalog for the current year may be obtained by writing the Order Section, 211 East Chicago Avenue, Chicago, Il 60611.

4. To prepare the patient to be better able to nurse the baby.
5. To provide the essential building materials for the developing fetus.
6. To protect and promote the health of the oral tissues of the mother.

B. **Dietary Needs of Pregnancy**

In the *Recommended Daily Dietary Allowances* from the Food and Nutrition Board of the National Research Council[9] the increased allowances during pregnancy and lactation are specified. Since the embryo or fetus is a parasite and thrives at the mother's expense, the mother's diet must be adequate to maintain her own nutritional status as well as to meet the needs of the fetus.

The particular needs of the fetus are:
1. Proteins, for general tissue construction.
2. Minerals, especially calcium and phosphorus, for bone and tooth calcification; and iron for blood corpuscles.
3. Vitamins.

C. **Dietary Adjustments**[10]

Foods from the four food groups (table 28–1, page 403) are selected. To meet the needs for calcium, phosphorus, and riboflavin, a quart of milk or its equivalent in milk products is sufficient except for the teen-age mother who needs a quart and one-half if her own maturing body requirements are to be met.

An added citrus fruit or other good source of vitamin C, a dark green or deep yellow vegetable daily for vitamin A, along with sources for iron, thiamine, and vitamin D are indicated. Proteins of high physiological value are important, that is, proteins from meat, eggs, fish, and fowl rather than of vegetable origin only. Calories may be increased in accord with exercise and tendency for weight gain. A decreased

use of foods containing sucrose is important in the prevention of dental caries.

III. **Dental Caries Control**

A. **Incidence During Pregnancy**

Certain patients believe that they have more dental caries during and because of pregnancy. Research has shown that this is not true, and that any relationship is an indirect one. Factors which result in dental caries formation are the same during pregnancy as at other times.

B. **Factors Which May Contribute to Apparent Increase in Dental Caries Rate**
1. Previous neglect: a patient may not have kept a regular appointment plan so that the existing dental caries during pregnancy represents an accumulation, possibly even of years.
2. Diet during pregnancy: possible increase in intake of fermentable carbohydrates.
   a. Unusual cravings may be for sweet foods.
   b. Frequency of eating: patient may be eating every few hours for prevention of nausea and these foods may be cariogenic.
3. Neglect of personal oral care procedures: lack of interest or laxity in toothbrushing or rinsing immediately following intake of fermentable carbohydrates.

C. **Calcium and the Mother's Teeth**[11,12]

There has been widespread misconception concerning the withdrawal of calcium from the mother's teeth and its relationship to dental caries. It is important to review the known facts and provide references for further reading on the subject since the patient's beliefs may need clarification. When discussing the problem a summary of the process of dental caries initiation can be helpful (pages 243–244).

1. Minerals contained in the erupted tooth enamel and dentin are not available and no removal of minerals can occur by way of the pulp.
2. Minerals contained within the alveolar bone are available as from other bones of the body. When the mother's diet does not contain sufficient calcium and phosphorus, her own reserve is utilized.
3. Majority of calcium and phosphorus of bones and teeth is added to the fetus during the third trimester. Incidence of dental caries in the mother is not different during that period although the carious lesions may be larger if the teeth have been neglected throughout the pregnancy.
4. There is a definite tendency for the teeth of the fetus to develop and calcify normally in spite of the diet of the mother since the reserve in her bones is used.

D. **Relationship of Fluoride**

There is no direct evidence to show that prenatal fluoride intake will influence the dental caries rate in the child.[13-16] When the community water supply is not fluoridated, dietary fluoride by prescription is advised for the baby after birth (pages 428–430).

References

1. Orban, B. J. and Wentz, F. M.: *Atlas of Clinical Pathology of the Oral Mucous Membrane,* 2nd ed. St. Louis, Mosby, 1960, pp. 110–111.
2. Glickman, I.: *Clinical Periodontology,* 4th ed. Philadelphia, Saunders, 1972, pp. 100–101, 148–149.
3. Grant, D. A., Stern, I. B., and Everett, F. G.: *Orban' Periodontics,* 4th ed. St. Louis, Mosby, 1972, pp. 217–220.
4. Goldman, H. M. and Cohen, D. W.: *Periodontal Therapy,* 5th ed. St. Louis, Mosby, 1973, pp. 231–232.
5. Löe, H.: Periodontal Changes in Pregnancy, *J. Periodont.,* 36, 209, May-June, 1965.
6. Cohen, D. W., Friedman, L., Shapiro, J., and Kyle, G. C.: A Longitudinal Investigation of the Periodontal Changes During Pregnancy, *J. Periodont.,* 40, 563, October, 1969.
7. McCarthy, P. L. and Shklar, G.: *Diseases of the Oral Mucosa.* New York, Blakiston Division, McGraw-Hill, 1964, pp. 247–248, 271–272.
8. Glickman: op. cit., pp. 797, 980–981.
9. Food and Nutrition Board: *Recommended Dietary Allowances,* 8th ed. Washington, D.C., National Academy of Sciences—National Research Council, 1974.
10. Nizel, A. E.: *Nutrition in Preventive Dentistry: Science and Practice.* Philadelphia, Saunders, 1972, pp. 279–282, 287–289.
11. Burket, L. W.: *Oral Medicine,* 6th ed. Philadelphia, Lippincott, 1971, pp. 323–327.
12. Bawden, J. W.: Calcium Metabolism During Pregnancy, *J. Dent. Child.,* 30, 93, 2nd Quarter, 1963.
13. Carlos, J. P., Gittelsohn, A. M., and Haddon, W. Jr.: Caries in Deciduous Teeth in Relation to Maternal Ingestion of Fluoride, *Pub. Health Rep.,* 77, 658, August, 1962.
14. Dale, P. P.: Prenatal Fluorides: the Value of Fluoride During Pregnancy, *J. Am. Dent. Assoc.,* 68, 530, April, 1964.
15. Horowitz, H. S. and Heifetz, S. B.: Effects of Prenatal Exposure to Fluoridation on Dental Caries, *Pub. Health Rep.,* 82, 297, April, 1967.
16. Katz S. and Muhler, J. C.: Prenatal and Postnatal Fluoride and Dental Caries Experience in Deciduous Teeth, *J. Am. Dent. Assoc.,* 76, 305, February, 1968.

Suggested Readings

American Dental Association, Council on Dental Therapeutics: *Accepted Dental Therapeutics,* 36th ed. Chicago, American Dental Association, 1975, pp. 85–86, 179, 290–291.

Arafat, A. H.: Periodontal Status During Pregnancy, *J. Periodont.,* 45, 641, August, 1974.

Buchman, M. L. and Fasano, J.: The Obstetrician's View of Dental Care in Pregnancy, *N.Y. J. Dent.* 36, 120, April, 1966.

Camilleri, A. P.: Dental Obstetrics, *Br. Dent. J.,* 124, 219, March 5, 1968.

Cheney, H. G.: The Dental Hygienist as a Health Educator in Prenatal Care, *Dent. Hyg.,* 48, 150, May-June, 1974.

Driscoll, W. S.: The Use of Fluoride Tablets for the Prevention of Dental Caries, in Forrester, D. J. ed.: *International Workshop on Fluorides and Dental Caries Reductions.* Baltimore, Maryland, 1974, pp. 33–40.

El-Ashiry, G. M., El-Kafrawy, A. H., Nasr, M. F., and Younis, N.: Comparative Study of the Influence of Pregnancy and Oral Contraceptives on the Gingivae, *Oral Surg.,* 30, 472, October, 1970.

Hatziotis, J. C.: The Incidence of Pregnancy Tumors and Their Probable Relation to the Embryo's Sex, *J. Periodont.*, *43*, 447, July, 1972.

Pearlman, B. A.: An Oral Contraceptive Drug and Gingival Enlargement; the Relationship Be-tween Local and Systemic Factors, *J. Clin. Periodont.*, *1*, 47, No. 1, 1974.

Raynor, J. F.: Socioeconomic Status and Factors Influencing the Dental Health Practices of Mothers, *Am. J. Public Health*, *60*, 1250, July, 1970.

Chapter 54

Emergency Care

It is relatively easy to be skillful in techniques which are repeated frequently. Emergency care through first aid measures is performed only occasionally, and in instances which involve lifesaving measures, may be performed once in many years. To be prepared for that rare moment is difficult, but the public expects an individual trained in a health profession to be able to act in an emergency. Periodic review of procedures is necessary if application is to be effective.

Emergencies may occur within or in the vicinity of the dental office or clinic. Readiness involves not only having knowledge of proper procedures but equipment kept in a convenient place. A quick, handy reference of first aid measures is important, preferably in the form of a posted chart which gives characteristic symptoms and related treatment.

The information included in this chapter is basic and presented without an attempt to mention all types of emergencies which may arise, particularly those of involved traumatic injuries. The principal objectives are to list the symptoms and treatment of the more common emergencies which can occur and to provide a list

of the equipment which should be readily available in every dental office. It is assumed that other references will be kept in the dental office and that all dental personnel will familiarize themselves with such sources of information.

As an auxiliary to the dentist, the dental hygienist needs to be familiar with all procedures required in emergencies. Resuscitation involving techniques such as drug injection or tracheotomy would be carried out by the dentist. Knowledge of procedures and required equipment or materials is necessary in order that the dentist may have immediate and efficient assistance.

I. Prevention of Emergencies

A. Understanding the Patient's Needs

1. *Patient History*

    The carefully prepared and regularly updated medical and personal history with adequate follow-up consultation with the patient's physician for integration of dental and medical care can prevent many emergencies by alerting dental personnel to the individual patient's needs and idiosyncrasies. Factors

723

which should be included in the patient's history have been listed in tables 6–1, 6–2, and 6–3 on pages 72–78 and include:

a. Knowledge of specific physical conditions which may lead to an emergency.

b. Knowledge of diseases for which the patient is or has been under the care of a physician and the type of treatment, particularly drugs, currently being prescribed.

c. Information concerning allergies or drug reactions.

2. *Previous Records*

Reference to records of previous appointment experiences with the particular patient.

3. *Patient's Physical and Mental State*

a. Record of vital signs (pages 81–88).

b. Extraoral inspection: general appearance as an indication of health.

B. **Preparation of the Patient for the Appointment**

1. Prevention of excess exertion on the part of a patient.

a. Arrange time of appointment in accord with personal health requirements.

b. Limit length of appointment.

2. Establishment of rapport; aid in allaying fears.

3. Use of premedication when indicated and recommended by physician and dentist.

4. Medications: patients who are subject to emergencies should be instructed to bring their own prescribed medicines, for example, the patient with asthma or one who is subject to attacks of angina pectoris.

II. General First Aid Procedures[1–3]

Life-endangering conditions must be treated first, namely, respiratory difficulty, bleeding, and shock. It is necessary to keep calm and act promptly but not hastily. The incorrect procedure may be more harmful than none at all. It is assumed that each dental hygienist will have participated in a detailed course in first aid.

A. **Examine**

Determine the most urgent problems:

1. Respiratory distress: evidenced by dilated pupils (figure 8–5, page 95), choking, coughing, gasping, weak respirations, or no respirations.

2. Severe bleeding.

3. Poisoning or ingestion of harmful chemicals.

4. Shock: with symptoms of pallor, clammy skin, feeble pulse, shallow breathing, chills.

5. Note state of consciousness and degree of orientation.

B. **Lay Patient Flat**

1. On a flat surface.

2. Exceptions. Certain patients are best placed on a side or otherwise positioned.

a. During pregnancy, particularly the last three or four months, place on side to prevent pressure on vena cava (table 53–1, page 717).

b. Person with severe facial injury with bone fractures and bleeding is best on side or at least with the head turned to lessen the danger of blood, debris, and displaced parts from falling toward the throat.[4]

c. When there is shortness of breath which accompanies certain cardiovascular diseases, patient must be kept in a sitting or semi-sitting position.

C. **Establish Airway**

Hyperextend head (one hand on forehead, one in back of neck and pull gently but firmly), and tilt head back.

D. **Breathing**
  1. Clear the airway: use fingers or suction to remove mucus, blood, debris, or vomitus; pull tongue forward.
  2. Administer artificial respiration by mouth-to-mouth resuscitation or oxygen for the breathing patient.

E. **Bleeding**
  1. Apply pressure directly to the area with a compress (clean cloth).
  2. Elevate the part when applicable, except when there are broken bones which could be displaced.
  3. Tourniquet: *never used* except for amputated, mangled, or crushed arm or leg or when profuse bleeding cannot otherwise be stopped. A tourniquet should not be released except when directed by a physician. For the physician's immediate reference: write "T" on the patient's forehead and note time of application.

F. **Shock**
  Shock is the result of an inadequate volume of circulating blood to furnish normal oxygen and nutrient needs to the tissues of the body. Causes include massive blood loss, plasma loss (occurs in burns), severe infection, anaphylaxis, severe dehydration (also related to blood loss), hyperinsulinism, marked psychic or physical trauma, or severe cardiac disease when the heart cannot pump sufficient blood.
  1. Lay patient flat and elevate legs except in head injuries, breathing difficulty, or pain when legs are moved.
  2. Treat the cause when possible: for example, keep airway open, control bleeding, elevate legs, place head lower than the body, immerse a first or second degree burn area in cold water (see table 54–1, page 732).

  3. Keep patient warm.
  4. Give fluids when patient is able to swallow. Never give alcoholic beverages.
  5. Reassure patient.

G. **First Aid for Specific Conditions**
  See table 54–1 (pages 729–733).

H. **Seek Assistance**
  As it is required by the nature of the emergency.
  1. When alone: judgment must be used to determine the proper moment to leave the patient to telephone a physician.
    a. Leave patient in a safe position.
    b. Perform immediate first aid when hemorrhage is present.
  2. When summoning dentist from another part of the dental office, care should be taken not to alarm other patients who may be present in the reception area or other operatory.

ARTIFICIAL RESPIRATION

Some form of artificial respiration should be started immediately when it is determined that the patient has stopped breathing or when breathing has been critically reduced. The mouth-to-mouth technique has been established as the most practical for emergency ventilation of an individual of any age.

The objectives are to obtain and maintain an open air passageway from the lungs to the mouth and to provide for an alternate increase and decrease in the size of the chest, internally or externally, to move air in and out.

I. **Mouth-to-Mouth Method**[1,4-6]

A. Clean debris from mouth; remove removable prostheses; bring tongue forward.

B. Place patient flat on back, neck extended, head back, with chin lifted.

C. To tilt head, place one hand under the neck and the other hand on the forehead. Lift neck and tilt head back.

D. Pinch nose closed with fingers of the hand which has been used on the forehead.

E. Apply wide open mouth tightly over the patient's mouth. For mouth-to-nose method, hold mouth closed and place open mouth tightly over the nose.

F. Blow or exhale firmly into the patient's mouth to expand his lungs. Watch chest rise: determine immediately whether there is an obstruction and proceed to recheck to dislodge.

G. Remove mouth, watch and listen for air escape; take another deep breath.

H. Repeat 12 times per minute for an adult and 18 to 20 times per minute for a child; maintain hold under patient's neck.

I. Child patient: take relatively shallow breaths depending on the size of the child.

II. Oxygen Administration

Oxygen resuscitation equipment consists of an oxygen tank, a reducing valve, a flow meter, tubing, mask, and a positive pressure bag. Directions for use should be attached to the equipment.

A. Clean debris from mouth; bring tongue forward.

B. Place patient on back, neck extended, head back, with chin lifted.

C. Fit mask over the patient's nose and mouth.

D. Hold mask with first two fingers; extend ring and little finger under chin to raise it up and forward to secure airway.

E. Adjust flow of oxygen to the rate that keeps the bag filled which may be 5 to 10 liters per minute.

F. When it is necessary to force oxygen into the lungs, compress bag intermittently at three to four second intervals to provide 15 to 20 respirations per minute. Watch chest rise and fall.

G. Watch skin color and respirations for return to normal.

H. Adaptation: when patient is breathing but respirations are shallow or otherwise deficient, compress bag in harmony with each inspiration of the patient to increase the depth and volume.

CARDIOPULMONARY RESUSCITATION

Sudden unexpected cessation of effective respiration and circulation must be treated immediately. Without heart action, oxygen cannot be carried to the cells, and a deficiency occurs immediately. The lack of oxygenated blood affects the pupils within a minute; therefore the eyes are tested promptly for response to light. Irreversible tissue damage can result within four to six minutes in the absence of oxygenated blood.

I. Objectives[5,6]

A. *Airway Opened*

B. *Breathing Restored*

C. *Circulation Restored*

D. *Definitive Therapy* (Medical care)

II. Establish Airway

A. Patient in supine position on hard firm surface.

B. Clean debris from mouth by suction or fingers; remove removable prostheses.

C. Hyperextend head; tilt head back.

D. Spontaneous breathing may be resumed after opening airway.

III. Respiratory Resuscitation

A. Begin mouth-to-mouth breathing (see above).

B. External cardiac compression must always be accompanied by artificial respiration.

IV. External Cardiac Compression

A. **Principle**

Rhythmic pressure applied over the lower half of the sternum compresses the heart to produce artificial circulation (figure 54–1).

B. **Position**
   1. Locate upper and lower borders of the sternum.
   2. Place the heel (not the palm) of one hand on the lower half of the sternum.
   3. Check area of pressure: do not apply to lower end (xiphoid) of sternum or to the ribs. Keep fingers parallel to ribs but not touching them.
   4. Place other hand on top of the first with fingers in same direction. Link and close the fingers.

C. **Compression**
   1. Lean forward over the placed hands: keep arms straight; pressure

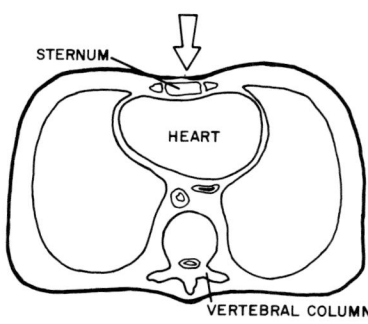

Figure 54–1. External cardiac compression. Cross section at level of heart to show relationship of sternum, heart, and vertebral column. Arrow points to sternum where intermittent rhythmic pressure is applied. The heart is compressed 60 times per minute between the sternum and the vertebral column. The patient should be placed in supine position on a hard flat surface. (Adapted from O'Day, R. A. and Driggs, R. L.: Cardiopulmonary Resuscitation in Dental Practice. *Dent. Clin. North Am. 17,* 329, April, 1973.)

on sternum comes from the muscles of the back.
   2. Use a firm, steady, vertical stroke (not a blow); sternum moves downward 1½ to 2 inches.
   3. Hold pressure at the bottom of each stroke for a brief fraction of a minute (allows heart to empty).
   4. Release: lighten pressure of hands and keep them in position; chest expands (heart refills).
   5. Repeat: a rate of 60 times per minute must be maintained. The compressions should be regular, smooth, and uninterrupted, with compression and relaxation being of equal duration. Under no circumstance should compression be interrupted for more than five seconds.[6]

V. Child Patient

A. Area for pressure slightly higher, near mid-sternum.

B. Judge pressure by size of child: for small child one hand is usually sufficient to prevent internal injury from too severe pressure.

VI. Length of Treatment

A. Signs of recovery: pupils constrict when exposed to light, normal skin color returns, patient may gasp or show other sign of breathing, and may move or wiggle his body.

B. Do not stop heart compressions while patient is being transported to the hospital for emergency treatment.

C. When circulation and breathing appear to have returned, do not leave patient: watch for need to continue first aid in case of relapse.

VII. Coordinated Activity

A. **Immediate Steps**
   1. Check for cessation of breathing.
   2. Begin mouth-to-mouth breathing with four quick lung inflations.

3. Check carotid pulse (at level with larynx). If no pulse or very weak pulse, start external cardiac massage.

B. **Lone Operator**
   1. Perform immediate steps listed above.
   2. Must alternate mouth-to-mouth breathing with cardiac massage.
   3. Establish rhythm of applying two quick lung inflations after each 15 chest compressions.
   4. Check carotid pulse and pupil response frequently.

C. **Two Operators**
   1. First person: perform immediate steps listed above.
   2. Second person: calls for ambulance and physician, then *promptly* takes over the mouth-to-mouth breathing.
   3. Establish coordinated rhythm of applying one quick lung inflation after every five compressions. *Do not* interrupt the rhythm of the compressions.
   4. Check carotid pulse and pupil response frequently.

D. **Three Operators**
   The third person seeks assistance through telephoning physician and ambulance, and aids the other two as necessary.

EMERGENCY MATERIALS AND PREPARATION

I. Reference Materials

A. **Books**
   1. American National Red Cross, *Standard First Aid and Personal Safety.*[1]
   2. American Dental Association, *Accepted Dental Therapeutics* (Current edition).
   3. American Medical Association, *First Aid Manual.*[2]

B. **Telephone Numbers**
   1. Number for each patient's physi-

cian in convenient reference place in permanent record.
   2. Numbers posted near telephone.
      a. Physicians who may be called when patient's physician is not available or distance is too great for immediate assistance.
      b. Fire department.
      c. Police department.
      d. Ambulance service.
      e. Nearest hospital.
      f. Poison Information Center.
   3. For clinic or specialized dental practice: telephone number for each patient's dentist.

II. Equipment for Use in an Emergency

Every dental office or clinic should have an emergency kit or cart;[7] and everyone in the office must be familiar with its contents. The kit should be in order and its contents replenished and old materials replaced as needed.

The emergency equipment should be portable and kept in a place readily accessible to the dental and dental hygiene operating rooms. Materials are kept separate from other office supplies and plainly marked. Materials included are selected by the dentist to fulfill emergency needs by preferred methods.

A. **Bandages and Dressings**
   Dressings are purchased in individual packages and maintained in the sealed sterile state.
   1. Adhesive bandages.
   2. Sterile dressings in sealed envelopes: 2″ × 2″, and 4″ × 4″.
   3. Roller bandage: One-inch (five yards); two-inch (five yards).
   4. Adhesive tape.
   5. Gauze sponges (4″ × 4″).
   6. Inflatable splints (assorted sizes).

B. **Instruments and Related Equipment**
   1. Blood pressure cuff and stethoscope.
   2. Sterile syringes: 2, 5, and 10 ml. capacities with disposable sterile

(text continues on page 734)

Table 54-1. Emergency Reference Chart

Emergency	Symptoms	Procedures

Hemorrhage	Prolonged bleeding
	  a. Spurting blood: artery
	  b. Oozing blood: vein
		Compression over bleeding area
		  a. Apply gauze pack with pressure.
		  b. Bandage pack into place firmly
		    where possible.
		Severe bleeding: digital pressure on
		  pressure point of supplying vessel

	Bleeding from tooth socket	Pack with folded gauze. Have patient bite down firmly.

	Bleeding of an extremity	Elevate the part: support with pillows or
		  substitute.
		Apply tourniquet only when limb is
		  amputated, mangled, or crushed.

	Nosebleed	Tell patient to breathe through mouth.
		Apply cold application to nose.
		Press nostril on bleeding side for a few
		  minutes.
		Plug nostril with gauze (not cotton);
		  leave end hanging out.
		Advise patient not to blow the nose for
		  an hour or more.

Respiratory Failure	Labored or weak respirations
	  or cessation of breathing
	Cyanosis or ashen white with
	  blood loss
	Pupils dilated
	Loss of consciousness
		Lay patient down flat: turn head to one
		  side.
		Check for and remove any foreign bodies
		  or obstruction in mouth.
		Pull tongue forward.
		Perform mouth-to-mouth breathing.
		May require tracheotomy.
		May need oxygen administration.

Shock	Pale skin, sometimes cyanotic
	Moist skin: cold, clammy
	Restless; sometimes
	  unconscious
	Dilated pupils
	Rapid, shallow breathing
	Pulse weak and thready
	Lowered blood pressure
		Patient position depends on injuries.
		  Generally place lying down (page
		  725).
		Keep airway open. Clear debris from
		  mouth; take out removable dental
		  appliances.
		Keep quiet and warm (body
		  temperature, not hot).
		Check vital signs and record time;
		  repeat at 15 minute intervals.
		Do not give fluids (water, tea, coffee)
		  unless medical assistance is exten-
		  sively delayed and patient is
		  conscious, neither vomiting nor
		  having convulsions or other condition
		  which might lead to aspiration of
		  fluids into the lungs.

Table 54-1.   Emergency Reference Chart *(Continued)*

Emergency	*Symptoms*	*Procedures*
Stroke (cerebrovascular accident)	*Premonitory* Dizziness, vertigo Transient paresthesia or weakness one side Transient speech defects *Serious* Headache (with cerebral hemorrhage) Breathing labored, deep, slow Paralysis one side of body Nausea, vomiting Convulsions Loss of consciousness (slow or sudden onset)	Turn patient on affected side. Elevate head slightly. Loosen clothing about the throat. Keep patient quiet, comfortable, warm May need oxygen. Do not give stimulant, sedative, or narcotic.
Syncope (fainting)	Pale, gray face Dilated pupils Weakness, giddiness, dizziness, faintness Profuse cold perspiration Rapid pulse at first, followed by slow pulse Shallow breathing Drop in blood pressure Loss of consciousness	Place in recumbent position with head lower than heart level and feet above heart level. Loosen tight clothing. Place cold damp towel on forehead. May require oxygen. Keep in supine position 10 minutes after recovery to prevent nausea and dizziness.
Cardiovascular Diseases	Symptoms vary depending on cause (pages 676–677).	*For all patients* Be calm and reassure patient. Keep patient warm and quiet; restrict effort. Call physician.
Angina Pectoris	Sudden, transient pain in the substernal area which may radiate to shoulder, neck and arms May have pallor, faintness, and breathing may be shallow Anxiety, fear	Place patient in upright position, as patient requests for comfortable breathing. Place nitroglycerin sublingually. Administer oxygen. Reassure patient. Without prompt relief from nitroglycerin, call physician. Patient suspected of or known to be subject to angina attacks should not be given adrenalin or ammonia.

Table 54-1. Emergency Reference Chart (Continued)

Emergency	Symptoms	Procedures
Myocardial Infarction	Sudden pain similar to angina pectoris which also may radiate, but of longer duration Pallor; cold, clammy skin Nausea Difficulty in breathing Marked weakness Anxiety, fear	Patient seated with head up. Symptoms are not relieved by nitroglycerin. Call physician and ambulance for transfer to a hospital. Administer oxygen. Make patient comfortable and alleviate anxiety.
Heart Failure	Difficult or labored breathing Pulmonary congestion with cough. May cough up blood. Rapid, weak pulse Dilated pupils May have chest pain	Call physician immediately. Place patient in sitting position. Make patient comfortable: cover with blanket. Administer oxygen.
Cardiac Arrest	No pulse Irregular heartbeat followed by no heartbeat Gasping, followed by no breathing Dilated pupils; no constriction with light Cyanosis	Place patient in supine position on a hard flat surface. Open airway; clear the mouth and remove dental appliances. Apply suction when excess saliva or blood is present. Restore breathing (mouth-to-mouth breathing). Restore circulation (external cardiac compression). Described in detail in text, page 727.
Insulin Reaction (Hyperinsulinism; hypoglycemia)	Hunger Nervousness; trembling Weakness Restlessness, anxiety Sweating; possible drooling Transient period of unconsciousness Dizziness	When conscious: feed patient sugar cubes, orange juice, or candy. When unconscious: call physician. No first aid procedures (pages 692–693).
Diabetic Coma (ketoacidosis)	Slow onset in comparison with insulin reaction Skin flushed and dry Breath with fruity odor Eyeballs soft and sunken Lack of appetite Dry mouth, thirst Drowsiness, lethargy, weakness Coma	Immediate professional care: hospitalization Keep patient warm. Give fluids to conscious patient. Insulin injection by physician.

Table 54-1. Emergency Reference Chart *(Continued)*

Emergency	*Symptoms*	*Procedures*
Epileptic Seizure	*Grand Mal* (page 634) Pale face: may become cyanotic Dilated pupils Muscular contractions Loss of consciousness	Lay patient flat; turn head to side. Do not force anything between the teeth. Prevent injury by clearing area around. Open airway: may need mouth-to-nose resuscitation. Do not move or attempt to restrain (page 639). Allow patient to sleep during post-convulsive period.
	Petit mal (page 634) Brief loss of consciousness Fixed posture Rhythmic twitching of eyelids, eyebrows, or head May be pale	Take objects from patient's hands to prevent dropping.
Burns	*First degree:* skin reddened *Second degree:* blisters *Third degree:* severe damage, skin burned off	*First and Second Degree:* immerse or cover with cool or cold water. Do not apply ointment, grease, or baking soda. *Third degree:* Call ambulance. Do not give sedative. Do not remove clothing. Cover loosely with nonadherent dressing to protect from air and dust while patient is transported. Elevate burned part.
	Chemical burn of oral mucous membrane	Flush with water. Have patient rinse with solution of bicarbonate of soda if burn was caused by acid; or solution of one teaspoonful vinegar in glass of water if burn caused by alkali. Advise bland diet during healing to minimize irritation.
Internal Poisoning	Nausea Evidence of empty container or information from patient	Give water or milk in large amounts to dilute the substance when the patient is conscious. Have patient swallow strong bicarbonate of soda solution to induce vomiting. Do not induce vomiting if strong acids, strong alkalis, or petroleum products have been ingested. Administer universal antidote.

Table 54-1.   Emergency Reference Chart *(Continued)*

Emergency	Symptoms	Procedures
Foreign Body in Eye	Tears Blinking	Wash hands. Ask patient to look down. Bring upper lid down over lower lid for a moment; move it upward. Turn down lower lid and examine: if particle is visible remove with moistened cotton applicator. Use eye cup: wash out eye with mild boric acid solution. When unsuccessful, seek medical attention: prevent patient from rubbing eye by placing gauze pack over eye and stabilizing with adhesive tape.
Dislocated Jaw	Mouth is open: patient is unable to close	Stand in front of seated patient. Wrap thumbs in towels and place on occlusal surfaces of mandibular posterior teeth. Curve fingers and place under body of the mandible. Press down and back with thumbs and at same time pull up and forward with fingers. As joint slips into place, quickly move thumbs outward. Place bandage around head to support jaw.
Facial Fracture	Pain, swelling Ecchymosis Deformity, limitation of movement Crepitus on manipulation Zygoma fracture: depression of cheek Mandibular fracture: abnormal occlusion	Place patient on side (see II. B.2., page 724). Support with bandage around face, under chin, and tied on the top of the head (Barton).
Tooth Forcibly Displaced (avulsed tooth)	Swelling, bruises, or other signs of trauma, depending on the type of accident	Instruct patient or parent to rinse tooth gently in cool water and place in water or wrap in wet cloth. Bring to the dental office or clinic *immediately.* The longer the time lapse between avulsion and replantation, the poorer the prognosis.
Choking	Violent coughing Gasping attempts at breathing Cyanosis Possible cessation of breathing and loss of consciousness.	Do not give anything by mouth. Pull tongue forward: use suction. Allow patient to cough. Call physician and/or ambulance. Do not "thump" back. When object swallowed has disappeared but there is no respiratory distress, refer promptly for examination to determine location of object, whether in digestive or respiratory tract.

needles for intravenous, intramuscular, and subcutaneous injections. Many emergency drugs are administered intravenously.

3. Oxygen administration equipment: tank of oxygen, regulator, mask, breathing bag.
4. Scissors.
5. Hemostat.
6. Cotton pliers.
7. Sterile suture and needle holder.
8. Rubber bite block (mouth prop).
9. Commercial cold packs (nonrefrigerated quick-forming ice bag).
10. Tourniquet (rubber tubing).
11. Eye rinsing cup.
12. Blanket and pillow.

C. **Drugs**

All dental personnel must be familiar with the emergency drugs which are maintained in the particular office or clinic. The purpose and method of administration for each should be clearly identified with the container. A compartmentalized clear plastic cabinet or box is particularly useful for this purpose since the labels and instructions can be seen from the outside and efficient selection made.

Drugs which are most frequently included relate to the major emergencies, for example, a *coronary dilator* (nitroglycerin or amyl nitrite for angina pectoris), an *anticonvulsant* (sedative such as Seconal or Nembutal), an *antihistamine* (Benadryl or aminophyllin for allergic reactions), and *epinephrine* for cardiac standstill and anaphylactic and allergic reactions.

The following household agents and drugs should be kept readily available with other first aid materials:

1. Sugar cubes, granulated sugar, or hard candies for insulin reaction.
2. Bicarbonate of soda.
3. Table salt.

4. Boric acid for eye wash.
5. Universal antidote.*

III. Practice and Drill

A. **Staff Instruction**

Each member of the clinic or office staff must be thoroughly familiar with the location, purpose, effect, and application of each item of equipment and the materials and their sources.

B. **Assignments**

Specific responsibilities are assigned to each staff member. Each must know the order of procedures in an emergency. Moments count, and there is no time for fumbling or discussion. Because of the possibility of a staff member being absent from the scene at the time of emergency, each person needs to know the duties of at least one other person in the group so that substitutions and doubling of duties can be made.

C. **Drills**

1. Regular reviews and rehearsals for each type of emergency should be made. These should be conducted on a "surprise" basis. The dentist can use a specific code call when there is an intercom, or other message system.
2. Practice in the use of oxygen, mouth-to-mouth breathing, and external cardiac compression, as well as patient positioning, is indicated.

D. **New Staff Member**

Assignment of duties and practice for the new member should be part of the first working day's orientation.

TECHNICAL HINTS

I. Vital signs, including blood pressure, should be recorded periodically dur-

---

*Universal antidote, available commercially, is composed of two parts activated charcoal, one part magnesium oxide, and one part tannic acid. For internal poisoning administer one tablespoon in a glass of warm water.

ing the emergency and sent to the hospital with the patient. Vital signs are outlined in Chapter 7, pages 81–89.

II. Post basic emergency procedures in outline form in a convenient place.

III. Care of materials
   A. Replace drugs in emergency kit at appropriate intervals. Check the shelf-life of each material: for example, nitroglycerin should be renewed at six months.
   B. Test the oxygen equipment on a regular plan to guard against leaks in the tubing and to insure a supply of oxygen.

IV. Identification for patients with medical problem: a metal emblem worn as a bracelet or a pendant is available to provide specific information pertinent to an emergency which may arise. Information about the emblems is available by writing the Medic Alert Foundation International, Turlock, California. In addition to noting patients who are wearing the identification and recording the fact along with other information in the patient history, other patients can be given information about the service.

V. Sources of Materials and Information:

   American Heart Association
   44 East 23rd Street
   New York, New York 10010
   American National Red Cross
   17th and D Streets
   Washington, D.C. 20006

References

1. American National Red Cross: *Standard First Aid and Personal Safety.* New York, Doubleday, 1973, pp. 11–90.
2. American Medical Association: *First Aid Manual,* Revised ed. Chicago, American Medical Association, 1967, pp. 2–14.
3. American Dental Association, Council on Dental Therapeutics: *Accepted Dental Therapeutics,* 36th ed. Chicago, American Dental Association, 1975, pp. 18–33.
4. McKelvey, L. E.: Maxillofacial Injuries, in McCarthy, F. M.: *Emergencies in Dental Practice,* 2nd ed. Philadelphia, Saunders, 1972, pp. 363–380.
5. American Heart Association and National Academy of Sciences—National Research Council: Standards for Cardiopulmonary Resuscitation (CPR) and Emergency Cardiac Care (ECC), *J. Am. Med. Assoc.,* 227, 833, February 18, 1974.
6. American National Red Cross: *Cardiopulmonary Resuscitation.* Washington, D.C., American National Red Cross, 1974, 41 pp.
7. Booth, D. F. and Dunn, M. J.: Systemic Emergencies, in Dunn, M. J., ed.: *Dental Auxiliary Practice,* Module 4. Baltimore, Williams and Wilkins, 1975, pp. 71–72.

Suggested Readings

Chue, P. W. Y.: Emergency Management of Cardiac Arrest, *Dent. Surv.,* 51, 36, April, 1975.
Chue, P. W. Y.: Emergency Management of Anaphylactic Reactions, *Dent. Surv.,* 51, 32, July, 1975.
Dempster, A. E.: Emergencies in Dental Practice, *J. Can. Dent. Assoc.,* 32, 1, January, 1966.
Frame, J. W.: An Emergency Drug Cabinet for Use in General Dental Practice, *Br. Dent. J.,* 132, 363, May 2, 1972.
Gaum, L. I.: Basic Steps in Cardiopulmonary Resuscitation, *J. Can. Dent. Assoc.,* 36, 158, April, 1970.
Glauda, N. M., Henefer E. P., and Super, S.: Nonfatal Anaphylaxis Caused by Oral Penicillin: Report of a Case, *J. Am. Dent. Assoc.,* 90, 159, January, 1975.
Hagen, J.: Oxygen Therapy, Pulse and Blood Pressure Determination, and Parenteral Drug Administration, in McCarthy, F. M.: *Emergencies in Dental Practice,* 2nd ed. Philadelphia, Saunders, 1972, pp. 214–231.
Harrison, J. B.: Faints and Spells, *Dent. Clin. North Am.,* 17, 461, July, 1973.
Hendler, B. H. and Rose, L. F.: Common Medical Emergencies: A Dilemma in Dental Education, *J. Am. Dent. Assoc.,* 91, 575, September, 1975.
Hooley, J. R. and Conn, R. D.: A Simplified Approach to the Treatment of Medical Emergencies in the Dental Office, *J. Am. Dent. Assoc.,* 73, 77, July, 1966.
Jastak, J. T. and Cowan, F. F.: Patients at Risk, *Dent. Clin. North Am.,* 17, 363, July, 1973.
Jones, R. C. and Shires, G. T.: Emergency Room Triage—Preliminary Lifesaving Methods, *J. Oral Surg.,* 27, 461, July, 1969.
Laskin, D. M.: Treatment of Common Emergencies of the Hospital Dental Patient, in Douglas, B. L., ed.: *Introduction to Hospital Dentistry,* 2nd ed. St. Louis, Mosby, 1970, pp. 103–128.
Mitchell, D. F., Standish, S. M., and Fast, T. B.: *Oral Diagnosis/Oral Medicine,* 2nd ed. Philadelphia, Lea & Febiger, 1971, pp. 421–436.
Needleman, H. L. and Berkowitz, R. J.: Electric Trauma to the Oral Tissues of Children, *J. Dent. Child.,* 41, 19, January-February, 1974.

O'Day, R. A. and Driggs, R. L.: Cardiopulmonary Resuscitation in Dental Practice, *Dent. Clin. North Am.*, 17, 329, April, 1973.

Panuska, H. J., Miller, H. D., and Yamane, G. M.: Major Medical Emergencies—Diagnosis and Management. A Manual for Dentists, *Northwest Dent.*, 48, 107, March-April, 1969.

Reeve, L. W.: Hemorrhage, in McCarthy, F. M.: *Emergencies in Dental Practice*, 2nd ed. Philadelphia, Saunders, 1972, pp. 381–409.

Roberts, M. W. and Morrill, G. S.: Medical Emergencies and a Standardized Emergency Kit for the Dental Office, *J. Acad. Gen. Dent.*, 20, 36, September, 1972.

Shira, R. B.: Emergency Treatment of Patients with Facial Trauma, in Douglas, B. L., ed.: *Introduction to Hospital Dentistry*, 2nd ed. St. Louis, Mosby, 1970, pp. 129–144.

Simon, W. J.: *Clinical Dental Assisting*. Hagerstown, Maryland, Harper & Row, 1973, pp. 163–167.

Smith, B. H.: The Unconscious Patient, *J. Oral Surg.*, 27, 709, September, 1969.

Staples, A. F.: Cardiopulmonary Crises in the Dental Office, *Dent. Clin. North Am.*, 17, 473, July, 1973.

Woodworth, J. V.: Recognition and Treatment of Medical Emergencies in the Dental Office, *J. Am. Dent. Assoc.*, 81, 887, October, 1970.

Local Anesthesia Complications

Ash, H. L.: Complications Associated with Office Anesthesia, *Dent. Clin. North Am.*, 17, 315, April, 1973.

Bennett, C. R.: *Monheim's Local Anesthesia and Pain Control in Dental Practice*, 5th ed. St. Louis, Mosby, 1974, pp. 154–196.

Booth, D. F. and Dunn, M. J.: Reactions to Local Anesthetic Agents, in Dunn, M. J., ed.: *Dental Auxiliary Practice*, Module 5. Baltimore, Williams and Wilkins, 1975, pp. 45–50.

Jorgensen, N. B. and Hayden, J.: Complications from Local Analgesia, in McCarthy, F. M.: *Emergencies in Dental Practice*, 2nd ed. Philadelphia, Saunders, 1972, pp. 274–284.

Kramer, H. S. and Mitton, V. A.: Complications of Local Anesthesia, *Dent. Clin. North Am.*, 17, 443, July, 1973.

Waldrep, A. C.: Complications of Local Anesthesia, in Goldman, H. M., Gilmore, H. W., Irby, W. B., and Olsen, N. H.: *Current Therapy in Dentistry*, Volume 5. St. Louis, Mosby, 1974, pp. 437–443.

Prefixes, Suffixes, and Combining Forms

a-, an- absence, lack, without, e.g. *a*morphous
ab- from, away, e.g. *ab*normal
ad- (change d to c,f,g,p,s, or t before words beginning with those consonants) to, toward, e.g. *ad*hesion, *ac*cretion
-algia pain, e.g. neur*algia*
ambi- on both sides, e.g. *ambi*dexterity
ana- up, excessive, again, e.g. *ana*bolism
angio- vessel, e.g. *angi*oma
anti- against, e.g. *anti*dote
aqu-, aqua- water, e.g. *aqu*eous
arthro-, arth- joints, e.g. *arthr*itis
-ase denotes an enzyme, e.g. dextrin*ase*
-asthenia weakness, e.g. my*asthenia* gravis
auto-, aut- self, e.g. *auto*transplant

bi- two, twice, double, e.g. *bi*furcation
bio-, bi- life, living, e.g. *bio*psy
-blast formative cell, e.g. osteo*blast*
brady- slow, e.g. *brady*cardia
bucc- cheek, e.g. *bucc*inator

calc- stone, calcium, lime, e.g. *calc*ification
cardio-, cardi- heart, e.g. *cardio*vascular
cata- down, against, e.g. *cata*bolism
cephalo-, cephal- head, e.g. *cephalo*metry
cerebro-, cerebr- large brain, e.g. *cerebr*al palsy
cheilo-, cheil- lip, e.g. *cheil*itis
chloro-, chlor- pale green, e.g. *chloro*phyll
chromo-, chromat- color, pigmentation, e.g. *chromo*genic
-cidal killing, e.g. bacteri*cidal*
-clast break up, divide into parts, e.g. osteo*clast*

-clus- shut, e.g. oc*clus*ion
co-, com-, con-, cor- with, together, e.g. *con*genital
coll- glue, e.g. *coll*oid
contra- opposite, e.g. *contra*lateral
cryo-, cry- cold, freezing, e.g. *cryo*therapy
cuti- skin, e.g. *cuti*cle
cyan- blue, e.g. *cyan*otic
-cyto-, -cyt- cell, e.g. leuko*cyte*

de- down, away from, separation, e.g. *de*calcification
denti-, dent- tooth, e.g. *dent*ition
-derm-, -derma- skin, e.g. hypo*derm*ic
di- twice, two, e.g. *di*plopia
dia- (drop *a* before words beginning with a vowel) through, apart, e.g. *dia*phragm
dis- separation, opposite, taking apart, e.g. *dis*infect
disto-, dist- posterior, distant from center, e.g. *disto*buccal
-drome course, e.g. syn*drome*
dur- hard, e.g. in*dur*ation
dys- bad, ill, difficult, e.g. *dys*trophy

ecto-, ect- without, outer side, e.g. *ecto*derm
-ectomy surgical removal, e.g. gingiv*ectomy*
-emia (-aemia) blood condition, e.g. bacter*emia*
en- in, on, into, e.g. *en*demic
endo- inside, e.g. *endo*dontics
entero-, enter- intestine, e.g. *entero*toxin
epi- upon, after, in addition, e.g. *epi*dermis
erythro-, eryth- red, e.g. *eryth*ema
ex- beyond, from, out of, e.g. *ex*udate

extra- outside of, beyond the scope of, e.g. *extra*cellular

faci- face, e.g. *faci*al
-ferent carry, bear, e.g. af*ferent*
fibro-, fibr- fibers, fibrous tissue, e.g. *fibro*blast
fract- break, e.g. *fract*ional

galacto-, galact- milk, e.g. *galact*ose
gastro-, gastr- stomach, e.g. *gastr*itis
-gen produced, e.g. glyco*gen*
genio- chin, lower jaw, e.g. *genio*plasty
germ- bud, early growth, e.g. *germ*inal
gero- old age, e.g. *gero*dontics
glosso-, gloss- tongue, e.g. *gloss*itis
gluco-, gluc- glucose, e.g. *gluco*neogenesis
glyco-, glyc- sweet, e.g. *glyc*erin
gnatho-, gnath- jaw, e.g. *gnath*odynamometer
-gnosis knowledge, e.g. prog*nosis*
-gram, -graph write, draw, e.g. radio*graph*ic
gran- grain, particle, e.g. *gran*uloma
gyn-, gyne-, gynec- woman, e.g. *gynec*ology

hemi- half, e.g., *hemi*section
hemo-, (haemo-) blood, e.g. *hemo*rrhage
hepato-, hepat- liver, e.g. *hepat*itis
hetero-, heter- other, different, e.g. *hetero*genous
histo-, hist- tissue, e.g. *histo*logy
homo-, homeo- like, similar, e.g. *homeo*stasis
hydro-, hydr- water, e.g. *hydro*cephalic
hyper- abnormal, excessive, e.g. *hyper*trophy
hypno-, hypn- sleep, e.g. *hypn*otic
hypo-, hyp- deficiency, lack, below, e.g. *hypo*tonic
hystero-, hyster- uterus or hysteria, e.g. *hyster*ectomy

-ia state or condition, e.g. glycosur*ia*
-ic of, pertaining to, e.g. gast*ric*
idio- one's own, separate, distinct, e.g. *idio*pathic
in- not, without, e.g. *in*activate
infra- beneath, below, e.g. *infra*orbital
inter- between, among, e.g. *inter*cellular
intra- within, into, e.g. *intra*oral
ischo-, isch- suppression, stoppage, e.g. *isch*emia
iso- equality, similarity, e.g. *iso*tonic
-ist one who practices, holds certain principles, e.g. hygien*ist*
-itis inflammation, e.g. derma*titis*

-ject- throw, e.g. in*ject*ion
juxta- next to, near, e.g. *juxta*position

karyo-, kary- nucleus of a cell, e.g. *karyo*lysis
kerato-, kerat- horny, keratinized tissue, e.g. *kerat*inization
kin- move, e.g. *kin*etic

labio- lip, e.g. *labio*version
lacto-, lact- milk, e.g. *lact*ation
laryngo-, laryn- larynx, e.g. *laryn*gitis
later- side, e.g. *later*oversion
leuko-, leuk- white, e.g. *leuko*plakia
linguo-, lingu- tongue, e.g. *lingu*al
lipo-, lip- fat, fatty, e.g. *lip*oma
-logy doctrine, science, e.g. periodonto*logy*
lympho-, lymph- lymph, e.g. *lymph*angioma
-lysin, -lysis, -lytic dissolving, destructive, e.g. hemo*lysis*

macro-, macr- enlargement, elongated part, e.g. *macro*dontia
mal- bad, ill, e.g. *mal*nutrition
melano- dark-colored, relating to melanin, e.g. *melano*genesis
meno- month, e.g. *meno*pause
mes-, medi-, mesio- middle, intermediate, e.g. *meso*derm
meta-, met- over, beyond, transformation, e.g. *meta*bolism
metro-, metra- uterus, e.g. *metro*fibroma
metry- measure, e.g. cephalo*metry*
micro-, micr- small, e.g. *micro*organism
mono- one, single, e.g. *mono*saccharide
morpho-, morph- form, shape, e.g. *morph*ology
muco-, muc- relating to mucous membrane, e.g. *muco*gingival
myo-, my- muscle, e.g. *myo*cardium

naso- nose, e.g. *naso*palatine
necr- death, e.g. *necr*otic
neo-, ne- new, recent, e.g. *neo*plasm
nephro-, nephr- kidneys, e.g. *nephr*itis
neuro-, neuri-, neur- pertaining to nerves, e.g. *neur*asthenia
nucleo-, nucle- pertaining to nucleus, e.g. *nucleo*protein

ob- (change b to c before words beginning with c) against, toward, e.g. oc*clusion
odonto-, odont- tooth, e.g. *odont*algia
-oid like, resembling, e.g. ameb*oid*
-oma swelling, tumor, e.g. lip*oma*
-opia, -opy sight, eye defect, e.g. my*opia*
oro- mouth, oral, e.g. *oro*nasal
ortho-, orth- straight, normal, e.g. *ortho*dontics
-osis condition, state, e.g. cyan*osis*
osteo-, oste- bone, e.g. *osteo*porosis

oto-, ot- ear, e.g. *oto*plasty
-ous full of, having, e.g. aque*ous*
ovi-, ovo-, ovu- egg, e.g. *ovu*lation

pan- all, every, general, e.g. *pan*acea
para- beyond, beside, near, e.g. *para*site
patho-, path- disease, e.g. *patho*gnomonic
pedia-, pedo- (paedo-) child, e.g. *pedo*dontics
per- throughout, completely, e.g. *per*cussion
peri- around, near, e.g. *peri*apical
phago- to eat, e.g. *phago*cytic
-phile, -phil loving, e.g. hemo*phil*ia
phlebo-, phleb- vein, e.g. *phleb*itis
-phobe, -phobia fear, dread, e.g. photo*phobia*
-plas- mold, shape, e.g. gingivo*plas*ty
plasmo-, -plasm form, e.g. cyto*plasm*
-plegia, -plexy paralysis, stroke, e.g. hemi-*plegia*
-pnea, (-pnoea) breathing, e.g. dys*pnea*
pneumo- air, lung, e.g. *pneumo*thorax
poly- many, much, e.g. *poly*saccharide
pont- bridge, e.g. *pont*ic
post- behind, after, e.g. *post*natal
pre- before, in front of, e.g. *pre*maxilla
pro- before, in front of, e.g. *pro*gnathic
proprio- one's own, e.g. *proprio*ceptive
proto- first, e.g. *proto*plasm
pseudo- false, deceptive, e.g. *pseudo*membrane
psycho-, psych- mind, mental processes, e.g. *psycho*somatic
pulmo- lung, e.g. *pulmo*nary
pur-, pyo- pus, e.g. *pur*ulent, *pyo*rrhea
pyro- fever, heat, e.g. *pyro*genic

re- back, again, e.g. *re*gurgitate
-renal kidney, e.g. ad*renal*
retro- back, backward, behind, e.g. *retro*molar

-rhage breaking, bursting forth, profuse flow, e.g. hemor*rhage*
-rhea, (-rhoea) flow, discharge, e.g. pyor*rhea*
rhino-, rhin- nose, e.g. *rhin*itis
rube- red, e.g. *rube*lla

sarco- flesh, muscle, e.g. *sarco*ma
-sclero- hard, e.g. *sclero*derma
-scopy examination, inspection, e.g. micros-*copy*
semi- half, e.g. *semi*permeable
sial-, sialo- saliva, e.g. *sial*ography
-some- body, e.g. chromo*some*
-squam- scale, e.g. des*quam*ative
stomat- mouth, e.g. *stomat*itis
sub- beneath, under, deficient, e.g. *sub*acute
super- above, upon, excessive, e.g. *super*numerary tooth
syn- with, together, e.g. *syn*drome

tachy- swift, e.g. *tachy*cardia
tact- touch, e.g. *tact*ile
thermo- heat, e.g. *thermo*phile
thrombo-, thromb- clot, coagulation, e.g. *thromb*in
trans- beyond, through, across, e.g. *trans*plantation
tropho-, -trophic, nutrition, nourishment, e.g. hyper*trophic*
-tropic turning toward, changing, e.g. hydro*tropic*

-ule diminutive, small, e.g. tub*ule*
-uria urine, e.g. glucos*uria*

vaso- blood vessels, e.g. *vaso*dilation
vita- life, e.g. *vita*min

xero- dry, e.g. *xero*stomia

Glossary

This brief glossary includes primarily the words which have been used but not defined in the text. Those defined in the text may be located through the Index. The meaning of words from the basic medical and dental sciences frequently can be determined from the list of word prefixes, suffixes, and combining forms of the previous pages. A medical dictionary should be an important adjunct to guide professional reading.

A.

Abscess: a localized collection of pus in a cavity formed by the disintegration of tissues.

Absorption: taking up of fluids or other substances by the skin or mucous surfaces; passage of substances to the blood, lymph, and cells from the alimentary canal after digestion.

Abutment: a tooth used for the support or retention of a fixed or removable prosthesis.

Accessory: subordinate, attached, or added for convenience.

Acid: a chemical substance which in aqueous solution undergoes dissociation with the formation of hydrogen ions; pH less than 7.0.

Acidogenic: acid-forming or producing.

Acne vulgaris: a chronic inflammatory disease of the sebaceous glands which appears on the face, back, and chest in the form of eruptions.

Acquired characteristics: those obtained after birth, as a result of environment.

Acuity: sharpness or clearness, especially of the vision.

Acute: having rapid onset, short, severe course, and pronounced symptoms; opposite of chronic.

Adsorption: a process believed to be physical in nature in which molecules of a gas or liquid condense or adhere on the surface of another substance.

Aerobe: a microorganism that requires free oxygen to exist.

Agar: gelatin extracted from seaweed used as a nutrient solidifying agent in bacteriologic culture media; constituent of a reversible hydrocolloid impression material.

Agglutination: state of being united; adhesion of parts; clumping, as bacteria or other cells.

Alkali: a strong water-soluble base; see **Base.**

Allergen: an antigenic substance that produces hypersensitivity which may be inhaled, ingested, or injected, or may produce a reaction upon contact with the skin.

Allergy: a hypersensitive state gained from exposure to a specific substance, re-exposure causes an altered capacity to react.

Alloy: a substance composed of two or more metals fused or melted together.

Amalgam: an alloy of two or more metals, one of which is mercury.

Dental amalgam: an alloy of silver, tin, copper, zinc, and mercury, used for dental restorations.

Ameloblast: epithelial cell of the enamel organ which functions in the formation of enamel.

Amorphous: lacking specific form or shape; unorganized.

Ampere: unit of quantity of electric current.

Amylase: an enzyme which converts starch into sugar.

Anaerobe: a microorganism that requires complete, or almost complete, absence of free oxygen to exist.

  Facultative anaerobe: microorganism that can exist under either aerobic or anaerobic conditions.

  Obligative anaerobe: microorganism that can exist only in the complete absence of free oxygen because oxygen is toxic to it.

Analgesia: absence of sensibility to pain; loss of sensibility to pain without loss of consciousness; first stage of general anesthesia.

Anaphylaxis: an acute, severe, allergic reaction characterized by sudden collapse, shock, or respiratory and circulatory failure following the injection of an allergen; increased susceptibility to an allergen resulting from previous exposure to it.

Anemia, nutritional: deficiency anemia; caused by some deficiency or fault in the diet or in nutrition.

Anesthesia: loss of feeling or sensation.

  General anesthesia: an irregular, reversible depression of the cells of higher centers of the central nervous system that makes the patient unconscious and insensible to pain.

  Local anesthesia: loss of sensibility to pain in a specific area, not accompanied by loss of consciousness.

  Topical anesthesia: a form of local anesthesia whereby free nerve endings in accessible structures are rendered incapable of stimulation by application of an anesthetic drug directly to the surface of the area.

Aneurysm: dilatation of an artery in which one or more layers of the vessel walls are distended.

Anhydrous: containing no water.

Ankylosis: union or consolidation of two similar or dissimilar hard tissues previously adjacent but not attached, as a tooth and its surrounding bone.

Anodontia: congenital absence of teeth; failure of teeth to form; may be partial or complete.

Anodyne: any agent which neutralizes or relieves pain.

Anomaly: deviation from the normal.

Anoxia: oxygen deficiency; a condition in which the cells of the body do not have or cannot utilize sufficient oxygen to perform normal function.

Antibiotic: a chemical substance produced by microorganisms which, in dilute solutions, can destroy or inhibit the growth of bacteria and other microorganisms; used in the treatment of infectious diseases of man, animals, and plants.

Antidote: a medicine or other remedy for counteracting the effects of poison.

Antiseptic: a substance that will inhibit the growth and development of microorganisms without necessarily destroying them; term is applied to human tissue.

Apatite: inorganic compound with a complex formula containing calcium and phosphate; makes up the inorganic portion of bones and teeth.

  Fluorapatite, containing fluoride radical.

  Hydroxyapatite, containing hydroxyl radical.

Aphasia: defect of loss of the power of expression by speech, writing, or signs, or of comprehending spoken or written language, due to injury or disease of the brain centers.

Aphtha: a little ulcer.

Aphthous ulcer: aphthous stomatitis; canker sore, vesicle which ruptures after one or two days and forms a depressed, spherical, painful ulcer with elevated rim.

Aqueous: watery; prepared with water.

Armamentarium: the equipment, such as books, medicines, and instruments, with which a practitioner supplies himself.

  Dental hygiene armamentarium: all the instruments and equipment used during a dental hygiene procedure.

  Dental hygiene instrumentarium: set of instruments used for a particular operation by the dental hygienist.

Articulation: the place where two or more bones of the skeleton join or unite; bony joint which may or may not be movable.

Artifact: in radiography, a substance or structure not naturally present in living tissues, but of which an authentic image appears in a radiograph; a blemish or an unintended radiographic image which is not an authentic appearance, such as may result from the faulty manufacture, manipulation, exposure, or processing of an x-ray film.

Asepsis: condition in which septic, infective, putrefactive material is absent; exclusion of microorganisms.

Asphyxia: suffocation or a temporary state of lifelessness as a result of cessation of breathing.

Aspirator: an apparatus employing suction.

Astringent: a substance which causes contraction or shrinkage and arrests discharges.

Atom: the smallest particle of an element which is capable of entering into a chemical reaction.

Atrophy: a defect or failure of nutrition manifested as a wasting or gradual reduction in the size of a cell, tissue, or organ; usually applied to wasting that is secondary to some known cause.

Attenuation: reducing, thinning, or weakening; reduction of the virulence of a virus or pathogenic microorganism as by successive culture or repeated inoculation in radiography, the process by which a beam of radiation is reduced in energy when passing through some material.

Attrition: gradual wearing away of tooth structure resulting from mastication.

Autism: the condition of being dominated by subjective, self-centered trends of thought or behavior; tendency to morbid concentration on oneself.

Autoclave: an apparatus for effecting sterilization by high temperature obtained from steam under pressure.

Autograft: an autologous graft in which the tissue is obtained from the same individual.

Autonomic (involuntary) nervous system: division of the nervous system which supplies the sensory innervation for the smooth muscles, heart, and glands. It is divided into the parasympathetic (craniosacral) and the sympathetic (thoracolumbar) systems.

Auxiliary: giving support; helping; aiding; assisting.

B.

Backscatter: radiation deflected by scattering processes at angles greater than 90 degrees to the original direction of the beam of radiation.

Bacteremia: presence of bacteria in the blood stream. It may be transient, intermittent, or continuous.

Bacterial spore: a resistant form of bacteria encapsulated by a thick cell wall which enables the cell to survive in environments unfavorable to immediate growth and division; not a reproductive mechanism.

Bactericidal: capable of destroying bacteria.

Bacteriostatic: capable of inhibiting the growth and multiplication of bacteria.

Barodontalgia (Aerodontalgia): the sudden acute pain response in a tooth under reduced barometric pressure, notably during space flight.

Base: a chemical substance that in solution yields hydroxyl ions and reacts with an acid to form a salt and water. A base turns red litmus paper blue and has a pH higher than 7.0.

Bevel: the inclination one line or surface makes with another when they are not at right angles.

Bifid: cleft into two parts or branches.

Biopsy: the removal and examination, usually microscopic, of a section of tissue or other material from the living body for the purpose of diagnosis.

Bite-wing radiographic survey: dental radiographs which show the coronal portions of maxillary and mandibular teeth, used for detecting deviations in the structure or form of the proximal surfaces of teeth or interdental bone.

Body mechanics: proper balance of the skeleton by muscular alignment which favors function with the least amount of expended energy; refers to a dynamic position as opposed to **posture** which is alignment in a rigid position.

Bruxism: the clenching and/or grinding of the teeth when the patient is not masticating or swallowing.

Buffer: any substance in a fluid which tends to lessen the change in hydrogen ion concentration (reaction) which otherwise would be produced by adding acids or alkalis.

Burnish: to make smooth and bright; to polish by friction.

C.

Calcification: the process by which organic tissue becomes hardened by a deposit of calcium and other inorganic salts within its substance.

Cancer: malignant and invasive neoplasm.

Canker sore: see **Aphthous ulcer.**

Carbohydrate: organic compound of carbon, hydrogen, and oxygen: includes starches, sugars, cellulose; formed by plants and used for growth and source of energy.

Carcinoma: a malignant neoplasm of epithelial origin.

Caries: see **Dental caries.**

Cariogenic: caries producing; conducive to caries.

Carious: affected with caries or decay; in dentistry, a carious lesion is a cavity in a tooth which is the result of dental caries.

Carrier: an infected person who harbors a specific infectious agent in the absence of discernible clinical disease and serves as a potential source of infection for man.

Cartilage: firm, elastic, flexible connective tissue which is attached to articular bone surfaces and which forms certain parts of the skeleton.

Cassette: light-tight container in which x-ray films are placed for exposure to x radiation; usually backed with lead to eliminate the effect of backscatter radiation.

Cataract: a clouding or opacity of the lens of the eye which leads to blurring of vision and eventual loss of sight.

Caustic: an agent which burns or corrodes; destroys living tissue; having a burning taste.

Cauterize: to burn, corrode, or destroy living tissue by means of a caustic substance, heated metal, or an electric current.

Central ray: a hypothetical x ray whose direction of travel corresponds to the geometric center of a useful beam of x radiation.

Cephalometer: an orienting device for positioning the head for radiographic examination and measurement.

Cephalometrics: scientific study of the measurements of the head.

Cephalometry: measurement of the bony structure of the head using reproducible lateral and anteroposterior radiographs.

Cheilosis: a condition marked by fissuring and dry scaling of the surface of the lips and angles of the mouth; characteristic of riboflavin deficiency.

Chronic: characterized by a long slow course as compared with acute.

Clean: freedom from or removal of all matter in which microorganisms may find favorable conditions for continued life and growth.

Clinic: an establishment where patients are admitted for study and treatment by a group of practitioners.

Clinical: pertaining to a clinic or to the actual observation and treatment of patients, as distinguished from theoretical or experimental.

Coagulation: changing of a soluble into an insoluble protein; process of changing into a clot.

Coaptation: proper adaptation or union of parts to each other, such as the ends of a fractured bone or the edges of a wound.

Col: concavity of the interdental gingiva; ridge-shaped depression between two peaks formed by the buccal and lingual papillae.

Communicable: capable of being transmitted from one person to another.

Compatible: capable of existing together in harmony; with medications, suitable for simultaneous administration.

Conduction: the transfer of sound waves, heat, nerve influences, or electricity.

Cone: an accessory device on a dental x-ray machine designed to indicate the direction of the central axis of its x-ray beam and to serve as a guide in establishing a desired source-to-film distance. Such "cones" may be conical or cylindrical in form; provision for beam collimation and/or added filtration may be incorporated in the construction of the "cone."

Congenital: existing at or before birth.

Contaminate: to render impure by contact or mixture; in sterile technique, to introduce microorganisms.

Contracture: shortening or distortion; permanent as from shrinkage of muscles, or temporary from sudden stimulus.

Convalescence: the gradual recovery of health and strength after illness.

Corrode: to eat away or wear away, as by rust, causing deterioration of a substance.

Crepitation: a crackling sound; noise made by rubbing together the ends of a broken bone.

Cryosurgery: surgery performed with the use of decreased temperature.

Cryotherapy: therapeutic application of cold.

Cryptogenic: of obscure, doubtful, or undeterminable origin.

Curet (Fr. curette): spoon-shaped instrument with its peripheral edges sharpened to facilitate removal of material.

Curettage: planned and systematic operation to remove the chronically inflamed, degenerated, and necrotic tissue lining the gingival wall of a periodontal pocket.

Current: the number of electrons per second passing a given point on a conductor. Electrons are negatively charged and move toward the positive.

Cuticle, primary: a delicate membrane covering the crown of a newly erupted tooth; produced by the ameloblasts after they produce the enamel rods. Also called Nasmyth's membrane.

Cyanosis: blueness of the skin often due to insufficient oxygenation of the blood.

Cyst: a sac, normal or pathologic, containing fluid or other material.

　Dentigerous cyst: formed by a dental follicle, containing one or more well-formed teeth.

　Radicular cyst: an epithelial-lined sac, formed at the apex of a pulpless tooth, containing cystic fluid.

D.

Debridement: removal of debris, foreign material, or devitalized tissue.

Decalcification: process by which calcium salts and other inorganic substances are removed.

Deglutition: the act of swallowing.

Dehiscence: isolated area in which a root is denuded of bone when the denuded area extends to the margin of the bone. Compare with **Fenestration.**

Dehydration: removal of water; the condition which results from undue loss of water.

Dental caries: a disease of the calcified structures of the teeth, characterized by decalcification of the mineral components and dissolution of the organic matrix.

Dental public health: see under **Public health.**

Denticle: a pulp stone; relatively large body of calcified substance in the pulp chamber of a tooth.

Dentition: the kind, size, and arrangement of the teeth.

Mixed dentition: combination of both primary and permanent teeth present in the oral cavity; state occurs when the first permanent molars erupt and extends until the last primary tooth is exfoliated.

Permanent dentition: the natural teeth which must function throughout the adult life.

Primary (deciduous) dentition: the first teeth; normally will be shed and replaced by permanent teeth.

Succedaneous dentition: permanent teeth that erupt in positions of exfoliated primary teeth.

Denture: an artificial substitute for missing natural teeth and adjacent tissues.

Complete denture: a dental prosthesis which is a substitute for the lost natural dentition and associated structures.

Fixed partial denture (bridge): a restoration of one or more missing teeth which cannot readily be removed by the patient or the dentist; it is permanently attached to natural teeth or roots which furnish the primary support of the appliance.

Removable partial denture: a dental prosthesis which supplies teeth and associated structures in a partially edentulous mouth and which can be removed and replaced at will.

Denudation: laying bare; surgical or pathological removal of epithelial covering.

Desensitization: process of removing the reactivity or sensitivity.

Desquamation: shedding or casting off, as of the superficial epithelium of mucous membrane or skin; a normal physiologic process.

Detergent: agent which cleanses.

Detritus: debris which adheres to tooth surfaces.

Devitalize: to deprive of vitality or of life; in dentistry, to destroy the vitality of the dental pulp.

Diagnosis: a scientific evaluation of existing conditions; the process of determining by examination the nature and circumstances of a diseased condition; the decision reached as to the nature of a disease.

Differential diagnosis: the art of distinguishing one disease from another.

Diastema: a space or cleft; in dentistry, a space between teeth.

Diet: the customary allowance of food and drink taken by a person from day to day.

Bland diet: meal plan in which all food that can cause chemical, mechanical, or thermal irritation is avoided.

Dietary: a regular or systematic scheme of diet.

Digital: of, pertaining to, or performed with a finger.

Dilate: to make wider or larger; cause to expand.

Dislocation: see **Luxation.**

Distilled water: water which has been subjected to a process of vaporization and subsequent condensation for purification.

Distortion: (radiographic) deviation of a radiographic image from the true outline or shape of an object or structure.

Donor site: area from which tissue is obtained for a graft.

Dorsum: the back surface or a part similar to the back in position.

Duct: a passage with well-defined walls; especially a tube for the passage of excretions or secretions.

Dyslexia: impairment in the ability to read.

Dysplasia: abnormal development or growth; an alteration in adult cells characterized by variation in their size, shape, and organization.

Dyspnea: difficult or labored breathing.

Dystrophy: defective or faulty nutrition within a tissue or organ manifested by wasting and atrophy.

E.

Ecchymosis: black and blue discoloration of the skin caused by the escape of blood from the vessels into the tissues; bleeding into the subcutaneous tissues.

Ecology: the science which deals with the study of the environment and the life history of organisms.

Ectopic: out of place. An **ectopic pregnancy** is one that occurs elsewhere than in the cavity of the uterus.

Edema: collection of abnormally large amounts of fluid in the intercellular spaces, causing swelling.

Pitting edema: pressure on edematous area causes pits which remain for prolonged period after pressure is released.

Edentulous: without teeth.

Emaciation: condition of excessive leanness or wasted body tissues.

Embolism: sudden blocking of an artery or vein by a clot or obstruction which has been brought to its place by the blood current.

Embryo: the fetus in its earlier stages of development, especially before the end of the second month.

Emesis basin: a basin, usually kidney shaped, used for receiving material expectorated or vomited.

Emollient: softening or soothing; an agent used to soften the skin or other body surface.

Endemic: present in a community or among a group of people; the continuing prevalence of a disease as distinguished from an epidemic.

Endocardium: the endothelial lining membrane of the heart.

Endodontics: that branch of dentistry concerned with the etiology, diagnosis, and treatment of diseases of the dental pulp and their sequelae.

Endometrium: the mucous membrane lining the uterus.

Enzyme: an organic compound, frequently protein in nature, which can accelerate or produce by catalytic action some change in a specific substance.

Ephebodontics: dentistry for the individual undergoing the transition from childhood to adulthood, that is, the period of life known as adolescence.

Epidemic: the occurrence in a community or region of a group of illnesses of similar nature, clearly in excess of normal expectancy and derived from a common source.

Epithelization: growth of epithelium over a raw surface.

Epithelize, epithelialize: to cover or become covered with epithelium.

Erosion: progressive loss of tooth structure by a chemical process without the aid of bacteria which appears as a sharply defined wedge-shaped depression in the cervical area of a tooth: area is smooth, hard, and polished.

Eruption: the act of breaking out, appearing or becoming visible; a visible pathological lesion of the skin, marked by redness, swelling, or both.

Tooth eruption: the combination of movements of a tooth both before and after the emergence of its crown into the oral cavity which serves to bring it and maintain it in occlusion with the tooth or teeth of the opposing arch.

Erythema: abnormal redness of the skin due to local congestion; may result from inflammation or excess exposure to x ray.

Erythrocyte: red blood corpuscle, specialized cell for the transportation of oxygen.

Escharotic: corrosive; capable of producing sloughing.

Ethics: the science of right conduct; a system of rules or principles governing the conduct of a professional group planned by them for the common good of man; the principles of morality.

Etiology: the science or study of the cause of disease; that which is known about the causes of a disease.

Euphoria: well-being; absence of pain or distress; in psychiatry, an abnormal or exaggerated sense of well-being.

Exfoliate: to fall off in scales or layers; in dentistry, to shed primary teeth.

Exodontics: that branch of dentistry concerned with the extraction of teeth.

Exostosis: a bony outgrowth from the surface of bone.

Extirpation: complete removal or eradication of a part; in dentistry, the removal of the dental pulp from the pulp chamber and root canal.

Exudate: the material composed of serum, fibrin, and white blood cells in variable amounts that escapes from blood vessels into a superficial lesion of an area of inflammation.

F.

Febrile: pertaining to fever; feverish.

Fenestration: isolated area in which a root is denuded of bone when the marginal bone is intact. Compare with **Dehiscence.**

Fermentable: term applied to a substance which is capable of undergoing chemical change as a result of the influence of an enzyme; usually applied to substances which break down to an acid or an alcohol; applied to carbohydrate breakdown to form acid in the dental plaque.

Fetus: the unborn offspring in the uterus after the second month.

Film badge: a pack containing a radiographic film or films to be used for the detection and measurement of radiation exposure in personnel monitoring.

Fistula: a narrow passage or duct leading from one cavity to another, as from a periapical abscess to the oral cavity.

Flora: the entire plant life of a geographic area; used to indicate the microorganisms which live together in a specific location.

Oral flora: the microorganisms which inhabit the oral cavity of an individual, usually saprophytic, and which live together in a symbiotic relationship.

Fluorescence: emission of radiation of a particular wave length by certain substances as the result of absorption of radiation of shorter wave length. The emission occurs only during the irradiation as contrasted to phosphorescence.

Fluoridization: application of fluoride solution to the teeth; compare with fluoridation in which the fluoride content of the community water supply is adjusted (page 424).

Fluoroscope: a fluorescent screen suitably mounted with respect to an x-ray tube for ease of observation and protection, used for the indirect visualization by means of x rays of internal structures in living organisms or inanimate objects.

Fog: darkening of the whole or part of a developed radiograph from sources other than the radiation of the primary beam to which the film was exposed.

Chemical fog: darkening due to imbalance or deterioration of processing solutions.

Light fog: darkening due to unintentional exposure to light to which the emulsion is sensitive, either before or during the processing.

Radiation fog: darkening due to radiation from sources other than intentional exposure to the primary beam, for example, scatter radiation, or film storage not protected from radiation.

Follicle (dental): the sac that encloses the developing tooth before its eruption.

Forceps: a two-bladed instrument with handles for pulling, compressing, or grasping.

Frenectomy: complete removal of a frenum.

Frenotomy: partial removal of a frenum.

Frenum: a narrow fold of mucous membrane passing from a more fixed to a movable part, as from the gingiva to the lip, cheek, or undersurface of the tongue, serving in a measure to check undue movement of the part.

Friable: easily broken or crumbled.

Furcation: area or region lying between and at the base of two or more normal anatomically divided roots.

G.

Germicide: anything that destroys bacteria; applied especially to chemical agents that kill disease germs, but not necessarily bacterial spores: applied to both living tissue and inanimate objects.

Gerodontics: that branch of dentistry which treats all problems peculiar to the oral cavity in old age and aging including clinical problems of senescence and senility.

Gingivectomy: the surgical removal of diseased gingiva to eliminate periodontal pockets.

Gingivoplasty: the surgical contouring of the gingival tissue to produce the physiologic architectural form necessary for the maintenance of tissue health and integrity.

Glaucoma: a disease of the eye marked by intense intraocular pressure, which can result in hardness of the eye, atrophy of the retina, cupping of the optic disk, and blindness.

Glossitis: inflammation of the tongue.

Gnathodynamometer: an instrument for measuring the force exerted in closing the jaws.

Graft: tissues transferred from one site to replace damaged structures in another site.

Free graft: tissue for grafting is completely removed from its donor site.

Pedicle graft: the graft remains attached to its donor site. See also **Autograft; Heterograft; Homograft.**

Grit: the size of abrasive particles determined by the number of particles which, end to end, equal one inch; fine, stony, hard particles used for grinding.

H.

Habilitation: application of measures which will assist a person in obtaining a state of health, efficiency, and independent action; make over in an improved form.

Half value layer (HVL): the thickness, or surface density, of a layer of a specified material which attenuates the beam to such an extent that the exposure rate is reduced to one-half, under narrow beam conditions.

Halitosis: offensive or bad breath, may be related to systemic disease or uncleanliness of the oral cavity.

Health: state of complete physical, mental, and social well-being, not merely the absence of disease.

Hemangioma: a benign tumor composed of newly formed blood capillaries filled with blood.

Hematoma: a blood clot formed from blood which has been released by trauma or pathology and which accumulates within a tissue.

Hemoglobin: the protein coloring matter of the red blood cells; conveys oxygen to the tissues; occurs as oxyhemoglobin in arterial blood and reduced hemoglobin in venous blood.

Hemorrhage: bleeding; an escape of blood from the blood vessels.

Hemostat: an instrument or other agent used to arrest the escape or flow of blood.

Hepatitis: inflammation of the liver.
  Infectious hepatitis: caused by a virus transmitted by fecal contamination.
  Serum hepatitis: caused by a virus transmitted by human blood.

Heredity: the inheritance of resemblance, physical qualities, or diseases from a familial predecessor; the passage of characteristics from one generation to its progeny by genetic linkage.

Heterograft: a heterologous graft in which the tissue is obtained from another species.

Homeostasis: the state of equilibrium in the living body with respect to various functions and to the chemical compositions of the fluids and tissues.

Homograft: a homologous graft in which the tissue is obtained from a different individual of the same species.

Hone: a fine grit stone used for sharpening a cutting instrument (noun); to sharpen (verb).

Hydrogen peroxide: clear, colorless liquid which is a strong oxidizing and bleaching agent.

Hygiene: the science which deals with the preservation of health.

Hyperkeratosis: abnormal increase in the thickness of the keratin layer (stratum corneum) of the epithelium. **Benign hyperkeratosis** is one of the most common white lesions of the oral mucous membrane.

Hyperplasia: increase in size of a tissue or organ caused by the increase in number of cells in normal arrangement.

Hypertension: Pathologic elevation of the blood pressure.

Hypertonic: having excessive tone, tonicity, or activity.
  Hypertonic solution: one which has a higher molecular concentration than another to which it is compared; of greater concentration than isotonic.

Hypertrophy: increase in size of a tissue or organ caused by the increase in size of its cells.

Hypnotic: inducing sleep.

Hypocalcification: deficiency in the mineral content of the enamel resulting from disturbance in the maturation phase during development; may be due to systemic, local, or hereditary factors; dental fluorosis is an example of a systemic cause.

Hypoplasia: defective or incomplete development; enamel hypoplasia results when the enamel matrix formation is disturbed.

Hypotonic: having diminished tone, tonicity, or activity.
  Hypotonic solution: one which has a lesser molecular concentration than another to which it is compared; of less concentration than isotonic.

I.

Iatrogenic: caused by inadvertent or erroneous diagnosis and/or treatment by a professional.

Idiopathic: self-originated; of unknown cause.

Idiosyncrasy: any tendency, characteristic, or the like, peculiar to an individual.

Immunity: an inherited, congenital, or naturally or artificially acquired ability to resist the occurrence and effects of a specific disease.
  Acquired immunity: that possessed as a result of having and recovering from a disease or from building up resistance against vaccines, toxins, or toxoids.
  Natural immunity: that inherited by the child from the mother or from the race.
  Passive immunity: that possessed as a result of injection of antibodies or antitoxins in serum from an immune individual or lower animal.

Implant: a material from any source which is grafted or inserted within body tissues.

Implantation: the placement within body tissues of a foreign substance, for example metal or plastic, for restoration by mechanical means. In dentistry, a foreign material placed into or onto the jawbone to support a crown, partial, or complete denture.

Incipient: beginning to exist; coming into existence.

Incubation: the keeping of a microbial or tissue culture in an incubator to facilitate development.

Incubation period: used to denote the time between exposure to a communicable disease and the appearance of clinical symptoms.

Inert: without intrinsic active properties; no inherent power of action, motion, or resistance.

Infarct: a circumscribed portion of tissue which has suddenly been deprived of its blood supply by embolism or thrombosis and which results in necrosis of the tissue.

Infection: invasion of the body by pathogenic microorganisms and the body's response to the microorganisms and their toxic products; transfer of disease from one part to another or one person to another.

Inflammation: reaction of living tissue to injury; a defense reaction of the body characterized by heat, redness, swelling, pain, and loss of function.

Inhibitor: a chemical substance which arrests or restrains the action of a tissue organizer or the growth of microorganisms.

Inoculation: introduction of microorganisms or some substance into living tissues or culture media; introduction of a disease agent into a healthy individual to induce immunity.

Inorganic: not characterized by organization of living bodies or vital processes; also, pertaining to compounds not containing carbon, except cyanides and carbonates.

Insidious: coming on gradually or almost imperceptibly, as a disease the onset of which is gradual with a more serious effect than is apparent.

Intensifying screen: a card or plastic sheet coated with fluorescent material, positioned in a cassette to contact the film in radiography, so that the visible light from its fluorescent image, when exposed to radiation, will add to the latent image being produced directly by radiation, on a film sensitive to both visible light and x rays.

In vitro: outside the living body: in a test tube or other artificial environment.

In vivo: in the living body of a plant or animal.

Ion: an electrically charged atom or group of atoms.

Anion: negatively charged ion which passes to the positive pole in electrolysis.

Cation: positively charged ion which passes to the negative pole in electrolysis.

I.Q.: Intelligence Quotient; the relationship between intelligence and chronological age.

Irrigation: the covering or washing out of anything with water or other liquid for the purpose of making it moist, diluting another substance present, or cleaning the area.

Ischemia: local decrease in the blood supply to tissues due to obstruction of inflow of arterial blood.

Isotonic: having a uniform tonicity or tension.

Isotonic solution: one which has the same molecular concentration as another to which it is compared.

J.

Jaundice: condition in which there are bile pigments in the blood and deposition of bile pigments in the skin and mucous membranes with resulting yellowish appearance.

Jurisprudence: the science of law, its interpretation and application.

K.

Kaolin: a fine white clay; used in pharmacy in ointments and for coating pills.

Keratin: a protein material formed as a transformation product of the cellular proteins of the flat cells on the surface of the epithelium; form of protective adaptation to function.

Keratinization: process of formation of a horny protective layer on the surface of stratified squamous epithelium of certain body surfaces including the epidermis and masticatory oral mucosa.

Kilovoltage: in x-ray machines, the potential difference between the anode and cathode of an x-ray tube.

L.

Laceration: a wound produced by tearing or irregular cutting.

Latent: concealed, not apparent, potential.

Lesion: an alteration of structure or of functional capacity due to injury or disease.

Lethargy: condition of drowsiness or sleepiness.

Leukocyte: white blood corpuscle; a formed element of the blood consisting of a colorless, granular mass of protoplasm, having ameboid movements and involved in the destruction of disease-producing microorganisms.

Leukoplakia: white plaque formed upon the oral mucous membrane from surface epithelial cells; potentially a premalignant surface lesion characterized by hyperkeratosis of the stratified squamous epithelium.

Local: restricted to one spot; not generalized.

Luxation: a dislocation. For example, dislocation of the temporomandibular joint occurs when the head of the condyle moves anteriorly over the articular eminence and cannot be returned voluntarily.

M.

Macroglossia: enlargement of the tongue.

Malaise: any vague feeling of illness, uneasiness, or discomfort.

Malignant: as applied to tumors, rapidly growing, infiltrate into normal structures, metastasize, and if untreated invariably lead to death.

Malnutrition: a condition of the body resulting from an inadequate supply or impaired utilization of one or more food constituents.

Mandrel: a spindle, axle, or shaft designed to fit a dental handpiece for the purpose of supporting a revolving instrument.

Manifestation: that which is made evident, especially to the sight and understanding.

Oral manifestation: a symptom or sign of a disease.

Manikin: model of the human body or a part; used for teaching purposes.

Massage: manipulation of tissues for remedial or hygienic purposes with the hand or other instrument; the systematic application of frictional rubbing and stroking to the gingival tissues for cleansing purposes, for increasing the circulation of blood through the tissues, and for increasing the keratinization of the surface epithelium.

Mastication: a series of highly coordinated functions which involve the teeth, tongue, muscles of mastication, lips, cheeks, and saliva, in the preparation of food for swallowing and digestion.

Matrix: the form or substance within which something originates, takes form, or develops; intercellular substance of a tissue.

Amalgam matrix: a thin metal form, usually stainless steel, adapted to a prepared cavity to supply the missing wall so the amalgam will be confined when condensed into the cavity preparation.

Maxillofacial: pertaining to the jaws and the face.

Maxillofacial prosthetics: the art and science of anatomic, functional, and cosmetic reconstruction, utilizing nonliving substitutes, of those regions in the maxillae, mandible, and face that are missing or defective.

Medication: use of medicine or medicaments for treatment of a disease.

Metabolism: the sum total of the chemical changes occurring in the body; chemical process of transforming foods into complex tissue elements and of transforming complex body substances into simple ones, along with the production of heat and energy.

Anabolism: the building up of tissue; maintenance and repair of the body.

Catabolism: the breaking down of tissue into simpler constituents for energy production and excretion.

Micron: unit of linear measurement; one-thousandth of a millimeter.

Milliliter: one-thousandth part of a liter, usually abbreviated **ml.** It is approximately equal to one cubic centimeter.

Miscible: capable of being mixed.

Morphology: the science which deals with form and structure without regard to function.

Mucin: secretion of the mucous or goblet cell; a polysaccharide protein which, combined with water, forms a lubricating solution called mucus; contained in saliva.

Myocardium: heart muscle; muscular substance of the heart.

N.

Nasmyth's membrane: see **Cuticle, primary.**

Necrosis: cell or tissue death within the living body.

Necrotizing ulcerative gingivitis: an acute, inflammatory, painful process with ulceration of the interdental papillae; the tissues bleed easily, a pseudomembrane may be present, and an offensive mouth odor is usually associated with the necrosis.

Neoplasm: a new growth comprised of an abnormal collection of cells, the growth of which exceeds and is uncoordinated with that of the normal tissues. See **Cancer** and **Malignant.**

Nidus: the point of origin or focus of a process.

Nostrum: a quack, patent, or secret remedy.

Nutrition: sum of processes by which an animal or plant absorbs, or takes in and utilizes, food substances; ingestion, digestion, absorption (of products of digestion) of food materials through mucous membranes of the alimentary tract, transportation by blood and lymph to body cells where they are used or stored.

O.

Obese: excessively fat.

Obstetrician: a physician who specializes in the management of pregnancy, labor, and the period of confinement after delivery.

Obtundent: having the power to dull sensibility or soothe pain; a soothing or partially anesthetic medicine.

Odontalgia: toothache; pain in a tooth.

Odontoblast: connective tissue cell which functions in the formation of dentin.

Olfactory: pertaining to the sense of smell.

Oncology: study or science of neoplastic growth.

Ophthalmologist: physician with specialized training and experience who specializes in the diagnosis and treatment of eye diseases; one versed in **ophthalmology,** the sum of knowledge concerning the eye and its diseases. (Obsolete term: oculist.)

Optician: technician who grinds and fits lenses; a maker of optical instruments or glasses.

Optometrist: one who practices **optometry,** the measurement of visual acuity and the fitting of glasses to correct visual defects; a term adopted by opticians who prescribe and fit glasses.

Oral surgery: that part of dental practice which deals with the diagnosis and surgical and adjunctive treatment of the diseases, injuries, and defects of the human jaws and associated structures.

Orthodontics: the clinical science that has for its objective the prevention and correction of dental and oral anomalies; that branch of dentistry concerned with the etiology, diagnosis, prevention, and correction of malocclusion of the teeth and associated dentofacial disharmonies.

Osmosis: the passage of a solvent through a semipermeable membrane into a solution of higher molecular concentration thus equalizing the concentrations on either side of the membrane.

Osteoblast: cell whose activity initiates the formation of new bone.

Osteoclast: large multinucleated cell which brings about the resorption of bone; found only during the process of active bone or root resorption.

Osteoectomy, ostectomy: removal of tooth-supporting bone for correction of pockets and nonphysiologic bony contours.

Osteomyelitis: acute or chronic inflammation of the bone marrow or of the bone and marrow.

Osteoplasty: reshaping of bone; plastic contouring of the alveolar process to achieve physiologic contours in the bone and gingival tissues.

Osteoporosis: abnormal decrease in density of bone by the enlargement of its canals or the formation of abnormal spaces.

Otolaryngologist: medical specialist who treats the ears, throat, pharynx, larynx, nasopharynx, and tracheobronchial tree.

P.

Palliative: affording relief but not cure.

Pallor: paleness.

Palpitation: rapid beating of the heart.

Parasympathetic nervous system: craniosacral division of the autonomic nervous system; composed of the ocular, bulbar, and sacral divisions.

Parenteral: route of administration other than by the alimentary canal, that is, by intravenous, intramuscular, or subcutaneous means.

Pathogenesis: the course of development of disease, including the sequence of processes or events from inception to the characteristic lesion or disease.

Pathogenic: causing disease: disease-producing.

Pathognomonic: a sign or symptom significantly unique to a disease to distinguish the disease from other diseases.

Pedodontics: that branch of dentistry concerned with the etiology, diagnosis, and treatment of oral diseases of children.

Periapical: around the apex of a tooth.

   Periapical tissues: the tissues surrounding the apex of a tooth, including the periodontal ligament (membrane), and the alveolar bone.

Pericardium: the membranous sac which contains the heart.

Pericoronitis: inflammation of the soft tissues surrounding the crown of an erupting tooth; frequently seen in association with erupting mandibular third molars and usually accompanied by infection.

Periodontal care: for the patient with periodontal disease: consists of effective treatment for the elimination of disease and the creation of conditions conducive to the maintenance of periodontal health.

   Periodontal care, maintenance phase: after or between phases of active therapy: requires close supervision to prevent recurrence of periodontal disease; includes control of calculus formation, diet, plaque control, and oral physical therapy supervision, follow-up radiographs, and complete operative care.

Periodontics: that branch of dental practice comprising the prevention, diagnosis, and treatment of diseases of the surrounding and supporting structures of the teeth.

Periodontium: the tissues which surround, support, and are attached to the teeth; includes gingiva, cementum, periodontal ligament (membrane), and alveolar bone.

Periodontology: the clinical science that deals with the periodontium in health and disease; that branch of dentistry concerned with the etiology, diagnosis, and treatment of diseases of the supporting structures of the teeth.

Petechia: minute hemorrhagic spot, of pinhead to pinpoint size, in the skin.

Petri plate: a small shallow dish of thin glass with a loosely fitting, overlapping cover, used for plate cultures in microbiology.

pH: symbol commonly used to express hydrogen ion concentration, the measure of alkalinity and acidity. Normal (neutral) pH is 7.0. Above 7.0 the solution is alkaline; below, acid.

Phosphorescence: emission of radiation by a substance as a result of previous absorption of radiation of shorter wave length; contrasts with fluorescence in that the emission may continue for a time after cessation of the ionizing radiation.

Physiologic saline solution: a 0.9 percent sodium chloride solution which exerts an osmotic pressure equal to that exerted by the blood, thus is compatible with blood.

Pipette: a slender graduated tube for measuring and transferring liquids from one vessel to another.

Plasma: fluid portion of the blood (serum and fibrinogen) without formed elements; fluid portion of the lymph without its corpuscles or cells.

Pontic: the suspended member of a fixed partial denture; it replaces the lost natural tooth, restores its functions, and usually occupies the space previously filled by the natural crown.

Precipitate: to cause a substance in solution to separate out in solid particles (verb); that which is separated out is called the precipitate (noun).

Predisposition: a concealed but present susceptibility to disease which may be activated under certain conditions.

Premaxilla: the intermaxillary bone situated in front of the maxilla proper; carries the incisor teeth.

Premedication: preliminary treatment, usually with a drug, to prevent untoward results which may be affected by the operation to be performed.

Prescribe: to designate or recommend a remedy for administration; to direct in writing the dosage, preparation, and dispensing of a remedy or drug.

Primate space: diastema or gap in tooth row occasionally observed in primary dentition. Characteristic of almost all species of primate except man. Maxillary primate spaces accommodate mandibular canines and mandibular primate spaces accommodate maxillary canines when teeth are in occlusion. Reduced length of canines accompanied man's evolution so canines no longer protruded beyond occlusal level and diastema was no longer functional.

Prognosis: a forecasting of the probable course and termination of a disease and response to treatment; the prospect of recovery from a disease as indicated by the nature and symptoms of the case.

Proliferation: reproduction or multiplication of similar forms.

Prone: flat, prostrate; **prone position,** lying flat.

Prosthesis: artificial replacement for a missing part.

Prosthodontics: prosthetic dentistry; that branch of dental art and science pertaining to the restoration and maintenance of oral function by the replacement of missing teeth and adjacent structures by artificial devices. See also **Maxillofacial prosthetics.**

Protective barrier: a barrier of radiation-absorbing material such as lead, concrete, or plaster which serves to reduce radiation hazards.

Protein: any one of a group of complex organic nitrogenous compounds widely distributed in plants and animals which form the principal constituents of cell protoplasm. They are essentially combinations of alpha amino acids and their derivatives.

Proteolytic: effecting the digestion of proteins.

Protoplasm: the only known form of matter in which life is apparent; it composes the essential material of all plant and animal cells.

Protrusion: condition of being thrust forward as the protrusion of the anterior teeth.

Psychiatry: that branch of medicine which deals with disorders of the mind.

Psychosomatic: pertaining to the mind-body relationship; having body symptoms of a psychic, emotional, or mental origin.

Ptyalin: an enzyme occurring in the saliva which converts starch into maltose and dextrose.

Public health: the science and art of preventing disease, prolonging life, and promoting physical health and efficiency through organized community efforts.

  Dental public health: art of preventing and controlling dental diseases and promoting oral health through organized community efforts.

Pulp stone: see **Denticle.**

Pulpectomy: removal of the pulp chamber and root canals of a tooth.

Pulpotomy: the removal of a portion of the pulp of a tooth, usually meaning the coronal portion.

Purpura: escape of blood into the skin and mucous membranes forming petechiae and ecchymoses.

Purulent: containing, consisting of, or forming pus.

Pyorrhea: a purulent discharge; discharge of pus. Formerly a name for advanced, severe periodontal disease.

Q.

Quadrant: any one of the four parts or quarters of the dentition with the dividing line of the maxillary or mandibular teeth at the midline between the central incisors.

R.

Radiation, ionizing: any electromagnetic or particulate radiation capable of producing ions, directly or indirectly, in its passage through matter.

Radiolucent: a substance, which because of its lack of density, permits the passage of x rays with only very light resistance; radiolucent objects appear dark on radiographs.

Radiopaque: a substance, which because of its density, resists the passage of x rays; radiopaque objects appear light on radiographs.

Radioresistant: relatively resistant to injury by ionizing radiation.

Radiosensitive: relatively susceptible to injury by ionizing radiation.

Raphe: a ridge, furrow, or seam-like union between two parts or halves of an organ or structure.

Rarefaction: being or becoming less dense.

Recession: gradual drawing away of a tissue or part from its normal position, as the progressive exposure of the root surface by an apical shift of the gingiva.

Rectification: conversion of alternating current to direct current.

Recurrent: returning after intermissions.

Rehabilitation: restoration to former state of health, efficiency, and independent action; regeneration.

Relative biological effectiveness (R.B.E.): a factor used to compare the biological effects of absorbed doses of differing types of ionizing radiation in a particular organism or tissue. The standard of comparison is medium voltage x rays delivered at about 10 rads/minute. The unit of R.B.E. is the **rem.**

Remission: a decrease or arrest of the symptoms of a disease; also the period during which such decrease occurs.

Replantation: replacement of a traumatically or otherwise removed tooth back into its own alveolar socket.

Resection: operation in which a part of a tissue or an organ is removed.

  Root resection: a root is removed from a multirooted tooth.

  Hemisection: half of a tooth is removed.

Resorption: removal of bone or tooth structure by pressure; gradual destruction of dentin and cementum of the root, as the primary teeth prior to shedding; in orthodontic tooth movement, bone formation on one side compensates for resorption of bone on the other side.

Resuscitation: restoration of life or consciousness; restoration of heartbeat and respiration.

Rh factor: agglutinogens of red blood cells responsible for isoimmune reactions such as occur in erythroblastosis fetalis and incompatible blood transfusions; erythroblastosis fetalis results when a mother is Rh negative and develops antibodies against the fetus which is Rh positive.

Rheostat: an appliance for regulating the resistance and thus controlling the amount of current entering an electric circuit; the dental unit control is located in a device operated by the foot.

Rheumatic: pertaining to or affected with **rheumatism** which is a general term pertaining to conditions characterized by inflammation or pain in muscles or joints.

Roentgen (R): an international unit of quantity of radiation based on the ability of x rays to ionize air.

Rubefacient: reddening of the skin; an agent that reddens the skin by producing active or passive hyperemia.

Ruga: ridge, wrinkle, fold.

Palatal rugae: the irregular ridges in the mucous membrane covering the anterior part of the hard palate.

S.

Sarcoma: malignant neoplasm of connective tissue elements.

Sclerosis: abnormal hardening or thickening of tissue, especially as a result of inflammation or disease of the interstitial substance.

Sedative: a remedy that allays activity, excitement, apprehension.

Senescence: process or condition of growing old; physiologic aging not necessarily related to chronologic age.

Senile: of or pertaining to old age; characteristic of old age.

Senility: old age; feebleness of body and mind occurring with old age.

Septum: a dividing wall, partition, or membrane.

Sequestrum: a piece of necrosed bone that has become separated from the surrounding bone; usually the necrosed bone is being expelled from the body.

Serrated: having a sawlike edge.

Serum: the clear, liquid part of blood separated from its more solid elements after clotting; the blood plasma from which fibrinogen has been removed in the process of clotting.

Shelf-life: the length of time a substance or preparation can be kept without changing its chemical structure or other properties.

Slough: a mass of dead tissue in, or cast out of, living tissue.

Sorbitol: a proprietary sugar solution which will mix with water and glycerin and is slightly soluble in alcohol; used as a moistener, softener, and binder in dental preparations.

Sordes: filth, dirt, especially crusts that accumulate on the teeth and lips in fever.

Space maintainer: a fixed or removable appliance used to replace missing primary teeth to prevent drifting of surrounding teeth until eruption of permanent teeth.

Splint: a rigid or flexible appliance for the fixation of displaced or movable parts.

Spore: see **Bacterial spore.**

Stabile: not moving, stationary, resistant; opposite of labile.

Heat stabile (thermostabile): resistant to moderate degrees of heat.

Stannous: containing tin.

Sterile: aseptic, free from microorganisms.

Stomatitis: inflammation of the oral mucosa, due to local or systemic factors. See also **Aphthous ulcer.**

Subclinical: without clinical manifestations; said of early stages or slight degree, of a disease.

Subluxation: partial or incomplete dislocation. See **Luxation.**

Submerged tooth: one which is below the line of occlusion and may be ankylosed; intrusion; infraocclusion.

Supernumerary tooth: extra tooth; one which is in excess of the normal number.

Suppuration: formation of, conversion into, or act of discharging pus.

Sympathetic nervous system: that part of the autonomic (involuntary) nervous system which arises in the thoracic and the first three lumbar segments of the spinal cord.

Syndrome: a group of symptoms and signs which when considered together characterize a disease or lesion.

Systemic: pertaining to or affecting the whole body.

T.

Tactile: pertaining to the touch; perceptible to the touch.

Tarnish: surface discoloration on a metal, usually the result of oxidation.

Therapeutic: pertaining to the treating or curing of disease; curative.

Therapy: the treatment of disease.

Threshold: that amount of stimulus which just produces a perceptible sensation.

Pain threshold: that amount of stimulus which just produces a sensation of pain.

Threshold exposure: the minimum exposure that will produce a detectable degree of any given effect.

Thrombosis: the formation, development, or presence of a thrombus.

Thrombus: a plug or clot in blood vessel or in one of the cavities of the heart formed by coagulation of the blood and remaining at the point of its formation.

Tic: an involuntary purposeless movement of muscle which usually occurs under emotional stress; a twitching, especially of facial muscles.

Tincture: an alcoholic solution of a drug or other chemical substance.

Tone: the normal degree of vigor and tension; a healthy state of a part.

Tonguetie: abnormal shortness of the frenum of the tongue resulting in limitation of the motion of that organ.

Tonus: the slight, continuous contraction of muscle, which in skeletal muscle aids in the maintenance of posture and the return of blood to the heart. See **Tone.**

Topical: on the surface; pertaining to a particular spot; local.

Topography: the detailed description and analysis of the features of an anatomical region or of a special part.

Toxin: any poisonous substance of microbic, vegetable, or animal origin which causes poisonous symptoms only after a period of incubation; can induce the elaboration of specific antitoxins in suitable animals.

Tracheotomy: surgical operation to provide an artificial opening into the trachea.

Transformer: an electrical device which increases or reduces the voltage of an alternating current by mutual induction between primary and secondary coils or windings.

Transplant: tissue removed from any portion of the body and placed at a different site.

Transplantation: replacement of a lost tooth by another tooth.

    Autotransplant: transfer of a tooth from one alveolus to another in the same mouth.

Trauma: an injury; damage; impairment; external violence producing body injury or degeneration.

Trauma from occlusion (traumatic occlusion): the injury to periodontal tissues caused by occlusal forces.

Treatment: the management and care of a patient for the purpose of curing a disease or disorder.

Tremor: involuntary trembling or quivering.

Trendelenburg position: supine, inclined at an angle of 45 degrees so that the pelvis is higher than the head and chest.

Trismus: motor disturbance of the trigeminal nerve, especially spasm of the masticatory muscles, which causes difficulty in opening the mouth.

U.

Urticaria: smooth, slightly raised patches of skin which are redder or paler than the surrounding skin and accompanied by intense itching; may be caused by systemic disturbance, allergy to certain foods, or emotion.

V.

Vehicle: a substance possessing little or no medicinal action, used as a medium to confer a suitable consistency or form to a drug.

Vincent's disease: trench mouth. See **Necrotizing ulcerative gingivitis.**

Virulent: capable of causing infection or disease.

Viscosity: stickiness; ability of a fluid to resist change in shape or arrangement during flow.

Volatile: tending to evaporate readily.

Volt: unit of electromotive force or potential difference, sufficient to cause a current of one ampere to flow through a resistance of one ohm.

Voltage: the potential or electromotive force of an electric charge, expressed in volts.

Vulcanite: a hard rubber prepared by vulcanizing India rubber with sulfur; formerly used for making removable dentures.

X.

Xerostomia: dryness of the mouth due to functional or organic disturbances of the salivary glands.

Appendix

Table A-1. Tooth Development and Eruption: Primary Teeth

		Hard Tissue Formation Begins (weeks in utero)	Enamel Completed (months after birth)	Emergence (months)	Root Completed (year)
Maxillary	Central Incisor	14	1½	10 (8–12)	1½
	Lateral Incisor	16	2½	11 (9–13)	2
	Canine	17	9	19 (16–22)	3¼
	First Molar	15½	6	16 (13–19 boys) (14–18 girls)	2½
	Second Molar	19	11	29 (25–33)	3
Mandibular	Central Incisor	14	2½	8 (6–10)	1½
	Lateral Incisor	16	3	13 (10–16)	1½
	Canine	17	9	20 (17–23)	3¼
	First Molar	15½	5½	16 (14–18)	2¼
	Second Molar	18	10	27 (23–31 boys) (24–30 girls)	3

From Lunt, R. C. and Law, D. B.: A Review of the Chronology of Eruption of Deciduous Teeth, *J. Am. Dent. Assoc.*, 89, 872, October, 1974.

Table A-2.   Tooth Development and Eruption: Permanent Teeth

		Hard Tissue Formation Begins	Enamel Completed (years)	Emergence (years)	Root Completed (years)
Maxillary	Central Incisor	3–4 mos.	4–5	7–8	10
	Lateral Incisor	10 mos.	4–5	8–9	11
	Canine	4–5 mos.	6–7	11–12	13–15
	First Premolar	1½–1¾ yrs.	5–6	10–11	12–13
	Second Premolar	2–2¼ yrs.	6–7	10–12	12–14
	First Molar	at birth	2½–3	6–7	9–10
	Second Molar	2½–3 yrs.	7–8	12–13	14–16
	Third Molar	7–9 yrs	12–16	17–21	18–25
Mandibular	Central Incisor	3–4 mos.	4–5	6–7	9
	Lateral Incisor	3–4 mos.	4–5	7–8	10
	Canine	4–5 mos.	6–7	9–10	12–14
	First Premolar	1¾–2 yrs.	5–6	10–12	12–13
	Second Premolar	2¼–2½ yrs.	6–7	11–12	13–14
	First Molar	at birth	2½–3	6–7	9–10
	Second Molar	2½–3 yrs.	7–8	11–13	14–15
	Third Molar	8–10 yrs.	12–16	17–21	18–25

From Wheeler, R. C.: *Dental Anatomy, Physiology and Occlusion*, 5th ed. Philadelphia, Saunders, 1974.

Table A-3.   Average Measurements of the Primary Teeth (in millimeters)

		Overall Length	Length of Crown	Length of Root	Width of Crown (mesial-distal at widest point)
Maxillary	Central Incisor	16.0	6.0	10.0	6.5
	Lateral Incisor	15.8	5.6	11.4	5.1
	Canine	19.0	6.5	13.5	7.0
	First Molar	15.2	5.1	10.0	7.3
	Second Molar	17.5	5.7	11.7	8.2
Mandibular	Central Incisor	14.0	5.0	9.0	4.2
	Lateral Incisor	15.0	5.2	10.0	4.1
	Canine	17.5	6.0	11.5	5.0
	First Molar	15.8	6.0	9.8	7.7
	Second Molar	18.8	5.5	11.3	9.9

From Black, G. V.: *Descriptive Anatomy of the Human Teeth*, ed. 4, Philadelphia, Pa., The S. S. White Dental Manufacturing Company, according to Zeisz, R. C. and Nuchols, J.: *Dental Anatomy*. St. Louis, Mosby, 1969, p. 458.

Table A-4. Average Measurements of the Permanent Teeth (in millimeters)

		Overall Length	Length of Crown	Length of Root	Width of Crown (mesial-distal at widest point)
Maxillary	Central Incisor	22.5	10.0	12.0	9.0
	Lateral Incisor	22.0	8.0	13.0	6.4
	Canine	26.5	9.5	17.3	7.6
	First Premolar	20.6	8.2	12.4	7.6
	Second Premolar	21.5	7.5	14.0	6.8
	First Molar	20.8	7.7	13.2	10.7
	Second Molar	20.0	7.2	13.0	9.2
	Third Molar	17.1	6.3	11.4	8.6
Mandibular	Central Incisor	20.7	8.8	11.8	5.4
	Lateral Incisor	21.1	9.6	12.7	5.9
	Canine	25.6	10.3	15.3	6.9
	First Premolar	21.6	7.8	14.0	6.9
	Second Premolar	22.3	7.9	14.4	7.1
	First Molar	21.0	7.7	13.2	11.2
	Second Molar	19.8	6.9	12.9	10.7
	Third Molar	18.5	6.7	11.8	10.7

From Black, G. V.: *Descriptive Anatomy of the Human Teeth,* ed. 4 Philadelphia, Pa., The S. S. White Dental Manufacturing Company, according to Zeisz, R. C. and Nuchols, J.: *Dental Anatomy.* St. Louis, Mosby, 1969, pp. 456–457.

INDEX

Body mechanics, assistant and, 55
  defined, 743
  hygienist and, 48
Boiling water disinfection, 32
  advantages and disadvantages, 33
  care of equipment, 33
  principles for action, 32
  procedure for use, 32
  time-temperature ratio, 32
  uses, 32
Bone, alveolar. See *Alveolar bone.*
Boric acid, first aid kit, 734
Boric acid solution, eye wash, 733
Breath odor. See *Halitosis.*
Bridge. See *Denture, fixed, partial.*
Bristle brushes. See *Brush, polishing.*
Bristles, toothbrush. See *Toothbrush, bristles.*
Brown pellicle, 262
Brush, clasp, 369
  denture, 365, 370
  polishing, dental lathe, for dentures, 550
    dentures, removable, cleaning, 549–560
    stroke and procedure, 546
    types, materials, 544
    uses, precautions, 545
  tooth. See *Toothbrush.*
Brushing plane of toothbrush, 308
Brushite, in calculus, 255
Bruxism, defined, 743
  epileptic patient and, 636
  occlusion and, 229
  patient history and, 78
Buccoversion, 225
Buffer, defined, 743
Bulla, defined, 94
Burn, chemical, 732
  symptoms, 732
Burnish, defined, 743
Burs, finishing, polishing amalgam, 552

C

CABINET, dental care of, 15–16
Calcification, defined, 743
  fluoride and, 421
Calcium, calculus composition, 255
  calculus formation and, 255
  diet, pregnant patient, 719–720
    fractured jaw, 611
  fluoride, 428
Calculus, 249–258
  acquired pellicle, 235, 252
  attachment, modes of, 254, 504
  classification, terminology, 249
  clinical characteristics, 250–252
  composition, 255
  control, 256
  defined, 236, 249
  dental plaque and, 253
  dentures, removable, 363
  factors to teach patient, 257
  formation, 252
    bacteriological factors, 253
  gingiva, reaction to, 252
  index, 275

inspection for, 199–201, 252, 497–499
matrix, 253
morphology, 251, 504
radiographs and, 205
removal. See *Instrumentation, Scalers, Scaling.*
submarginal, 250, 251
  clinical characteristics, 251
  distribution, 251
  occurrence, 250
  other names for, 250
supramarginal, 249, 251
  characteristics, 249
  distribution, 249
  occurrence, 250
  other names for, 250
Cancer. See also *Tumor.*
  biopsy and, 100–101
  defined, 743
  early lesions, 100
  exfoliative cytology, 101–103
  gerodontic patient, 591
  inspection for, 93–99
  oral, 615–623. See also *Oral cancer.*
  warning signs, 103
Canker sore. See *Aphthous ulcer.*
Carbohydrate, defined, 743
  fermentable, dental caries and, 243, 410
    dietary analysis and, 400, 410
    fluoride and, 443
    hypersensitive tooth and, 563, 565
  galactosemia, 642
  intake, diabetes mellitus and, 696
  sucrose. See *Sucrose.*
  use during pregnancy, 719
Carcinoma. See *Cancer.*
Cardiac disease. See *Cardiovascular disease.*
Cardiopulmonary resuscitation, 726–728
Cardiovascular disease, 675–682
  acute myocardial infarction, 677, 731
  angina pectoris, 677, 730
  anticoagulant drug and, 679
  arteriosclerotic heart disease, 677
  chronic illness and, 578
  classification, 676
  complications, arrhythmia, congestive heart failure, 676
  congenital heart disease, 676
    mongoloid and, 646
  coronary heart disease, 677
  diabetes and, 694
  first aid for, 730
  heart failure, symptoms, 676, 731
  hypertension, 86, 677
  incidence, 676
  patient history, 75, 675
    record, 79
  psychological factors, 678
  recall frequency, 574
  rheumatic heart disease, 75, 677, 681
Cardiovascular system, aging and, 588
Caries, dental. See *Dental caries.*
Caries control study. See *Dental caries control study.*
Cariogenic, defined, 743

porte polisher for, 559, 565
technical hints for, 566
Desquamation, defined, 745
Desquamative gingivitis, 710
Detergent, defined, 745
dentifrices, 345
Detergent foods. See *Foods.*
Detritus, defined, 745. See also *Debris.*
Developer, processing radiographs, 134
Development, oral, cleft lip and palate and, 626
teeth, diet in pregnancy and, 719–720
fluoride uptake, 422–423
Devitalize, defined, 745
Dexterity, development by exercises, 469
technical hints for development, 471
toothbrushing and, 310, 387
manual and automatic compared, 321
Dextrostix, 700
Diabetes mellitus, 689–700
categories, 691
complications, 692
dental hygiene care, 697–699
defined, 690
diet and, 696
emergencies, 692, 693, 731
glucose tolerance test, 690(n), 700
incidence, 689
infection and, 694
oral relationships, 697
patient history, 75, 698, 700
records, 79
pregnancy and, 692, 694
psychological, 694
recall frequency, 574
screening tests, 700
signs, symptoms, 690–693
treatment, 695–697
uncontrolled, premedication, 71, 698
Diagnosis, 294. See *Oral diagnosis.*
Diagnostic work-up, 57
following acute necrotizing ulcerative gingivitis, 603
parts, 57–58
patient care and, 10
preparation for instrumentation, 497
purposes, 58
Diamond sharpening stone, 480
Diastema, defined, 745
Diet, acute necrotizing ulcerative gingivitis, 598
adolescent patient, 707
analysis. See *Dietary analysis.*
defined, 399, 745
dental caries control, 410–411
diabetes mellitus control, 699
fluorides in, 421, 428, 594, 720
fractured jaw patient, 611
gerodontic patient, 592–594
hypersensitive teeth and, 565
liquid, 611
for cleft lip and palate surgery, 631
for necrotizing ulcerative gingivitis, 602
physical character, consistency, 400
postoperative procedures and, 571
pregnant patient, 718
selection deposit retention and, 271

sucrose control, 410
tissue healing, 608, 610
Diet instruction, acute necrotizing ulcerative gingivitis, 602
adolescent patient, 707
blood disease patient, 683
cardiovascular disease patient, 680
cleft lip and palate patient, 631
diabetic patient, 699
epileptic patient, 638
fractured jaw patient, 611
gerodontic patient, 594
handicapped patient, 657
menopause, patient during, 711
mentally retarded patient, 650
oral cancer patient, 621
oral surgery patient, 608
pregnant patient 718–720
Dietary. See also *Diet, Diet instruction, Foods.*
daily, patient history and, 74
defined, 745
Dietary analysis, 402–410
forms, 406–408
objectives, 402
procedure for, 404
qualitative, 402
quantitative, 402
summary and analysis, 405
Dietary habits. See *Habits, dietary.*
Differential diagnosis, 294, 745
Diffuse, defined, 745
gingival enlargement, 170
Digestive system, aging and, 588
Digital, defined, 745
Dilantin hyperplasia. See *Diphenylhydantoin-induced hyperplasia.*
Dilate, defined, 745
Diphenylhydantoin-induced hyperplasia, 635
occurrence, 635
treatment, 636
Disability, physical, chronic disease, defined, 578
handicaps, physical. See *Handicapped patient.*
major causes, 578
Disclosing agents, 381–384
application technique, 383
child and, 394
evaluation plaque control, 388, 389, 391, 392
factors to teach the patient, 384
names and formulae, 382–383
patient hygiene performance index, 280
purposes, 381
selection factors, 381–382
tablets, 383
technical hints for, 384
uses, 381
Discrete, defined, 94
Disease, chronic. See *Chronic disease.*
Disinfectant, chemical, sanitization charting implements, 286
compared with antiseptic, 29
handpiece, 19
Disinfection, 32–36
boiling water, 32. See also *Boiling water disinfection.*

Emesis basin, bedridden patient and, 582
  defined, 746
Emollient, defined, 746
Emotional disturbances, deposit retention and, 271
  problems, patient history and, 76
Emulsion, oil and water, instrument protection
    during autoclaving, 30
  x-ray film, 112, 134, 136
Enamel, anatomy cementoenamel junction, 181
  calcification, percent, 255
  decalcification, 243
  dental caries in, 212
  erosion, 211
  fluoride penetration, 423
  hypoplasia, defined, 210
    hereditary amelogenesis imperfecta, 264
    local, defined, 264
    mongoloid and, 646
    systemic, defined, 264
  mode attachment calculus to, 254
  mottled. See *Fluorosis, dental.*
  tooth development and, 757, 758
  trauma to. See *Trauma, tooth.*
Enamel pellicle. See *Pellicle.*
Endemic, defined, 746
Endocarditis, bacterial. See *Subacute bacterial endocarditis.*
Endocardium, defined, 746
  heart disease and, 676
Endocrine glands, 703
  dysfunction, cause diabetes, 692
    cause mental deficiency, 642
    patient history and, 76
  hormones. See *Hormones.*
Endodontics, defined, 746
  treatment, intrinsic stain and, 263
Endogenous stains, 259
Endometrium, defined, 746
  menstruation, and 708
End-to-end bite, 222, 223
Engine belt, care of, 18
  high-speed transmission, 543, 544
Enlargement of gingiva. See *Gingival enlargement.*
Enzyme, amylase, 742
  defined, 746
Ephebodontics, defined, 746
Epidemic, defined, 746
Epilepsy, defined, 633
  etiology, 635
  incidence, 633
  patient, 633–639
    dental hygiene care, 637–639
    diphenylhydantoin-induced hyperplasia, 636
    history and, 76
    oral characteristics, 635
    physical symptoms, 633–634
    plaque control, 636, 638
    psychological characteristics, 636
    seizure, *grand mal*, symptoms, 634, 732
      petit mal, symptoms, 634, 732
Epithelial attachment, 166. See *Junctional epithelium.*
Epithelium, absorption topical anesthetic, 512
  aging and, 588, 589, 590

exfoliative cytology, 101–102
  emergency care, 638, 732
  healing and, 508, 523
  keratinization and massage, 304
  stratified squamous on gingiva, 164, 165
  trauma to. See *Trauma, gingival.*
Epithelization, defined, 746
Equipment, chair. See *Chair, dental.*
  dental, care of, 15–16
  light adjustment, 54. See also *Light, dental.*
  operating stool, 49–53
  oxygen administration, 726
  portable, for bedridden patient, 581
  preparation for appointment, 47
  ultrasonic unit, 509–510
  x-ray machine, 107. See also *X-ray machine.*
Erosion, defined, 211, 746
  oral inspection and, 208
  soft tissue, 95
  tooth surface irregularity, 181
Eruption, chronology of, 757, 758
  defined, 746
Erythema, defined, 94, 746
  exposure, x-ray, 112. See also *Radiation.*
Erythrocyte, defined, 746
  red blood cells, anemia, 682–683
Erythrosin, disclosing agent, 383
Escharotic, defined, 746
Estrogen, 704
Ethics, defined, 746
  Principles of, American Dental Hygienists' Association, 4
Ethyl alcohol, compared with isopropyl, 36
Etiology, calculus, 252–254
  defined, 746
  dental caries, 243
  dental plaque, 239–240
  periodontal pocket, 177–178
Euphoria, defined, 746
  multiple sclerosis and, 663
Evacuation equipment, care, 16
  four-handed dentistry and, 54–55
Evaluation, dental caries control study, 418
  explorer sharpness, 196, 491
  gingiva, for scaling, 497, 570
  gingival health, follow-up, 572
  instrumentation, 570, 572–573
  plaque control, 391, 392, 573
  scaler sharpness, 481
  teaching aids, 395–396
  ultrasonic scaling, 511
Examination, 58–60
  cancer, 91, 95–103
  frena, attachment, 180, 193
  gingiva, 163–181
  instrumentation, 496–499
  instruments for, 183–201
  intraoral, extraoral, 91–104
  methods, 59, 92
  mobility of teeth, 201–202
  pockets, 188–193
  pulpal vitality, 217–219
  radiographic, 137, 202–205, 216, 289–290
  tactile, 198, 497, 499, 570. See also *Tactile sense.*
  teeth, 198, 207–219